AF443485

ANNALS OF THE NEW YORK ACADEMY OF SCIENCES

Volume 832

EDITORIAL STAFF

Executive Editor
BILL BOLAND

Managing Editor
JUSTINE CULLINAN

Associate Editor
MARY KATHERINE BRENNAN

The New York Academy of Sciences
2 East 63rd Street
New York, New York 10021

PHAGOCYTES
BIOLOGY, PHYSIOLOGY, PATHOLOGY, AND PHARMACOTHERAPEUTICS

ANNALS OF THE NEW YORK ACADEMY OF SCIENCES

Volume 832

PHAGOCYTES

BIOLOGY, PHYSIOLOGY, PATHOLOGY, AND PHARMACOTHERAPEUTICS

Edited by Rodolfo Paoletti, Antonia Notario,
and Giovanni Ricevuti

The New York Academy of Sciences
New York, New York
1997

Library of Congress Cataloging-in-Publication Data

Phagocytes : biology, physiology, pathology, and pharmacotherapeutics
 : edited by Rodolfo Paoletti, Antonia Notario, and Giovanni
Ricevuti.
       p.   cm. — (Annals of the New York Academy of Sciences, ISSN
0077-8923 ; v. 832)
    "The results of a conference . . . held in Pavia, Italy, September
5–7, 1996"—contents p.
    Includes bibliographical references and index.
    ISBN 1-57331-102-2 (alk. paper : cloth). — ISBN 1-57331-103-0
(paper : alk. paper)
    1. Phagocytes—Congresses.   I. Paoletti, Rodolfo.   II. Notario,
A. (Antonia)   III. Ricevuti, G. (Giovanni)   IV. Series.
    [DNLM: 1. Phagocytes—physiology—congresses.   W1AN626YL v.832
1997]
    Q11.N5   vol.832
    [QR185.8.p45]
    500 s—dc21
    [616.07'99]
    DNLM/DLC
    for Library of Congress   97-43318
                                                                  CIP

ANNALS OF THE NEW YORK ACADEMY OF SCIENCES

Volume 832
December 15, 1997

PHAGOCYTES: BIOLOGY, PHYSIOLOGY, PATHOLOGY, AND PHARMACOTHERAPEUTICS[a]

Editors
RODOLFO PAOLETTI, ANTONIA NOTARIO, AND GIOVANNI RICEVUTI

CONTENTS

I. Technical Workshop

Inflammation and Anti-inflammation: Gating of Cell/Cell Adhesion at the Level of Mitogen-activated Protein Kinases. *By* MICHAEL H. PILLINGER, CONSTANCE CAPODICI, GENE HAN, AND GERALD WEISSMANN 1

Defective Neutrophil Oxidative Metabolism in Polycythemia Vera Is Associated with an Impaired Activation of Phospholipase D. *By* JAN SAMUELSSON AND JAN PALMBLAD 13

Triple-Labeling Cytofluorimetric Quantitative and Qualitative Evaluation of Phagocytic Activity of Monocytes and Polymorphonuclear Cells. *By* E. MANCA, V. ARANGINO, S. LOMBARDINI, A. GHIANI, D. MUSU, B. AMBROSINI, S. R. DEL GIACCO, AND G. S. DEL GIACCO 21

Evaluation of Neutrophil Motility by Image Analysis. *By* ANTONIO AZZARÀ ... 29

A Flow Cytometric Method for the Analysis of Phagocytosis and Killing by Polymorphonuclear Leukocytes. *By* M. SARASELLA, K. RODA, L. SPECIALE, D. TARAMELLI, E. MENDOZZI, F. GUERINI, AND P. FERRANTE 53

II. Physiology

Development of Neutrophil Granule Diversity. *By* NIELS BORREGAARD 62

Phagocyte Chemoattractant Receptors. *By* F. BOULAY, N. NAIK, E. GIANNINI, M. TARDIF, AND L. BROUCHON 69

[a]This volume is the result of a conference entitled **Phagocytes: Biological and Clinical Aspects—Biology, Physiology, Pathology and Pharmacotherapeutics** held by the University of Pavia, the IRCCS Policlinico San Matteo, and the Lorenzini Foundation in Pavia, Italy on September 5–7, 1996.

The NADPH Oxidase: Lessons from Chronic Granulomatous Disease
Neutrophils. *By* ARTHUR J. VERHOEVEN 85

Endothelial Activation by Cytokines. *By* ALBERTO MONTOVANI,
SILVANO SOZZANI, AND MARTINO INTRONA 93

Evidence of Differential Mycobacterial Growth and Modulation of
Mycobactericidal Property by Glucoaminylmuramyl Dipeptide in Murine
Macrophages. *By* NANDAGOPAL VENKATAPRASAD 117

Effects of Carbamazepine on Human PMN Function: Possible Role of
Peripheral Benzodiazepine Receptors. *By* E. CALDIROLI, A. M. FIETTA,
F. DE PONTI, M. COSENTINO, F. MARINO, M. TADDEI, S. LECCHINI, AND
G. M. FRIGO 130

Human and Bovine Endothelial Cell Monolayers Are Differentially Activated
for Neutrophil Transmigration by Human Plasma. *By* CHRISTIAN J.
WIEDERMANN, PETER SCHRATZBERGER, STEFAN DUNZENDORFER,
STEFAN KIECHL, NORBERT REINISCH, CHRISTIAN M. KÄHLER, AND
JOHANN WILLEIT 135

The Cathelicidin Family of Antimicrobial Peptide Precursors: A Component
of the Oxygen-Independent Defense Mechanisms of Neutrophils. *By*
MARGHERITA ZANETTI, RENATO GENNARO, AND DOMENICO ROMEO 147

Cytokine Activation of Human Endothelial Cells Stimulates Neutrophils To
Become Cytotoxic: The Role of Nitric Oxide. *By* JOHANN BRATT AND
JAN PALMBLAD 163

Osteoclastic Bone Resorption: Normal and Pathological.
By IGOR SCHEPETKIN 170

Ultrastructural Changes of Neutrophils following IL-2 Treatment *in Vivo*.
By R. NANO, E. CAPELLI, S. BARNI, AND G. GERZELI 194

III. Pathology

Network Analysis of Arachidonic Acid Pathophysiology in Human Phagocytes
and Primary Brain Tumors. *By* H. A. LEAVER, J. R. WILLIAMS, S. R. CRAIG,
A. GREGOR, J. W. IRONSIDE, I. R. WHITTLE, B. H. SU, AND P. L. YAP 200

The NADPH Oxidase of Phagocytic Leukocytes. *By* ANTHONY W. SEGAL
AND KAROLYN P. SHATWELL 215

Influence of Interleukin-1 Receptor Antagonist on [³H]Serotonin and Histamine
Release by Rat Basophilic Leukemia-2H3 Cells. *By* PIO CONTI, RENATO C.
BARBACANE, MIRTO TRAKATELLIS, FERNANDA C. PLACIDO, IVANA CATALDO, AND
MARCELLA REALE 223

Cytokine Expression and Release by Neutrophils. *By* MARCO A. CASSATELLA,
SARA GASPERINI, AND MARIA PIA RUSSO 233

Phagocytes in Ischemia Injury. *By* KEITH A. YOUKER, HOLLY H. BIRDSALL,
NIKOLAOS FRANGOGIANNIS, AJITH G. KUMAR, MERRY L. LINDSEY,
CHRISTIE M. BALLANTYNE, C. WAYNE SMITH, ROGER D. ROSSEN, AND
MARK L. ENTMAN 243

Phagocytes and Acute Lung Injury: Dual Roles for Interleukin-1. *By* BROOKS M. HYBERTSON, YOUNG M. LEE, AND JOHN E. REPINE 266

Histiocytic Activation following Neutron Irradiation of Boron-Enriched Rat Liver Metastases. *By* R. NANO, S. BARNI, G. GERZELI, T. PINELLI, S. ALTIERI, F. FOSSATI, U. PRATI, L. ROVEDA, AND A. ZONTA 274

Expression of Lymphocyte Function-Associated Antigen-1 (LFA-1) in Glioblastoma Patients: A Flow Cytometric Analysis. *By* E. CAPELLI, R. NANO, M. CIVALLERO, K. MARINU-AKTIPI, AND M. CERONI 279

IV. Clinical Aspects

Interaction *in Vivo* between Tumor Cells and Phagocytes. *By* ANTONIA NOTARIO, IOLANDA MAZZUCCHELLI, GIANLUCA FOSSATI, AND MARIA LAURA ROLANDI 284

Cationic Protein-Rich Supernatants of Cultured Eosinophils from IL-2-Treated Patients Have No Cytotoxic Activity on Human Renal Cell Carcinoma and Melanoma Cells: A Preliminary Report. *By* M. MORONI, C. PORTA, D. GRITTI, M. DEAMICI, O. GIACOBBE, E. BOBBIO-PALLAVICINI, AND A. NOTARIO 295

Phagocytes and the Lung. *By* PETER A. WARD 304

Leukocyte-Endothelial Cell Interactions in Ischemia-Reperfusion Injury. *By* ROBERT K. WINN, CHANDRA RAMAMOORTHY, NICHOLAS B. VEDDER, SAM R. SHARAR, AND JOHN M. HARLAN 311

Pharmacological Control of Phagocyte Function: Inhibition of Cholesterol Accumulation. *By* R. PAOLETTI, S. BELLOSTA, AND F. BERNINI 322

V. Late Papers

Pentoxifylline Differently Regulates Migration and Respiratory Burst Activity of the Neutrophil. *By* STEFAN DUNZENDORFER, PETER SCHRATZBERGER, NORBERT REINISCH, CHRISTIAN M. KÄHLER, AND CHRISTIAN J. WIEDERMANN 330

Activation of Human Neutrophils by Soluble Immune Complexes: Role of FCγRII and FCγRIIIb in Stimulation of the Respiratory Burst and Elevation of Intracellular Ca^{2+}. *By* STEVEN W. EDWARDS, FIONA WATSON, LAKHDAR GASMI, DALE A. MOULDING, AND JULIE A. QUAYLE 341

Phagocytic Activity of Bronchoalveolar Lavage Neutrophils in Intensive Care Unit Patients on Mechanical Ventilation. *By* E. PIVA, S. DE TONI, G. SERVIDIO, P. BORIN, AND M. PLEBANI 358

Respiratory Burst of Neutrophils in Diabetic Patients with Periodontal Disease. *By* S. DE TONI, E. PIVA, A. LAPOLLA, G. FONTANA, D. FEDELE, AND M. PLEBANI 363

G-Protein-Coupled Receptor–Mediated Activation of PI-3 Kinase in Neutrophils. *By* MARCUS THELEN AND SVETLANA A. DIDICHENKO 368

Influence of Heat Inactivation of Human Serum on the Opsonization of
Streptococcus mutans. By MICHELLE A. MOORE, ZAID W. HAKKI,
RICHARD L. GREGORY, LINDA E. GFELL, WAN K. KIM-PARK, AND
MICHAEL J. KOWOLIK 383

Activation of the Neutrophil Respiratory Burst Requires Both Intracellular and
Extracellular Calcium. *By* W. K. KIM-PARK, M. A. MOORE, Z. W. HAKKI,
AND M. J. KOWOLIK 394

The Phagocyte in Human Gliomas. *By* LORENZO LORUSSO AND M. L. ROSSI ... 405

Host Tissue Damage by Phagocytes. *By* GIOVANNI RICEVUTI 426

Index of Contributors 449

Preface

The study of phagocytes has attained considerable relevance in clinical and experimental medicine and has attracted the interest of a great number of researchers. Because phagocytes perform a pivotal role in many human diseases, the range of conditions in which they are involved is wide and encompasses many disciplines, be it clinical, biochemical, or genetic.

Phagocytes are the main players in the process of inflammation and in the defense of the body against a variety of noxae.

Impairment of their function, for example during pharmacological treatment or from extrinsic or genetic causes, may trigger and/or worsen diseases such as atherosclerosis, arthritis, autoimmune diseases, and myocardial and cerebral ischemia, and may play a role in cancerogenesis. Phagocytes may even participate to the aging process.

Their absence, whether physical or functional, as in leukemia and neoplasms, may lead to death due to infection.

Some phagocyte defects require bone marrow transplantation and genetic therapy to be alleviated or cured.

This volume contains selected papers from the proceedings of the Second International Congress entitled Phagocytes: Biological And Clinical Aspects—Biology, Physiology, Pathology And Pharmacotherapeutics, held in Pavia, Italy.

The volume is a compendium of recent knowledge relating to the biology, pathophysiology, pharmacology, and genetics of phagocytes as of 1996, and thus represents state-of-the-art insight into these topics. The present volume updates the information presented in *The Biology of Phagocytes in Health and Disease*,[a] which summarized the status of knowledge on phagocytes in 1986 as highlighted in a prior congress, also held in Pavia, and entitled The Biological and Clinical Aspects of Phagocyte Function. The 1986 congress was organized by Profs. Carlo Mauri, Salvatore C. Rizzo, and myself.

The aim of the congress was to stimulate the broadening of existing knowledge on phagocytes and to identify directions for future research. This, I believe, was achieved through the participation of the recognized experts in the field presenting numerous enticing and forward-looking presentations. We were honored to have with us Prof. Bengt Samuelson, who received the Nobel Prize for Medicine in 1982.

It is hoped that the thread of inquiry into phagocytes will be further lengthened with exciting new research and lead to the organization of more meetings of this kind.

ACKNOWLEDGMENTS

The organization of the Phagocyte Conference in Pavia was the result of teamwork of a small group of dedicated people. Our gratitude goes to all those behind the

[a]Edited by C. Mauri, S. C. Rizzo, and G. Ricevuti and published by the Pergamon Press in 1987.

scenes who have contributed so much of their time and talent and who made both the congress and this volume possible.

We would particularly like to thank the congress presidents Profs. Antonia Notario (Pavia) and Rodolfo Paoletti (Milan), who made the congress a reality by inspiring the organizing committee and providing the necessary support even in the moments of greatest difficulty.

We would also very much like to thank Prof. Marco Baggiolini (Bern), Prof. Gerald Weissmann (New York), and Dr. Marco L.M. Rossi (Liverpool) for their extremely helpful advice and assistance in the preparation of the congress and this volume.

Many other colleagues have also lent us a strong helping hand and we are grateful. These include Dr. Andrea Baldi, Dr. Iolanda Mazzucchelli, Dr. GianLuca Fossati, Dr. Donatella Gritti, Dr. Cristina Pistone, Dr. Monica Montagna, and Dr. Claudia Canale. They contributed to the production of materials for the congress and as liaisons for the researchers attending the congress.

Graphics and the very original congress logo on the program are the handiwork of Mr. Michele Moscato. Congress information provided via the internet was made possible by the efforts of Dr. Pietro Micheletti. The information thus provided was greatly appreciated by a multitude of participants.

Finally we would like to thank the very competent editorial staff of the New York Academy of Sciences, and particularly Mary K. Brennan, for seeing this volume through the press.

Giovanni Ricevuti, M.D.
Secretary of the Congress

Inflammation and Anti-inflammation: Gating of Cell/Cell Adhesion at the Level of Mitogen-activated Protein Kinases[a]

MICHAEL H. PILLINGER,[b,c] CONSTANCE CAPODICI,[c] GENE HAN, AND GERALD WEISSMANN

Department of Medicine
New York University School of Medicine
New York, New York 10016

INTRODUCTION

Eicosanoids and related compounds play a variety of roles in mediating and moderating inflammation. Leukotriene B_4 (LTB_4), generated by the action of lipoxygenase on arachidonic acid, engages G protein–linked receptors on human neutrophils to stimulate aggregation, chemotaxis, degranulation, and superoxide anion (O_2^-) generation, contributing to the cellular component of the inflammatory response. Prostaglandins, derived from arachidonic acid by cyclooxygenase enzymes and acting as local hormones, engage G protein–linked receptors on endothelial cells to stimulate vasodilation and increase vascular permeability. In contrast to their inflammatory effect on vascular endothelium, stable prostaglandins of the E series (PGEs) contribute to the inhibition of a variety of neutrophil responses, including aggregation and O_2^- generation.[1] Interestingly, arachidonic acid itself stimulates neutrophil responses including aggregation, degranulation, and O_2^- generation.[2–4] Although some effects of prostaglandins, leukotrienes, and arachidonic acid on neutrophils have been well described, the mechanisms of their actions remain incompletely elucidated. Moreover, little or no information is available on the importance of cross-talk between eicosanoid and arachidonic acid signaling pathways in neutrophil activation.

The mitogen-activated protein kinases (MAPKs) p44[erk1] and p42[erk2] are serine/threonine protein kinases that have been shown to play roles in cell growth and division.[5] However, we and others have demonstrated that in neutrophils, post-mitotic cells with no capacity for division, MAPK is activated in response to chemoattractants such as formylmethionyl-leucyl-phenylalanine (FMLP), LTB_4, and the complement split product C5a.[6–9] Activation of neutrophil MAPK by chemoattractants resembles MAPK activation by protein tyrosine kinase receptors (PTKRs) in mitotic

[a]This work was supported by grants from the National Chapter of the Arthritis Foundation and the American Cancer Society (M.H.P.), and by National Institutes of Health Grants AI-36224, AR11949, and HL19721 (G.W.).

[b]Address correspondence to: Michael H. Pillinger, Division of Rheumatology NB16N1, New York University Medical Center, 550 First Avenue, New York, NY 10016. Phone, 212-263-6404. Fax, 212-263-8804.
[c]These authors contributed equally to this work.

cells, in that chemoattractant-stimulation of neutrophil MAPK depends, at least in part, on the activation of the low-molecular weight GTP–binding protein p21^{ras}.[10,11] Activated, GTP-bound p21^{ras} initiates a signaling cascade in which the kinases Raf-1, MEK, and MAPK are sequentially phosphorylated and activated.[12–14] In contrast to FMLP-stimulated O_2^- generation, which appears to be independent of MAPK activation,[15] we have observed an association between MAPK activity and homotypic aggregation of human neutrophils.[6]

In the present study we have examined the effects of arachidonic acid on neutrophil MAPK activity. Because (*1*) PGEs raise intracellular levels of cyclic adenine monophosphate (cAMP) in neutrophils,[16,17] (*2*) cAMP inhibits growth factor–stimulated activation of MAPK,[18,19] and (*3*) adenine and guanine cyclic nucleotides modulate chemoattractant-stimulated neutrophil functions,[20–23] we also studied the effects of PGE$_1$, cAMP, and cyclic guanine monophosphate (cGMP) on neutrophil MAPK activity in response to arachidonic acid. Finally, we tested the effects of acetylsalicylic acid (ASA) and sodium salicylate (NaS)—potent and poor cyclooxygenase inhibitors, respectively—on neutrophil MAPK activity in response to both arachidonic acid and FMLP. Our data indicate that arachidonic acid stimulates, whereas PGE$_1$, cAMP, and salicylates inhibit, MAPK activity in human neutrophils. The effects of these agents on MAPK were concordant with their effects on homotypic aggregation, supporting a role for MAPK signaling in stimulus-response coupling in these cells. Consistent with previous reports on the inhibition of neutrophil responses by salicylates and other NSAIDs, inhibition of both MAPK and homotypic aggregation by salicylates was not dependent upon inhibition of cyclooxygenase activity.

EXPERIMENTAL PROCEDURES

Materials

Except where otherwise noted, reagents were purchased from Sigma Chemical Co. (St. Louis, MO). Accuprep™ was from Accurate Scientific, Inc. Dextran T500 was from Pharmacia LKB Biotechnology Inc. Myelin basic protein (MBP) substrate peptide (MBPp) was from Upstate Biotechnology Incorporated. MBPp control peptide (valine substituted for threonine) was synthesized by Chiron Mimotopes. Antisera specific for p44^{erk1} (*sc-93*) and p42^{erk2} (*sc-154*) were from Santa Cruz Biotechnology. Rabbit anti-mouse and rabbit anti-rat antisera were from Organon Teknika Corporation (Cappel). ATP was from Boerhinger Mannheim. [γ-^{32}P]ATP was from Amersham. Pertussis toxin was from List Biologicals. [^{3}H]Arachidonic acid was purchased from Moravek Biochemicals. Phosphocellulose papers and GF/C glass microfiber filters were purchased from Whatman.

Neutrophil Isolation

Neutrophils were isolated from whole blood from volunteer donors by density sedimentation, dextran sedimentation, and hypotonic lysis according to the method of Boyum,[24] except that Accuprep Lymphocytes™ was substituted for Ficoll-Hypaque during density sedimentation. Microscopic examination confirmed that these preparations contained ≥90% neutrophils.

MBPp Kinase Activity Assay

Neutrophils (2×10^8/ml) were incubated in the absence or presence of various concentrations of arachidonic acid or FMLP at 37°C for the times indicated in the RESULTS section. In some experiments, neutrophils were preincubated in the absence or presence of potential inhibitors or enhancers of MAPK activation for 10 min at 37°C prior to stimulation as above. Reactions were stopped by addition of lysis buffer (20 mM Tris pH 7.4, 1 mM NaEGTA, 2 mM sodium vanadate, 25 mM sodium fluoride, 0.5% Triton-X, 2 mM PMSF, 10 KU/ml aprotinin, and 10 μg/ml each of chymostatin, antipain, and pepstatin). Neutrophil lysates were centrifuged (14,000 g × 10 min at 4°C) to remove nuclei. Lysates were kept on ice for 15 min, followed by incubation for 15 min at 37°C in a buffer (25 mM Tris pH 7.4, 12.5 mM $MgCl_2$, 125 mM NaEGTA, 1.25 mM sodium fluoride, 2 mM dithiothreitol, 220 μM ATP, and 25 μCi/ml [^{32}P]ATP) containing 500 μM MBPp or a control peptide in which valine was substituted for threonine. Reactions were stopped by the addition of formic acid to a final concentration of 6%. The lysates were spotted onto phosphocellulose papers, which were washed thoroughly with distilled water and quantitated by scintillation counting. Duplicate assays in the absence of MBP peptide were performed to determine non-MAPK background kinase activities.

Immunodepletion of MAPK from Neutrophil Lysates

Neutrophils were incubated for 2 min at 37°C in the absence or presence of 100 mM FMLP or 20 μM arachidonic acid, followed by the addition of lysis buffer. Lysates were incubated overnight with equimolar amounts of antisera to p44^{erk1} and p42^{erk2} or a control antiserum in varying concentrations (expressed as the ratio of antisera added versus neutrophil equivalents) in the presence of protein A–agarose beads. The beads were removed by centrifugation and MAPK activity was measured as described above and expressed as MAPK activity in supernatants immunodepleted with anti-MAPK antibodies relative to MAPK activity in the control supernatants.

Neutrophil Aggregation

Neutrophil (1.25×10^7/ml) aggregation was monitored as the increase in transmission of light through stirred suspensions in a platelet aggregometer (Payton Industries) as previously described.[25] Aggregation curves were quantitated as the area under the curve in the first 2 min following stimulation.

Binding of [³H]Arachidonic Acid to Neutrophils

Neutrophils (4×10^5 cells/ml) were incubated with [³H]arachidonic acid (210 Ci/mmol) in the absence or presence of 100-fold excess of unlabeled arachidonic acid for 1 h at 0°C. The reaction was stopped by diluting the samples 40-fold with ice-cold wash buffer (150 mM NaCl, 0.01% bovine serum albumin, and 20 mM Tris, pH 7.4). The cells were trapped by filtration on GF/C glass microfiber filters, which were washed extensively and counted. To obtain specific binding, values obtained from cells incubated with both tritiated and unlabeled arachidonic acid were subtracted from values obtained from cells incubated with [³H]arachidonic acid alone.

RESULTS

Arachidonic Acid Stimulates MAPK Activity in Human Neutrophils

MAPK activity was determined as the ability of lysates of unstimulated, FMLP, or arachidonic acid–stimulated neutrophils to phosphorylate a nonapeptide containing the specific sequence of myelin basic protein (MBP) phosphorylated by MAPK (PRTP).[26] Consistent with our previous observations,[6] stimulation with FMLP (100 nM) for 1 min at 37°C resulted in a fivefold upregulation of neutrophil MAPK activity as measured by this assay (FIG. 1, A). Stimulation with arachidonic acid (20 μM–40 μM) also resulted in significant MAPK activation, though less than that of FMLP (FIG. 1, B). Stimulation with lower and higher concentrations of arachidonic acid resulted in lesser degrees of stimulation (not shown). In contrast to stimulation with arachidonic acid (20:4 *cis*), stimulation with other fatty acids [arachidic (20:0), linoleic (18:2 *cis*), and linolelaidic (18:2 *trans*)] had little or no effect on MAPK in neutrophils. To confirm that the counts measured represented specific phosphorylation of the target peptide, phosphorylation events in neutrophil lysates were also measured in the presence of a control peptide in which valine was substituted for tyrosine. In these assays, the number of phosphorylation events were identical to background levels (FIG. 1, A and B). To confirm that the enzyme(s) phosphorylating the target peptide was MAPK, we immunodepleted FMLP- and arachidonic acid–stimulated lysates with antibodies to p44^{erk1} and p42^{erk2} prior to phosphorylation of MBPp (FIG. 1, C). In these experiments MBPp phosphorylation declined in inverse relation to the concentration of anti-MAPK antibodies employed during immunodepletion, and at maximal antibody concentrations greater than 95% of FMLP- or arachidonic acid–stimulated MBPp phosphorylation was depleted. These data confirm the specificity of our assay for MAPK activity and demonstrate that both FMLP and arachidonic acid are capable of stimulating MAPK activity in human neutrophils. Consistent with the effects of FMLP and arachidonic acid on MAPK activity, arachidonic acid stimulation of neutrophil homotypic aggregation was reduced relative to that of FMLP (FIG. 1, D). However, AA stimulation of MAPK was preserved relative to aggregation.

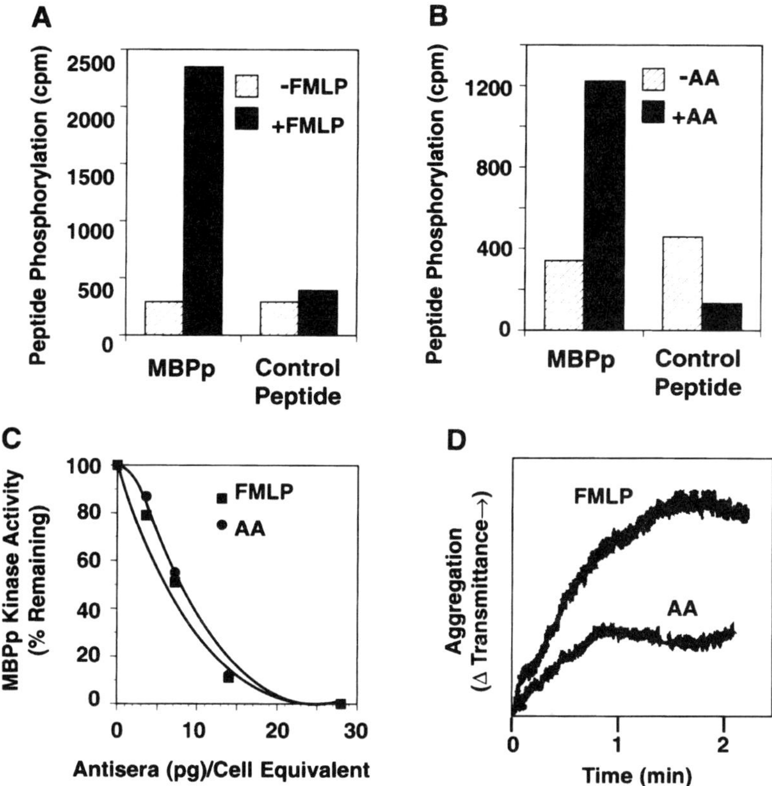

FIGURE 1. FMLP and arachidonic acid stimulate MAPK activation in human neutrophils. (**A**) Neutrophils were incubated for 2 min in the absence or presence of FMLP, lysed, and assayed for MAPK activity as the capacity to phosphorylate MBPp, a nonapeptide substrate of MAPK. Lysates from FMLP-stimulated neutrophils failed to phosphorylate a control peptide in which valine was substituted for tyrosine. (**B**) Neutrophils were incubated for 2 min in the absence or presence of arachidonic acid (AA), then assayed for MAPK activity against MBPp or the control peptide as in **A**. (**C**) Neutrophils were stimulated with FMLP or arachidonic acid, lysed, and the lysates were immunodepleted overnight with varying concentrations of antisera to Erk1 and Erk2 prior to assaying for MAPK activity. (**D**) Neutrophils were stimulated with FMLP or arachidonic acid and homotypic aggregation was measured on-line as described in EXPERIMENTAL PROCEDURES. Data shown are representative of three experiments.

Effects of ASA and NaS on MAPK Activity

Salicylates and other nonsteroidal antiinflammatory drugs (NSAIDs) inhibit a variety of FMLP-stimulated neutrophil responses including aggregation, degranulation, and O_2^- generation. Our observation that FMLP stimulation of neutrophil MAPK is consistent with a role for MAPK in mediating neutrophil homotypic aggregation

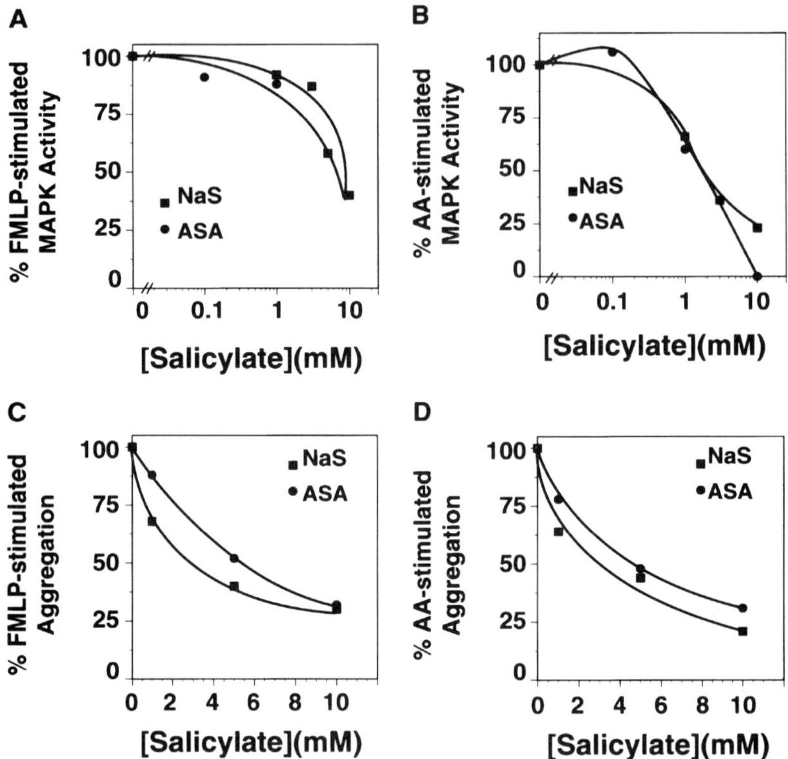

FIGURE 2. ASA and NaS inhibit neutrophil MAPK activity and aggregation in response to FMLP and arachidonic acid. Neutrophils were preincubated in the absence or presence of ASA or NaS. Neutrophil MAPK activity (**A** and **B**) and homotypic aggregation (**C** and **D**) were measured following stimulation for 2 min with FMLP (**A** and **C**) or arachidonic acid (**B** and **D**). Data shown are representative of three experiments.

suggested that salicylates might also inhibit MAPK activity. This hypothesis was confirmed. Preincubation of neutrophils with either ASA or NaS for 10 min inhibited MAPK activation by both FMLP and arachidonic acid (FIG. 2). The concentrations required for these effects were similar to those required for inhibition of FMLP- and arachidonic acid–stimulated neutrophil homotypic aggregation (FIG. 2) and for inhibition of other FMLP-stimulated functions, but were several orders of magnitude higher than those required for inhibition of neutrophil cyclooxygenase activity by ASA.

Effect of cAMP and PGE₁ on Arachidonic Acid–Stimulated MAPK Activity

cAMP and agents that raise intracellular concentrations of cyclic AMP inhibit a variety of FMLP-stimulated neutrophil responses. However, the mechanisms of these effects remain unclear. We have recently observed that the cell-permeable analog dibutyryl cAMP (Bt$_2$cAMP) inhibits both MAPK activation and aggregation of neutrophil cytoplasts, but not neutrophils themselves, in response to FMLP.[6] These observations led us to propose the existence of an FMLP signaling pathway for homotypic aggregation, observable in cytoplasts but not neutrophils, that is MAPK dependent and cAMP sensitive. We now extend these observations by demonstrating that, in contrast to FMLP, arachidonic acid stimulation of MAPK activity in intact neutrophils is sensitive to Bt$_2$cAMP (FIG. 3). Consistent with a role for MAPK in neutrophil adhesive function, Bt$_2$cAMP also inhibited arachidonic acid–stimulated neutrophil aggregation (not shown). We have also observed that, like Bt$_2$cAMP, PGE$_1$ inhibits FMLP-stimulated MAPK activity in enucleate neutrophil cytoplasts.[27] We now extend this observation by testing the effects of PGE$_1$ on arachidonic acid–stimulated MAPK activity in intact neutrophils. Preincubation of intact neutrophils with PGE$_1$ markedly inhibited arachidonic acid–stimulated MAPK activity (FIG. 3).

Effect of cGMP and Carbachol on Arachidonic Acid–Stimulated MAPK Activity

In contrast to cAMP, cGMP and agents that raise intracellular cGMP levels enhance FMLP stimulation of several neutrophil functions. However, the mechanisms of these effects, like those of cAMP, remain unknown. We therefore tested the effects of the cell-permeable cGMP analog, dibutyryl cGMP (Bt$_2$cGMP) on arachidonic acid–stimulated MAPK activity. Whereas Bt$_2$cGMP alone had no effect on basal levels of neutrophil MAPK activity, preincubation with 1 mM Bt$_2$cGMP for 10 min at 37°C prior to stimulation resulted in a $\geq$90% increase in neutrophil MAPK activity in response to arachidonic acid (FIG. 3). Carbachol, a muscarinic acid receptor agonist that raises intracellular cGMP levels in neutrophils, also had no effect by itself but enhanced arachidonic acid–stimulated MAPK activity by $\geq$45% (FIG. 3).

Pertussis Toxin Sensitivity of FMLP- and Arachidonic Acid–Stimulated MAPK Activity in Neutrophils

FMLP stimulates neutrophils via engagement of a G protein–linked, seven-transmembrane-domain receptor. In contrast, arachidonic acid has been reported to have a variety of effects on human neutrophils, including stimulating phospholipase A$_2$ and protein kinase C activities and serving as a substrate for neutrophil lipoxygenase.[28,29] Our laboratory has reported that GTP-binding to neutrophil plasma membranes is stimulated by arachidonic acid, suggesting a role for G protein activation in arachidonic acid stimulation of neutrophil responses.[4] Moreover, we have also reported that pertussis toxin, which inhibits G protein activation by stimulating ADP-ribosylation of the alpha subunit of heterotrimeric G proteins, inhibits arachidonic acid–stimulated neutrophil superoxide anion generation.[4] To determine whether FMLP- and arachidonic acid–stimulated MAPK activity in neutrophils were also G protein dependent, we tested the effects of pertussis toxin on MAPK activity. Consistent with previous reports, preincubation with pertussis toxin inhibited FMLP-stimulated MAPK activity in neutrophils by $\geq$33%. Arachidonic acid–stimulated MAPK activa-

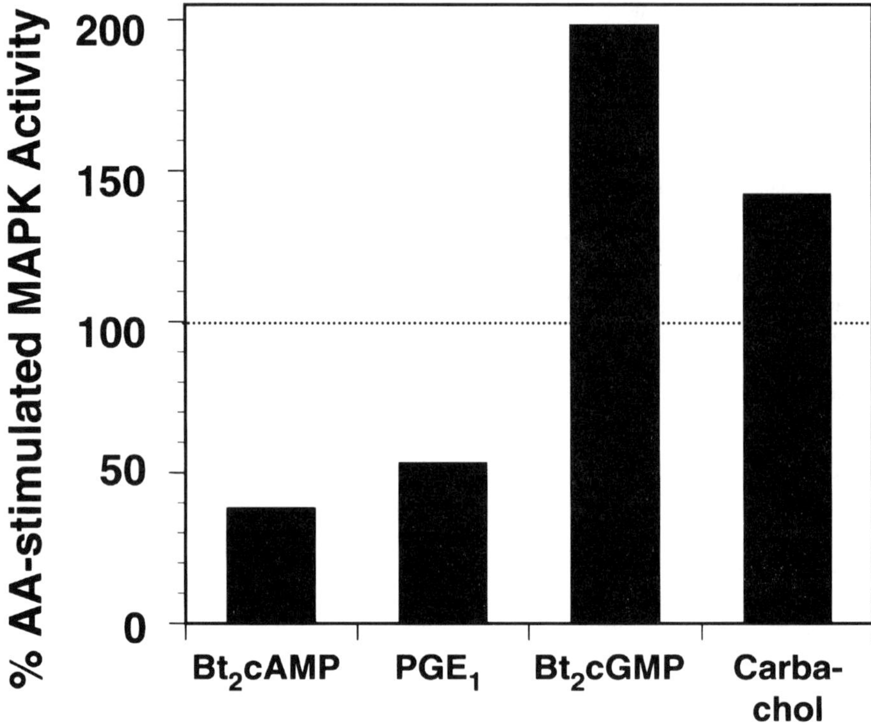

FIGURE 3. Effects of cyclic nucleotides on arachidonic acid–stimulated MAPK activity. Neutrophils were incubated for 10 min in the absence or presence of Bt_2cAMP (1 mM), PGE_1, Bt_2cGMP (1 mM), or carbachol, followed by incubation for 2 min in the absence or presence of arachidonic acid, and assayed for MAPK activity. Data shown are representative of three experiments.

tion was even more sensitive to pertussis toxin than FMLP ($\geq$45% inhibition). These data suggest that arachidonic acid stimulates MAPK activity, at least in part, through stimulation of a membrane-associated G protein(s). They further suggest that arachidonic acid stimulation of MAPK may proceed, as in the case of FMLP, through the ligation of a G protein–linked receptor. To examine this possibility we studied the binding of [^{14}C]arachidonic acid to intact neutrophils (FIG. 4, C). However, these studies failed to demonstrate a saturable component of arachidonic acid binding.

DISCUSSION

In this study we examined the role of cyclic nucleotides, prostaglandin E_1, and its precursor arachidonic acid on the activation of MAPK in human neutrophils. Our data suggest that cross-talk between lipid signaling pathways at the level of MAPK may play a critical role in regulating at least one neutrophil function, stimulated homotypic aggregation. Our data further indicate that ASA, recognized for its ability to block cyclooxygenase activity, inhibits MAPK activation in neutrophils. However, the mechanism of MAPK inhibition by ASA, like its effect on a variety of other neutrophil functions, is unlikely to depend upon cyclooxygenase inhibition.

Arachidonic acid is most commonly regarded as a substrate for cyclooxygenase and lipoxygenase activities, resulting in prostaglandin and leukotriene production, respectively. However, neutrophils retain little cyclooxygenase activity. Moreover, although they possess lipoxygenase, neutrophils under commonly observed resting or stimulatory conditions generate little or no LTB_4.[30] Nonetheless, when exposed to arachidonic acid at various concentrations, neutrophils aggregate, degranulate, and produce O_2^-. The mechanisms by which arachidonic acid stimulates neutrophil responses are likely to be various. Exposure of neutrophils to arachidonic acid induces activation of both protein kinase C[29] and phospholipase A_2 (measured as generation of arachidonic acid).[28] Whereas in cell-free preparations arachidonic acid at high concentrations is capable of directly activating the O_2^- generating system,[2] the concentrations of arachidonic acid required to stimulate intact neutrophils approximate the critical micellar concentration for arachidonic acid and raise the possibility that complex fatty acid structures may be required to activate neutrophils via receptor-based interactions. This hypothesis may be supported by previous studies from our

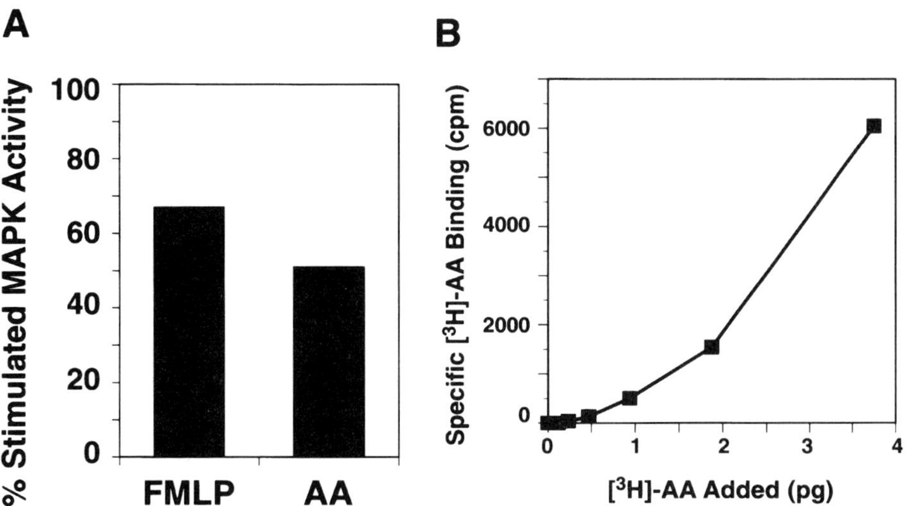

FIGURE 4. Pertussis toxin inhibits FMLP- and arachidonic acid–stimulated MAPK activity in neutrophils. (**A**) Neutrophils were incubated with pertussis toxin for 1 h at 37°C, followed by stimulation with FMLP or arachidonic acid and assay for MAPK activity. (**B**) Arachidonic acid binding to neutrophils fails to demonstrate saturation. [^{14}C]arachidonic acid binding to neutrophils was measured in the presence or absence of excess unlabeled arachidonic acid, and specific binding to neutrophils was calculated and expressed as described in EXPERIMENTAL PROCEDURES. Data shown are representative of three experiments.

own laboratory, demonstrating a probable role for a membrane-associated G protein(s) in arachidonic acid stimulation of O_2^-.

Our observation that arachidonic acid activates MAPK in neutrophils extends the repertoire of neutrophil responses to this agent and suggests a mechanism for arachidonic acid stimulation of at least some neutrophil functions. We have previously observed that FMLP stimulates MAPK activation in neutrophils in a manner consistent with a role for MAPK in neutrophil homotypic aggregation. Like FMLP, arachidonic acid activation of MAPK was rapid and transient, with kinetics concordant with arachidonic acid–stimulated aggregation. However, in comparison with FMLP, arachidonic acid stimulation of MAPK was preserved relative to neutrophil aggregation. This observation may be consistent with our previous suggestion that MAPK activity is necessary but not sufficient for aggregation, i.e., that MAPK serves a gating function in the regulation of PMN responses. Like FMLP, arachidonic acid–stimulated MAPK activity was sensitive to pertussis toxin, supporting the observation that at least some effects of arachidonic acid on PMN may be G protein dependent.[4] However, our binding studies did not support the saturable interaction of arachidonic acid with a receptor on intact PMN. The failure of arachidonic acid binding to demonstrate a saturable component may be due to technical limitations involved in measuring the specific binding of a fatty acid that can directly intersperse in the plasma membrane.[31] However, it is also possible that arachidonic acid activates a G protein(s) via a receptor-independent mechanism, through either membrane perturbations or direct interaction with the G protein(s) itself. Experiments to resolve this apparent paradox between pertussis toxin sensitivity and binding studies are ongoing in our laboratory.

Our studies on the effects of cyclic nucleotides and E series prostaglandins on MAPK activation by arachidonic acid support a MAPK-dependent mechanism of regulatory cross-talk among lipid-dependent signaling pathways. The best-elucidated pathway for MAPK activation involves the sequential activation of the low molecular weight GTP-binding protein p21^{ras}, and the kinases Raf-1 and MEK. cAMP and agents that raise intracellular cAMP levels have been shown to inhibit MAPK activation by stimulating PKA-dependent phosphorylation of Raf-1, inhibiting p21^{ras}/Raf-1 interactions.[18,19] It is likely that Bt_2cAMP and PGE_1 inhibit arachidonic acid–stimulated MAPK activation by a similar mechanism, suggesting that arachidonic acid stimulation of MAPK is dependent on p21^{ras}/Raf-1. In contrast, the failure of Bt_2cAMP to inhibit FMLP-stimulated MAPK activation in intact neutrophils suggests that arachidonic acid and FMLP act on MAPK via divergent signaling pathways, or, as we have previously proposed, that FMLP stimulation of MAPK occurs via two or more redundant pathways, not all of which are sensitive to cAMP.[6] It has long been appreciated that cAMP and cGMP can have opposing effects on neutrophil responses, such as chemokinesis and O_2^- generation,[21,23] but the mechanisms of such effects have remained unclear. Our preliminary observation that Bt_2cGMP and carbachol enhance MAPK stimulation by FMLP and arachidonic acid suggests for the first time a MAPK-dependent mechanism for cGMP enhancement of neutrophil responses. However, the effect of carbachol on neutrophil MAPK must be interpreted with caution, since carbachol has been shown to stimulate MAPK in mitotic cells by increasing the activity of Ras-GRF/CDC25^{Mm}, a guanine nucleotide exchange factor that activates p21^{ras}.[32] The failure of cGMP to enhance FMLP- and arachidonic acid–stimulated aggregation suggests, once again, that MAPK activity may be necessary but not sufficient for neutrophil adhesive function.

Although western medicine has appreciated for centuries the antiinflammatory effects of salicylates, no explanation for their mechanism of action was proposed until 1971, when Vane demonstrated that ASA and other NSAIDS inhibit the production of prostaglandins by cells.[33] However, ASA inhibition of neutrophil responses is unlikely to be due to effects on cyclooxygenase activity, since (*1*) neutrophils retain little or no cyclooxygenase, (*2*) the concentrations of ASA required to inhibit neutrophils exceed, by several orders of magnitude, those required to inhibit cyclooxygenase, and (*3*) NaS, a poor cyclooxygenase inhibitor, is as potent as ASA at inhibiting stimulated neutrophil responses. Our observation that both ASA and NaS inhibit MAPK activity at concentrations consistent with those required for inhibition of neutrophil homotypic aggregation suggests a mechanism of action for salicylates. At similar concentrations, salicylates may affect neutrophil plasma membrane viscosity,[34] enhance post–FMLP-stimulation intracellular cAMP levels,[35] and interfere with G protein–coupled receptor signaling.[36] Whether salicylates inhibit MAPK by these or by other means remains to be determined. Schwenger and colleagues have recently reported that NaS inhibits TNF-stimulated MAPK activity in FS-4 fibroblasts, but the mechanism of that action has also not yet been elucidated.[37]

MAPK has been most fully studied in cells in culture, in which MAPK stimulated in response to mitogens and growth factors translocates to the nucleus, where it phosphorylates and activates transcription factors such as c-*fos* and c-*jun*. In contrast, rapid MAPK activation in neutrophils, post-mitotic cells with limited capacity for protein synthesis, is unlikely to participate in transcriptional regulation. The ability of FMLP and arachidonic acid to stimulate both MAPK activity and acute neutrophil responses argues a role for MAPK in neutrophil function. The ability of PGEs and cAMP to inhibit both MAPK activity and homotypic aggregation in response to arachidonic acid supports such a view. We are currently exploring the mechanism(s) by which MAPK, stimulated by extracellular agonists, may mediate aggregation and other aspects of neutrophil response.

REFERENCES

1. KITSIS, E. A., G. WEISSMANN & S. B. ABRAMSON. 1991. J. Rheum. **18**(10): 1461–1465.
2. CURNUTTE, J. T., J. A. BADWEY, J. M. ROBINSON, M. J. KARNOVSKY & M. L. KARNOVSKY. 1984. J. Biol. Chem. **259**: 11851.
3. SMITH, R. J., L. M. SAM, J. M. JUSTEN, K. L. LEACH & D. VAN EPPS. 1987. Br. J. Pharmac. **91**: 641.
4. ABRAMSON, S. B., J. LESZCZYNSKA-PIZIAK & G. WEISSMANN. 1991. J. Immunol. **147**: 231–236.
5. COBB, M. H., J. E. HEPLER, M. CHENG & D. ROBBINS. 1994. Sem. Cancer Biol. **5**(4): 261–268.
6. PILLINGER, M. H., A. S. FEOKTISTOV, C. CAPODICI, B. SOLITAR, J. LEVY, T. T. OEI & M. R. PHILIPS. 1994. J. Biol. Chem. **271**(20): 12049–12056.
7. TORRES, M., F. L. HALL & K. O'NEILL. 1993. J. Immunol. **150**: 1563–1578.
8. WORTHEN, G. S., N. AVDI, A. M. BUHL, N. SUZUKI & G. L. JOHNSON. 1994. J. Clin. Invest. **94**: 815–823.

9. BUHL, A. M., N. AVDI, G. S. WORTHEN & G. L. JOHNSON. 1994. Proc. Natl. Acad. Sci. USA **91:** 9190–9194.
10. BUDAY, L. & J. DOWNWARD. 1993. Cell **73:** 611–620.
11. LOWENSTEIN, E. J., R. J. DALY, A. G. BATZER, W. LI, B. MARGOLIS, R. LAMMERS, A. ULLRICH, E. Y. SKOLNIK, D. BAR-SAGI & J. SCHLESSINGER. 1992. Cell **70:** 431–442.
12. LEEVERS, S. J., H. F. PATERSON & C. J. MARSHALL. 1994. Nature **369:** 411–414.
13. KYRIAKIS, J. M., H. APP, X.-F. ZHANG, P. BANERJEE, D. L. BRAUTIGAN, U. R. RAPP & J. AVRUCH. 1992. Nature **358:** 417–421.
14. CREWS, C. M. & R. L. ERIKSON. 1992. Proc. Natl. Acad. Sci. USA **89:** 8205–8209.
15. YU, H., S. J. SUCHARD, R. NAIRN & R. JOVE. 1995. J. Biol. Chem. **270**(26): 15719–15724.
16. ZURIER, R. B., G. WEISSMANN, S. HOFFSTEIN, S. KAMMERMAN & H. H. TAI. 1974. J. Clin. Invest. **53:** 297–309.
17. CALI, J. J., E. A. BALCUEVA, I. RYBALKIN & J. D. ROBISHAW. 1992. J. Biol. Chem. **267:** 24023–24027.
18. COOK, S. J. & F. MCCORMICK. 1993. Science **262:** 1069–1072.
19. WU, J., P. DENT, T. JELINEK, A. WOLFMAN, M. J. WEBER & T. W. STURGILL. 1993. Science **262:** 1065–1068.
20. HARVATH, L., J. D. ROBBINS, A. A. RUSSELL & K. B. SEAMON. 1991. J. Immunol. **146**(1): 224–232.
21. ERVENS, J., G. SCHULTZ & R. SEIFERT. 1991. Biochemical Soc. Trans. **19:** 59–63.
22. SMOLEN, J. E., S. J. STOEHR & B. KUCZYNSKI. 1991. J. Leuk. Biol. **49:** 172–179.
23. ELFERINK, J. G. R. & B. M. DE KOSTER. 1993. Eur. J. Pharmacol. **246**(2): 157–161.
24. BOYUM, A. 1968. Scand. J. Clin. Lab. Invest. **21** (Suppl 97): 77–78.
25. PHILIPS, M. R., J. P. BUYON, R. WINCHESTER, G. WEISSMANN & S. B. ABRAMSON. 1988. J. Clin. Invest. **82:** 495–501.
26. ERIKSON, A. K., D. M. PAYNE, P. A. MARTINO, A. J. ROSSOMANDO, J. S. SHABANOWITZ, M. J. WEBBER, D. F. HUNT & T. W. STURGILL. 1990. J. Biol. Chem. **265**(32): 19728–19735.
27. PILLINGER, M. H., M. R. PHILIPS, A. FEOKTISTOV & G. WEISSMANN. 1995. Adv. Prostaglandin Thromboxane Leukotriene Res. **23:** 311–316.
28. WINKLER, J. D., C.-M. SUNG, W. C. HUBBARD & F. H. CHILTON. 1993. Biochem. J. **291:** 825–831.
29. MCPHAIL, L. C., C. CLAYTON & R. SNYDERMAN. 1984. Science **224:** 622–626.
30. HAINES, K. A., K. N. GIEDD, A. M. RICH, H. M. KORCHAK & G. WEISSMANN. 1987. Biochem. J. **241:** 55–62.
31. CLANCY, R. M., C. A. DAHINDEN & T. E. HUGLI. 1984. Proc. Natl. Acad. Sci. USA **81:** 729–734.
32. MATTINGLY, R. R. & I. G. MACARA. 1996. Nature **382:** 268–272.
33. VANE, J. R. 1971. Natl. New Biol. **231**(25): 232–235.
34. ABRAMSON, S. B., B. CHERKSEY, D. GUDE, J. LESZCZYNSKA-PIZIAK, M. R. PHILIPS, L. BLAU & G. WEISSMANN. 1990. Inflammation **14:** 11–30.
35. ABRAMSON, S. B., H. KORCHAK, R. LUDEWIG, H. EDELSON, K. HAINES, R. I. LEVIN, R. HERMAN, L. RIDER, S. KIMMEL & G. WEISSMANN. 1985. Proc. Natl. Acad. Sci. USA **82:** 7227–7231.
36. ABRAMSON, S. B., J. LESZCZYNSKA-PIZIAK, R. M. CLANCY, M. R. PHILIPS & G. WEISSMANN. 1994. Biochem. Pharmacol. **47:** 563–572.
37. SCHWENGER, P., E. Y. SKOLNIK & J. VILCEK. 1996. J. Biol. Chem. **271**(14): 8089–8094.

Defective Neutrophil Oxidative Metabolism in Polycythemia Vera Is Associated with an Impaired Activation of Phospholipase D[a]

JAN SAMUELSSON[b] AND JAN PALMBLAD

Department of Medicine
Hematology Section
Centre for Inflammation Research
Karolinska Institute
Stockholm Söder Hospital
S-118 83 Stockholm, Sweden

INTRODUCTION

Studies using X-chromosome-linked gene probes have revealed that circulating polymorphonuclear neutrophil granulocytes (PMN) are derived from the transformed stem cell in the vast majority of polycythemia vera (PV) patients,[1–6] making PMN an accessible source of malignant cells for the study of biochemical changes associated with the clonal transformation. Since the beginning of the 1970s papers describing the "activated phagocyte in PV" have appeared in the literature. We therefore conducted a series of studies where we instead found an impaired PMN oxidative metabolism associated with a defective activation of phospholipase D. However, in recent years reports on phagocytosis and expression of certain surface markers of cell activation have also indicated that PV PMN indeed are activated. This paper describes the current knowledge, and some controversies, regarding PMN function in PV, which are summarized in TABLE 1.

NEUTROPHIL FUNCTIONS THAT APPEAR NORMAL IN POLYCYTHEMIA VERA

The qualitative production, maturation, and transit of PMN in PV are similar to that seen in normal controls,[7] whereas the number of myeloid progenitors in DNA

[a]This work was supported by the King Gustav V Jubilee Fund, The Cancer Society of Stockholm, the Swedish Medical Research Council (grants 16X-105, 19X-05991, and 19P-9851), the Swedish Society of Medicine, the Swedish Work Environment Fund, the Funds of Robert Lundberg, Magnus Bergwall, and Claes Groschinsky, as well as the Research Funds of the Karolinska Institute and Stockholm Söder Hospital

[b]Address correspondence to: Dr. Jan Samuelsson, Department of Hematology, Huddinge University Hospital, 14186 Huddinge, Sweden. Telephone, 46-8-58582597; Fax, 46-8-7748725.

TABLE 1. Neutrophil Response Aberrations in PV

↑ *Increased glycogen stores* (34,35,36)	*Leukotriene generation* → normal (20)
Expression of surface receptors ↑ increased FcR (16), CD64 and CD14 (41) → normal fMLP-R (22), CD11b (19)	*PMN migration (skin window, Boyden chambers)* → normal (10,14,15) ↓ reduced (11,12,13)
Adherence ↑ enhanced (16-18, assessed on whole blood) → normal (15,18, in isolated PMN)	*Aggregation* ↑ enhanced due to a plasma factor (37)
Phagocytosis ↑ enhanced (23,39,41) → normal (12,13,40) ↓ reduced (38)	*Granule content and mobilization* → normal (19,21)
Superoxide ion generation ↑ enhanced (23[a]) → normal (24,[a] 26,[b] 15,[b] 21,[b] 22,[b] 28[b]) ↓ reduced (12,[a] 13,[a] 26,[b] and 15,[c] 21,[c] 22,[c] 28[c])	*Phospholipase (PL) activation* → normal PL-A (20), PL-C (22) ↓ reduced PL-D (22)

Note: Numbers in parentheses refer to references. The stimuli used were latex beads([a]), PMA ([b]), and fMLP and other surface receptor–dependent stimuli ([c]).

synthesis is increased,[8] resulting in PV patients having a total body PMN pool five times the normal mean value.[9] Earlier studies of PMN functions in PV have often yielded conflicting results, which to some extent can be explained by studies being performed using whole blood or impure PMN preparations, as well as the often unphysiological stimuli that were utilized in order to evoke a functional response from the cells.

Migration of PMN has been evaluated *in vivo* using the skin window technique. Ghosh and colleagues[10] found a significantly greater percentage of PMN in skin windows and a corresponding reduction of macrophages, but Jungi and colleagues,[11] employing the same technique, found a markedly diminished leukocyte mobilization. In accordance with this, neutrophil random migration, tested on whole blood in a capillary tube system, was reported to be reduced in PV.[12,13] However, when isolated PMN were studied in a Boyden chamber, a normal migratory response to serum complement stimulation was reported.[14] We have documented that both spontaneous migration and chemotaxis [induced by n-formyl-methionyl-leucyl-phenylalanine (fMLP) and leukotriene B$_4$ (LTB$_4$)] were normal in the Boyden system.[15] Similar results have been published regarding PMN adherence, which was first reported to be augmented when assayed in whole blood filtered through nylon fiber columns.[16] It was later clearly demonstrated that the presence of erythrocytes and platelets increased the adherence of normal PMN in glass bead columns,[17] and a subsequent investigation showed that adherence of isolated PV PMN was normal.[18] We were able to corroborate these findings by showing that spontaneous and fMLP-stimulated adherence to a plastic dish was normal.[15] Finally, it has been shown that incorporation of the β-2 integrin CD11b into the plasma membrane during stimulation was normal in PV PMN.[19] Therefore, it seems safe to state that PMN migration and adherence is normal when pure PMN preparations are investigated. Other measures of neutrophil activation found to be intact include the production of leukotrienes,[20] the extrusion of secondary granule constituents, e.g., lactoferrin,[21] as well as mobilization of neutrophil granule subsets.[19] Finally, the activation of phospholipase C (PLC) was also normal,[19,22] which will be further detailed below.

IMPAIRED NEUTROPHIL OXIDATIVE METABOLISM IN POLYCYTHEMIA VERA

A few earlier studies evaluating oxidative metabolism of PV PMN have been published. Cooper and colleagues[23] demonstrated that latex particle–stimulated PMN had an increased hexose-monophosphate shunt activity, an increased oxygen consumption, and an increased NBT reduction. However, the same group later reported that NBT reduction was normal in PV PMN,[24] and two other studies found that NBT reduction after stimulation with latex particles was impaired.[12,13] When we stimulated PV PMN with various soluble stimuli with defined as well as discrete pathways for activation of the cell an impairment of the oxidative metabolism of PV PMN was discovered, and this has been the topic of a recent extensive review.[25] Briefly, chemiluminescence, NBT reduction, and superoxide anion production were significantly reduced when induced by fMLP, LTB_4 and platelet-activating factor (PAF) in PV PMN,[15,20,22] but normal when the response was elicited by the calcium ionophore A23187 or phorbol myristate acetate (PMA). A normal NADPH oxidase activity, measured photometrically in PV PMN after stimulation with PMA has also been described by Piva and coworkers.[26] In that study, two PV patients were further analyzed with the microscopic NBT assay and those patients had a reduced NBT reduction after PMA stimulation, in contrast to our findings. However, since a very limited amount of patients were investigated and the NBT analysis was performed on whole blood by Piva and colleagues, interactions between PMN and other blood cells may have influenced their results. In accordance with this assumption, it has been reported that increasing concentrations of platelets can hamper PMN oxidative metabolism in healthy controls and, but to a lesser degree, in patients with essential thrombocythemia.[27] Finally, we also described that the intracellular generation of hydrogen peroxide, measured in single cells by flow cytometry, was reduced in PV PMN after stimulation with fMLP, but normal after PMA stimulation.[28] Interestingly, the same defective response to fMLP was also seen in PV monocytes. The flow cytometry analysis failed to detect any subpopulation of less responsive PMN or monocytes.

Since platelets do not express the NADPH oxidase, we investigated platelet aggregation in PV and found it to be subnormal when induced by PAF but normal after PMA stimulation.[29] This dampened aggregatory response was shown to exist in single PV platelets and associated with an impaired interaction of fibrinogen with its receptor on PV platelets.[30] Thus, we found evidence for a defect of oxidative metabolism present in *single* PV PMN and monocytes, as well as a defect of *single* platelet aggregation, after stimulation with surface receptor–dependent stimuli.

THE STIMULUS-RESPONSE COUPLING FOR OXIDATIVE METABOLISM IN PV PMN

Which, then, is the step in the stimulus-response coupling responsible for the defective oxidative response to fMLP in PV PMN? A summary of results obtained in our group is depicted in FIGURE 1. We demonstrated that there was no difference between PV and control PMN in the total number or binding affinity of the fMLP receptor.[22] The cells from PV patients displayed an intact activation of the PLC-mediated metabolism of phosphoinositides as evidenced by a normal generation of 1,4,5-inositoltrisphosphate and a normal subsequent increment of intracellular calcium.[22] Since oxidative metabolism induced by fMLP, LTB_4, and PAF is dependent on the activation of PLD,[31,32] the reduced response to these stimuli pointed towards an impaired activation of PLD in PV PMN. We found that fMLP-induced generation of phosphatidylethanol, formed in ethanol-treated PMN by a reaction unique for PLD and giving an indirect measurement of the production of phosphatidic acid, was reduced in PV PMN. In contrast, PMA activated PLD to the same extent in PV as in normal PMN.[22] Since there is a consensus that phosphatidic acid is the important second messenger for activation of the respiratory burst in PMN, this hampered PLD function is likely to be causally related to the defective oxidative response to fMLP in PV PMN. The proposed impairment of fMLP-induced activation of PLD needs to be characterized at the molecular level, but is a novel and perhaps unique finding, pertaining to the clone of cells originating from a malignant precursor cell. A similar reduction of fMLP oxidative metabolism has also recently been described in a subgroup of patients suffering from myelodysplastic syndromes, but investigation of PLD activation was not performed in that study,[33] and no analysis of single cell function was employed.

AN ACTIVATED STATE OF THE NEUTROPHIL IN PV?

One constant finding suggesting an activated state of PV PMN is the increased content of neutrophil alkaline phosphatase,[19] which is also elevated in bacterial infections as well as during treatment with granulocyte colony-stimulating factor. There is a consensus in the literature that PV PMN have an increased glycogen content and an elevated rate of glycogenolysis.[34–36] Moreover, it has been suggested that spontaneous PMN aggregation is increased in untreated PV patients due to an ill-defined plasma factor, while after treatment aggregation becomes normal.[37]

The phagocytic activity of PV PMN was first reported to be subnormal,[38] but this study was performed in whole blood and it was later proven that the presence of erythrocytes reduces PMN phagocytosis.[39] Two studies on purified PV PMN showed an increased phagocytosis of latex particles.[23,39] whereas other investigators found a normal phagocytic activity in the same assay system,[12,13] and yet another study indi-

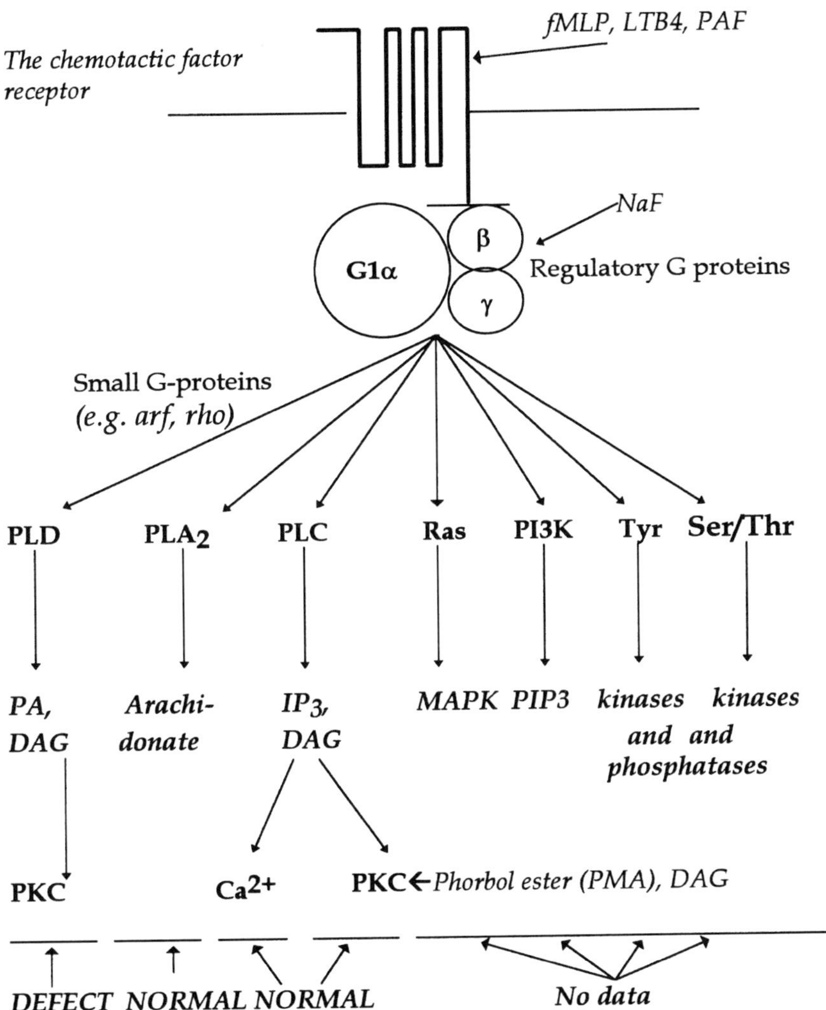

FIGURE 1. The stimulus response coupling in a PMN and possible defects in PV (according to the Stockholm Söder Hospital hypothesis). PLD, phospholipase D; PLA2, phospholipase A2; PLC, phospholipase C; PI3K, phosphatidyl inositol-3-kinase; Tyr, tyrosine; Ser/Thr, serine/threonine kinases; PA, phosphatidic acid; DAG, diacylglycerol; IP3, inositol trisphosphate; MAPK, MAP kinase; PKC, protein kinase C.

cated a normal phagocytosis and killing of *Staphylococcus aureus* and *Pseudomonas aeruginosa*.[40] Still, a recent study employing a more sensitive flow cytometry technique convincingly demonstrated a larger percentage of PV PMN and monocytes having an increased expression of the high affinity receptor for IgG, CD64, and of CD14+ PMN, compared to controls.[41] The percentage of PMN undergoing phagocytosis induced by immunoglobulin-opsonized *Escherichia coli* was also significantly higher in PV than in controls.

In summary, the neutrophil in polycythemia vera displays a complex phenotype that is indeed intriguing. Some cellular functions, i.e. migration and adherence, decidedly appear normal. At the same time, oxidative metabolism and PLD activation is impaired, while phagocytosis and expression of certain surface markers indicate an activated state of the cell. Obviously, this is an area that requires further investigation in order to explain the nature of the underlying molecular aberrations responsible for these divergent aspects of neutrophil function in PV and to see if any of the changes have a relation to prognosis.[42]

REFERENCES

1. ADAMSON, J. W., P. J. FIALKOW, J. MURPHY, J. F. PRCHAL & L. STEINMANN. 1976. Polycythemia vera stem cell and probable clonal origin of the disease. N. Engl. J. Med. **295:** 913–916.

2. RASKIND, W. H., R. JACOBSON, S. MURPHY, J. W. ADAMSON & P. J. FIALKOW. 1985. Evidence for the involvement of B lymphoid cells in polycythemia vera and essential thrombocythemia. J. Clin. Invest. **75:** 1388–1390.

3. LUCAS, G. S., R. A. PADUA, G. S. MASTERS, D. G. OSCIER & A. JACOBS. 1989. The application of X-chromosome gene probes to the diagnosis of myeloproliferative disease. Br. J. Haematol. **72:** 530–533.

4. ANGER, B., J. W. G. JANSSEN, H. SCHREZENMEIER, R. HEHLMANN, H. HEIMPEL & C. R. BARTRAM. 1990. Clonal analysis of chronic myeloproliferative disorders using X-linked DNA polymorphism. Leuk. Res. **4:** 258–261.

5. GILLILAND, D. G., K. L. BLANCHARD, J. LEVY, S. PERRIN & H. F. BUNN. 1991. Clonality in myeloproliferative disorders using X-linked DNA polymorphism. Proc. Natl. Acad. Sci. USA **88:** 6448–6452.

6. TSUKAMOTO, T., K. MORITA, T. MAEHARA *et al.* 1994. Clonality in chronic myeloproliferative disorders defined by X-chromosome linked probes: Demonstration of heterogeneity in lineage involvement. Br. J. Haematol. **86:** 253–258.

7. WALKER, R. I., J. C. HERION, W. B. HERRING & J. G. PALMER. 1964. Leukocyte kinetics in hematological disorders studied by DNA-phosphorus labeling. Blood **23:** 795–810.

8. RICHARD, K. A., R. D. BROWN, T. WILKINSON & H. KRONENBERG. 1979. The colony forming cell in the myeloproliferative disorders and aplastic anaemia. Scand. J. Haematol. **22:** 121–128.

9. ATHENS, J. W., O. P. HAAB, S. O. RAAB *et al.* 1965. Leukokinetic studies. XI. Granulocyte kinetics in polycythemia vera, infection and myelofibrosis. J. Clin. Invest. **44:** 778–788.

10. GHOSH, M. L., G. HUDSON & E. K. BLACKBURN. 1975. Skin window studies in polycythaemia rubra vera. Br. J. Haematol. **29:** 461–467.

11. JUNGI, W. F., G. MEURET & H. J. SENN. 1974. Granulocytenclearence and granulozytenkinetik bei myeloproliferativen syndromen. Schweiz Med. Wschr. **104:** 133–135.

12. CORBERAND, J., P. LAHARRAGUE, B. DE LARRAD, F. NGUYEN & J. PRIS. 1980. Phagocytosis in myeloproliferative disorders. Am. J. Clin. Pathol. **74:** 301–305.

13. LAHARRAGUE, P. F., J. X. CORBERAND, G. FILLOLA, B. P. BONEU & J. F. PRIS. 1984. Simultaneous study of platelets and phagocytes in myeloproliferative disorders. Biomed. Pharmacother. **38:** 462–465.

14. McCALL, C. E., J. CAVES, R. COOPER & L. DeCHATELET. 1971. Functional characteristics of human toxic neutrophils. J. Infect. Dis. **124:** 68–75.

15. SAMUELSSON, J., P. LINDSTRÖM & J. PALMBLAD. 1988. Stimulus-specific defect in oxidative metabolism of polymorphonuclear granulocytes in polycythemia vera. Eur. J. Haematol. **41:** 454–458.

16. GILBERT, H. S. & L. WARD. 1976. Augmented granulocyte adherence: An intrinsic abnormality in polycythemia vera. Blood **48:** 971a.

17. HOPEN, G. 1979. Retention in glass bead columns as a measure of leukocyte adhesiveness. II. Influence of platelets and erythrocytes. Scand. J. Haematol. **22:** 226–234.

18. HOPEN, G. 1981. Granulocyte and platelet adhesiveness in malignant paraproteinemia, leukemia and myeloproliferative diseases. Scand. J. Haematol. **27:** 339–345.

19. BORREGAARD, N., L. KJELDSEN & H. SENGELOV. 1993. Mobilization of granules in neutrophils from patients with myeloproliferative disorders. Eur. J. Haematol. **50:** 189–199.

20. STENKE, L., J. SAMUELSSON, J. PALMBLAD, L. DABROWSKI, P. REIZENSTEIN & J. Å. LINDGREN. 1990. Elevated white blood cell synthesis of leukotriene C4 in chronic myelogenous lekaemia but not in polycythaemia vera. Br. J. Haematol. **74:** 257–63.

21. SAMUELSSON, J. & A. BERG. 1991. Further studies of the defective stimulus-response coupling for the oxidative burst in neutrophils in polycythemia vera. Eur. J. Haematol. **47:** 239–245.

22. SAMUELSSON, J., A. HANSSON, K. ROSENDAHL & J. PALMBLAD. 1993. Superoxide anion production and phospholipase D mediated generation of diacylglycerol are subnormal after N-formyl-methionyl-leucyl-phenylalanine stimulation of polymorphonuclear granulocytes in polycythemia vera. J. Lab. Clin. Med. **121:** 310–319.

23. COOPER, M. R., L. R. DeCHATELET, C. E. McCALL & C. L. SPURR. 1972. The activated phagocyte of polycythemia vera. Blood **40:** 366–374.

24. ASHBURN, P., M. R. COOPER, C. E. McCALL & L. R. DeCHATELET. 1973. Nitroblue tetrazolium reduction: False positive and false negative results. Blood **41:** 921–925.

25. SAMUELSSON, J. 1995. Impaired activation of phospholipase D in polycythaemia vera—implications for the pathogenesis of the disease. Leuk. Lymphoma **19:** 21–26.

26. PIVA, E., S. DE TONI, A. CAENAZZO, M. PRADELLA, F. PIETROGRANDE & M. PLEBANI. 1995. Neutrophil NADPH oxidase activity in chronic myeloproliferative and myelodysplastic diseases by microscopic and photometric assays. Acta Haematol. **94:** 16–22.

27. CARULLI, G., S. MINNUCCI, M. L. GIANFALDONI, C. ANGIOLINI, A. AZZARÀ & F. AMBROGI. 1995. Interactions between platelets and neutrophils in essential thrombocythaemia. Effects on neutrophil chemiluminescence and superoxide anion generation. Eur. J. Clin. Invest. **25:** 929–934.

28. SAMUELSSON, J., J. FORSLID, J. HED & J. PALMBLAD. 1994. Studies of neutrophil and monocyte oxidative responses in polycythaemia vera and related myeloproliferative disorders. Br. J. Haematol. **87:** 464–470.

29. LE BLANC, K., A. BERG, J. PALMBLAD & J. SAMUELSSON. 1994. Stimulus-specific defect in platelet aggregation in polycythemia vera. Eur. J. Haematol. **53:** 145–149.

30. LE BLANC, K., T. LINDAHL, K. ROSENDAHL & J. SAMUELSSON. 1996. Impaired activation of the fibrinogen receptor on polycythaemia vera platelets after platelet activating factor stimulation. Br. J. Haematol. **93**(Suppl 2): 168a.

31. BALSINDE, J. & F. MOLLINEDO. 1991. Platelet-activating factor synergizes with phorbol myristate acetate in activating phospholipase D in the human promonocytic cell line U937. Evidence for different mechanisms of activation. J. Biol. Chem. **266:** 18726–18730.

32. KANAHO, Y., H. KANAHO, K. SAITOH & Y. NOZAWA. 1991. Phospholipase D activation by platelet activating factor, leukotriene B4, and formyl-methionyl-leucyl-phenylalanine in

rabbit neutrophils. Phospholipase D activation is involved in enzyme release. J. Immunol. **146:** 3536–3541.

33. Lowe, G. M., Y. Dang, F. Watson, S. W. Edwards & D. W. Galvani. 1994. Identification of a subgroup of myelodysplastic patients with a neutrophil stimulation-signaling defect. Br. J. Haematol. **86:** 761–766.

34. Wagner, R. 1947. Studies on the physiology of white blood cells. The glycogen content of leukocytes in leukemia and polycythemia. Blood **2:** 235–243.

35. Luganova, I. S. & I. E. Seitz. 1963. Glycogen content and normal metabolism in normal and leukemic human leukocytes. Fed. Proc. Transpl. Suppl. **22:** 1058–1061.

36. Gahrton, G. 1966. The periodic acid-Schiff reaction in neutrophil leukocytes in chronic myeloproliferative diseases. A microspectrophotometric study. Scand. J. Haematol. **3:** 106–116.

37. Fischer, H. 1985. Leukergie stimulierende faktoren bei polyzythaemia vera. Folia Hematol. **112:** 580–586.

38. Feher, L. & J. Komaromi. 1956. Uber phagozytose der leukozyten bei verschiedenen hämatologischen erkrankungen. Folio Hematol. **73:** 301–306.

39. Brandt, L. 1967. Studies on the phagocytic activity of neutrophil leukocytes. Scand. J. Haematol. **67**(Suppl 2): 54–64.

40. Sbarra, A. J., W. Shirley, R. J. Selvaraj, R. J. McRipley & E. Rosenbaum. 1965. The role of the phagocyte in host-parasite interactions. III. The phagocytic capabilities of leukocytes from myeloproliferative and other neoplastic disorders. Cancer Res. **25:** 1199–1206.

41. Westwood, N. B., E. R. Copson, L. A. Page, A. R. Mire-Sluis, K. A. Brown & T. C. Pearson. 1995. Activated phenotype in neutrophils and monocytes from patients with primary proliferative polycythaemia. J. Clin. Pathol. **48:** 525–530.

42. Mazzone, A., G. Ricevuti, M. Rossi & S. C. Rizzo. 1986. Prognostic significance of functional defects of granulocytes in myeloproliferative disease. Oncology **43:** 176–182.

Triple-Labeling Cytofluorimetric Quantitative and Qualitative Evaluation of Phagocytic Activity of Monocytes and Polymorphonuclear Cells

E. MANCA, V. ARANGINO, S. LOMBARDINI, A. GHIANI, D. MUSU,
B. AMBROSINI, S. R. DEL GIACCO, AND G. S. DEL GIACCO

Internal Medicine Department
School of Medicine
Cagliari University
Via S. Giorgio 12
09124 Cagliari, Italy

INTRODUCTION

Polymorphonuclear cells (PMNs) play an important role in the control of bacterial and mycotic infection and, partially, in the control of some viral infectious and some neoplasias.[1] A nonsecondary role in the pathogenesis of several noninfectious diseases is also played. The study of PMN functions is needed to evaluate their activity in various immunodeficiencies. In other diseases, useful information about their activation state can also be learned.

The main limits to the study of PMN function so far have been: the need to isolate the cells from peripheral blood (or other biological fluids); the need to use large blood volumes; the tests' complexity; the time-consuming nature of the tests; and the difficulty in processing many samples at the same time. The traditional tests to evaluate phagocytosis are impaired by several technical limitations. For direct microscopy these are: subjective judgment; difficulty in discriminating between intracellular and membrane-bound extracellular targets; low amount of neutrophils available for evaluation in a single test; and long time of reading. Also, the technical limitations for ra-

TABLE 1. Materials Used in Triple-Labeling Test

Reagents	Supplier
E. coli FITC	Orpegen
Quenching solution	Orpegen
CD14 PE	Becton Dickinson
CD15 PE	Becton Dickinson
CD45 Per CP	Becton Dickinson
Lysing solution	Ortho Immune System
Washing solution	Orpegen
Paraformaldehyde 1%	Polysciences

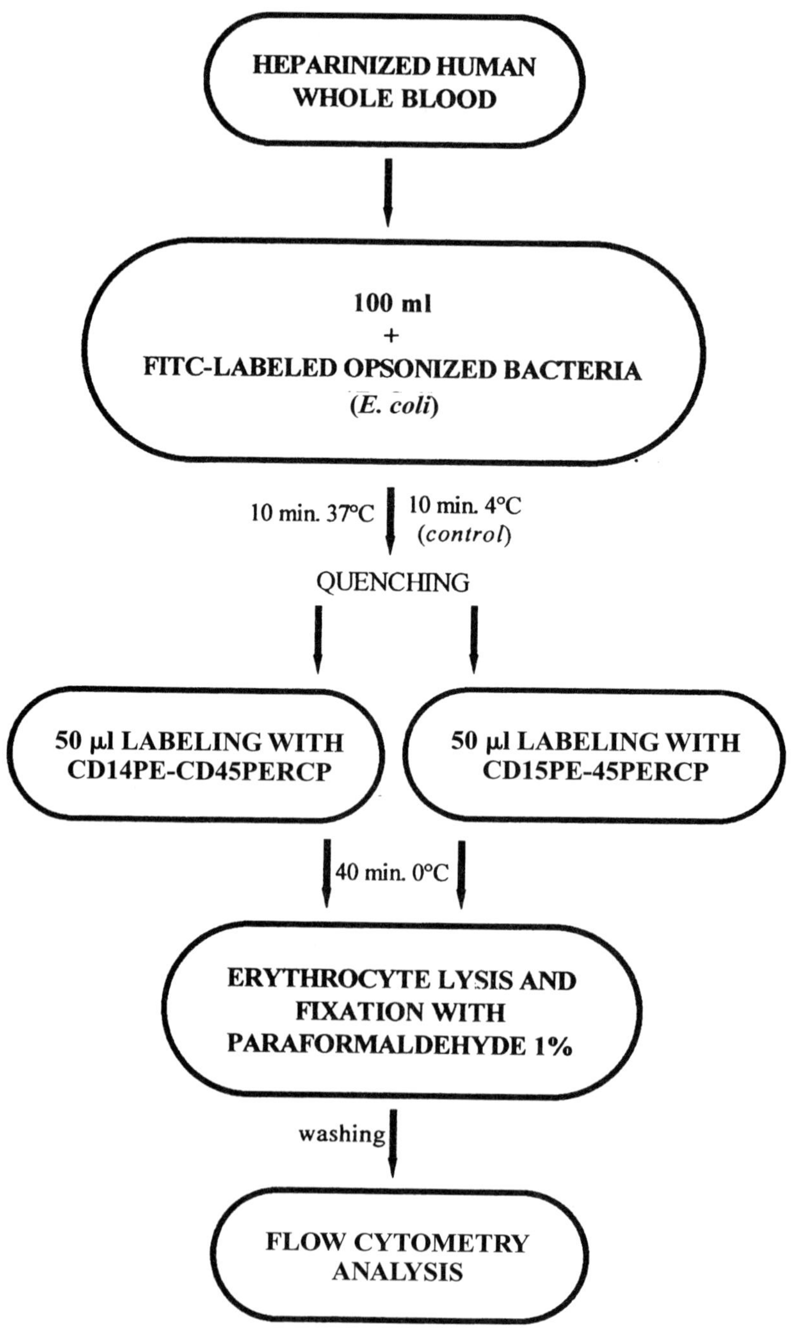

FIGURE 1. Triple-labeling method.

dionuclide tests are the use of radioactive substances and the global evaluation of phagocytosis.

A relevant improvement to routine tests for the evaluation of PMNs comes from methods employing whole blood. Flow cytometry, because of its specific technical peculiarities, provides the opportunity to study many different PMN functions[2] in a new and interesting way. Flow cytometry has certain advantages: the possibility to employ whole blood[3,4] (according to scatter characteristics using specific electronic gates); a large amount of cells to evaluate (8–10,000 events can be acquired during routine flow-cytometry analysis); evaluation of percentage of phagocytes and of phagocyted targets; and high specificity. In the present work, a flow-cytometry test with triple labeling has been employed to study phagocytic cells. In comparison to other alternative methods, based on propidium iodide incorporation in DNA,[5] our technique has many advantages: it requires small volumes of whole blood, it is fast, and it differentiates among monocytes, PMNs, and bacteria using monoclonal antibodies labeled for the second and third fluorescence detector.

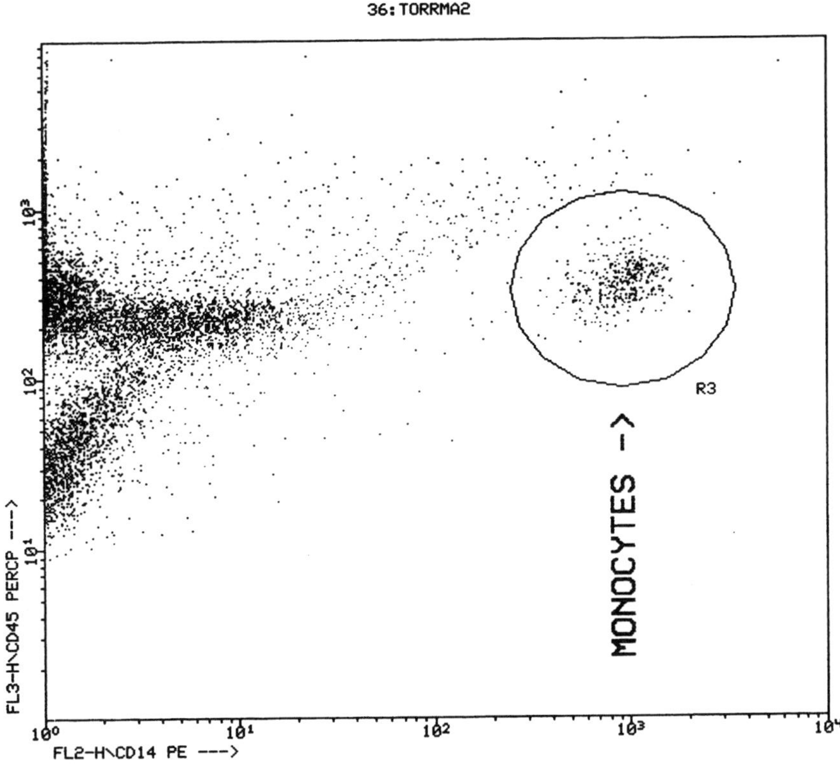

FIGURE 2. Gate R3 shows monocytes (double-positive cells for CD14 PE and CD45 PerCP).

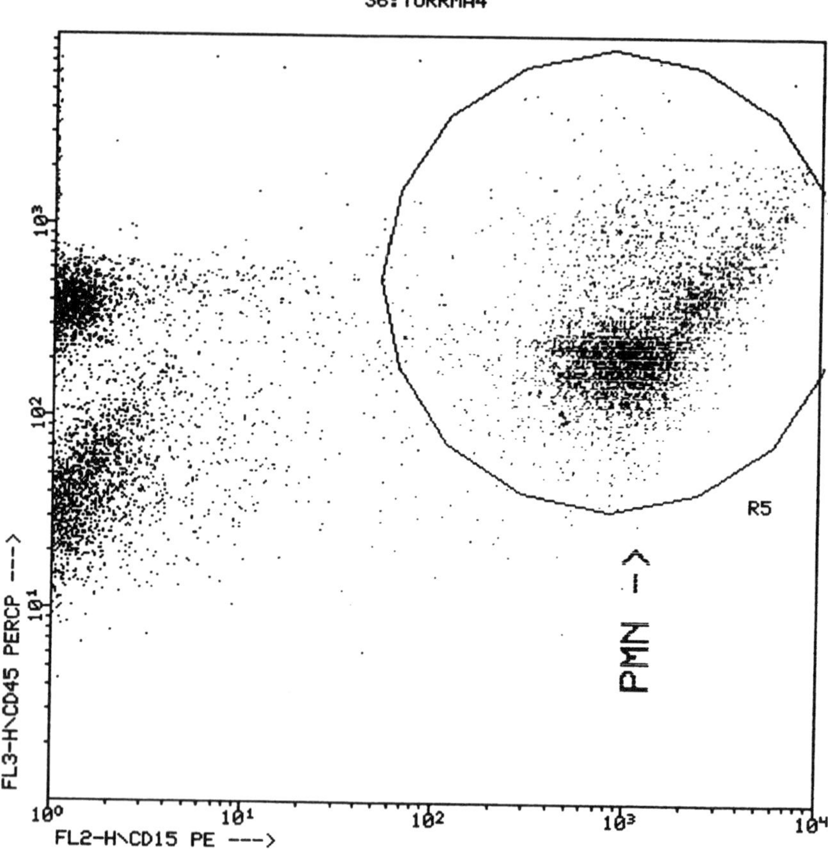

FIGURE 3. Gate R5 shows PMNs (double-positive cells for CD15 PE and CD45 PerCP).

MATERIAL AND METHODS

In this study, the phagocytosis of PMN and monocytes in whole blood of normal human subjects (20 males, 20 females, age 30±10 years) has been evaluated. A 100-µl aliquot of heparinized whole blood is incubated for 10 min at 37°C with 20×10⁶ *E. coli*[5] labeled with FITC (fluorescein-isothiocyanate) and opsonized with antibody and complement (control sample has been kept in ice during the same time). Then 100 µl of quenching solution[5] are added to eliminate the fluorescence of non-ingested bacteria. After several washings the cells are labeled to identify monocytes with CD14 PE (phycoerythrin) and CD45 PerCP (phycobiliprotein) and PMNs with CD15 PE and CD45 PerCP. After a 40-min incubation at 0°C, the red cells are lysed (1 ml

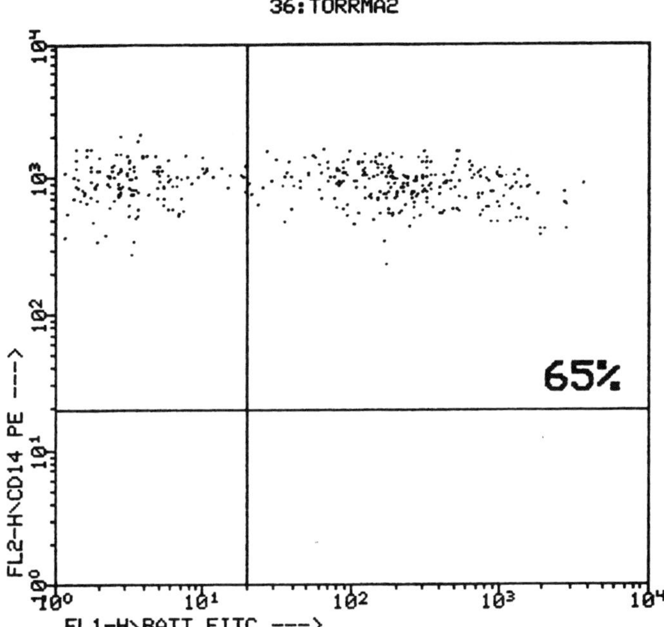

FIGURE 4. The upper right quadrant shows the percentage of monocyte phagocytosis.

of Ortho Lysing Solution for 20 min) and the remaining cells are fixed in 1% paraformaldehyde (TABLE 1). The analysis of results has been made with FACScan Cytofluorimeter (Becton Dickinson) (FIG. 1).

RESULTS

In order to evaluate the results by flow cytometry, lymphocytes have to be separated from monocytes and from PMNs by using corresponding surface markers. The percentage of phagocytic cells (PMNs and monocytes) and their mean fluorescence intensity (number of phagocytized *E. coli*)[6] are analyzed. For this purpose a gate around the white cells (first monocytes and then granulocytes) on the cytogram FL2 (fluorescence 2)/FL3 (fluorescence 3) has been placed (FIGS. 2 and 3) and the corresponding gate on a cytogram FL1 (fluorescence 1)/FL2 has been analyzed (FIGS. 4 and 5). The percentage of double-labeled cells indicates the percentage of phagocytic cells compared to non-phagocytic control cells. Our study performed on a control group (20 males and 20 females) shows that the phagocytosis values in monocytes are 55–65% and in PMNs 60–90% (FIGS. 6 and 7).

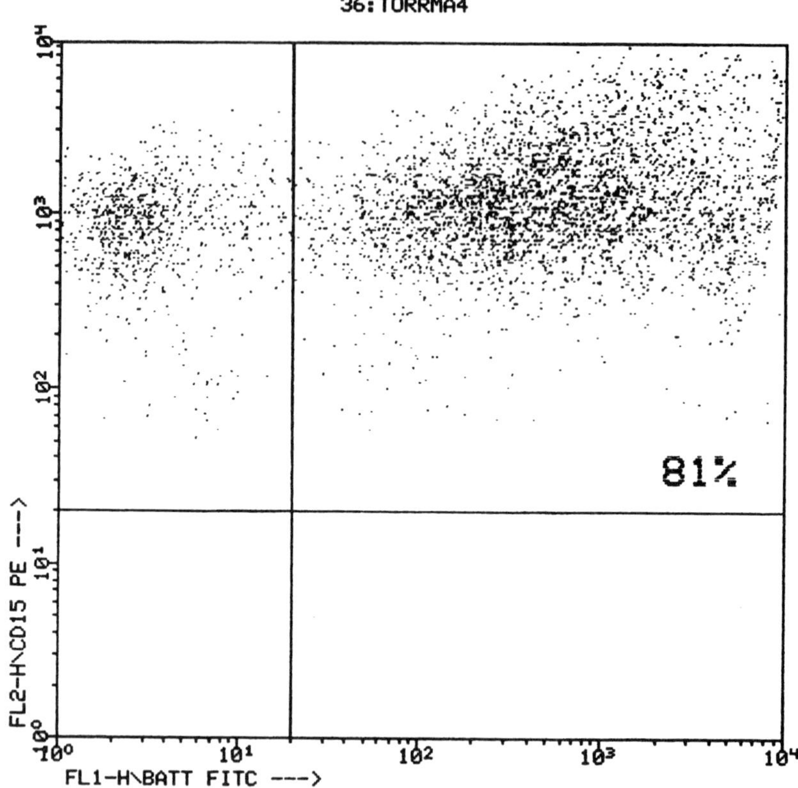

FIGURE 5. The upper right quadrant shows the percentage of PMN phagocytosis.

DISCUSSION

Because of the relevant role played by phagocytes in the control of bacterial and mycotic infections, several techniques to evaluate their functional activity are necessary.[7] The triple-labeling test allows the determination of the percentage of phagocytic monocytes and granulocytes. It also makes possible differentiation among monocytes, PMN, and bacteria by means of surface markers.

Alternative methods, based on incorporation of propidium iodine in DNA,[5] do not differentiate among monocytes, PMNs, and lymphocytes because monoclonal antibodies labeled for second and third fluorescence detector cannot be employed. Therefore, PMNs and monocytes are identified using light-scatter parameters, with a consequent less accurate determination of phagocytosis values. The flow cytometry with triple-labeling test is particularly interesting because with a single test, provided that suitable technical devices[2] are adopted, multiple biological and functional parameters can be studied.

Moreover, the triple-labeling test is extremely convenient, sensible, and repro-

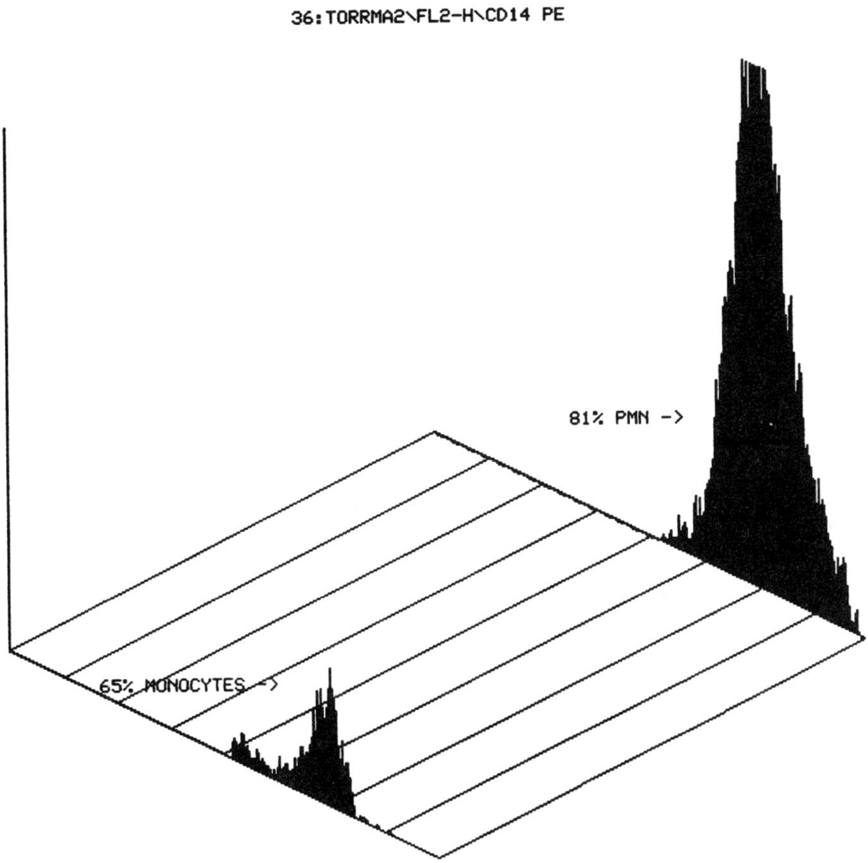

FIGURE 6. Percentage of phagocytosis of monocytes and PMN in a control subject.

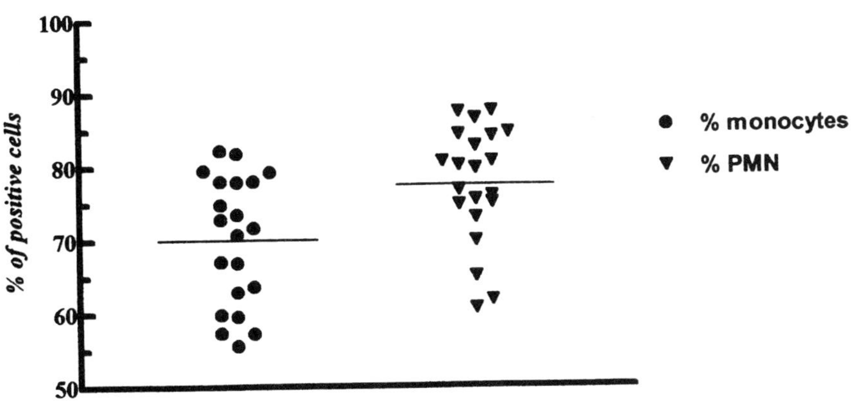

FIGURE 7. Percentage of phagocytosis in normal subjects.

ducible and would work well to evaluate phagocytosis in appropriate clinical contexts.[8]

REFERENCES

1. MALECH, H. L. & J. I. GALLIN. 1987. Neutrophils in human diseases. N. Engl. J. Med. **317:** 687–694.
2. CARULLI, G., S. MINNUCCI, R. VANACORE & F. AMBROGI. 1995. Il ruolo della citometria a flusso nello studio della fisiopatologia dei granulociti neutrofili. Rec. Progr. Med. **86(5):** 208–216.
3. BASSOE, C. F., J. SOLSVIK & O. D. LAERUM. 1980. Quantitation of single cell phagocytic capacity by flow cytometry. Acta. Pathol. Microbiol. Scand. Sect. A. **274:** 170–174.
4. HASUI, M., Y. HIRABAYASHI & Y. KOBAYASHI. 1989. Simultaneous measurement by flow cytometry of phagocytosis and hydrogen peroxide of neutrophils in whole blood. J. Immunol. Meth. **117:** 53–58.
5. ORPEGEN PHAGOTEST® Kit Operators Manual. 1992.
6. SHAPIRO, H. M. 1988. Practical Flow Cytometry. A. R. Liss. New York.
7. PERTICARARI, S., G. PRESANI & E. BANFI. 1994. A new flow cytometric assay for the evaluation of phagocytosis and the oxidative burst in whole blood. J. Immunol. Methods **170(1):** 117–124.
8. DONABEDIAN, H. D. Congenital and acquired neutrophil abnormalities. *In* Phagocytes and Disease. M. M. S. Klempner, B. Styrt & J. Ho, Eds. Kluwer, Dordrecht.

Evaluation of Neutrophil Motility by Image Analysis

ANTONIO AZZARÀ[a]

Unit of Hematology
Department of Oncology
University of Pisa
56100 Pisa, Italy

INTRODUCTION

Polymorphonuclear leukocytes (PMN) motility dysfunction may play an important role in a lot of diseases. Both primary[1–3] and secondary defective functions[4–6] or excessive functions[7–9] may be involved. Many of these disease entities have been widely investigated, but little information is available on the behavior of cell propagation in different pathologies. One of the main techniques currently used to explore PMN motility, namely micropore filters in a chemotactic chamber,[10] usually provides the distance traveled by the cells in a given time by the so-called leading front method,[11] which may be performed in a relatively short time, but is characterized by errors due to the dishomogeneity of the migration front itself. More information is provided by also evaluating the number of migrating cells at given distances,[12] but this method is characterized by numerous and tedious microscopic observations. In both cases the subjectivity of the operator and the increasing range of error due to multiple observations must be taken into account.

Some modifications have been proposed to ameliorate weaknesses of micropore filter technique: one of these[13] employs two overlapped filters (with different pore size) and three different ways of counting, so further tedious microscopic counts are needed. Other modifications evaluate PMN motility by indirect means: such as a spectrophotometric assay,[14] which quantitates the number of cells on the lower surface of the filters from the amount of stain extracted from those cells, and a cytochemical assay,[15] which measures PMN chemotaxis from the quantitation of myeloperoxidase in the lower compartment. The main problems with these indirect techniques are the difficulty in obtaining uniform exposure to the staining solution and the necessity of a complete removal of cells (or cellular debris) attached to the surfaces of the filter. Other authors have proposed the use of ^{51}Cr-labeled PMN in chambers equipped with a double micropore-filter system[16] or even the infusion of autologous ^{111}In-labeled PMN in a skin-window system,[17] with the aim of measuring the PMN migration by the radioactivity level in the filters. These methods, even if reliable and objective, have obvious limitations especially if a routine use is needed.

Both the conventional microscopic techniques and the more complex ones are unable to give information concerning the kinetics of migration in times suitable for

[a]Address correspondence to Dr. Antonio Azzarà, Unita Operativa di Ematologia, Ospedale S. Chiara, Via Rome 67, 56100 Pisa, Italy. Phone, 039-50-992185 and Fax, 039-50-502617.

current diagnostic use, even though some authors have clearly demonstrated the relevance of performing a mathematical analysis of the PMN distribution. In particular, we refer to the theoretical models of behavior of PMN moving randomly or under chemotactic stimuli through microporous filters,[18] which has been recently developed[19] as an extension of the model applied to the under-agarose assay.[20] So some modern approaches capable of acquiring and analyzing more data have been proposed, including computer-assisted systems. In some cases they were applied to densitometry[21,22]; in some others, to image analysis devices. Most of image analysis devices[23,24] have been applied in agarose assays[25] or were used to detect the orientation of a single cell or a small number of cells in experimental models.[26] Very rarely has image analysis been applied to the micropore method in assays evaluating only one optical plane (the lower surface of a 10-μm thin polycarbonate membrane)[27] or few optical planes in the final portion of the filters.[28]

Recently we have described an image processing workstation, designed for applications in both research work and in current diagnostic use, for the automatic evaluation of human PMN motility in micropore filters.[29] The workstation is able to measure many parameters in a reliable, reproducible, and rapid fashion. In particular, our algorithm recognizes and counts cells in several fields and focal planes throughout the whole filter; correlates counts and depth values; performs a statistical analysis of data; calculates the true value of PMN migration; determines the distribution of cells; and displays the migration pattern. These results may be stored in a database and printed, together with data about the patient or assay under study.

More recently, we have described a study in which PMN migration behavior in normal, healthy donors has been investigated by the use of the abovementioned workstation.[30] The mean propagation curve and the range of propagation were obtained for both spontaneous random migration and chemotaxis. In particular, we were able to confirm the previously hypothesized theoretical models of PMN random motility behavior and to identify a very typical behavior pattern of PMN under chemotactic stimuli.

In this paper, we report data (most of which were previously unreported) regarding some studies about migration kinetics of PMN from normal donors under different conditions (in particular, different incubation time, different chemoattractant stimuli, different chemoattractant concentrations). We also provide some examples of the potential use of our device in pathology. In particular, we report data regarding patients with migration defects (both congenital and acquired). Moreover, data about "*in vivo*" drug interference, undetectable by conventional methods, are reported: we refer to the effects of old and new drugs widely investigated and used to correct many kinds of neutropenia, such as lithium and rhG-CSF.[31,32] Finally, preliminary data regarding different migration patterns displayed by PMN from patients affected by myelodysplastic syndromes are reported.

MATERIALS AND METHODS

Chemotactic Assay

Neutrophils from donors or patients (obtained using 10 ml venous heparinized blood, 10 units heparin/ml), were sedimented with dextran 4:1 (vol/vol), centrifuged at $160 \times g$ for 10 min, resuspended and washed twice in phosphate-buffered saline Dulbecco solution at $160 \times g$ for 5 min, sedimented on a sodium metrizoate Ficoll density gradient, and centrifuged at $400 \times g$ for 30 min, treated by a buffered solution of NH_4Cl 0.87%. The cell suspension, which was composed of 97–98% of neutrophils, was adjusted in Dulbecco solution to final suspension of 750×10^5/ml (while the final suspension used in some of our previous experiments was 1×10^6/ml). Neutrophil viability was always greater than 98%. All the isolation steps were performed at 4°C to avoid aspecific surface molecule activation.[33] When PMN from patients were evaluated (Shwachman-Diamond syndrome, lymphomas under chemotherapy and rhG-CSF, myelodysplastic syndromes), blood smears were also observed by means of light microscopy after May-Grunwald-Giemsa staining, in order to detect the presence of band cells or more immature leukocytes.

The chemotactic assay was performed according to a modified Boyden method[34] with minor modifications, as elsewhere widely described.[29] Briefly, neutrophil random motility and chemotaxis were assessed in perspex chemotactic chambers (B.M. Strumentazione Biomedica, Milan, Italy); mixed-ester filters, diameter 13 mm, pore size 3 μm (Millipore Corporation, Bedford, MA) were used between the two compartments. A "crude" supernatant of *E. coli* culture (10%) or lipopolysaccharide (LPS) from *E. coli* Serotype 055:B5 (Sigma Chemicals, St. Louis, MO) at concentration ranging from 50 to 150 μg/ml, or formyl-methionyl-leucyl-phenylalanine (fMLP) (Sigma Chemicals, St. Louis, MO) at concentrations ranging from 10^{-8} to 10^{-7} M were used as attractant to evaluate chemotaxis. Dulbecco solution was used in the lower compartment to evaluate random migration. The chambers were incubated in a humid atmosphere with 5% CO_2 at 37°C for a standard time of 60 min (whereas the incubation time used in some of our previous experiments was 120 min). In some experiments the incubation was stopped after 20, 30, 40, 50, or 60 minutes. Then, the filters were removed, fixed in 95% ethyl alcohol, stained with Harris Hematoxylin, treated with 0.05% HCl and blueing agent, dehydrated in 95% ethyl alcohol and absolute isopropyl alcohol, cleared in xylol, and mounted on slides. In experiments exploring drug interference, although the automatic image analysis does not involve the operator's subjectivity, each slide was marked with a conventional sign by the laboratory staff and stored. The final evaluation was carried out "blind," in a single session by the staff involved in the image analysis workstation.

Computer-Assisted Image Analysis

The method, which was widely described elsewhere[29] provides a completely new approach for the evaluation of cell migration throughout microporous filters.

Hardware Components

The filters to be examined are mounted on the table of a Leitz Hortolux microscope. The focal plane of the 10× objective is imaged onto a solid-state TV-camera (Javelin JE7362 CCD B/W, Javelin Electronics, Torrance, CA) mounted on top of the microscope. The video signal produced by the TV camera is sent to a video board (PIP-1024B, Matrox Electronic System, Dorval, Canada), which can store up to four digital images defined by 512×512 pixels with 256 grey levels. Input images are acquired via an 8-bit analog to digital video converter while processed images are loaded from the host computer. The board drives on RGB (red, green, blue) monitor (FA-345L9ATKE Mitsubishi Electronic Corporation, Tokyo, Japan) for the display of digital images. The dimensions of the microscopic field acquired by the TV camera are 480 μm × 340 μm (horizontal resolution = 0.94 μm and vertical resolution = 0.66 μm). The area imaged onto the TV camera is equal to four conventional microscopic fields. The screw of the micrometric regulation of the microscope focusing is connected to a step-motor (M061-LS08 Slo-Syn, Superior Electric, Bristol, CO). The motor resolution is 1.8 degrees (200 steps per revolution): as a complete micrometric turn corresponds to 100 μm table movement along the optical axis of the microscope (Z axis) and one motor step corresponds to 0.5 μm displacement of the focused plane. The motor is driven by a 230-T Slo-Syn translator (Superior Electric, Bristol, CO), which in turn is controlled via an I/O interface.

Software Components

Dedicated software based on the photometric analysis has been especially developed by Istituto di Elaborazione dell'Informazione (CNR-Pisa, Italy) to detect and count the cells throughout the filter. Briefly, the digital image resulting from the acquisition of each focal plane is composed of a 512×512 matrix, defined by luminance elements (L) that range in value from 0 to 255 and depend on the amount of light reaching the TV camera. Each matrix element corresponds to a picture element (pixel); pixels located on cell images (dark objects on white background) display values lower than the background pixels, and corresponds to negative peaks on the matrix rows obtained by means of a line-scan technique. This signal variation is measured over a constant derivative distance (D), which specifies both the number of adjacent elements L and the interval over which the slope of the input signal is measured. By processing the acquisition matrix and using a decision process based on a detection threshold (T), the software takes into account only the contours of well-focused cells lying in the plane under study. After the detection of a reference value (corresponding to the "noise" count), the first plane (Z_0) is analyzed. Each row of the acquired matrix is processed and a counter is incremented whenever the absolute value of the difference between two consecutive elements L_0 of the row is greater than a predefined threshold value. This way, the final count C_0, relative to the plane Z_0, depends on the number of the detected-edge points of the cell images and is proportional to the number of cells contained in the focused field. Then the microscopic table is shifted along the optical axis so that a plane at distance Z_1 from the filter surface is focused and an image is acquired and processed, with a final count C_1. The table is shifted again and the process is repeated, while the software performs a progressive and automatic adjustment of the detection threshold (T) for each plane, until cells are found in focused planes. The set of values C_n is then interpolated and the continuous curve $C_{(z)}$, which represents the migration of PMN through the filter, is calculated and displayed. In the meantime, the software (*1*) calculates the sum of the counts and transforms them into percentage values for each plane; (*2*) calculates the logarithms of the measuring sequences and the square value of depth; (*3*) finds the linear regression between the two variables; (*4*) calculates the constant term, the gradient, and the correlation index (adjusted R^2) of the line interpolating the values; (*5*) identifies the intersection point with depth axis (corresponding to a decrease of two logarithmic units in the count axis) and calculates the square root of this value (this point, expressed in μm, is the true "Final plane" value, FP, reached by the cells; (6) builds the interpolating curve that describes the kinetics of cell propagation throughout the filter; and (7) displays it on the monitor. The whole sequence of operations and data processing is performed in a few seconds by a personal computer (PC), equipped with a VGA video board and a color monitor for the display of alphanumeric data or graphs, and a printer. The software, written in C language, requires about 300 Kbytes on disk.

Statistics

FP values of each sample were calculated by the software according to the above-mentioned procedure. Means and standard error of the mean of the obtained FP values were calculated, when necessary, by conventional methods and differences between means were calculated according to Student *t*-test for paired samples.

Subjects Studied

Donors

More than 100 assays on filters using samples from 18 donors were carried out in order to identify the values of the D and T parameters which best fit with the results obtained by conventional microscopic evaluation. These parameters had been tested initially during previous simulation studies[35] performed on microphotographs digitized by means of a high-resolution *xy* scanner (MFA/36, S. Salvadori srl, Firenze, Italy) and then applied in our workstation. Moreover, the stability of the system and the reproducibility of the single values obtained and of whole sequences of measurement, were controlled.

Samples from 21 donors were examined in order to assess the normal curves of PMN random motility and chemotaxis.

Patients

PMN from a child affected by Shwachman-Diamond syndrome (a congenital syndrome[3] characterized, apart from other important symptoms, by neutropenia and neutrophil motility defects[36]) were evaluated in basal condition, after 15 days and 30 days of lithium therapy (30 mg/kg/day), on the basis of previous studies showing the drug activity *in vitro*.[37]

PMN from seven patients affected by intermediate and high grade non-Hodgkin's lymphoma and undergoing chemotherapy were evaluated in order to investigate the interference of rhG-CSF with neutrophil motility. The study was carried out as far as possible from any direct effect of chemotherapy, that is, immediately before G-CSF administration (5 μg/kg/day for 5 days, subcutaneously) and 24 h after G-CSF interruption.

PMN from 11 patients affected by myelodysplastic syndrome were evaluated in order to identify specific motility patterns related to the degree of malignity. According to a French-American-British cooperative group, they were classified as: four cases of refractory anemia (RA); one case of refractory anemia with ringed sideroblasts (RARS); two cases of refractory anemia with excess blasts (RAEB); two cases of refractory anemia with excess blasts in leukemic transformation (RAEB-t); and two cases of chronic myelomonocytic leukemia (CMMoL) 2. All patients were studied at diagnosis; underlying infectious diseases were not evident. They were not being treated with cytotoxic drugs or other drugs that might have influenced neutrophil morphology or function.

RESULTS

Measurement Reproducibility

The best D and T parameters and in particular the suitable automatic progressive threshold variation capable of detecting cells only in the plane under observation with exclusion of the others, were identified with a good correlation ($r = 0.960$, $p < 0.001$) between conventional optical evaluation (performed plane by plane) and the computer-assisted evaluation. A very good correlation ($r = 0.999$, $p < 0.0001$) was also found when the stability of the system was controlled by measuring the same fields in different days without touching the filter and the workstation (data not shown).[29] This aspect was better defined by more accurate experiments with the "noise" associated with the component of the device (variation due to the light source and the TV camera and variation due to the movement of the microscope table). The first one was measured by repeated acquisition and analysis (12 times per 6 different depths: $N = 72$) of fixed focal planes and by blocking the table motor. The relative coefficient of variation was in the range 0.16–0.47%. The second one was evaluated by repeated (12 times per 6 different depths) sequences of measurement of the same field and by automatic repetition of the whole sequence without any manual correction. The relative coefficient of variation was found in the range 0.49–1.01%. The precision of the measurement can thus be estimated on the order of 1% (data not shown).[30]

Moreover, the reproducibility of the count using different depth progression (with adjustment of the related threshold) was studied, in order to evaluate the possibility of speeding up the automatic reading by doubling the depth increment (from 10 to 20 μm), thus halving the number of planes to be analyzed and achieving a very good correlation ($r = 0.999$, $p < 0.0001$) (TABLE 1). All these tests were performed by analyzing filters of leukocyte migration for 120 min. These tests allowed us to evaluate not only distance traveled by the migrating PMN, but also the migration curve profile. As regards random motility, it was perfectly comparable to a gaussian model, whereas a particular curve characterized by a "wave" was found as regards stimulated migration (FIG. 1).

The time required for the whole measurement sequence depends on the characteristics of the PC. When the first tests were carried out by a 286 20 MHz processor, 6 min and 35 sec were necessary to perform, for example, the evaluation on three

TABLE 1. Comparison of the Sequences of Counts Obtained at Depth Interval of 10 µm Versus Counts Obtained at Depth Interval of 20 µm in the Same Microscopic Field for Migration Time of 120 Minutes

Filter Depth (µm)	Count (pixel) $T_0 = 36$; $A_1 = 17\%$; $A_2 = 7\%$	Count (pixel) $T_0 = 36$; $A_1 = 23\%$; $A_2 = 14\%$
0	11273	11429
10	8574	—
20	4016	4190
30	2263	—
40	2915	3094
50	3668	—
60	4058	4250
70	3677	—
80	2910	3180
90	2289	—
100	1911	2168
110	1556	—
120	1250	1380
130	970	—
140	650	766
150	422	—
160	212	289

Note: T_0 (Initial threshold), A_1 (first threshold reduction), and A_2 (further progressive reduction of A_1) are parameters automatically applied by the workstation for specific depth intervals. $r = 0.999$ and $p < 0.0001$.

fields (corresponding to 12 conventional fields!) of a 160 µm stimulated migration. Today, using a PC equipped with a Pentium 60 MHz processor, the whole measurement sequence is performed in only 1 min and 32 sec!

Migration Values and Patterns in Normal Donors

In order to study the possibility of also speeding up the preliminary phase of the assay, the subsequent experiments were carried out halving the incubation time to 60 minutes. Using this model we also confirmed that the random migration propagation is defined by a gaussian curve. Its tangent intercepts the depth axis at a point that corresponds to a variation of two units in the logarithm transformation of counts (that is a variation of two decades in the counts). The square root of this value corresponds to the distance traveled by the cells. For random migration the normal interval between two standard deviations of the values for the final depth was 77–102 µm, whereas the average value for the final depth was 86.5 µm. Performing a linear regression on the average values of logarithms of counts, we obtained a line with corrected $R^2 = 0.993$.

In the case of chemotaxis, our data showed a very typical pattern. It could have been expected that the cell distribution throughout the filter would only be characterized by a higher intercept value with respect to the random migration values. On the

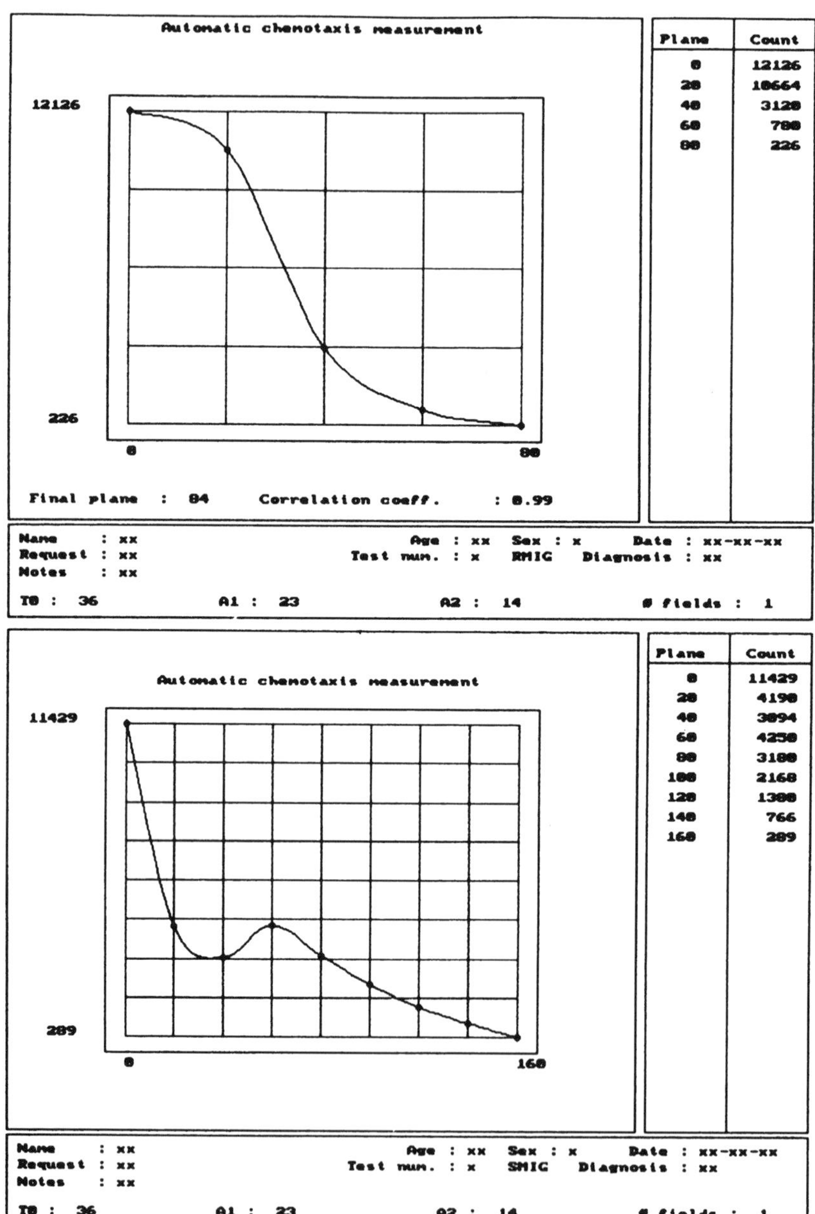

FIGURE 1. Printouts of results obtained in the analysis of a filter obtained under condition of random migration (*top*) and chemotaxis (*bottom*) for 120 minutes. In the first one, the plot obtained by interpolation of measurement points fits a gaussian function; in the second one, the plot describes a typical migration wave.

contrary, the measuring sequences displayed a maximum located around the depth of 20 μm rather than on the initial plane. The analysis of this trend of density of PMN within the filter would need a combination of very complex non-linear functions.[27] Anyway, taking into account the square value of the number that corresponds to this "shift," it was possible, with good approximation, to interpolate the values of the logarithms of the counts by a linear function. So, for chemotaxis the normal interval between two standard deviation of the values for the final depth was 117–162 μm, whereas the average value for the final depth was 134 μm. Performing a linear regression on the average values of logarithms of counts, we obtained a line with corrected $R^2 = 0.994$. The migration patterns and the intersection bands obtained after by mathematical analysis of data related to random motility and chemotaxis of normal donors' PMN are depicted in FIGURE 2. An example of printouts routinely available after the application of these models to our workstation is shown in FIGURE 3.

Migration Patterns under Different Conditions

Chemoattractants

The first experiments were carried out using a "crude" supernatant of *E. coli* culture (10%) (obtained by ultrafiltration after an overnight culture in TC 199 medium, in the same laboratory conditions and rapidly stored in small aliquots at –20°C) in the lower compartment of the chemotactic chamber. In order to obtain more reproducibility, LPS at concentrations of 50, 100, and 150 μg/ml were used. We found that only the highest concentration produced migration value (FP = 126 μm) in the normal range, whereas the lowest one produced values comparable to those of random motility (FP = 88 μm) (with intermediate values for intermediate concentration, FP = 109 μm). It must be pointed out that all concentrations were able to induce the typical stimulation peak previously obtained with the "crude" chemoattractant. So, the stimulation pattern is always detectable and, even for very low final distances, it cannot be confused with a random pattern (FIG. 4). The same results were obtained when we began to use fMLP (which is now the chemoattractant currently used in our laboratory). The concentration that best fitted with the normal migration range (FP = 138 μm) and displayed a migration pattern perfectly in the normality bands, was 10^{-7} M, while the concentration of 10^{-8} M (which is currently used in most laboratories) induced lower migration values (FP = 100 μm). Also in this case the typical stimulation peak was always present (FIG. 5).

Time of Incubation

In order to define better the kinetics of migration, two experiments performed in triplicate were carried out allowing the cells to migrate for 20, 30, 40, 50, 60 min under stimulated conditions (by fMLP 10^{-7} M). Every set of filters, when removed from the incubation, was immediately fixed and processed for the image analysis. The final planes reached were, respectively, 54, 75, 85, 107, 138 μm, and this result was expected. The most important result is that the typical migration peak (corresponding to the highest PMN concentration) appears early (between 20 and 30 min),

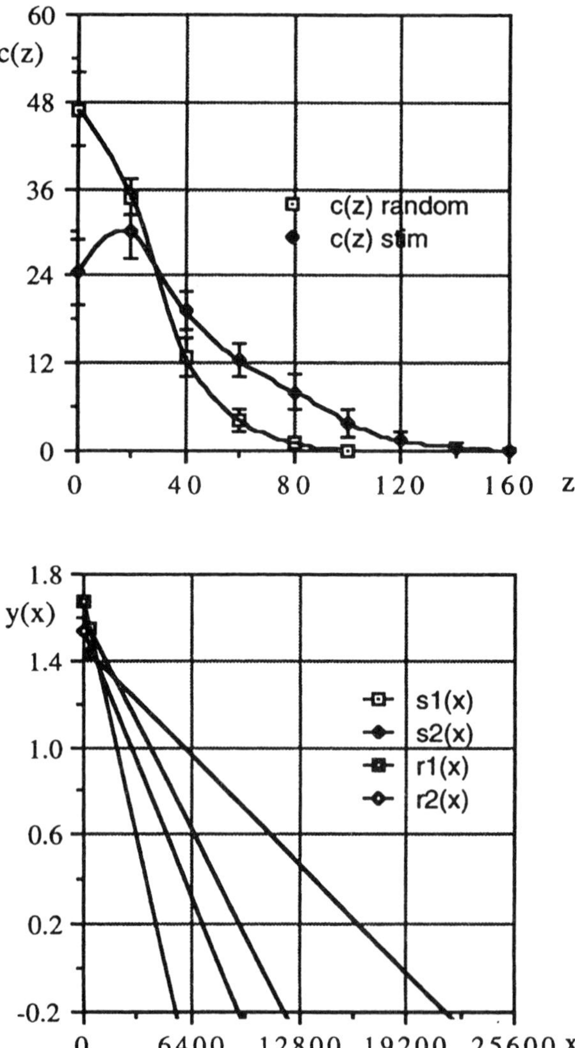

FIGURE 2. (*Top*) Plot of the interpolating curves of the average values for random migration (characterized by a gaussian model: adj. R^2 relative to the linear regression = 0.980 ± 0.03) and chemotaxis (characterized by a peculiar "peak" in the depth 0–40 μm interval) of PMN from normal donors ($N = 21$). The abscissa is given in μm, the ordinate in percentages. (*Bottom*) Plot of the regression extreme lines r_1 and r_2 (for random migration), and of the regression extreme lines s_1 and s_2 (for chemotaxis), after decimal logarithm transformation of counts (ordinate) and square transformation of depth (abscissa). The square root of the interception values on the abscissa (given in μm²), obtained when the logarithm value decreases of two units, gives the normal FP bands.

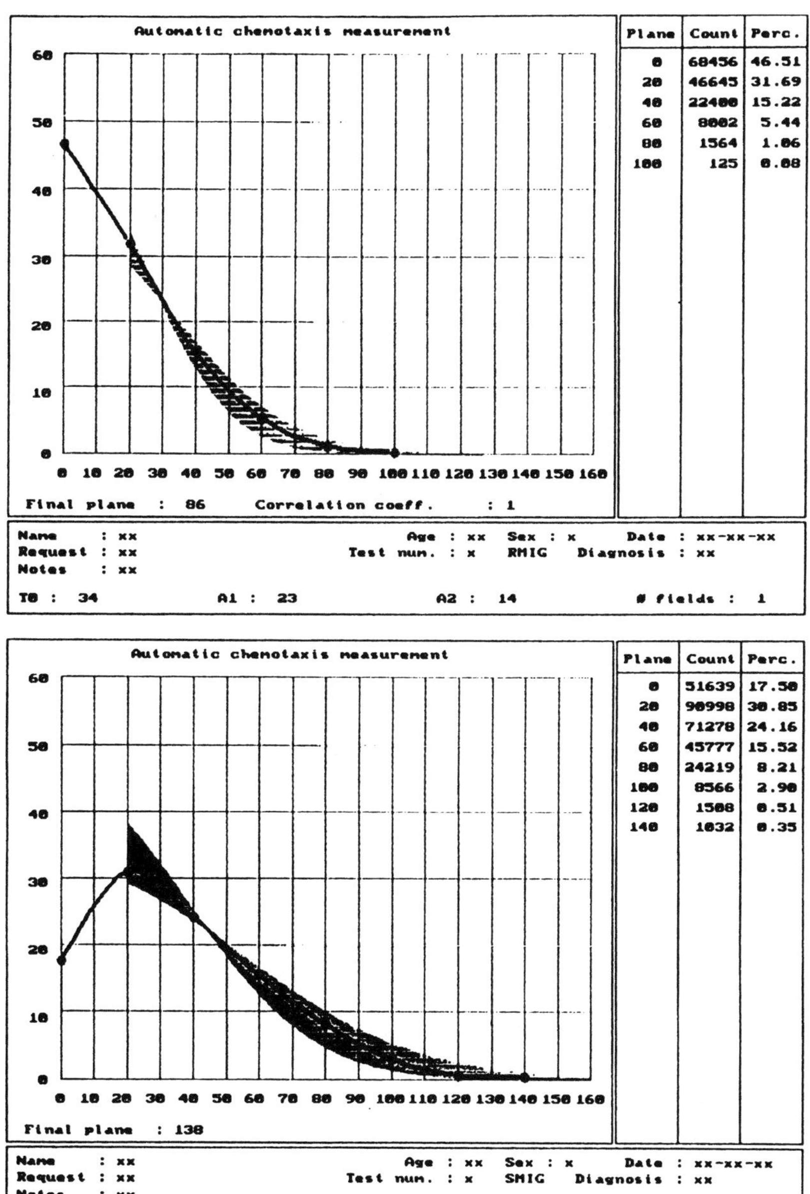

FIGURE 3. Examples of printouts of random migration (*top*) and of chemotaxis (*bottom*) routinely available by our workstation. Ancillary information (normality bands, plane under study, count of pixels, percentage transformation, final plane, threshold used, data about patient are displayed.

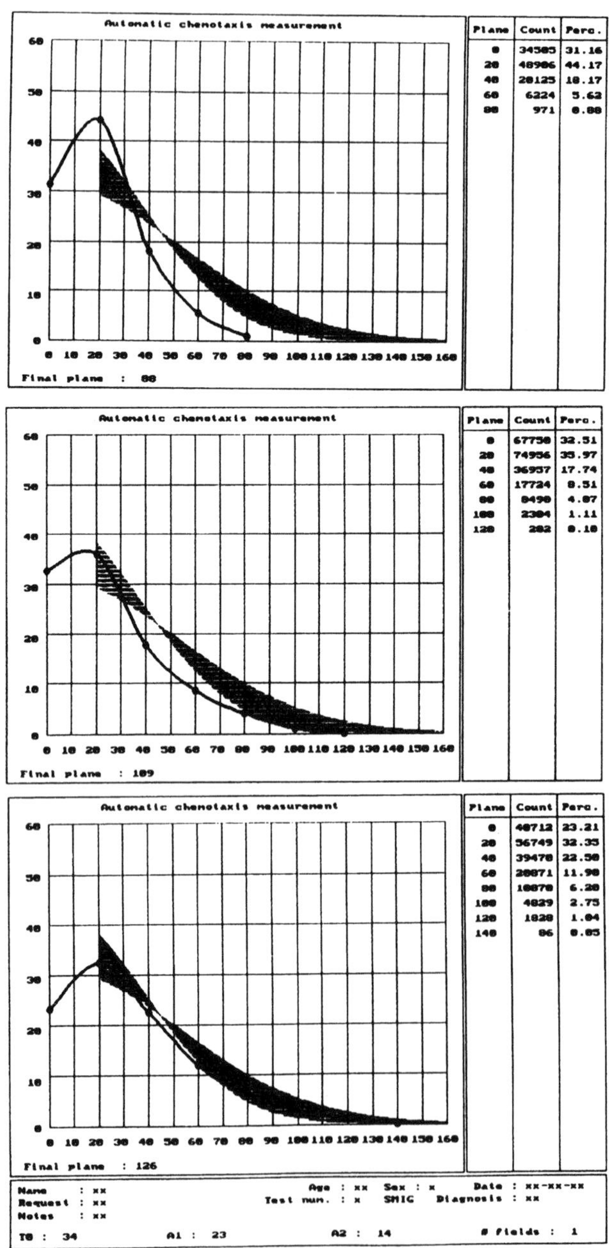

FIGURE 4. Printouts of chemotaxis curves displayed by normal PMN under stimulus by LPS at concentrations of 50 µg/ml (*top*), 100 µg/ml (*middle*), 150 µg/ml (*bottom*). All the concentrations are able to induce the typical stimulation peak, even if with different FP values.

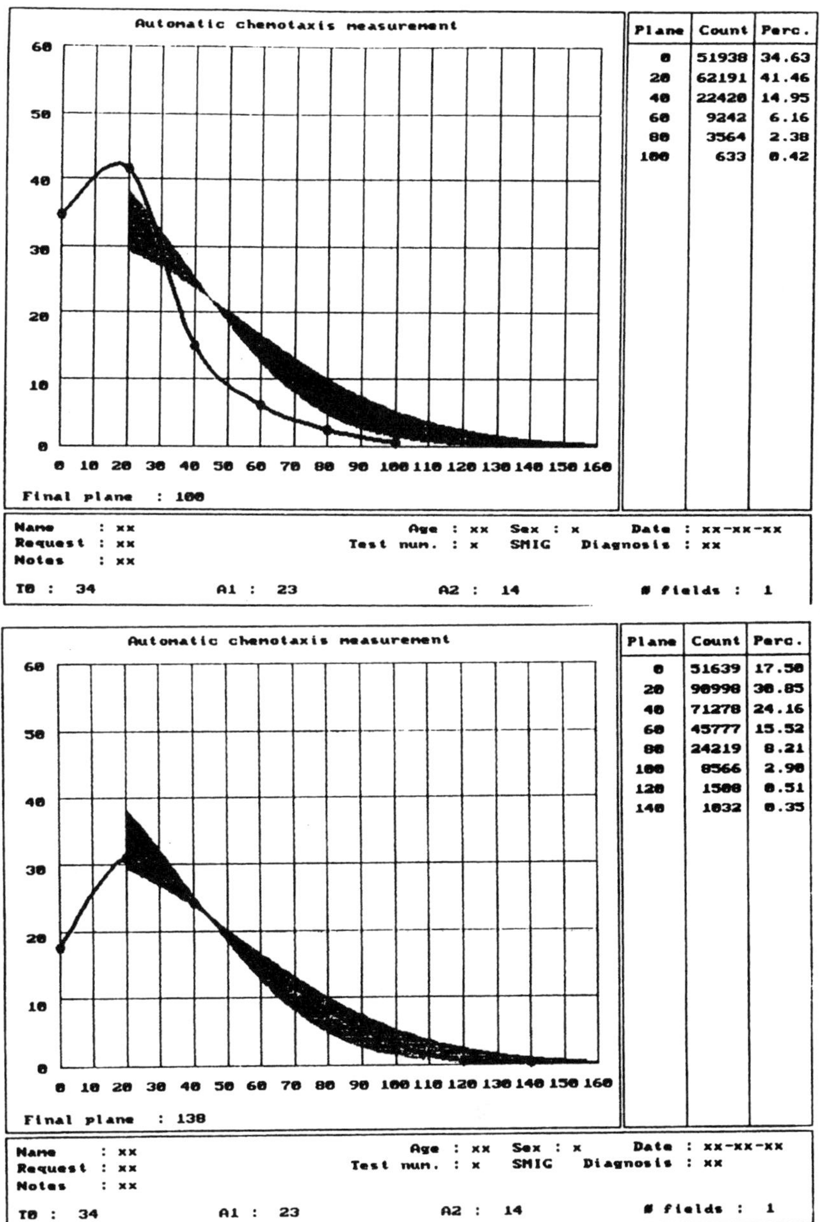

FIGURE 5. Printouts of chemotaxis curves displayed by normal PMN under stimulus by fMLP at concentrations of 10^{-8} M (*top*) and 10^{-7} M (*bottom*). Both concentrations are able to induce the typical stimulation peak, even if with different FP values.

and remains in a thin slice of the filter at a depth between 10 and 30 μm, in a dynamic way. In fact, after 20 min, only about 50% of cells remain on the upper face of the filter. A high percentage (44.29%) rapidly moves to a near plane and is continuously substituted (with a progressive slight reduction of the peak: 44.2, 40.5, 39.8, 33.1, 30.8%, respectively) by a lot of cells coming from the upper level whose percentage progressively decreases (51.3, 34.1, 31.8, 26.8, 17.5%, respectively), while, on the contrary, only few faster cells (the leading front) move to the lower face of the filter (FIG. 6).

Patients with Migration Defects and Drug Interference

As an example of the kind of information that may be supplied by our device in pathology, we report data about patients with migration defects (both congenital and acquired) and data about drug interference.

Lithium Effects on PMN Migration in Shwachman-Diamond Syndrome

The study, carried out in 1991, had shown by conventional methods that lithium carbonate did not interfere with random motility, which was normal in basal conditions (70 ± 6 μm), after 10 days therapy (65 ± 5 μm), and after 30 days therapy (76 ± 6 μm) (n.v. 70.6 ± 13 μm). On the contrary, it was able to enhance PMN chemotaxis, which was strongly inhibited in basal conditions (77 ± 8 μm), up to 102 ± 5 μm after 10 days therapy, and up to 111 ± 7 μm after 30 days therapy (n.v. 109 ± 5 μm).[38] Obviously, no information was available about the kinetics of migration.

When the same filters were examined later by the image analysis workstation, we had confirmation of the data about random migration, which moreover always exhibited a normal gaussian pattern. However, some interesting data were obtained about chemotaxis. In fact, while the measures of the distance traveled by the cells were very similar to those obtained in a conventional way (76, 104, 115 μm, respectively), neither the normal migration patterns, nor a gaussian pattern—which would have indicated an aspecific enhancement of chemokinesis—was obtained, indicating that the improvement probably belonged to a small PMN subpopulation, while most of cells remained always blocked on the initial plane (FIG. 7).

rhG-CSF on PMN Migration in Lymphoma under Chemotherapy

In this study, the mathematical analysis of data performed in real time by the algorithm of our workstation allowed us to solve some important controversies about the effects of this important growth factor on PMN motility.[39] In fact, as regards PMN random motility, the linear regression between the logarithms of the measuring sequences and the square depth values before and after rhG-CSF administration identified FP of 73.86 ± 7.65 μm and 54.71 ± 5.16 μm, respectively (p = 0.033). Nevertheless, even if the migration was reduced, the normal gaussian pattern was still present in the curve that refers to migration after rhG-CSF administration. In particular, the values of adj. R^2 relative to the linear regression confirmed an exponential trend (0.974 before and 0.980 after, n.v. = 0.980 ± 0.03). For PMN chemotaxis, the mean

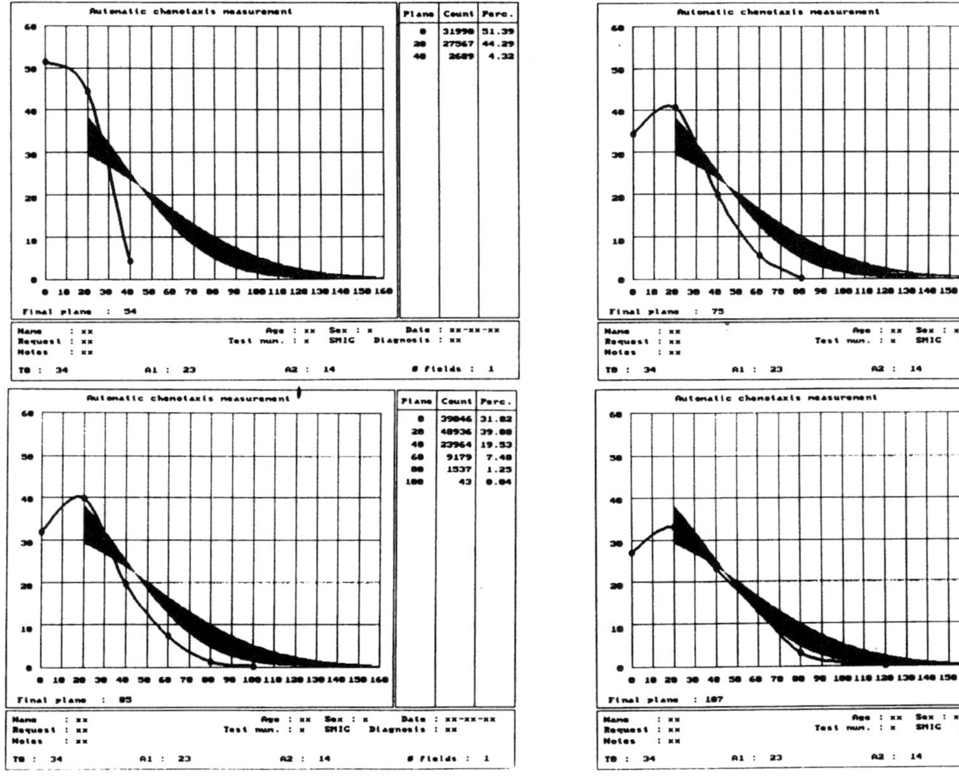

FIGURE 6. Printouts of chemotaxis curves displayed by normal PMN under stimulus by fMLP at 10^{-7} M, allowed to migrate for 20 min (*top, left*), 30 min (*top, right*), 40 min (*bottom, left*), 50 min (*bottom, right*), 60 min (not shown: see FIG. 4). The chemotactic peak appears between 20 and 30 min.

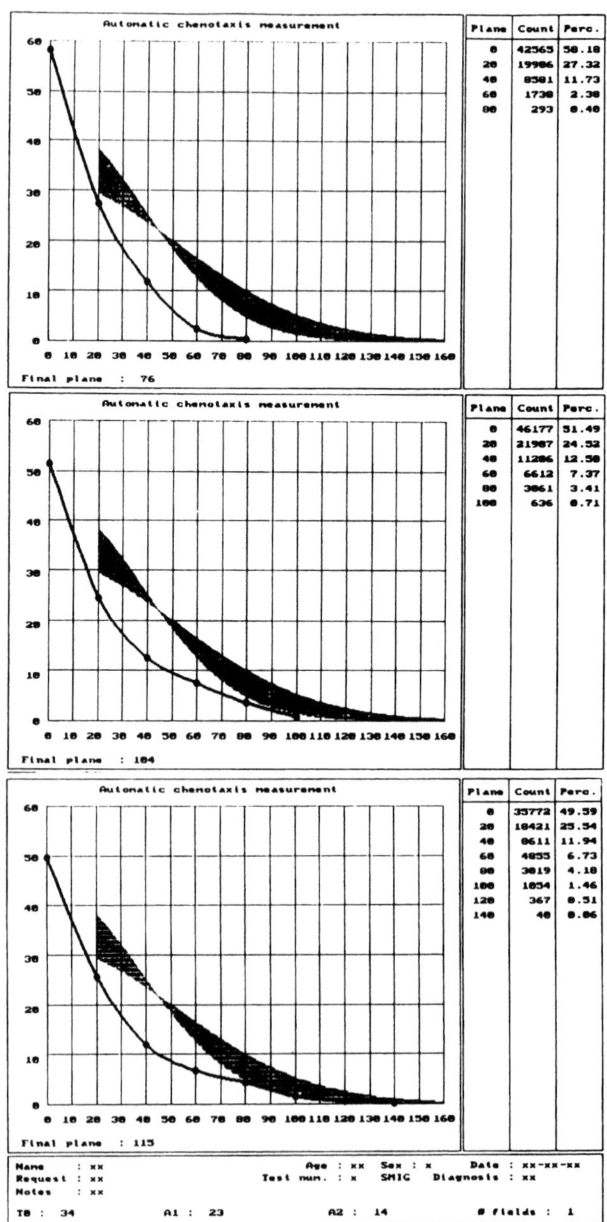

FIGURE 7. Printouts of chemotaxis curves displayed by PMN from a child affected by Shwachman-Diamond Syndrome evaluated in basal condition (*top*), after 15 days of therapy (*middle*), and after 30 days of therapy (*bottom*) with lithium carbonate (30 mg/kg/day). Despite a progressive enhancement of FP values, the normal chemotactic pattern is never achieved.

migration lines before and after rhG-CSF administration intercepted the depth axis at FP of 126.86 ± 16.52 μm and 102.50 ± 14.51 μm, respectively ($p = 0.016$). Moreover, the peak of maximal cell density was no longer present in the curve obtained after rhG-CSF administration. On the contrary, this curve displayed a typical gaussian pattern, just like a curve of random motility (FIG. 8).

Myelodysplastic Syndromes

PMN random motility was strongly inhibited, showing a mean FP of 62.82 ± 2.75 μm (normal range: 77–102 μm). A reduced value of FP was reached by PMN from 10 of 11 patients, but if we consider the other important normality parameter provided by our workstation, it must be pointed out that PMN from 7 of these 10 patients still displayed a normal gaussian motility pattern. PMN from only one patient showed a normal behavior both for the distance traveled and the migration curve. Also, PMN chemotaxis was strongly inhibited, showing mean values of 104.36 ± 9.48 μm (normal range: 117–162 μm). PMN from six patients showed a reduced value of FP, but it must be pointed out that PMN from four of these six patients still displayed a typical chemotactic pattern, while only in two cases did PMN with normal FP also have a normal curve. Thus, in conclusion, PMN from only 2 patients of 11 showed a normal behavior for both the distance traveled and the migration curve. No correlation is possible with the degree of malignity because of the low number of patients. Nevertheless, if the patients are divided in two groups (low grade: RA, RARS, $N = 5$ versus high grade: RAEB, RAEB-t, CMMoL, $N = 6$), an unexpected trend can be noted. In spite of a slight difference in the FP values (respectively, 61.6 μm versus 63.8 μm for random migration and 100.8 μm versus 107.3 μm for chemotaxis) an abnormal random curve is detectable in 40% of low grade syndromes and only in 17% of high grade syndromes. In the same way, an abnormal chemotaxis curve is detectable in 60% of low grade syndromes and only in 33% of high grade syndromes. All these data are reported in TABLE 2.

DISCUSSION

When a micropore filter is observed, cell shapes may appear quite different (round, oval, stretched) during the migration, because of the irregular direction of filter channels in which the cell is examined. Furthermore, other kinds of irregular shapes may be due to the partial overlapping of cells in very near focal planes. Finally, the true problem is to discriminate images of cells in focus from cells out of focus belonging to planes different from the plane under study. All these problems were resolved using a monodimensional processing system that performs a mobile difference by discrete steps on each line; in addition, each focal plane was identified by a specific threshold.

Our simple algorithm for the processing of acquired images, even if not planned for a real-cell recognition and count, supplies results statistically more reliable than those achieved by conventional microscopic methods. Furthermore, it calculates, by analysis of vectors, a migration value that is statistically the nearest to the true distance traveled by the cells and supplies information about PMN migration kinetics in

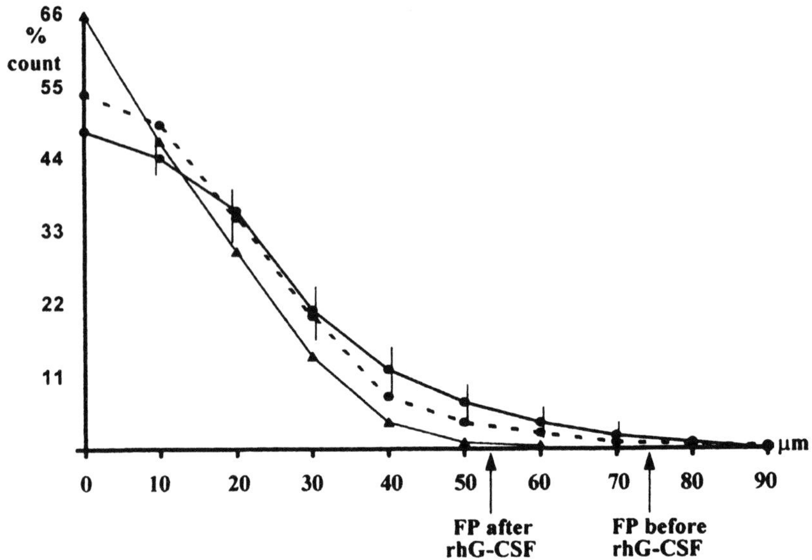

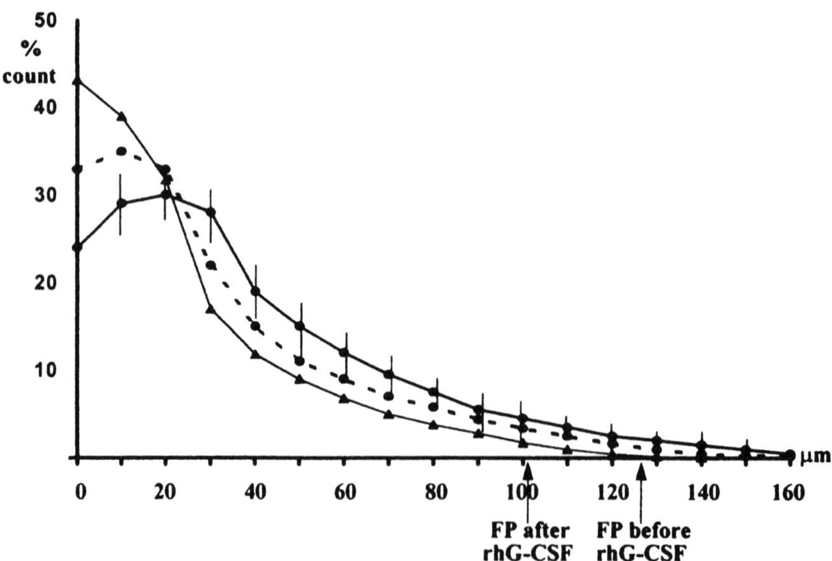

FIGURE 8. Plots of the interpolating curves of random migration (*top*) and chemotaxis (*bottom*) of rhG-CSF–induced PMN from patients affected by lymphoma under chemotherapy ($N = 7$). Dotted curve: kinetics of migration before rhG-CSF administration. Continuous curve with triangles: kinetics of migration after rhG-CSF administration. Continuous curve with circles and vertical bars: kinetics of migration (± SD) in normal donors. The arrows show the final migration plane (FP) calculated by the linear regression procedure depicted in FIG. 2.

TABLE 2. Random Motility and Chemotaxis of PMN from 11 Patients Affected by Myelodysplastic Syndrome

Patient	Diagnosis	Age	Sex	Random Motility Value (μm)[a]	Gaussian Pattern	Chemotaxis Value (μm)[b]	Chemotactic "Peak"
S.F.	RA	57	M	58	No	79	No
G.N.	RAEB-t	83	F	55	Yes	63	Yes
L.E.	RARS	72	M	**79**	**Yes**	**122**	**Yes**
M.S.	CMMoL	70	M	63	No	138	No
G.O.	RAEB	72	F	61	Yes	63	Yes
G.S.	RA	74	M	65	Yes	136	No
M.M.	RA	76	M	45	No	85	No
B.R.	RAEB	81	F	75	Yes	149	No
C.A.	RA	72	M	61	Yes	82	Yes
B.B.	CMMoL	74	F	64	Yes	104	Yes
T.O.	RAEB-t	72	F	65	Yes	**127**	**Yes**

Note: RA: refractory anemia; RARS: refractory anemia with ringed sideroblasts; RAEB: refractory anemia with excess blasts; RAEB-t: refractory anemia with excess blasts in leukemic transformation; CMMoL: chronic myelomonocyte leukemia. Bold characters: cases with both distance traveled and migration curve in the normal range (1/11 for random motility; 2/11 for chemotaxis).
[a]62.82 ± 2.75 μm (n.v.: 77–102 μm).
[b]104.36 ± 9.48 μm (n.v.: 117–162 μm).

a time markedly shorter (about 1/60!) than the time needed just for the microscopic counts.

Our results regarding migration values and patterns in normal donors indicated a PMN behavior that agrees with the results obtained by other authors who have performed a mathematical and statistical analysis of PMN kinetics in various systems under different conditions.[40–42] In our case, the better fitting with the theoretical model describing PMN chemotaxis[43] is probably due to the improvement in data collection offered by our system.

The parameters calculated in the procedure provided a complete definition of the migration pattern with a low number of automatic counts: because of PMN dimension, the detection of cells in focal planes every 20 μm is sufficient to build a reliable migration curve.

Moreover, a brief incubation time is sufficient to let PMN display their specific motility patterns. An important (50%) reduction of incubation time with respect to our first studies still allows a clear difference between random and stimulated motility (the bands delimited by the extreme lines for the two types of migration do not overlap), and an important difference in the curve profile is detectable, surely confirming that chemotactic motility is something more and something different than an enhanced spontaneous migration.

This important "marker" does not depend on the kind of chemoattractants, because in our hands it was induced both by "crude" bacterial supernatants and by standardized commercial kits, by choosing the optimal concentration. In fact, our results demonstrate that if the concentration is not sufficient, the FP may be lower, but the chemotactic curve is always detectable.

Other important information was supplied by the "time-response" experiments: they clearly indicate that the important difference in the curve profile appears very early (between 20 and 30 minutes) and remains (with a detectable shift) during the entire migration process.

We would like to point out that our system is also able to reveal situations of excessive PMN motility function, often undetectable by conventional methods. In fact, the algorithm is able to calculate, with statistical significance, even the projection of the possible distance that neutrophils with enhanced motility might travel in filters of suitable thickness, and also to display the curve profile of such an abnormally stimulated situation (see FIG. 9, referring to a patient with multiple skin abscesses and fever, where PMN could have been able to migrate up to 193 μm in 60 minutes, and even a double migration wave was detectable). In a conventional way, using the leading front technique, this case could have been classified in the normal range.

The migration profile can identify pathological situations, even when the distance traveled by the cells is in the normal range, as demonstrated, in particular, by the ob-

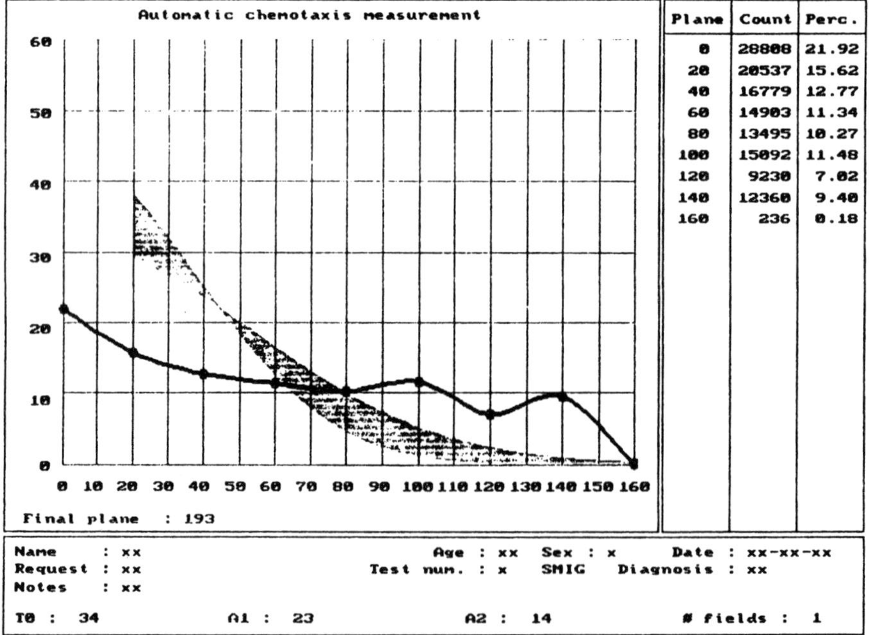

FIGURE 9. Printouts of a chemotaxis curve displayed by PMN from a patient with multiple skin abscesses and fever, under stimulus by fMLP at 10^{-7} M. The leading front technique would have indicated a migration value of about 150 μm in 60 min. (that is the maximum level achievable, considering the thickness of the filter). The linear regression procedure (depicted in FIG. 2) shows that PMN are able to migrate up to 193 μm. Moreover, a double migration wave is detectable.

servations in Shwachman-Diamond syndrome. A PMN cytoskeleton impairment has been hypothesized in this pathology.[44] Our data, in agreement with classical studies demonstrating that leukocytes with disassembled microtubules lose their directional movement, whereas they still move at random,[45] might sustain the hypothesis of a microtubule impairment, but might also indicate that only a PMN subpopulation is defective. So lithium (which has been demonstrated to modulate the PMN microtubular system in an opposite strictly dose-dependent way),[46,47] while it corrects this subpopulation, might block the normal one by an excessive microtubule assembly. We are now trying to find the optimum drug dosage for this patient.

The study performed on rhG-CSF–induced PMN also supplied information in this field. As regards random motility, our data seem to show that this function, even if reduced, displays a normal pattern before and after rhG-CSF. As regards chemotaxis, our data show that not only the actual distance traveled is reduced after rhG-CSF, but that the cells seem unable to give a normal chemotactic response. On the contrary, this curve displays a typical gaussian pattern, just like a curve of random motility. It is known that chemotaxis is conditioned by the capacity of neutrophils to synthesize and assemble microtubules[48] and that an increased polymerization of microtubules is needed by neutrophils migrating through micropore filters.[49] Moreover, membrane deformability strictly depends on a well-assembled cytoskeletal system, and it is known that membrane deformability increases during PMN maturation.[50] So our data might sustain the assertion that a defect in the structural cell maturation (an imperfect cytoskeletal assembly due to the accelerated bone marrow transit) may cause the reduced PMN motility. So maybe that, apart from the uninfluent number of band cells, rhG-CSF–induced PMN are "morphologically" mature, but "structurally" altered, because of the short maturation time. Probably, the best dosage useful both to correct the PMN number and to preserve the PMN functional status must be better investigated.

Only some preliminary conclusions may be drawn by the study carried out in myelodysplastic syndromes, apart from the data, statistically confirmed, of a strong inhibition of PMN motility capacity. Once again, we want to point out the importance of evaluating the migration pattern rather than the simple migration values. We want to underline the unexpected trend, according to which the most defective patterns seem to be found in the low malignancy-grade group, rather than in the high grade group. These data must be confirmed during the study, which is on going.

In conclusion, we think that our workstation is very useful in improving the investigation of the complex aspects of cell motility (time required, subpopulations involved, specific cell defects) so that many known pathologies might be re-evaluated (or new pathologies might be detected). We also think that it may also be particularly useful in the study of excessive PMN function not otherwise detectable or in the study of drug interference in many fields, such as hematology, oncology, immunology, and vascular pathology.

REFERENCES

1. HILL, H. R., H. D. OCHS, P. G. QUIE, H. F. PABST, S. J. KLEBANOFF & R. J. WEDGWOOD. 1974. Defect in neutrophil granulocyte chemotaxis in Job's syndrome of recurrent "cold" staphylococcal abscesses. Lancet **ii:** 617–619.

2. AGGETT, P. J., N. P. C. CAVANAGH, D. J. MATTHEW, J. R. PINCOTT, J. SUTCLIFFE & J. T. HAR-
   RIS. 1980. Shwachman syndrome. A review of 21 cases. Arch. Dis. Child. **55:** 331–347.
3. WILKINSON, P. C. 1993. Defects of leukocyte locomotion and chemotaxis: Prospects, assays, and lessons from Chediak-Higashi neutrophils. Eur. J. Clin. Invest. **23:** 690–692.
4. SIEGBAHAN, A., P. VENGE, K. NILSSON & B. SIMONSON. 1982. Identification of a chemoki-
   netic inhibitor in serum from patients with chronic lymphocytic leukaemia. Scand. J.
   Haematol. **28:** 122–131.
5. AZZARÀ, A., L. RUOCCO, R. POLIDORI, M. PETRINI, B. GRASSI & F. AMBROGI. 1985.
   Hodgkin's disease serum interference with human leukocytes locomotion. J. Exp. Clin.
   Cancer Res. **4:** 153–160.
6. ANKLESARIA, P. N., S. A. ADVANI & A. N. BHISEY. 1985. Defective chemotaxis and adherence in granulocytes from chronic myeloid leukemia (CML) patients. Leukemia Res. **9:**
   641–648.
7. COOPER, P. H., H. F. FRIERSON & K. E. GREER. 1983. Subcutaneous neutrophilic infiltrates
   in acute febrile neutrophilic dermatosis. Arch. Dermatol. **119:** 610–611.
8. WEISMAN, G. H. & H. KORCHAK. 1984. Rheumatoid arthritis. The role of neutrophil activation. Inflammation **8:** 3–14.
9. RICEVUTI, G., A. MAZZONE, D. PASOTTI, S. DE SERVI & G. SPECCHIA. 1991. Role of granulocytes in endothelial injury in coronary heart disease in humans. Atherosclerosis **91:**
   1–14.
10. BOYDEN, S. V. 1962. The chemotactic effect of mixtures of antibody and antigen on poly-
    morphonuclear leukocytes. J. Exp. Med. **115:** 453–466.
11. ZIGMOND, S. H. & J. G. HIRSH. 1973. Leukocyte locomotion and chemotaxis: New meth-
    ods for evaluation and demonstration of a cell-derived chemotactic factor. J. Exp. Med.
    137: 387–410.
12. MADERAZO, E. G. & C. L. WORONICK. 1978. A modified micropore filter assay of human
    granulocyte leukotaxis. *In* Leukocyte Chemotaxis: Methods, physiology, and clinical im-
    plication. J. I. Gallin & P. G. Quie, Eds.: 43–55. Raven Press. New York.
13. KELLER, H., J. H. WISSLER, B. DAMERAU, M. H. HESS & H. COTTIER. 1980. The filter tech-
    nique for measuring leukocyte locomotion in vitro. Comparison of three modifications.
    J. Immunol. Methods **36:** 41–53.
14. GROTENDORST, G. R. 1987. Spectrophotometric assay for the quantitation of cell migration
    in the Boyden chamber chemotaxis assay. Methods Enzymol. **147:** 144–152.
15. SOMERSALO, K., O. P. SALO & F. BJÖRKSTEN. 1990. A simplified Boyden chamber assay for
    neutrophil chemotaxis based on quantitation of myeloperoxidase. Anal. Biochem. **185:**
    238–242.
16. GALLIN, J. I., R. A. CLARK & E. J. GOETZL. 1978. Radioassay of leukocyte locomotion: A
    sensitive technique for clinical studies. *In* Leukocyte Chemotaxis: Methods, physiology,
    and clinical implication. J. I. Gallin & P. G. Quie, Eds.: 79–86. Raven Press. New York.
17. PINCHING, A. J., A. M. PETERS & S. H. SAVERYMUTTU. 1990. Quantification of radiolabeled
    granulocyte migration *in vivo*. J. Immunol. Methods **126:** 7–11.
18. ZIGMOND, S. H. 1978. A model for understanding Millipore filter assay system. *In* Leuko-
    cyte Chemotaxis: Methods, physiology, and clinical implication. J. I. Gallin & P. G. Quie,
    Eds.: 87–96. Raven Press. New York.
19. BUETTNER, H. M., D. A. LAUFFENBURGER & S. H. ZIGMOND. 1989. Measurement of leuko-
    cyte motility and chemotaxis parameters with the Millipore filter assay. J. Immunol.
    Methods **123:** 25–35.
20. TRANQUILLO, R. T., S. H. ZIGMOND & D. A. LAUFFENBURGER. 1988. Measurement of the
    chemotaxis coefficient for human neutrophils in the under-agarose migration assay. Cell
    Motil. Cytoskeleton **11:** 1–15.
21. KLOMP, J. P. J., A. A. TE VALDE & C. G. FIGDOR. 1989. Rapid densitometric determination

of cell migration and cell adhesion in a microchemotaxis chamber. J. Immunol. Methods **118:** 47–52.

22. MISSO, N. L. A., T. L. KANG, M. J. PHILLIPS & P. J. THOMPSON. 1992. Assessment of neutrophil chemotaxis by laser and video densitometry. J. Immunol. Methods **149:** 183–187.

23. DONOVAN, R. M., E. GOLDSTAIN, Y. KIM, W. LIPPERT, E. KAILATH, T. T. AOKI *et al.* 1987. A computer-assisted image-analysis system for analyzing polymorphonuclear leukocyte chemotaxis in patients with diabetes mellitus. J. Infect. Dis. **155:** 737–741.

24. PEDERSEN, J. O., L. HASSING, N. GRUNNET & C. JERSILD. 1988. Real-time scanning and image analysis. A fast method for the determination of neutrophil orientation under agarose. J. Immunol. Methods **109:** 131–137.

25. NELSON, R. D., P. G. QUIE & R. L. SIMMONS. 1975. Chemotaxis under agarose: A new and simple method for measuring chemotaxis and spontaneous migration of human polymorphonuclear leukocytes and monocytes. J. Immunol. **115:** 1650–1656.

26. MACFARLANE, G. D., M. C. HERZBERG & R. D. NELSON. 1987. Analysis of polarization and orientation of human polymorphonuclear leukocytes by computer-interfaced video microscopy. J. Leukocyte Biol. **41:** 307–317.

27. HARVATH, L., W. FALK & E. J. LEONARD. 1980. Rapid quantitation of neutrophil chemotaxis: Use of a polyvinylpyrrolidone-free polycarbonate membrane in a multiwell assembly. J. Immunol. Methods **37:** 39–45.

28. JENSEN, P. & A. KHARAZMI. 1991. Computer-assisted image analysis assay of human neutrophil chemotaxis *in vitro.* J. Immunol. Methods **144:** 43–48.

29. AZZARÀ, A., M. CHIMENTI, L. AZZARELLI, E. FANTINI, G. CARULLI & F. AMBROGI. 1992. An image processing workstation for automatic evaluation of human granulocyte motility. J. Immunol. Methods **148:** 29–40.

30. AZZARÀ, A., M. CHIMENTI, G. CARULLI, A. RIZZUTI-GULLACI & F. AMBROGI. 1995. An image processing procedure for the assessment of normality curves of motility of human granulocytes in micropore filters. Scand. J. Clin. Lab. Invest. **55:** 399–408.

31. SHOPSIN, B., R. FRIEDMANN & S. GERSHON. 1971. Lithium and leukocytosis. Clin. Pharmacol. Ther. **12:** 923–928.

32. LIESCHKE, G. J. & A. W. BURGESS. 1992. Granulocyte colony-stimulating factor and granulocyte-macrophage colony-stimulating factor (second of two parts). N. Engl. J. Med. **327:** 99–106.

33. FEARON, D. T. & L. A. COLLINS. 1983. Increased expression of C3b receptors on polymorphonuclear leukocytes induced by chemotactic factors and by purification procedures. J. Immunol. **130:** 370–375.

34. CATES, K. L., C. E. RAY & P. G. QUIE. 1978. Modified Boyden chamber method of measuring polymorphonuclear leukocyte chemotaxis. *In* Leukocyte Chemotaxis: Methods, physiology, and clinical implication. J. I. Gallin & P. G. Quie, Eds.: 67–71. Raven Press. New York.

35. AZZARÀ, A., M. CHIMENTI, O. SALVETTI, L. AZZARELLI, M. PETRINI & F. AMBROGI. 1989. Automatic evaluation by image analysis of chemotactic functions of human granulocytes. A preliminary study. Proc. Fourth Annual Meeting "Clinical Applications of Cytometry" (Charleston, South Carolina, September 13–16, 1986).

36. AGGETT, P. J., J. T. HARRIES, B. A. M. HARVEY & J. F. SOOTHILL. 1979. An inherited defect of neutrophil mobility in Shwachman syndrome. J. Pediatr. **94:** 391–394.

37. AZZARÀ, A., G. CARULLI, M. PETRINI, L. RUOCCO, A. MARINI, B. GRASSI & F. AMBROGI. 1988. *In vitro* restoration by lithium of defective chemotaxis in Shwachman-Diamond syndrome (case report). Br. J. Haematol. **4:** 502.

38. AZZARÀ, A., G. CARULLI, M. CECCARELLI, C. PUCCI, R. RAGGIO & F. AMBROGI. 1991. *In vivo* effectiveness of lithium on impaired chemotaxis in Shwachman-Diamond syndrome. Acta Haematol. **85:** 100–102.

39. AZZARÀ, A., G. CARULLI, A. RIZZUTI-GULLACI, S. MINNUCCI, E. CAPOCHIANI & F. AMBROGI. 1996. Motility of rhG-CSF induced neutrophils in patients undergoing chemotherapy: Evidence for inhibition detected by image analysis. Br. J. Haematol. **92:** 161–168.
40. SCHREINER, A. & D. VAULA. 1978. Kinetics of locomotion of human granulocyte populations. Acta Pathol. Microbiol. Scand. C **86:** 205–209.
41. SCHREINER, A. & D. VAULA. 1980. Kinetics of locomotion of human granulocyte populations in a double-filter system. Acta Path. Microbiol. Scand. C **88:** 83–88.
42. SCHREINER, A., T. KALAGER & D. VAULA. 1980. Leukocyte migration in different systems. Effect of colchicin. Kinetics of migration under agarose. Acta Path. Microbiol. Scand. C **88:** 89–96.
43. ROSEN, G. 1976. Chemotactic transport theory for neutrophil leukocytes. J. Theor. Biol. **59:** 371–380.
44. ROTHBAUN, R. J., D. A. WILLIAMS & C. C. DAUGHERTY. 1982. Unusual surface distribution of concanavalin A reflects a cytoskeletal defect in neutrophils in Shwachman syndrome. Lancet **ii:** 800–801.
45. WILKINSON, P. C. & R. B. ALLAN. 1978. Assays systems for measuring leukocyte chemotaxis: An overview. *In* Leukocyte Chemotaxis: Methods, physiology, and clinical implication. J. I. Gallin & P. G. Quie, Eds.: 1–24. Raven Press. New York.
46. AZZARÀ, A., G. CARULLI, L. RUOCCO, A. MARINI, M. PETRINI & F. AMBROGI. 1986. Human neutrophil microtubular system: *In vitro* and *in vivo* evidence of lithium interference. Hemat. Rev. Commun. (Suppl) **1:** 48 (Abstract, International Congress on the Biological and Clinical Aspects of Phagocyte Function, Pavia Sept. 1986)
47. AZZARÀ, A., G. CARULLI, M. PETRINI, L. RUOCCO, A. MARINI, B. GRASSI & F. AMBROGI. 1987. Effects of lithium on human leukocyte chemotaxis. Indirect evidence from the use of potassium and vinblastine concerning the modulation of microtubular system. Haematologica **72:** 121–127.
48. GALLIN, J. I., E. K. GALLIN, H. L. MALECH & E. B. KRAMER. 1978. Structural and ionic events during leukocyte chemotaxis. *In* Leukocyte Chemotaxis: Methods, physiology, and clinical implication. J. I. Gallin & P. G. Quie, Eds.: 123–140. Raven Press. New York.
49. GALLIN, J. I. & A. S. ROSENTHAL. 1974. The regulatory role of divalent cations in human granulocyte chemotaxis: Evidence for an association between calcium exchanges and microtubule assembly. J. Cell Biol. **62:** 594–609.
50. MARSHALL, A. & M. D. LICHTMAN. 1970. Cellular deformability during maturation of the myeloblasts: Possible role in marrow egress. N. Engl. J. Med. **283:** 943–948.

A Flow Cytometric Method for the Analysis of Phagocytosis and Killing by Polymorphonuclear Leukocytes

M. SARESELLA,[a] K. RODA, L. SPECIALE, D. TARAMELLI,[b]
E. MENDOZZI, F. GUERINI, AND P. FERRANTE[b]

Don C. Gnocchi Foundation
IRCCS
Biology Laboratory
Via Capecelatro 66
I-20148 Milan, Italy

[b]*Institute of Medical Microbiology*
University of Milan
Via Pascal, 36
I-20133 Milan, Italy

INTRODUCTION

Phagocytes represent the first line of defense against invasive microorganisms as they are capable of rapid phagocytosis and killing of bacteria and fungi. A rapid evaluation of both the number and function of the human polymorphonuclear leukocyte (PMN) population could be of fundamental importance in defining the immunological defects of patients with recurrent or persistent infections. Moreover, any technical modifications that could improve the clinical screening of PMNs function would be advantageous for the treatment of many disease states. Flow cytometry can be adopted for routine monitoring of the immune functions of human polymorphonuclear leukocytes (PMNs) in several disease states.[1–4]

In this study, we describe a fast, reliable, and inexpensive method for studying the phagocytosis and killing of *Candida albicans* blastospores by fresh human polymorphonuclear cells, using flow cytometry (FCM). We have modified previously described methods[5] in order to achieve the reproducibility and speed necessary for testing several samples in the diagnostic laboratory. This assay is capable of distinguishing adherent blastospores from those that have been ingested and permits an evaluation of intracellular killing as well. Briefly summarized, the advantages offered by this assay are (*1*) more rapid PMN preparation; (*2*) the staining procedure involves less time, thereby contributing to a faster assay; (*3*) the *C. albicans* to PMN ratio is 2:1, which allows an accurate estimation of truly phagocytic PMN; (*4*) fluorescence-labeled *C. albicans* blastospores can be frozen and used when needed without loss of fluorescence; and (*5*) this assay also measures killing. The technique can be easily

[a]Address correspondence to: Marina Saresella, Ph.D, Laboratorio di Biologia, Via Capecelatro, 66, I-20148 Milan, Italy. Fax, (39) (2) 40092297 and Phone, (39) (2) 40308211.

adapted to monitor the immune reactivity of PMNs against different pathogens, including bacteria and filamentous fungi.

MATERIALS AND METHODS

Blastospores

Candida albicans (C. Albicans CM2 strain) blastospores were grown in Sabouraud broth with 2% dextrose (Difco Laboratories, Detroit, MI) at 37°C for 18–24 h. The blastospores were then washed three times and resuspended in phosphate-buffered saline (PBS). They were then counted with a STKS hemocytometer (Coulter Electronics, Inc., Miami Lakes, FL) and checked for viability by trypan blue exclusion (Sigma Chemical Co., St. Louis, MO). Viability proved to be greater than 90%.

For the killing assays, *C. albicans* blastospores were resuspended in PBS to a final concentration of 10^7 blastospore cells/ml and then labeled with fluorescein isothiocyanate (FITC; Sigma Chemical Co.) (0.1 mg/ml) in a 0.5 M carbonate/bicarbonate buffer (pH 9.5) for 1 h with agitation at room temperature and in a light-protected environment. Following incubation, the blastospores were washed twice in PBS and divided into aliquots of 10^6 blastospores each.

For the phagocytosis assay, *C. albicans* blastospores were ethanol-fixed (70% ethanol for 1 h at room temperature) and washed twice in PBS. They were then labeled with FITC (0.01 mg/ml; Sigma Chemical Co.) in a 0.5 M carbonate/bicarbonate buffer (pH 9.5) for 30 min with agitation, in a light-protected environment. The labeled blastospores were washed and stored in 2×10^6 aliquots at -80°C until use.

Preparation of Human Polymorphonuclear Cells

Human leukocytes were obtained from the heparinized whole blood of healthy donors after lysis of red blood cells by hypotonic shock with ammonium chloride. Total and differential leukocyte counts were made using a Coulter STKS Counter (Coulter Electronics, Inc., Miami Lakes, FL) and the PMN concentration was adjusted to 3×10^6 cells/ml, washed again in PBS, and then divided into three aliquots of 10^6 cells each.

Opsonization and Phagocytosis

Prior to the phagocytosis and cytotoxicity assays, the opsonization of the aliquots of live or ethanol-fixed FITC-labeled *C. albicans* blastospores was achieved by suspension in 200 μl of patient serum for 30 min at 37°C. They were then washed several times in PBS and resuspended in 200 μl of PBS. For the phagocytosis assay, 2×10^6 opsonized ethanol-fixed FITC-*C. albicans* blastospores were incubated in 1×10^6 PMNs for 30 min at 37°C in a water bath with continuous agitation and in a light-protected environment, to a final volume of 400 μl with a PMN to blastospore cell ratio of 1:2.

After several assays, this ratio proved to be optimal for the discrimination between adherent and ingested blastospores. The samples were centrifuged at 500*g* and resuspended in 1 ml of cold PBS containing 0.02% ethylenediamine tetraacetic acid (EDTA) to stop phagocytosis. Finally, ethidium bromide (EtBr) was added to a concentration of 10 μg/ml. The FCM analysis of the samples was carried out immediately following the addition of EtBr.

FCM Measurement of Phagocytosis

The PMNs were selected by means of forward and side scatter (FSC and SSC) and displayed as a biparametric graph. The energy transfer method was used to provide a distinction between adherent and ingested blastospores.[5,6] This procedure is based on the observation that FITC-labeled *C. albicans* blastospores lose their green fluorescence and acquire red fluorescence after staining with EtBr through the phenomenon of resonance energy transfer.[4] Therefore, internalized *C. albicans* blastospores remain green, whereas adherent and non-phagocytized blastospore cells turn red. The percentage of phagocytizing PMNs was equal to the number of green and double-labeled (green and red) fluorescent PMNs divided by the total number of leukocytes multiplied by 100.

The Killing Assay

The cytotoxicity assay was performed by adding 2×10^6 live FITC-labeled *C. albicans* blastospores to 1×10^6 PMNs from the test sample. Only live FITC-*C. albicans* blastospores were used as controls. Both samples were incubated at 37°C in a water bath with continuous agitation for 2.5 h. The PMNs were then lysed by hypotonic shock. To remove extracellular DNA released from the lysed PMNs, 1 ml of a warm (37°C) DNase solution (2 mg deoxyribonuclease I from bovine pancreas = 4000 Kunitz units dissolved in 100 ml of PBS) was added and the PMNs were incubated for 5 min with periodic agitation. The samples were then repeatedly washed in PBS and incubated with 200 μl of propidium iodide (PI; 100 μg/ml) for 30 min at 4°C in a light-protected environment. The PI penetrates killed blastospore cells and stains DNA, yielding red fluorescence.

FCM Measurement of Intracellular Killing

To analyze the percentage of killed FITC-labeled *C. albicans* blastospores, the green and red fluorescence biparametric graph of the double-labeled blastospores was evaluated. The following formula was adopted to calculate the percentage of killed blastospores in the samples analyzed: % killed blastospores = % double-labeled blastospores of sample − % double-labeled blastospores of control.

Flow Cytometry

The cytometric analysis of phagocytosis and killing was performed using a FAC-Star cytofluorimeter (Becton Dickinson FACS Systems, San Jose, CA) equipped with a water-cooled 2 W argon ion laser operating at 488 nm, interfaced with a Hewlett Packard 300 series computer (Hewlett-Packard Company, Roseville, CA). Multiparametric data were acquired for 10,000 events and analyzed using Fac-StarPlus software supported by the PC-LYSYS program (Becton Dickinson, San Jose, CA). Red fluorescence from PI (FL2) was collected through a 620 nm long pass filter, green fluorescence from FITC (FL1) through a 530 nm band pass filter, and finally the fluorescence from EtBr (FL3) was measured through a 630 nm band pass filter.

Data were collected using linear amplifiers for FSC and SSC and logarithmic amplifiers for FL1, FL2, and FL3. Samples were first run using single fluorochrome-stained preparations for color compensation. The FSC threshold was set at 50 to measure the killing function and was raised to 100 to acquire data on phagocytosis.

RESULTS

Fluorescein-labeling of Candida albicans

Homogeneous bright fluorescent staining should also be homogeneous in intensity to obtain correct cytometric readings of *C. albicans* blastospores. For this reason, the fluorescence was checked by fluorescence microscopy for staining uniformity, before reliable cytometric results were obtained. Incubation of ethanol-fixed blastospores with FITC (0.01 mg/ml) for 15 min showed highly heterogeneous staining of the cells, rendering further quantification of *C. albicans* blastospore ingestion by PMNs impossible. Extension of the incubation time to 30 min yielded a more uniform staining and this was the procedure used in all the subsequent tests.

Several concentrations of EtBr were also tested to select an optimal concentration capable of completely extinguishing the green fluorescence, while leaving a low background of red fluorescence. In fact, the green fluorescence did not completely disappear at solutions containing concentrations of 5 or 7 μg/ml and the red fluorescence remained very low. On the contrary, EtBr solutions of 30 or 50 μg/ml produced a strong red fluorescent background. Thus, an intermediate EtBr solution of 10 μg/ml was chosen in the end.

When live *C. albicans* blastospores were used in the killing assay, a different staining procedure was employed. An incubation period of 1 h and a FITC solution of 0.1 mg/ml proved necessary to obtain homogeneous labeling and a suitable stain intensity. In the preliminary trials, FITC was also used at 0.01 mg/ml for 1 h, but *C. albicans* blastospore labeling was not uniform at this concentration. Several trials were also necessary to establish the optimal PI concentration needed to quantify the percentage of killed *C. albicans* blastospores. When 100 μg/ml of PI were used at 4°C for 30 min, upon microscopic observation, the ethanol-fixed FITC-labeled blastospores appeared to be completely stained red inside with an outer green fluorescence. Concentrations of 50 and 200 μg/ml produced a red fluorescence that was either too low or too high, with respect to the green fluorescence of the external blastospores.

Phagocytosis of FITC-labeled C. albicans *by PMNs*

The analysis of PMN phagocytosis according to cytometric readings is visualized in correlated double-parameter contour plots. Four distinct PMN subsets were distinguishable on the basis of the fluorescence emitted. FIGURE 1 illustrates typical trial results: region 1 (4%) contains PMNs with adherent blastospore particles only, region 2 (12%) shows PMNs with ingested and adherent FITC-labeled *C. albicans* blastospores, whereas PMNs with no interactions with particles appear in region 3

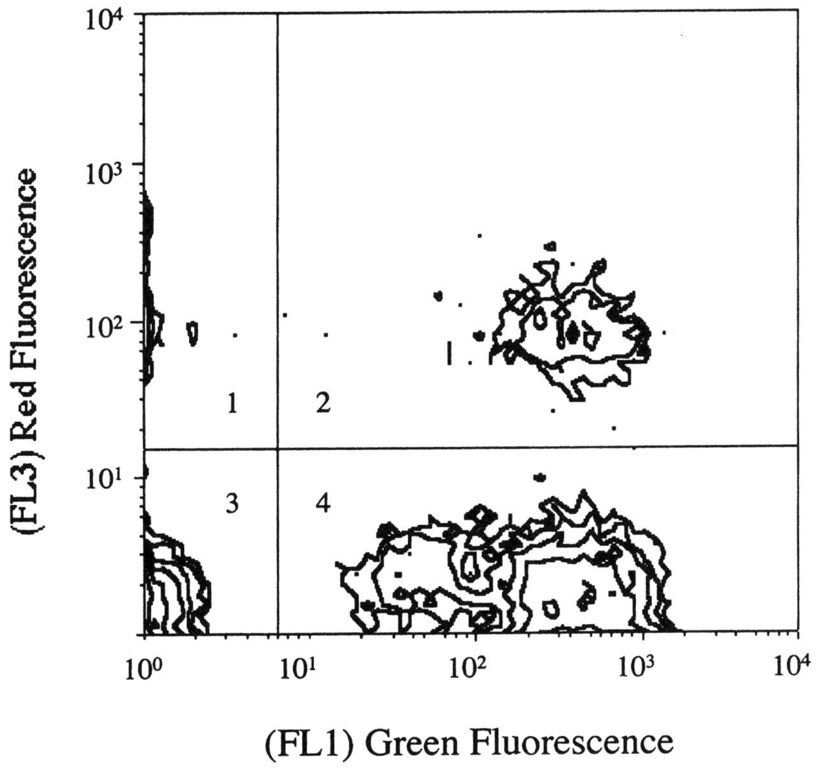

FIGURE 1. Contour plot of green (FL1) and red (FL3) fluorescence of PMNs incubated with ethanol-fixed fluorescein-labeled *C. albicans* blastospores at 37°C after the addition of EtBr. In this experiment, 4% (region 1) were PMNs with only membrane-bound blastospores, 55% (region 4) were PMNs with ingested FITC-labeled *C. albicans*, 12% (region 2) were PMNs with both ingested and adherent FITC-labeled *C. albicans* blastospores, and 27% (region 3) were PMNs without any interactions with blastospore cells.

TABLE 1. Phagocytosis and Killing Function of PMNs

	% PMN (Mean ± SD; $N = 15$)
PMNs/FITC-labeled *C. albicans* Fluorescence/Interaction[a]	
Adherence	9±6%
Adherence and ingestion	15±10%
Ingestion	50±14%
No interaction	26±13%
PMN Killing Function[b]	
	% Killed FITC-labeled *C. albicans*
	33±19

[a]Percentage of phagocytes with adherent and/or ingested FITC-labeled *C. albicans* blastospores after incubation with opsonized FITC-labeled *C. albicans* blastospores at 37°C for 30 min with continuous agitation.

[b]Killing function of PMNs expressed as percentage of killed FITC-labeled *C. albicans* blastospores after incubation with opsonized FITC-labeled *C. albicans* at 37°C for 2.5 h with continuous agitation.

(27%), and PMNs with only ingested FITC-labeled *C. albicans* blastospores are found in region 4 (55%).

TABLE 1 provides a summary of the analysis of phagocytosis and adherence conducted on blood samples obtained from 15 healthy donors. The table reports the means and standard deviations of the percentages of PMNs that ingested FITC-labeled *C. albicans* blastospores, as well as those with adherent and phagocytized FITC-labeled *C. albicans* blastospores.

Killing of FITC-labeled C. albicans by PMNs

The cytometric analysis of the percentage of blastospores killed by PMNs is represented in a two-color biparametric graph: green fluorescence and red fluorescence (FIG. 2). Dead FITC-labeled *C. albicans* blastospores are visible in region 2 among the double-labeled cells. In fact, the killed blastospores proved to be red inside due to PI penetration of the cell and green outside due to FITC. FIGURE 2 (A and B) illustrates a representative killing assay. FIGURE 2 (A) shows the fluorescence of live *C. albicans* blastospore before the killing assay. The percentage of killed blastospores proved to be 30% and was calculated by comparing the results of the analysis of region 2 of FIGURE 2(A) and (B). Residual live FITC-labeled *C. albicans* blastospores are visible in region 4 of FIGURE 2(B). Moreover, dead FITC-labeled *C. albicans* blastospores were easily discriminated from leukocyte debris by cytogram simultaneously evaluating their different FSC and SSC properties. The means and standard deviations for the percentages of dead FITC-labeled *C. albicans* blastospores following incubation with PMNs from the peripheral blood samples collected from the 15 healthy donors were 33±19.

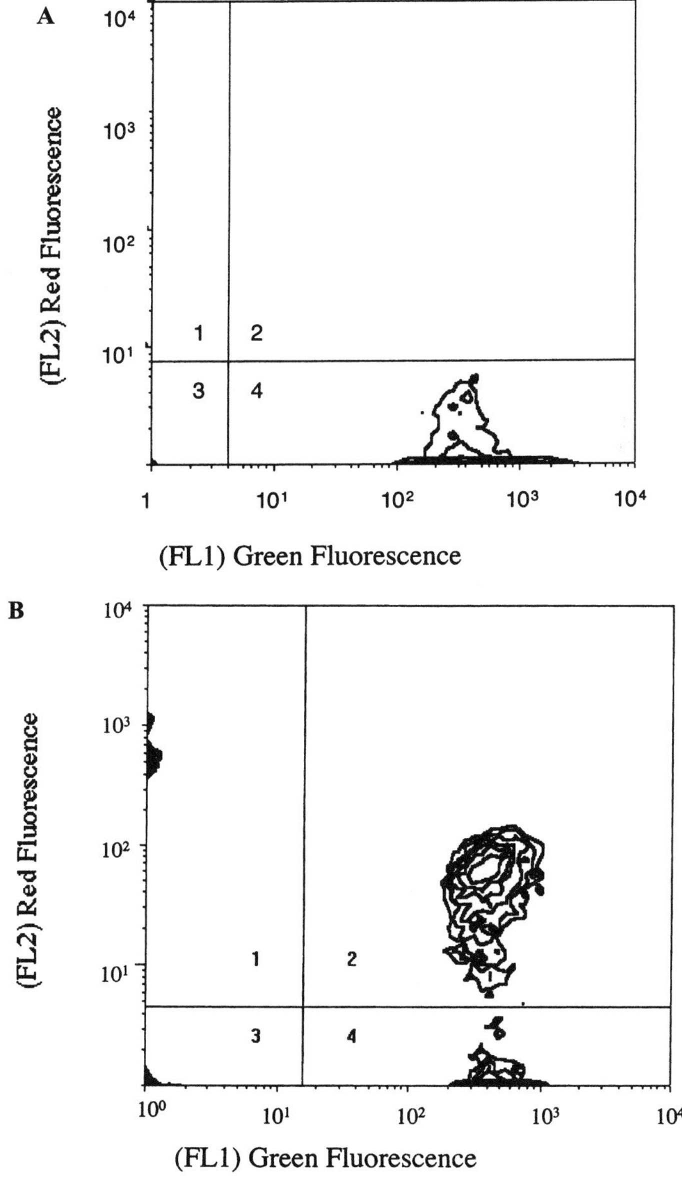

FIGURE 2. (**A**) Contour plot of green (FL1) and red (FL2) fluorescence of control FITC-labeled *C. albicans*. The percentage of living blastospore cells was 98% (region 4). (**B**) Contour plot of FL1 and FL2 fluorescence of killed FITC-labeled *C. albicans* blastospores after incubation at 37°C for 90 min with PMNs. The percentage of killed blastospore cells was 30% (region 2).

DISCUSSION

We have described a quick and reliable method for the analysis of phagocytosis and killing of *Candida albicans* blastospores by human PMNs using flow cytometry. This assay offers several advantages compared to previous microscopic and/or cytometric techniques. First of all, it confirms that it is possible to utilize unseparated PMNs, which can be easily distinguishable from the leukocyte population by selection on the basis of their FSC and SSC properties. This reduces the time normally required for the preparation of specimens for routine assays because in this case, only the lysis of red blood cells is required for the preparation of the phagocytosis and killing assays.

In addition, unlike microscopic or microbiological techniques, this method is less time-consuming and more precise: it allows for the detection of about 10,000 *C. albicans* blastospores or phagocytes in less than 2 min and with a yield of accurate and reproducible data.

The reason for the selection of *C. albicans* blastospores as a marker of phagocytosis and killing lies not only in the prevalence of this pathogen among opportunistic agents, but also in the practical advantages it provides. *C. albicans* blastospores present good flexibility *in vitro:* they are easily grown in culture broth; they can be easily opsonized by human serum; they can be labeled with FITC in a shorter time period than *A. fumigatus* conidia; they do not lose fluorescence after freezing at −70°C; and, finally, they can be used for both phagocytosis and killing assays. We now know that this assay can be easily adapted to evaluate the phagocytosis and the killing of *A. fumigatus* conidia by macrophages (Taramelli and Saresella, unpublished report). Therefore, we believe that it may be possible to adapt it to other fungi as well, provided that they can be consistently and quickly labeled with FITC.

One of the primary technical problems encountered in this study was the discrimination between adherent and internalized blastospores. This distinction is necessary to avoid overestimating the phagocytosis function of PMNs. Ethidium bromide, which transforms FITC-green fluorescence into red fluorescence[5] was used for this purpose. This phenomenon can be explained as an energy transfer between the two fluorochromes. In this case, EtBr is the donor, while FITC is the electron acceptor.[7] However, EtBr does not enter the living cells, and ingested FITC-labeled *C. albicans* blastospores thus retain their green fluorescence, whereas extracellular blastospores turn red. To further optimize the assay and reduce the number of non-ingested particles, a low phagocyte to blastospore ratio (1:2) was used. This ratio allows a better estimation of ingested versus membrane-bound yeasts, because it minimizes the crowding effect due to an excess of yeasts.

These results are a variation of what has been reported by others.[1,5,6] However, a careful examination of the data shows that the total number of phagocytic PMNs is quite similar among different reports, whereas the number of non-phagocytic cells or cells with ingested and adherent yeasts varies considerably.[5] This confirms a strong interference of free yeasts in the assay.

The possibility of using frozen FITC-labeled *C. albicans* blastospores without finding substantial changes in fluorescence intensity made the phagocytosis assay faster because it was possible to maintain frozen aliquots of FITC-labeled *C. albicans* for quite some time and to have the blastospores readily available for the assay.

This is particularly advantageous for routine assays, when several PMN samples have to be checked at one time. Furthermore, the use of the same preparation of FITC-labeled *C. albicans* blastospores reduces variability when follow-up monitoring of the recovery or the loss of PMN function for a individual patient is required. It was not possible to utilize frozen FITC-labeled *C. albicans* for the killing assay, because the percentage of killed blastospore cells in the control group samples increased, especially after thawing. Therefore, live *C. albicans* blastospores had to be labeled with FITC immediately prior to testing. Thanks to the brief incubation time required, the method was fairly rapid. The distinction between live and killed *C. albicans* blastospores was made possible by the use of PI, which does not penetrate the plasma membrane of living cells.[8] Thus, live *C. albicans* blastospores do not stain with PI, however, killed blastospores turn red.[6] As PI binds to DNA, it is very important that external DNA is destroyed by means of DNase treatment before PI is added.[8] Elimination of residual DNA from PMNs and the subsequent gate designed around the blastospores to eliminate debris, allow for a reliable calculation of the percentage of killed FITC-labeled *C. albicans* blastospores. Killed FITC-labeled *C. albicans* blastospores appear as double-labeled and emit both red and green fluorescence, thereby rendering them unmistakably distinct upon the cytometric reading in a biparametric graph showing two fluorescences in the common region.

A simple quantitative cytometric assay for the combined kinetic study of PMN phagocytosis and the intracellular killing of *C. albicans* blastospores has been presented here. The method may be useful for rapid automatic screening of phagocyte function in infectious diseases, hematological disorders, and in cases of immunosuppression.

REFERENCES

1. MARTIN E. & S. BHAKDI. 1991. Quantitative analysis of opsonophagocytosis and of killing of *Candida albicans* by human peripheral blood leukocytes by using flow cytometry. J. Clin. Microbiol. **29:** 2013–2023.
2. STEINKAMP, J.A., J.S. WILSON, J.C. SAUNDERS & C.C. STEWART. 1982. Phagocytosis: flow cytometric quantitation with fluorescent microspheres. Science **215:** 64–66.
3. STEWART, C.C., B.E. LEHNERT & J.A. STEINKAMP. 1986. *In vitro* and *in vivo* measurement of phagocytosis by flow cytometry. Methods Enzymol. **132:** 183–192.
4. WILSON, R.M., A.M. GALVIN, R.A. ROBINS & W.G. REEVES. 1985. A flow cytometric method for the measurement of phagocytosis by polymorphonuclear leukocytes. J. Immunol. Methods **76:** 247–253.
5. FATTOROSSI, A., R. NISINI, J.C. PIZZOLO & R. D'AMELIO. 1989. New, simple flow cytometry technique to discriminate between internalized and membrane bound particles in phagocytosis. Cytometry **10:** 320–325.
6. BJERKNES, R. 1984. Flow cytometric assay for combined measurement of phagocytosis and intracellular killing of *Candida albicans*. J. Immunol. Methods **72:** 229–241.
7. SZOLLOSI, J., L. TRÒN, S. DAMJANOVICH, S.H. HELLIWELL, D. ARNDT-JOVIN & T.M. JOVIN. 1984. Fluorescence energy transfer measurements on cell surfaces: a critical comparison of steady-state fluorimetric and flow cytometric methods. Cytometry **5:** 210–216.
8. BUSCHMANN, H. & M. WINTER. 1989. Assessment of phagocytic activity of granulocytes using laser flow cytometry. J. Immunol. Methods **124:** 231–234.

Development of Neutrophil Granule Diversity

NIELS BORREGAARD

The Granulocyte Research Laboratory
Division of Hematology
The Finsen Center
Rigshospitalet
Copenhagen, Denmark

INTRODUCTION

The granules of the human neutrophil have long been recognized for their content of proteolytic and bactericidal proteins.[1] During the last 10–15 years it has become clear that the membrane of granules also contributes to the function of the neutrophil as a store of membrane proteins that become incorporated into the plasma membrane during mobilization of granules and exocytosis of their content.[2] The human neutrophil contains a variety of granules, that at least to some extent should be regarded as a continuum from granules that contain myeloperoxidase to granules that are particularly rich in the matrix metalloproteinase gelatinase.[3] The neutrophil granules are traditionally classified into peroxidase-positive and peroxidase-negative granules based on their content of myeloperoxidase.[4] This has been convenient since myeloperoxidase can be detected by an enzymatic reaction and thus provides an easy method of detection by histochemistry. If one wanted to classify on the basis of lysozyme, only one type of granule would be observed, since all neutrophil granules contain lysozyme.[5] Alternatively, one could pick a membrane protein for classification of granules. The b-cytochrome or the β_2-integrin, Mac-1, would distinguish also between two types of granules: Those that do not contain these proteins, which would be congruent with the peroxidase-positive granules, and those that contain these membrane proteins. These would include not only the peroxidase-negative granules,[6,7] but also the secretory vesicles,[8] which are specialized endocytic structures that contain plasma proteins in their lumen[9] and whose membrane is particularly rich in receptors (CR1, CR3, Fc-γ, fMLP receptor, among others).[8,10–13]

Why should we care about the classification of human neutrophil granules? If the neutrophil has organized its granules in a highly diversified but ordered way and furthermore carefully controls the order of mobilization of its granules, then we should be able to learn important lessons by studying the neutrophil and asking the following questions: Why does the neutrophil have these many different granules? How does the neutrophil control the individual mobilization of these granules? How does the neutrophil control the targeting of the correct proteins into the different types of granules?

WHY DOES THE NEUTROPHIL HAVE SUCH A DIVERSITY OF GRANULES?

One reason for putting different proteins into different granules could be that this would permit a differential exocytosis of granular proteins, if the mobilization of the different granule subsets differs. Another reason could be that some proteins cannot exist together in the same granule, and thus have to be segregated. The first question one must ask to address these possibilities is, does the neutrophil mobilize its granules in a differential fashion? The answer is unequivocally yes. In this context it must be mentioned that the secretory vesicles are mobilized rapidly and completely by stimulation with inflammatory mediators. It is believed that secretory vesicles are mobilized during rolling of neutrophils along the endothelium and provide the structural basis for the subsequent firm adhesion. This is supported by the fact that secretory vesicles are rapidly and completely mobilized by inflammatory mediators such as GM-CSF, PAF, IL-8, fMLP, that are relevant for the interaction of neutrophils with endothelial cells, and these stimuli have been shown to convert the neutrophil from a selectin-presenting cell to a CD11b-presenting cell.[14,15] This concept is supported by the finding that neutrophils isolated from a skin window chamber have mobilized their secretory vesicles completely.[16] Although unable to mobilize the marker proteins of the traditional granules—lactoferrin from specific granules and myeloperoxidase from azurophil granules—these stimuli (G-CSF, PAF, IL-8, fMLP) are capable of causing a significant release of the cellular content of gelatinase from intact neutrophils.[17] This makes sense, since gelatinase is a collagenase of type IV collagen, the collagen of basement membranes that constitute the first barrier for the neutrophil after emigration through endothelial cells. The differential exocytosis of lactoferrin and gelatinase can only be explained if these proteins are localized in different granules that are mobilized differently.[18,19] Furthermore, stimulation of neutrophils with a variety of stimuli, the most powerful being the calcium ionophore, Ionomycin, have shown that there is a fundamental difference between peroxidase-negative and peroxidase-positive granules, since the peroxidase-negative granules can be mobilized almost completely, in contrast to peroxidase-positive granule of which at most 30% of granule content can be found extracellularly.[20] Furthermore, during phagocytosis, peroxidase-positive granules are mobilized only to the phagosome, in contrast to peroxidase-negative granules.[21] Classification of neutrophil granules with regards to their content of peroxidase and the two marker proteins lactoferrin and gelatinase therefore makes sense from a functional point of view.

CLASSIFICATION OF GRANULES

Subcellular fractionation provides a simple and powerful method of classification of granules as seen in FIGURE 1, where the localization of marker proteins is given in a Percoll density gradient. Although some myeloperoxidase is observed in the fractions that also contain specific granules, myeloperoxidase and lactoferrin are completely segregated in two different granule subsets.[22] On the other hand, the separation between lactoferrin and gelatinase seems almost complete, yet, in approximately 50% of peroxidase-negative granules both lactoferrin and gelatinase are present in

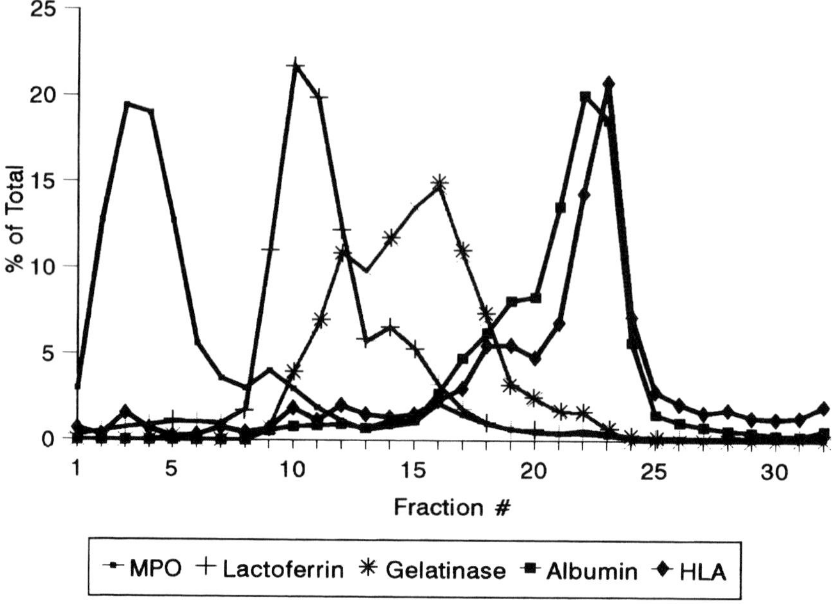

FIGURE 1. Subcellular distribution of proteins characteristic for the plasma membrane, secretory vesicles, and granules of the human neutrophil. Subcellular fractionation was performed as described in Kjeldjen and coworkers.[19] Azurophil granules were identified by myeloperoxidase. Specific granules by lactoferrin, gelatinase granules by gelatinase, secretory vesicles by albumin, and plasma membranes by HLA class I.

the same granule, as determined by double-labeling electron microscopy.[18] Many other proteins co-localize completely with either of these markers. β-Glucuronidase co-localizes with myeloperoxidase, elastase and cathepsin G, BPI, azurocidin likewise, whereas defensins only are present in a subset of the peroxidase-positive granules.[23–25] NGAL (neutrophil gelatinase associated lipocalin) and hCAP-18 co-localize with lactoferrin.[26,27] This again underscores that the neutrophil sorts proteins as groups into the different types of granules, which are mobilized differentially to provide the neutrophil with a structural basis for responding to activation in a differentiated way and to optimize its response to the physiological surrounding, be it adhesion to endothelium, diapedesis, migration through tissue, or phagocytosis.

HOW DOES THE NEUTROPHIL CONTROL THE DIFFERENTIAL MOBILIZATION OF GRANULES?

The signaling pathways that control the differential exocytosis of individual granule subpopulations have not been identified. Since the granules differ in size, one possibility could be that smaller granules are mobilized more rapidly and extensively, because they have a larger surface-to-mass ratio than have larger granules. More force would be generated per unit mass if the force for movement applied is proportional to the surface area. Also, smaller granules would be expected to meet less resistance from the cytoskeleton during movement. The size of granules is inversely proportional to the mobilization of granules,[18,28] but this of course does not prove a causal relationship.

It has recently been observed that the distribution of a fusion protein belonging to the v-SNARE family of proteins, VAMP-2 is in agreement with the known propensity for mobilization of the individual granules,[29] and it is possible, although as yet only a hypothesis, that exocytosis of the individual granule subsets is a stochastic process, the outcome of which is determined by the likelihood that any granule subset is docked to the plasma membrane, which again may be determined by the amount of v-SNARE present on the membrane of the granule.

HOW DOES THE NEUTROPHIL CREATE ITS DIVERSITY OF GRANULES?

It has long been known that peroxidase-positive granules are formed at the promyelocyte stage and peroxidase-negative granules at the myelocyte stage.[4] Realizing that it is functionally important to subdivide the peroxidase-negative granules into granules that are high in their content of gelatinase versus lactoferrin, the question arose whether the segregation of these two proteins into different granules could be explained solely by differences in the timing of biosynthesis. We were able to confirm that this is indeed the case[30] and have forwarded the hypothesis that the heterogeneity of neutrophil granules is explained solely by the timing of synthesis of each individual granule protein, without the need for any sorting between individual granule subsets (FIG. 2). This hypothesis could be tested by transfecting HL-60 cells with the cDNA of a granule protein that is expressed only at the metamyelocyte stage in normal neutrophil precursors, and completely co-localized with lactoferrin in specific granules of the mature neutrophil.[26] NGAL was transfected under the control of a constitutively active CMV promoter to secure that NGAL protein was expressed in the HL-60 cells, although these are developmentally arrested at the promyelocyte stage and only generate peroxidase-positive granules. NGAL was localized to the azurophil granules in these cells, but was unable to resist the proteolytic milieu of azurophil granules and was eventually degraded, however, providing evidence that neutrophil granule proteins co-localize, if synthesized at the same time, before degradation became effective.[31] Thus showing, that in addition to the need for differential mobilization of granule contents, segregation of granule proteins into different granule subsets is needed because some proteins cannot co-exist in the same granule. These experiments show that the heterogeneity of granules is explained by the differential timing of granule protein synthesis. This, of course, does not exclude the possibility that differences may exist in the efficiency by which individual granule proteins may be sorted to the pathway of regulated storage granules as opposed to the pathway of constitutive secretion.

It is possible that the timing of biosynthesis may even determine the amount of v-SNARE on the membrane of granules and thus provide a link between content and control of exocytosis.

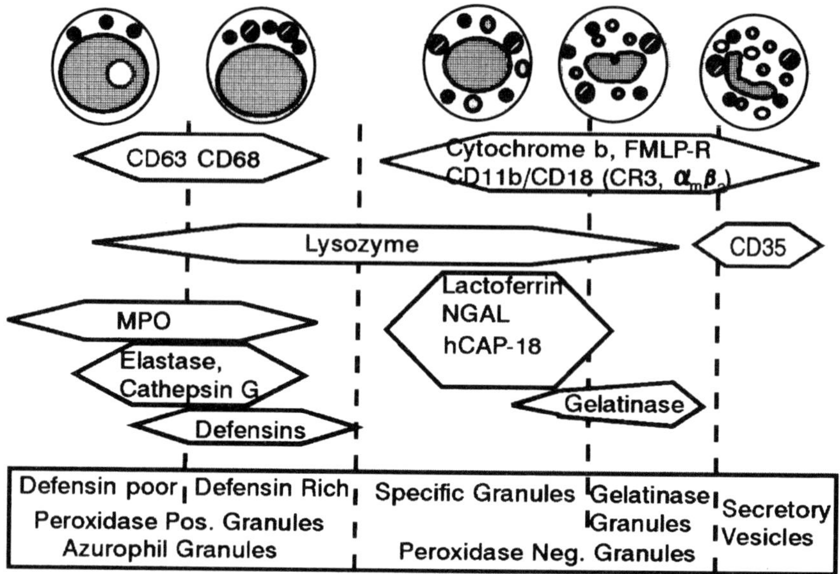

FIGURE 2. Targeting of granule proteins by controlled timing of biosynthesis. The biosynthetic window of granule proteins is indicated in relation to the stage of maturation of the cells in the bone marrow.

SUMMARY

The neutrophil has intracellular stores of both membrane proteins and soluble proteins that may be incorporated into the plasma membrane and exocytosed, respectively, at different times to meet the demands for assisting the neutrophil in adhesion to endothelium (secretory vesicles), for migration through basement membranes (gelatinase granules), and for phagocytosis, killing, and digestion of microorganisms (specific granules and azurophil granules). One reason for segregating the proteins into different subpopulations of granules is that some proteins cannot exist in the same compartment (NGAL digested if present in azurophil granules). Another reason is that the content of the different granules is needed at different times and places. The background for the diversity of neutrophil granules is the timing of biosynthesis, which again most likely is the result of transcriptional control, although this is not yet proven. It is possible that the control of exocytosis is also determined by the same mechanism—a carefully controlled timing of biosynthesis of fusion proteins that ties the content of granules to the likelihood that a given stimulus will result in exocytosis of that individual granule subset.

REFERENCES

1. WELSH, I.R.H. & J.K. SPITZNAGEL. 1971. Distribution of lysosomal enzymes, cationic proteins, and bactericidal substances in subcellular fractions of human polymorphonuclear leukocytes. Infect. Immun. **4:** 97–102.

2. BORREGAARD, N., J.M. HEIPLE, E.R. SIMONS & R.A. CLARK. 1983. Subcellular localization of the b-cytochrome component of the human neutrophil microbicidal oxidase: Translocation during activation. J. Cell Biol. **97:** 52–61.

3. BORREGAARD, N. 1996. Current opinion about neutrophil granule physiology. Curr. Opin. Hematol. **3:** 11–20.

4. BAINTON, D.F., J.L. ULLYOT & M. FARQUHAR. 1971. The development of neutrophilic polymorphonuclear leukocytes in human bone marrow. J. Exp. Med. **143:** 907–934.

5. LOLLIKE, K., L. KJELDSEN, H. SENGELOV & N. BORREGAARD. 1995. Lysozyme in human neutrophils and plasma. A parameter of myelopoietic activity. Leukemia **9:** 159–164.

6. JESAITIS, A., E.S. BUESCHER, D. HARRISON, M.T. QUINN, C.A. PARKOS, S. LIVESEY & J. LINNER. 1990. Ultrastructural localization of cytochrome b in the membrane of resting and phagocytosing human granulocytes. J. Clin. Invest. **85:** 821–835.

7. BAINTON, D.F., L.J. MILLER, T.K. KISHIMOTO & T.A. SPRINGER. 1987. Leukocyte adhesion receptors are stored in peroxidase-negative granules of human neutrophils. J. Exp. Med. **166:** 1641–1653.

8. CALAFAT, J., T.W. KUIJPERS, H. JANSSEN, N. BORREGAARD, A.J. VERHOEVEN & D. ROOS. 1993. Evidence for small intracellular vesicles in human blood phagocytes containing cytochrome b_{558} and the adhesion molecule CD11b/CD18. Blood **81:** 3122–3129.

9. BORREGAARD, N., L. KJELDSEN, K. RYGAARD, L. BASTHOLM, M.H. NIELSEN, H. SENGELOV, O.W. BJERRUM & A.H. JOHNSEN. 1992. Stimulus-dependent secretion of plasma proteins from human neutrophils. J. Clin. Invest. **90:** 86–96.

10. SENGELOV, H., L. KJELDSEN, M.S. DIAMOND, T.A. SPRINGER & N. BORREGAARD. 1993. Subcellular localization and dynamics of Mac-1 ($\alpha_m\beta_2$) in human neutrophils. J. Clin. Invest. **92:** 1467–1476.

11. SENGELOV, H., F. BOULAY, L. KJELDSEN & N. BORREGAARD. 1994. Subcellular localization and translocation of the receptor for N-formyl-methionyl-leucyl-phenylalanine in human neutrophils. Biochem. J. **299:** 473–479.

12. SENGELOV, H., L. KJELDSEN, W. KROEZE, M. BERGER & N. BORREGAARD. 1994. Secretory vesicles are the intracellular reservoir of complement receptor 1 in human neutrophils. J. Immunol. **153:** 804–810.

13. DEHAAS, M., J.M. KERST, C.E. VANDERSCHOOT, J. CALAFAT, C.E. HACK, J.H. NUIJENS, D. ROOS, R.H.J. VANOERS & A.E.G.K. VONDEMBORNE. 1994. Granulocyte colony-stimulating factor administration to healthy volunteers: analysis of the immediate activating effects on circulating neutrophils. Blood **84:** 3885–3894.

14. BORREGAARD, N., L. MILLER & T.A. SPRINGER. 1987. Chemoattractant-regulated mobilization of a novel intracellular compartment in human neutrophils. Science **237:** 1204–1206.

15. BORREGAARD, N., L. KJELDSEN, H. SENGELOV, M.S. DIAMOND, T.A. SPRINGER, H.C. ANDERSON, D.F. BAINTON & T.K. KISHIMOTO. 1994. Changes in the subcellular localization and surface expression of L-selectin, alkaline phosphatase, and Mac-1 in human neutrophils during stimulation with inflammatory mediators. J. Leuk. Biol. **56:** 80–87.

16. SENGELOV, H., P. FOLLIN, L. KJELDSEN, K. LOLLIKE, C. DAHLGREN & N. BORREGAARD. 1995. Mobilization of granules and secretory vesicles during in vivo exudation of human neutrophils. J. Immunol. **154:** 4157–4165.

17. KJELDSEN, L., O.W. BJERRUM, J. ASKAA & N. BORREGAARD. 1992. Subcellular localization and release of human neutrophil gelatinase, confirming the existence of separate gelatinase-containing granules. Biochem. J. **287:** 603–610.

18. KJELDSEN, L., D.F. BAINTON, H. SENGELOV & N. BORREGAARD. 1993. Structural and functional heterogeneity among peroxidase-negative granules in human neutrophils: Identification of a distinct gelatinase containing granule subset by combined immunocytochemistry and subcellular fractionation. Blood **82:** 3183–3191.

19. KJELDSEN, L., H. SENGELOV, K. LOLLIKE, M.H. NIELSEN & N. BORREGAARD. 1994. Isolation

and characterization of gelatinase granules from human neutrophils. Blood **83:** 1640–1649.

20. SENGELOV, H., L. KJELDSEN & N. BORREGAARD. 1993. Control of exocytosis in early neutrophil activation. J. Immunol. **150:** 1535–1543.

21. GANZ, T. 1987. Extracellular release of antimicrobial defensins by human polymorphonuclear leukocytes. Infect. Immun. **55:** 568–571.

22. CRAMER, E., K.B. PRYZWANSKY, J.-C. VILLEVAL, U. TESTA & J. BRETON-GORIUS. 1985. Ultrastructural localization of lactoferrin and myeloperoxidase in human neutrophils by immunogold. Blood **65:** 423–432.

23. GANZ, T., M. SELSTED, D. SZKLAREK, S.S.L. HARWIG, K. DAHER, D.F. BAINTON & R.I. LEHRER. 1985. Defensins. Natural peptide antibiotics of human neutrophils. J. Clin. Invest. **76:** 1427–1435.

24. RICE, W.G., T. GANZ, J.M. KINKADE, M.E. SELSTED, R.I. LEHRER & R.T. PARMLEY. 1987. Defensin-rich dense granules of human neutrophils. Blood **70:** 757–765.

25. BORREGAARD, N., K. LOLLIKE, L. KJELDSEN, H. SENGELOV, L. BASTHOLM, M.H. NIELSEN & D.F. BAINTON. 1993. Human neutrophil granules and secretory vesicles. Eur. J. Haematol. **51:** 187–198.

26. KJELDSEN, L., D.F. BAINTON, H. SENGELOV & N. BORREGAARD. 1994. Identification of NGAL as a novel matrix protein of specific granules in human neutrophils. Blood **83:** 799–807.

27. COWLAND, J.B., A.H. JOHNSEN & N. BORREGAARD. 1995. hCAP-18, a cathelin/bactenecin like protein of human neutrophil specific granules. FEBS Lett. **368:** 173–176.

28. LOLLIKE, K., N. BORREGAARD & M. LINDAU. 1995. The exocytotic fusion pore of small granules has a conductance similar to an ion channel. J. Cell Biol. **129:** 99–104.

29. BRUMELL, J.H., A. VOLCHUK, H. SENGELOV, N. BORREGAARD, A.M. CIEUTAT, D.F. BAINTON, S. GRINSTEIN & A. KLIP. 1995. Subcellular distribution of docking/fusion proteins in neutrophils, secretory cells with multiple exocytic compartments. J. Immunol. **155:** 5750–5759.

30. BORREGAARD, N., M. SEHESTED, B.S. NIELSEN, H. SENGELOV & L. KJELDSEN. 1995. Biosynthesis of granule proteins in normal human bone marrow cells. Gelatinase is a marker of terminal neutrophil differentiation. Blood **85:** 812–817.

31. LE CABEC, V., J.B. COWLAND, J. CALAFAT & N. BORREGAARD. 1996. Targeting of proteins to granule subsets determined by timing not by sorting: the specific granule protein NGAL is localized to azurophil granules when expressed in HL-60 cells. Proc. Natl. Acad. Sci. USA **93:** 6454–6457.

Phagocyte Chemoattractant Receptors

F. BOULAY,[a] N. NAIK,[b] E. GIANNINI, M. TARDIF,
AND L. BROUCHON

Commissariat á l'Energie Atomique/Grenoble
Département de Biologie Moléculaire et Structurale
Laboratoire de Biochimie et Biophysique des Systèmes Intégrés
(Unité Mixte de Recherche 314, CEA/CNRS)
17 rue des Martyrs
38054 Grenoble cedex 9, France

INTRODUCTION

Phagocytic leukocytes are capable of migrating by active amoeboid movements along a chemical gradient to inflammatory sites and/or sites of infection. This phenomenon known as chemotaxis is essential for host defense against bacterial and fungal infections and for wound healing. The directed locomotion of phagocytes is triggered by specific substances, termed chemoattractants, that were pharmacologically and structurally characterized during the past 25 years. Study of the classical chemotactic agents began in the 1970s when a variety of ligands were recognized as chemoattractants for phagocytic leukocytes. These include: (*1*) the C3a and C5a anaphylatoxins generated by cleavage of the complement proteins C3 and C5, respectively; (*2*) the N-formylated peptides (fMLF) that may derive from bacterial cells as well as mitochondrially encoded proteins; (*3*) the platelet-activating factor (PAF) that is released from platelets, neutrophils, and related phagocytic cells; (*4*) the leukotriene B4 (LTB4), which belongs to a family of compounds that derive from arachidonic acid. Since the mid 1980s, a new class of structurally related chemotactic cytokines (chemokines) of 8 to 10 kD proteins has emerged. They are secreted by activated leukocytes and chemoattract and activate a variety of cells that are involved in inflammation. This growing family is divided in two groups according to sequence similarity and the position of the first two cysteine residues; the C-X-C family (or α chemokines) in which the two cysteine residues are separated by a single amino acid and the C-C family (β chemokines) where the first two cysteine residues are adjacent.[1,2] Most C-X-C chemokines, such as interleukin-8, MGSA/Gro-α, and NAP-2, act on neutrophils but not on monocytes, while the C-C chemokines, including MIP-1α, MIP-β, and RANTES (*R*egulated on *A*ctivation, *N*ormal *T* cell *E*xpressed and *Se*creted), potently activate monocytes and T lymphocytes but not neutrophils.[1]

The chemotactic agents bind to cell surface receptors that are coupled to G-proteins. As a result, phagocytic cells rearrange their cytoskeleton, morphologically po-

[a]Address correspondence to F. Boulay, CEA/Grenoble, DBMS/Biochimie (CNRS/URA 1130), 17 rue des Martyrs, 38054 Genoble cedex 9, France. Telephone, 33-76-88-31-38; Fax, 33-76-88-51-85.

[b]Present address: Cell Biology Division, Cancer Research Institute, Tata Memorial Centre, Dr. Ernest Borges Road, Parel, Bombay-400012 India.

larize, and move to sites of infection. Cells ultimately phagocytize and kill invading pathogens through the release of degradative enzymes and the production of superoxide anions by NADPH oxidase. These microbicidal and cytotoxic functions of phagocytes are evoked at chemoattractant concentrations 10- to 100-fold higher than that required for chemotaxis.[3] In addition to these well-characterized functions, leukocyte chemoattractants can also produce or exacerbate inflammatory disorders as they have been shown to trigger the release of inflammatory cytokines[4,5] and induce the activation of the transcription factor NF-kB.[6] More recently, several C-C chemokines, including MIP-1α, MIP-1β, and RANTES, have been found to potently inhibit replication of HIV-1 in peripheral blood leukocytes. Understanding the regulation of chemotactic receptor function and signaling pathways, as well as the intracellular trafficking of these receptors in leukocytes, is therefore of particular interest and clinical relevance. Here, we will briefly summarize the current understanding of the structure/function, signaling, and regulation of the G protein–coupled chemoattractant receptors. The reader is referred to several recent reviews on these topics.[1,7–11]

MOLECULAR CLONING AND STRUCTURE OF CHEMOATTRACTANT RECEPTORS

Major progress toward the understanding of neutrophil activation was achieved by cloning the cDNAs encoding chemoattractant receptors. The application of new molecular cloning techniques (ectopic expression and homology hybridization strategies) led to the characterization of the primary structure of receptors for classical chemoattractants and chemokines. These receptors have a predicted heptahelical structure typical of G protein–coupled receptors (GPCR) with a number of remarkable peculiarities: (*1*) they are similar in length (350–360 aa); (*2*) the third intracellular loop is short and rich in lysine and arginine residues; (*3*) with the exception of the PAF receptor (PAFR), the C-terminal region of chemoattractant receptors does not contain a cysteine residue, which is generally conserved and palmitoylated in other GPCRs; and (*4*) a stretch of residues, DRYLAIVHA, is invariably observed at the end of the third transmembrane domain of chemokine receptors. The reader interested in the structure and function of leukocyte chemoattractant receptors is referred to a recent review by Ye and Boulay.[10]

The Classical Chemoattractant Receptors: FPR, C5aR, C3aR, and PAFR

With the exception of the LTB$_4$ receptor, the receptors for the aforementioned classical chemoattractants have been cloned (TABLE 1). A strategy relying on the ability of functional receptors to confer high affinity fMLF binding to COS-7 cells allowed the isolation of two human cDNAs encoding two 350-amino acid long allelic receptors (FPR).[12] Subsequently, two genes encoding human FPR-like receptors (*FPRL1* and *FPRL2*) were described.[13–15] They encode proteins that are highly homologous to the human FPR (FPRH1 and FPRH2, respectively). The gene product of *FPRL1* (351 aa) shares 69% sequence identity with the human FPR, but despite this high level of amino acid identity, fMLF was found to be a poor agonist.[16] In 1994, it has been reported that Chinese hamster ovary cells expressing the *FPRL1* gene product displayed specific and high-affinity binding sites for lipoxin A_4.[17] However, attempts to induce phosphorylation of FPRH1 with high concentrations of fMLF or lipoxin A_4 have remained unsuccessful (Boulay, unpublished data). The gene *FPRL2* encodes a protein (353 aa) with 56% amino acid identity to the human FPR and 83% amino acid identity with FPRH1. While the transcripts for FPR and FPRH1 are abundant in neutrophils, the FPRH2 transcript is observed in monocytes but not in neutrophils.[18] Expression of FPRH2 in *Xenopus* oocytes does not result in transient calcium mobilization in response to fMLF.[18]

Elucidation of the C5a receptor amino acid sequence was independently achieved by two groups using different strategies.[19,20] The overall amino acid identity of C5aR (350 aa) with the FPR is 34%, with the greatest sequence similarity in the hydrophobic transmembrane regions. Cloning of C5a receptor from different species revealed a striking divergence between species in the putative extracellular regions. However, despite a marked sequence divergence, the mouse and dog receptors both bind human C5a with high affinity.[8] In contrast to the human FPR, no polymorphism has been reported for the human C5aR, suggesting a strong selective pressure for the maintenance of a conserved structure. In this context it is worth noting that most mutant C5aRs generated *in vitro* are not functional in transfected cells.[21] Recently, Ye and coworkers have isolated an orphan receptor, named AZ3B, from a differentiated HL-60 cDNA library using the human FPR cDNA as probe.[22] The AZ3B protein is most homologous to the sequences of C5aR and FPR, but has the unique feature to contain a large second extracellular loop (~172 amino acids) between the fourth and the fifth transmembrane regions. Using an expression cloning strategy to isolate the

TABLE 1. Ligand Specificity and Tissue Distribution of Classical Chemoattractant Receptors

Receptor	Ligand	Antagonist	Tissue Distribution
FPR	f-M-L-F (K_d ~1 nM) Ac-M-Nle-L-F-F	tBOC-peptides Cs H[a]	N, M, HepG2, Astrocyte
FPRH1	f-M-L-F (K_d > 0.4 μM) Lipoxin A4		N, M, HL-60
FPRH2	n.d.		M, Lung
C5aR	C5a	LRANISHK-DMQLGR[b]	N, M, Eo, HepG2, Ba, MØ
AZ3B/C3aR	C3a		N, M, En, Raji, Heart, Lung, Placenta
PAFR	PAF	WEB2086 L-659,989	N, M, Eo, Fb, Placenta, Lung

[a]Cyclosporine H (CsH) proved to be a potent antagonist for fMLF-mediated responses in neutrophils with a K_i value of 0.1 μM.[92]

[b]The multi-antigen form of the last 14 C-terminal amino acids of C5a behaves as an antagonist for C5a-mediated β-hexoaminidase release in U937 cells.[93]

Abbreviations: N, neutrophil; M, monocyte; n.d., not determined; Eo, eosinophil; Ba, basophil; MØ, macrophage; En, endothelial cells; HepG2 cell line; Raji cell line; Fb, fibroblast.

receptor for C3a from a differentiated U937 cDNA library, Bautsch and coworkers have independently isolated a cDNA with a sequence almost identical to that of AZ3B.[23] Competitive binding experiments using membranes of HEK293 cells transfected with AZ3B cDNA revealed the presence of a high affinity receptor for human C3a ($K_d \sim 5$ nM). Moreover, an intracellular accumulation of [^{3}H]phosphoinositides was observed in response to C3a in Chinese hamster ovary cells cotransfected with the cDNAs for AZ3B and Gα-16.[23] Thus, the AZ3B orphan receptor is likely to be the receptor for C3a.

The structure of PAFR was originally elucidated by Shimizu's group from a cDNA isolated from a guinea pig lung cDNA library.[24] The human counterpart was subsequently cloned.[25,26] Both the guinea pig and the human cDNAs encode a 342-amino acid protein that transduces signal in response to subnanomolar concentrations of PAF. Although a single gene has been unequivocally identified, two different transcripts with distinct tissue distribution have been detected. One is preferentially found in peripheral leukocytes, the differentiated eosinophilic cell line EoL-1, and brain, while both transcripts are detected in heart, lung, spleen, and kidney.[27]

Surprisingly, although the classical chemoattractant receptors FPR and C5aR were traditionally thought to be restricted to myeloid cells, in particular to neutrophils, they have recently been found in non myeloid cells. The N-formylpeptide and C5a anaphylatoxin receptors are expressed in liver hepatocytes, endothelial cells, lung bronchial and alveolar cells, astrocytes, and microglia.[28–31] In the hepatoma-derived cell line HepG2, fMLF and C5a mediate acute-phase gene regulation, as evidenced by the production of α1-antitrypsin and α1-antichymotrypsin.[32,33] Moreover, it has recently been reported that dendritic cells, a heterogeneous system of professional antigen presenting cells involved in the initiation of immune responses, respond to fMLF and C5a.[34] Thus, the activation of these chemoattractant receptors may play an important role in modulating the inflammatory and immune responses.

The C-X-C Chemokine Receptors

Affinity cross-linking experiments and competitive ligand binding studies with ^{125}I-labeled human interleukin-8, NAP-2, and MGSA/Groα led Moser and coworkers to anticipate the existence of two IL-8 receptors with overlapping pharmacological profiles.[35] The concept of "shared receptors" was further supported by the cloning of two distinct human IL-8 receptors (IL-8RA and IL-8RB) sharing 76% amino acid identity (FIG. 1).[36,37] Cells expressing IL-8RA (350 aa) displayed high-affinity binding sites for IL-8 ($K_d \sim 2$ nM) and low-affinity binding sites for NAP-2 and MGSA/Groα ($K_d \sim 450$ nM), whereas cells transfected with the cDNA encoding IL-8RB (360 aa) exhibited high-affinity binding sites for all three chemokines.[1] The two receptors mainly differ in the N- and C-terminal regions. Studies on the receptor structure-function relationships have revealed that the N-terminal domain is one of the major determinants for MGSA/Groα and NAP-2 selectivity. Divergence in the C-terminal domain may result in a differential regulation. Consequently, the functions of the type A and type B IL-8 receptors may be functionally different as suggested by several reports. Possible differences in the ability of IL-8RA and IL-RB to induce chemotaxis were assessed with receptor-specific antibodies by several laboratories.[38,39]

Opposite conclusions were reached, suggesting both receptors are able to elicit chemotaxis. Responses such as changes in intracellular Ca^{2+} concentration and release of granule enzymes seem to be mediated by both receptors.[40] However, IL-8 has been shown to stimulate phospholipase D activity and NADPH oxidase, while NAP-2 and MGSA/Groα do not despite the fact both receptors are equally expressed in neutrophils. This suggests that the respiratory burst and the activation of phospholipase D depend exclusively on the activation of IL-8RA.[40,41]

Interestingly, the herpesvirus saimiri was found to contain a gene (*ECRF3*) encoding a 321–amino acid long GPCR-like protein with a high degree of amino acid identity with the human IL-8 receptors.[42] Using the *Xenopus* oocyte expression system, Ahuja and Murphy have further found that the *ECRF3* gene product is a functional receptor for C-X-C chemokines.[43] Likewise, a gene (*US28*) encoding a promiscuous viral homologue of the C-C chemokine receptor 1 (CC CKR1) was found within the genome of the human cytomegalovirus. The open reading frame of *US28* encodes a heptahelical G protein–coupled receptor that functionally responds to MIP-1α, MIP-1β, MCP-1, and RANTES.[44] It does not respond to C-X-C chemokines such as inter-

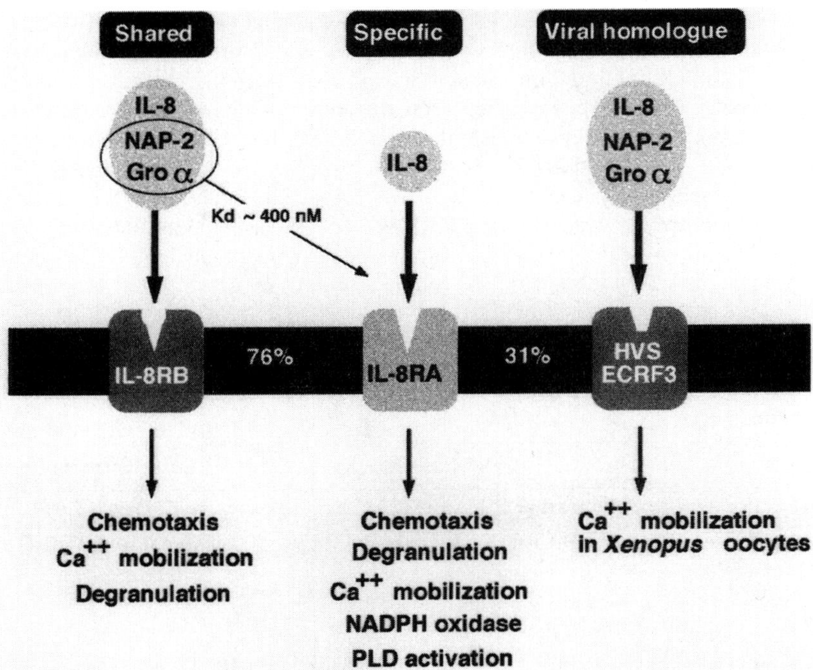

FIGURE 1. Agonist-mediated responses and ligand specificity for the two IL-8 receptors, IL-8RA and IL-8RB, and the structurally related homologue receptor ECRF3 from herpesvirus saimiri origin. The amino acid identity between the two IL-8 receptors and between the viral homologue and IL-8RA is 76% and 31%, respectively. (NAP-2, neutrophil activation peptide 2; Groα, growth-regulated oncogene α.)

leukin-8. At present, it is not known whether ECRF3 and US28 proteins have any physiological function. It remains to be determined whether infected cells expressed these viral homologues and, if so, to what extent the expression of ECRF3 or US28 protein benefits the virus.

The C-C Chemokine Receptors

Receptors with high affinity for MCP-1, MIP-1α, MIP-1β, and RANTES had been identified on monocytes, T lymphocytes, and basophils. Competition binding and cross-desensitization studies had also revealed a complex pattern of interactions between these chemokines, suggesting the existence of shared receptors. The recent cloning of five C-C chemokine receptors (CC CKRs) has clarified the complex relationship between these receptors and the different C-C chemokines (TABLE 2). CC CKR1 is specific of MIP-1α, RANTES, and MCP-3.[45–47] Although MIP-1β and MCP-1 bind to CC CKR1 with a better affinity than RANTES, they are poor agonists for calcium mobilization.[45,46] CC CKR2 does not respond to chemokines other than MCP-1 and MCP-3, despite its strong relatedness to CC CKR1 (51% amino acid identity).[47,48] Quite uncommon in the chemoattractant receptor family whose genes are usually intronless in the coding sequences, two CC CKR2 isoforms are generated by alternative splicing in the carboxyl terminal tail. This may have functional consequences in terms of receptor regulation and G protein coupling (see next section). CC CKR3 is found on eosinophils and binds with high affinity eotaxin, an eosinophil-selective C-C chemokine, and with a lower affinity RANTES and MCP-3. Calcium mobilization assays indicate that eotaxin and RANTES, and to a lesser extent MCP-3, activate CC CKR3.[47,49] A fourth receptor, CC CKR4, is found on basophils and functionally responds to MIP-1α, RANTES, and MCP-1.[50] Last but not least, a fifth receptor designated CC CKR5 has recently been cloned and identified in lymphoid organs, including thymus and spleen, and in blood leukocytes such as macrophages and T lymphocytes.[51,52] Transfected cells expressing this receptor bind

TABLE 2. Ligand Specificity and Tissue Distribution of Cloned C-C Chemokine Receptors

Receptor	Agonist	Tissue Distribution
CKR1 (355 aa)	MIP-1 α, RANTES, MCP-3	M, N, T, THP-1, U937
CKR2 Type A (374 aa) Type B (356 aa)	MCP-1, MCP-3	M, MonoMac6, THP-1
CKR3 (355 aa)	Eotaxin, RANTES	Eo
CKR4 (360 aa)	MIP-1 α, RANTES, MCP-1	Ba
CKR5 (352 aa)	MIP-1 α/β, RANTES	M, THP-1, T(CD4+, CD8+)

Note: The two isoforms of CC CKR2 are generated by alternative splicing in the carboxyl terminal tail.

Abbreviations: M, monocyte; N, neutrophil; THP-1 cell line; MonoMac6 cell line; Eo, eosinophil; Ba, basophil; T, T lymphocyte.

MIP-1α, MIP-1β, and RANTES with high affinity and functionally respond to these chemokines.

Of particular interest is the finding that CC CKR5 is the principal coreceptor for the entry of primary non-syncytium-inducing HIV-1 strains into CD4+ T cells and macrophages.[53,54] This corroborates the finding by Cocchi and colleagues that MIP-1α, MIP-1β, and RANTES inhibit HIV-1 replication in peripheral blood leukocytes.[55] CC CKR3 has been reported to facilitate infection by a more restricted subset of primary viruses.[56] Fusin, another GPCR that does not respond to C-C chemokines has been found to promote the entry of syncytium-inducing primary HIV-1 strains.[57] The amino acid sequence of fusin is identical to an orphan receptor previously characterized by Loetscher and colleagues, which they named LESTR (*LE*ukocyte-derived *S*even *T*ransmembrane domain *R*eceptor).[58] This receptor is more homologous to the human IL-8 receptors (36% amino acid identity) than to C-C chemokine receptors, but it does not bind IL-8 and related molecules. LESTR/Fusin is now known as a receptor for stromal cell-derived factor 1 (SDF-1).[94,95]

G PROTEIN COUPLING AND SIGNALING

G Protein Coupling

In neutrophils, the biochemical and functional responses to a number of chemoattractants, including fMLF, C5a, and IL-8 are largely inhibited by pertussis toxin (PTX), a bacterial toxin that inactivates the α subunit of the G_i class but not the α subunit of the Gq class (Gαq, Gα11, Gz, and Gα16). The mechanism involved in pertussis-sensitive signal transduction remained unclear until recently. Although the α subunit of G_{i2} was originally thought to activate phosphoinositide-specific phospholipase C (PI-PLC), a series of studies have recently established that it is actually the Gβγ subunit that regulates the myeloid cell–specific PI-PLCβ2.[59,60] However, the pattern of G proteins activated in response to chemoattractant binding is dependent on the background of the cells in which chemoattractant receptors are expressed. For instance, the responses to PAF are not inhibited by PTX in platelets[61] nor in COS-7 cells that transiently express PAFR.[62] In COS-7 cells, the transfected PAFR most likely couples to endogenous pertussis-insensitive G proteins, presumably $G_{q/11}$, which activate PI-PLCβ1. In contrast, the other chemoattractant receptors fail to transduce signal in COS-7 cells. This deficiency is attributable to the fact that most chemoattractant-bound receptors do not couple to $G_{q/11}$. Even though they activate endogenous G_i proteins, the released Gβγ subunits are unable to activate PI-PLCβ1 or PI-PLCβ4 as shown by cotransfection assays in COS-7 cells.[60,63] However, a pertussis toxin–sensitive activation of phospholipase C can be reconstituted in COS-7 cells by coexpression of the C5a or fMLF receptor with PI-PLCβ2.[64]

A pertussis toxin–resistant pathway for the fMLF, C5a, and IL-8 receptors has been reconstituted in COS-7 cells without the need of PI-PLCβ2, provided the chemoattractant receptors are cotransfected with Gα16, a pertussis-insensitive G protein whose expression is restricted to a subset of hematopoietic cell progenitors.[62,64,65] Although G16 is a rather promiscuous G protein that can couple to a variety of receptors, coupling of chemoattractant receptors to G16 is not a rule. CC CKR1 and CC-CKR2A are unable to couple to G16, whereas the splicing variant CC CKR2B can.[66] The physiological relevance of this pathway in mature leukocytes is unclear however, as the expression of G16 dramatically decreases after differentiation to neutrophil.[67] Therefore, in mature neutrophils, the G_i pathways seems to be the predominant one. However, one cannot exclude that G16 may play a role in monocytic cell activation since G16 is expressed in cell line differentiated to monocyte. Thus, both G16 and G_i pathways could be used by C-C chemokine receptors that are preferentially expressed in monocytes (FIG. 2).

Chemoattractant Signaling

Activation of neutrophil functions by chemoattractant was originally thought to result from their ability to induce the breakdown of phosphatidyl 4,5-biphosphate (PIP_2) by PI-PLC to form inositol triphosphate (IP_3) and diacylglycerol (DAG). These two messengers regulate the mobilization of Ca^{2+} from intracellular stores and the activation of various isoforms of protein kinase C (PKC), respectively. The reader is referred to a recent review by Bokoch on chemoattractant receptor signaling.[68]

Although the increase of intracellular calcium concentration and PKC activation are clearly two important events accounting for various neutrophil functions, several recent studies have provided evidence that additional pathways are activated by chemoattractant receptors. Many studies have shown that several proteins are transiently phosphorylated on tyrosine residues upon chemoattractant binding. Two of these proteins with an apparent molecular weight of ~42 to 44 kD were identified as members of the family of mitogen-activated protein kinases (MAPKs, also known as ERK-1 and ERK-2).[69,70] In neutrophils, the activation of MAP kinases by fMLF, C5a, or IL-8 appears to occur through the GTP-binding protein Ras and the activation of Raf and MEK-1.[71–73] The molecular mechanisms that lead to Ras activation through chemoattractant receptors are still imperfectly characterized. Several recent studies have provided evidence that G_i protein–coupled receptors mediate Ras activation through a series of steps involving the $\beta\gamma$ subunit of G_i, the activation of Src-like tyrosine kinases, and the phosphorylation of the Shc adapter protein, which contains SH2 and SH3 domains.[74–76] A Shc-Grb2-Sos complex is formed and Ras activation ensues. In addition, phosphatidylinositol-3 kinase activity has recently been demonstrated to be essential in the $G\beta\gamma$-mediated MAP kinase signaling pathway at a point upstream of the Sos and Ras activation.[77]

In neutrophils, it has recently been demonstrated that fMLF induced the activation of Lyn, a Src-related tyrosine kinase, that in turn tyrosine-phosphorylated the Shc adapter protein.[78] The mechanism by which $\beta\gamma$ activates Lyn is still unclear and a recent study by Torres and Ye[79] with FPR-transfected fibroblasts suggests that the activation of the MAP kinase pathway occurs in the absence of Lyn and tyrosine phosphorylation of Shc (FIG. 3). Although the participation of other Src-related kinases is not excluded, this second pathway may involve other activators, such as protein kinase C isoforms and the novel catalytic isoform of PI-3 kinase ($P110\gamma$), that can be directly activated by $G\beta\gamma$.[80]

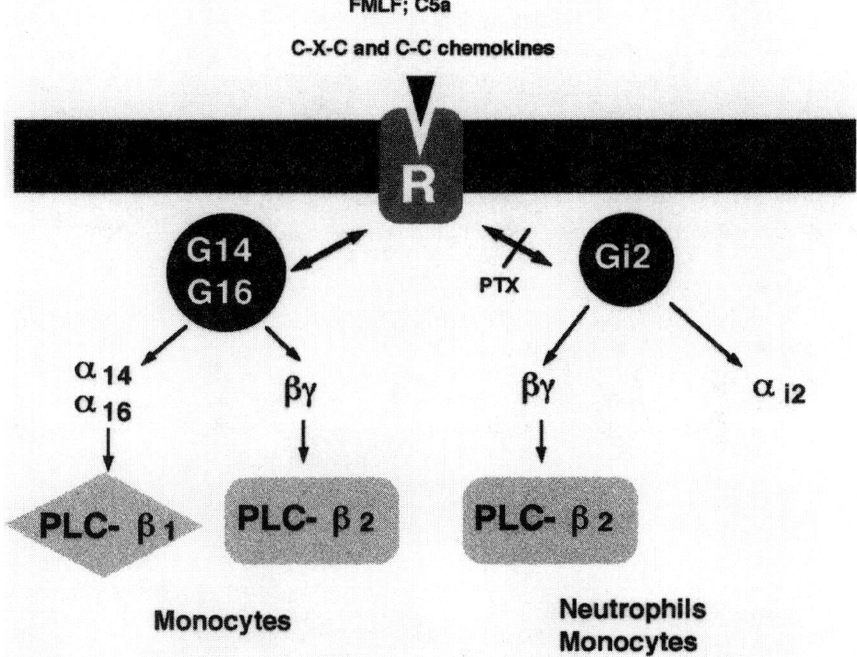

FIGURE 2. Chemoattractant receptor activation of PI-PLCβ isoforms. Chemoattractant receptors can couple to both pertussis toxin–sensitive and –insensitive G proteins. Both pathways may be activated in monocytes, whereas functional responses are largely inhibited by pertussis toxin in neutrophils (see text for details).

REGULATION OF CHEMOATTRACTANT RECEPTORS

Phosphorylation and Internalization

As a rule, the cellular responses to chemoattractants are transient and cells become refractory to a second stimulation with the same agonist. This phenomenon, common to many signaling systems, is termed homologous desensitization and involves the phosphorylation and the internalization of the agonist-occupied receptor. In addition, cells can become refractory to an agonist in response to the activation of other receptors or signaling pathways. This phenomenon, termed heterologous desensitization, may result from the phosphorylation of unoccupied receptors and/or effector enzymes by second messenger–activated kinases. The observation that fMLF, C5a, and IL-8 desensitize one another, while their are not desensitized by ATP-γS or lipid chemoattractants, led Snyderman and coworkers to the description of a third form of regulation known as class-specific cross-desensitization.[81,82] The underlying mechanisms appear to be complex. A cross-phosphorylation of the receptors does not

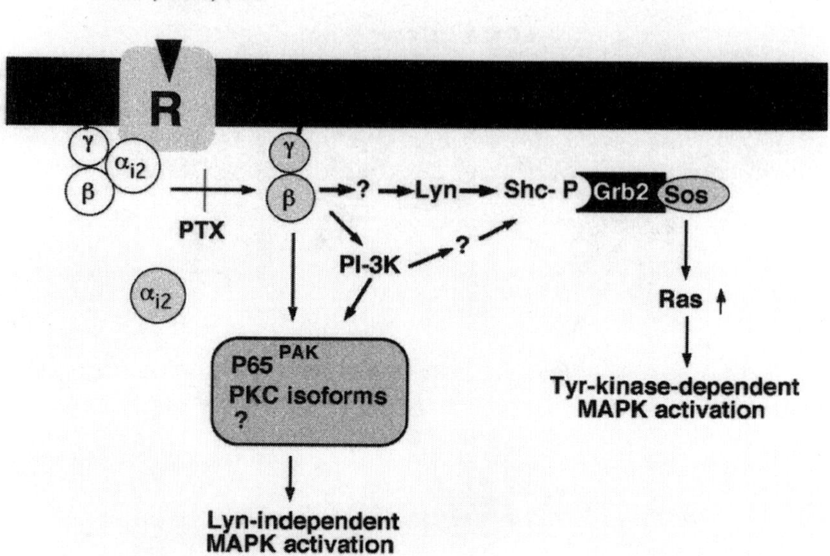

FIGURE 3. Schematic representation of chemoattractant-mediated activation of MAP kinases. In neutrophils, chemoattractant receptor occupancy results in the activation of Lyn, a Src-related tyrosine kinase, and in the phosphorylation of the adapter protein Shc. The complex formed with Grb2 and Sos results in Ras stimulation and activation of the MAP kinase pathway. In FPR-transfected fibroblasts, MAP kinases can be activated in a Lyn-independent manner.[79] Both pathways may require the stimulation of PI-3 kinase activity.

seem to be required since both C5a and IL-8 do alter the ability of FPR to mobilize intracellular Ca^{2+}, even though they are unable to induce the phosphorylation of FPR.

We and others have demonstrated that the receptors for fMLF, C5a, PAF, and IL-8 are rapidly phosphorylated upon agonist binding.[83–88] Activation of PKC by phorbol 12-myristate 13-acetate (PMA) induce the phosphorylation of C5aR, IL-8R and PAFR, but not of FPR, in the absence of agonist binding. Both PMA- and chemoattractant-mediated phosphorylations have been correlated with an inhibition of the GTPase activity associated with the membrane of chemoattractant-treated cells.[81,84,88] A sustained elevation of inositol 1,4,5-triphosphate was observed in cells transfected with the PAFR mutants in which potential phosphorylation sites in the cytoplasmic tail had been mutated.[89] This result supports the notion that receptor phosphorylation is essential to attenuate the cellular responses. The precise mechanism by which the interaction between the phosphorylated chemoattractant receptors and the G protein is impaired is not well understood, but it is likely to involve accessory proteins, such as arrestin.

The phosphorylation of C5aR, PAFR, and IL-8R is strongly enhanced by phorbol esters, but the activation of PKC does not seem to be essential to the agonist-mediated phosphorylation process under physiological conditions. Staurosporine, a potent

PKC inhibitor, partially inhibits the agonist-mediated phosphorylation of C5aR, PAFR, and IL-8R.[83,84,87] Moreover, the disruption of the signaling pathway by PTX does not impair the agonist-mediated phosphorylation of C5aR.[90] Although participation of PKC is not excluded, the dominant kinase is likely to be a member of G protein–coupled receptor kinase family (GRK family). Prossnitz and coworkers have shown that, *in vitro,* FPR could be efficiently phosphorylated in the C-terminal domain by GRK2, which is most abundant in leukocytes. It remains unclear however whether GRK2 is the isotype that phosphorylates FPR, C5aR, and IL-8R in neutrophils.

Phosphorylation sites have been localized on serine residues of the carboxyl terminal tail of C5aR for both C5a- and PMA-mediated phosphorylation.[91] Although all six serine residues could be phosphorylated upon C5a binding, the substitution of alanine for serine residues at positions 332, 334, and 338 results in a dramatic reduction of basal as well as C5a- and PMA-mediated phosphorylation (FIG. 4). This suggests a hierarchical phosphorylation process. Serine residues at positions 332, 334, and 338 are likely to be the key residues in the regulation of C5aR.

Stably transfected cell lines were used to characterize the intracellular trafficking of the C5a receptor. Upon agonist bonding, C5aRs are rapidly phosphorylated and, then, internalized in a perinuclear endosomal compartment (FIG. 5). Under conditions of persistent stimulation with C5a, and in the absence of protein synthesis, the receptors were not degraded but appeared to continuously cycle between the plasma membrane and the perinuclear endosomal compartment. Similar studies with non-phosphorylable mutants of C5aR suggested that phosphorylation may be a prerequisite for the agonist-mediated phosphorylation of chemoattractant receptors (Naik and coworkers, manuscript in preparation). Thus, phosphorylation appears to be a key event that regulates the biological function of the C5a receptor. It is likely that other chemoattractant receptors are regulated in a similar manner.

CONCLUDING REMARKS

The discovery that several chemokine receptors are cofactors for HIV entry is going to boost efforts for the development of small, nonpeptidic molecules that could block viral access to the chemokine receptors or down-regulate the coreceptor. Chemoattractant receptors are undoubtedly the primary targets for the development of anti-inflammatory molecules in the form of receptor antagonists. However, this approach may be complicated by the redundancy of the system, because inflammatory cells express multiple chemoattractant receptors. Understanding the mechanisms of chemoattractant signaling and receptor regulation in greater detail is therefore essential for the development of new therapeutic strategies with broader anti-inflammatory effects.

SUMMARY

Myeloid cells are attracted and activated by a variety of chemoattractants that bind to G protein–coupled receptors. In the past few years, the receptors for the classical

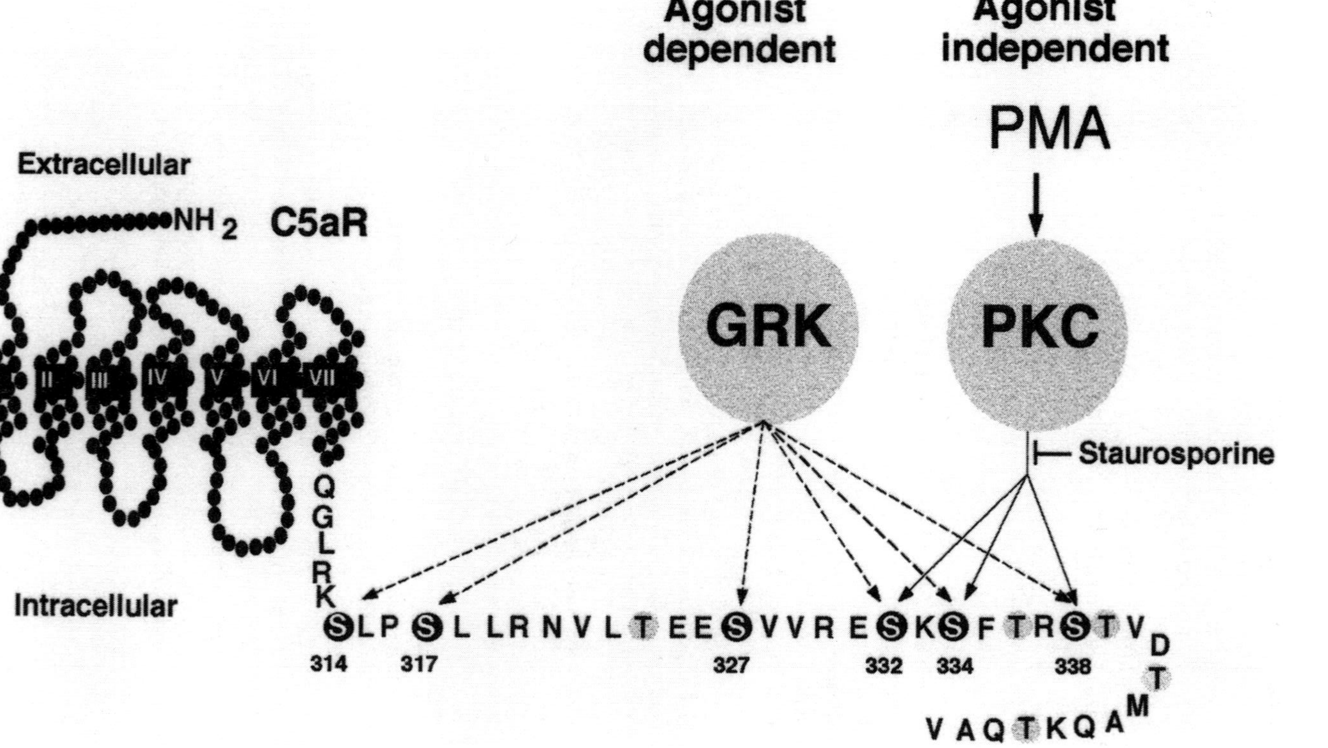

FIGURE 4. Localization of the phosphorylation sites in the C-terminal domain of C5aR. All six serine residues can be phosphorylated in an agonist-dependent manner by a kinase(s) largely insensitive to the protein kinase C inhibitor staurosporine. The key kinase is likely to be a member of the G protein–coupled receptor kinase family (GRK). Phorbol esters can induce the phosphorylation of C5aR in the absence of agonist. Alanine substitution for serine residues at positions 332, 334, and 338 inhibits both agonist- and PMA-dependent phosphorylation of C5aR.

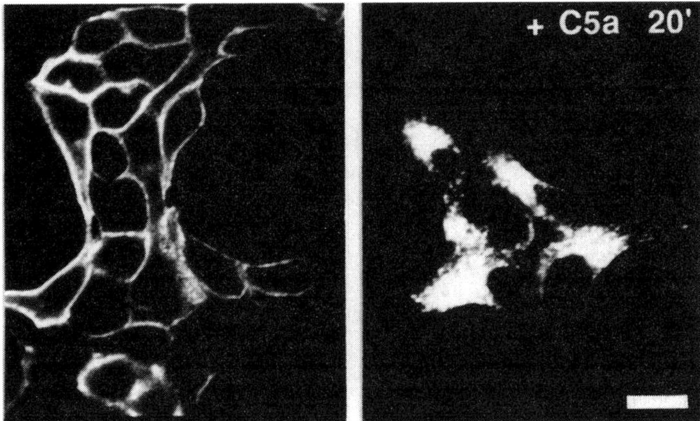

FIGURE 5. C5a-mediated internalization of the C5a receptor in stably transfected insulinoma cells. Confocal immunofluorescent microscopic images of C5aR in the absence of C5a (*left*) or after stimulation with C5a (*right*). Bar = 10 μm.

chemoattractants (fMLF, C5a, PAF) and the chemotactic cytokines, known as C-X-C and C-C chemokines, have been cloned from myeloid cells. This review briefly describes recent advances in structure-function relationships of chemotactic receptors in human leukocytes as well as activation of signaling pathways and regulation of receptor function. In neutrophils, the binding of chemoattractants mainly activates the G_{i2} protein inducing PIP_2 hydrolysis and activation of the MAP kinase pathway. The C-C chemokine receptor, CC CKR5, and a chemokine receptor homologue, named fusin, have been shown to be the major cofactors for HIV-1 entry in macrophages and T cells. Recent studies suggest that the phosphorylation of chemoattractant receptors is a key event that regulates their biological function.

ACKNOWLEDGMENTS

We are grateful to Drs. Ruth Griffin and M. J. Rabiet for critically reading the manuscript.

REFERENCES

1. BAGGIOLINI, M., B. DEWALD & B. MOSER. 1994. Adv. Immunol. **55:** 97–179.
2. BAGGIOLINI, M., P. LOETSCHER & B. MOSER. 1995. Int. J. Immunopharmacol. **17:** 103–108.
3. SNYDERMAN, R. & R. J. UHING. 1992. Inflammation: Basic Principles and Clinical Correlates. 2nd edit. J. I. Gallin, I. M. Goldstein & R. Snyderman, Eds.: 421–439. Raven Press, Ltd. New York.
4. GOODMAN, M. G., D. E. CHENOWETH & W. O. WEIGLE. 1982. J. Exp. Med. **156:** 912–917.
5. CASSATELLA, M. A., F. BAZZONI, M. CESKA, I. FERRO, M. BAGGIOLINI & G. BERTON. 1992. J. Immunol. **148:** 3216–3220.

6. KRAVCHENKO, V. V., Z. PAN, J. HAN, J. M. HERBERT, R. J. ULEVITCH & R. D. YE. 1995. J. Biol. Chem. **270:** 14928–14934.
7. MURPHY, P. M. 1994. Annu. Rev. Immunol. **12:** 593–633.
8. GERARD, C. & N. P. GERARD. 1994. Annu. Rev. Immunol. **12:** 775–808.
9. BEN-BARUCH, A., D. F. MICHIEL & J. J. OPPENHEIM. 1995. J. Biol. Chem. **270:** 11703–11706.
10. YE, R. & F. BOULAY. 1996. Adv. Pharmacol. **39:** 221–289.
11. BATES, P. 1996. Cell **86:** 1–3.
12. BOULAY, F., M. TARDIF, L. BROUCHON & P. VIGNAIS. 1990. Biochemistry **29:** 11123–11133.
13. YE, R. D., S. L. CAVANAGH, O. QUEHENBERGER, E. R. PROSSNITZ & C. G. COCHRANE. 1992. Biochem. Biophys. Res. Commun. **184:** 582–589.
14. MURPHY, P. M., T. OZCELIK, R. T. KENNEY, H. L. TIFFANY, D. MCDERMOTT & U. FRANCKE. 1992. J. Biol. Chem. **267:** 7637–7643.
15. BAO, L., N. P. GERARD, R. EDDY, JR., T. B. SHOWS & C. GERARD. 1992. Genomics **13:** 437–440.
16. QUEHENBERGER, O., E. R. PROSSNITZ, S. L. CAVANAGH, C. G. COCHRANE & R. D. YE. 1993. J. Biol. Chem. **268:** 18167–18175.
17. FIORE, S., J. F. MADDOX, H. D. PEREZ & C. N. SERHAN. 1994. J. Exp. Med. **180:** 253–260.
18. DURSTIN, M., J.-L. GAO, H. L. TIFFANY, D. MCDERMOTT & P. M. MURPHY. 1994. Biochem. Biophys. Res. Comm. **201:** 174–179.
19. GERARD, N. P. & C. GERARD. 1991. Nature **349:** 614–617.
20. BOULAY, F., L. MERY, M. TARDIF, L. BROUCHON & P. VIGNAIS. 1991. Biochemistry **30:** 2993–2999.
21. KOLAKOWSKI, L. F., B. LU, C. GERARD & N. GERARD. 1995. J. Biol. Chem. **270:** 18077–18082.
22. ROGLIC, A., E. R. PROSSNITZ, S. L. CAVANAGH, Z. PAN, A. ZOU & R. YE. 1996. Biochim. Biophys. Acta **1305:** 39–43.
23. CRASS, T., U. RAFFETSEDER, U. MARTIN, M. GROVE, A. KLOS, J. KÖHL & W. BAUTSCH. 1996. Eur. J. Immunol. **26:** 1944–1950.
24. HONDA, Z., M. NAKAMURA, I. MIKI, M. MINAMI, T. WATANABE, Y. SEYAMA, H. OKADO, H. TOH, K. ITO, T. MIYAMOTO & T. SHIMIZU. 1991. Nature **349:** 342–346.
25. NAKAMURA, M., Z. HONDA, T. IZUMI, C. SAKANAKA, H. MUTOH, M. MINAMI, H. BITO, Y. SEYAMA, T. MATSUMOTO, M. NOMA *et al.* 1991. J. Biol. Chem. **266:** 20400–20405.
26. YE, R. D., E. R. PROSSNITZ, A. ZOU & C. G. COCHRANE. 1991. Biochem. Biophys. Res. Commun. **180:** 105–111.
27. MUTOH, H., H. BITO, M. MINAMI, M. NAKAMURA, Z. HONDA, T. IZUMI, Y. NAKATA, A. TERANO & T. SHIMIZU. 1993. FEBS Lett. **322:** 129–134.
28. HAVILAND, D. L., R. L. MCCOY, W. T. WHITEHEAD, H. AKAMA, E. P. MOLMENTI, A. BROWN, J. C. HAVILAND, W. C. PARKS, D. H. PERLMUTTER & R. A. WETSEL. 1995. J. Immunol. **154:** 1861–1869.
29. GASQUE, P., P. CHAN, M. FONTAINE, A. ISCHENKO, M. LAMACZ, O. GÖTZE & B. P. MORGAN. 1995. J. Immunol. **155:** 4882–4889.
30. LACY, M., J. JONES, S. R. WHITTEMORE, D. L. HAVILAND, R. A. WETSEL & S. R. BARNUM. 1995. J. Neuroimmunol. **61:** 71–78.
31. FOREMAN, K. E., A. A. VAPORCIYAN, B. K. BONISH, M. L. JONES, K. J. JOHNSON, M. M. GLOVSKY, S. M. EDDY & P. A. WARD. 1994. J. Clin. Invest. **94:** 1147–1155.
32. MCCOY, R., D. L. HAVILAND, E. P. MOLMENTI, T. ZIAMBARAS, R. A. WETSEL & D. H. PERLMUTTER. 1995. J. Exp. Med. **182:** 207–217.
33. BUCHNER, R. R., T. E. HUGLI, J. A. EMBER & E. L. MORGAN. 1995. J. Immunol. **155:** 308–315.
34. SOZZANI, S., F. SALLUSTO, W. LUINI, D. ZHOU, L. PIEMONTI, P. ALLAVENA, J. VAN DAMME, S. VALITUTTI, A. LANZAVECCHIA & A. MANTOVANI. 1995. J. Immunol. **155:** 3292–3295.

35. MOSER, B., C. SCHUMACHER, V. VON-TSCHARNER, I. CLARK-LEWIS & M. BAGGIOLINI. 1991. J. Biol. Chem. **266:** 10666–10671.

36. MURPHY, P. M. & H. L. TIFFANY. 1991. Science **253:** 1280–1283.

37. HOLMES, W. E., J. LEE, W. J. KUANG, G. C. RICE & W. I. WOOD. 1991. Science **253:** 1278–1280.

38. CHUNTHARAPAI, A. & K. J. KIM. 1995. J. Immunol. **155:** 2587–2594.

39. HAMMOND, M. E., G. R. LAPOINTE, P. H. FEUCHT, S. HILT, C. A. GALLEGOS, C. A. GORDON, M. A. GIEDLIN, G. MULLENBACH & P. TEKAMP-OLSON. 1995. J. Immunol. **155:** 1428–1433.

40. JONES, S. A., M. WOLF, S. QIN, C. R. MACKAY & M. BAGGIOLINI. 1996. Proc. Natl. Acad. Sci. USA **93:** 6682–6686.

41. L'HEUREUX, G. P., S. BOURGOIN, N. JEAN, S. R. MCCOLL & P. H. NACCACHE. 1995. Blood **85:** 522–531.

42. NICHOLAS, J., K. R. CAMERON & R. W. HONESS. 1992. Nature **255:** 362–365.

43. AHUJA, S. K. & P. M. MURPHY. 1993. J. Biol. Chem. **268:** 20691–20694.

44. GAO, J. L. & P. M. MURPHY. 1994. J. Biol. Chem. **269:** 28539–28542.

45. NEOTE, K., D. DIGREGORIO, J. Y. MAK, R. HORUK & T. J. SCHALL. 1993. Cell **72:** 415–425.

46. GAO, J. L., D. B. KUHNS, H. L. TIFFANY, D. MCCERMOTT, X. LI, U. FRANCKE & P. M. MURPHY. 1993. J. Exp. Med. **177:** 1421–1427.

47. COMBADIERE, C., S. AHUJA & P. M. MURPHY. 1995. J. Biol. Chem. **270:** 16491–16494.

48. CHARO, I. F., S. J. MYERS, A. HERMAN, C. FRANCI, A. J. CONNOLLY & S. R. COUGHLIN. 1994. Proc. Natl. Acad. Sci. USA **91:** 2752–2756.

49. DAUGHERTY, B. L., S. J. SICILIANO, J. A. DEMARTINO, L. MALKOWITZ, A. SIROTINA & M. S. SPRINGER. 1996. J. Exp. Med. **183:** 2349–2354.

50. POWER, C. A., A. MEYER, K. NEMETH, K. B. BACON, A. J. HOOGEWERF, A. E. I. PROUDFOOT & T. N. C. WELLS. 1995. J. Biol. Chem. **270:** 19495–19500.

51. RAPORT, C. J., J. GOSLING, V. L. SCHWEICHART, P. W. GRAY & I. F. CHARO. 1996. J. Biol. Chem. **271:** 17161–17166.

52. SAMSON, M., O. LABBE, C. MOLLEREAU, G. VASSART & M. PARMENTIER. 1996. Biochemistry **35:** 3362–3367.

53. DENG, H., R. LIU, W. ELLMEIER, S. CHOE, R. UNUTMAZ, M. BURKHART, D. MARZIO, S. MARMON, R. E. SUTTON, C. M. HILL, C. B. DAVIS, S. C. PEIPER, T. J. SCHALL, D. R. LITTMAN & N. R. LANDAU. 1996. Nature **381:** 661–666.

54. DRAGIC, T., V. LITWIN, G. H. ALLAWAY, S. R. MARTIN, Y. HUANG, K. A. NAGASHIMA, C. CAYANAN, P. J. MADDON, R. A. KOUP, J. P. MOORE & W. A. PAXTON. 1996. Nature **381:** 667–673.

55. COCCHI, F., A. L. DEVICO, A. GARZINO-DEMO, S. K. ARYA, R. C. GALLO & P. LUSSO. 1995. Science **270:** 1811–1815.

56. CHOE, H., M. FARZAN, Y. SUN, N. SULLIVAN, B. ROLLINS, P. D. PONATH, L. WU, C. R. MACKAY, G. LAROSA, W. NEWMAN, N. GERARD, C. GERARD & J. SODROSKI. 1996. Cell **85:** 1135–1148.

57. YU, F., C. C. BRODER, P. E. KENNEDY & E. A. BERGER. 1996. Science **272:** 872–877.

58. LOETSCHER, P., M. SEITZ, I. CLARK-LEWIS, M. BAGGIOLINI & B. MOSER. 1994. FEBS Lett. **341:** 187–192.

59. CAMPS, M., A. CAROZZI, P. SCHNABEL, A. SCHEER, P. J. PARKER & P. GIERSCHIK. 1992. Nature **360:** 684–689.

60. KATZ, A., D. WU & M. I. SIMON. 1992. Nature **360:** 686–689.

61. HWANG, S.-B. 1988. J. Biol. Chem. **263:** 3225–3233.

62. AMATRUDA, T. D., N. P. GERARD, C. GERARD & M. I. SIMON. 1993. J. Biol. Chem. **268:** 10139–10144.

63. JIANG, H., D. WU & M. I. SIMON. 1994. J. Biol. Chem. **269:** 7593–7596.

64. WU, D., G. J. LAROSA & M. I. SIMON. 1993. Science **261:** 101–103.

65. AMATRUDA, T. T., S. DRAGAS-GRAONIC, R. HOLMES & H. D. PEREZ. 1995. J. Biol. Chem. **270:** 28010–28013.
66. KUANG, Y., Y. WU, H. JIANG & D. WU. 1996. J. Biol. Chem. **271:** 3975–3978.
67. AMATRUDA, T. T., D. A. STEELE, V. Z. SLEPAK & M. I. SIMON. 1991. Proc. Natl. Acad. Sci. USA **88:** 5587–5591.
68. BOKOCH, G. 1995. Blood **86:** 1649–1660.
69. TORRES, M., F. L. HALL & K. O'NEILL. 1993. J. Immunol. **150:** 1563–1578.
70. GRINSTEIN, S. & W. FURUYA. 1992. J. Biol. Chem. **267:** 18122–18125.
71. WORTHEN, S. G., N. AVDI, A. M. BUHL, N. SUZUKI & G. L. JOHNSON. 1994. J. Clin. Invest. **94:** 815–823.
72. BUHL, A. M., N. AVDI, G. S. WORTHEN & G. L. JOHNSON. 1994. Proc. Natl. Acad. Sci. USA **91:** 9190–9194.
73. KNALL, C., S. YOUNG, J. A. NICK, A. M. BUHL, G. S. WORTHEN & G. L. JOHNSON. 1996. J. Biol. Chem. **271:** 2832–2838.
74. van BIESEN, T., B. E. HAWES, D. LUTTRELL, K. M. KRUGER, K. TOUHARA, E. PORFIRI, M. SAKAUE, L. M. LUTTRELL & R. J. LEFKOWITZ. 1995. Nature **376:** 781–784.
75. OHMICHI, M., T. SAWADA, Y. KANDA, K. KOIKE, K. HIROTA, A. MIYAKE & A. R. SALTIEL. 1994. J. Biol. Chem. **269:** 3783–3788.
76. CAZAUBON, S. M., R.-M. F., S. FISCHER, F. SCHWEIGHOFFER, A. D. STROSBERG & P.-O. COURAUD. 1994. J. Biol. Chem. **269:** 24805–24809.
77. HAWES, B. E., L. M. LUTTRELL, T. van BIESEN & R. J. LEFKOWITZ. 1996. J. Biol. Chem. **271:** 12133–12136.
78. PTASZNIK, A., A. TRAYNOR-KAPLAN & G. M. BOKOCH. 1995. J. Biol. Chem. **270:** 19969–19973.
79. TORRES, M. & R. YE. 1996. J. Biol. Chem. **271:** 13244–13249.
80. STOYANOV, B., S. VOLINIA, T. HANCK, I. RUBIO, M. LOUBTCHENKOV, D. MALEK, S. STOYANO-VA, B. VANHAESEBROECK, R. DHAND, B. NÜRNBERG, P. GIERSCHIK, K. SEEDORF, J. J. HSUAN, M. D. WATERFIELD & R. WETZKER. 1995. Science **269:** 690–693.
81. TOMHAVE, E. D., R. M. RICHARDSON, J. R. DIDSBURY, L. MENARD, R. SNYDERMAN & H. ALI. 1994. J. Immunol. **153:** 3267–3275.
82. RICHARDSON, R. M., H. ALI, E. D. TOMHAVE, B. HARIBABU & R. SNYDERMAN. 1995. J. Biol. Chem. **270:** 27829–27833.
83. TARDIF, M., L. MERY, L. BROUCHON & F. BOULAY. 1993. J. Immunol. **150:** 3534–3545.
84. ALI, H., R. M. RICHARDSON, E. D. TOMHAVE, J. R. DIDSBURY & R. SNYDERMAN. 1993. J. Biol. Chem. **268:** 24247–24254.
85. ALI, H., R. M. RICHARDSON, E. D. TOMHAVE, R. A. DUBOSE, B. HARIBABU & R. SNYDER-MAN. 1994. J. Biol. Chem. **269:** 24557–24563.
86. MUELLER, S. G., W. P. SCHRAW & A. RICHMOND. 1994. J. Biol. Chem. **269:** 1973–1980.
87. MUELLER, S. G., W. P. SCHRAW & A. RICHMOND. 1995. J. Biol. Chem. **270:** 10439–10448.
88. RICHARDSON, R. M., R. A. DUBOSE, H. ALI, E. D. TOMHAVE, B. HARIBABU & R. SNYDER-MAN. 1995. Biochemistry **34:** 14193–14201.
89. TAKANO, T., Z.-I. HONDA, C. SAKANAKA, T. IZUMI, K. KAMEYAMA, K. HAGA, T. HAGA, K. KUROKAWA & T. SHIMIZU. 1994. J. Biol. Chem. **269:** 22453–22458.
90. GIANNINI, E. & F. BOULAY. 1995. J. Immunol. **154:** 4055–4064.
91. GIANNINI, E., L. BROUCHON & F. BOULAY. 1995. J. Biol. Chem. **270:** 19166–19172.
92. WENZEL-SEIFERT, K. & R. SEIFERT. 1993. J. Immunol. **150:** 4591–4599.
93. KANEKO, Y., N. OKADA, L. BARANYI, T. AZUMA & H. OKADA. 1995. Immunology **86:** 149–154.
94. BLEUL, C. C., M. FARZAN, H. CHOE, C. PAROLIN, I. CLARK-LEWIS, J. SODROSKI & T. A. SPRINGER. 1996. Nature **382:** 829–833.
95. OBERLIN, E., A. AMARA, F. BACHELERIE, C. BESSIA, J-L. VIRELIZIER, F. ARENZANA-SEISDE-DOS, O. SCHWARTZ, J. M. HEARD, I. CLARK-LEWIS, D. F. LEGLER, M. LOETSCHER, M. BAZZIOLINI & B. MOSER. 1996. Nature **382:** 833–836.

The NADPH Oxidase:
Lessons from Chronic Granulomatous
Disease Neutrophils

ARTHUR J. VERHOEVEN[a]

Central Laboratory of the Netherlands Red Cross Blood Transfusion Service
Laboratory for Experimental and Clinical Immunology
University of Amsterdam
1066 CX Amsterdam, The Netherlands.

INTRODUCTION

NADPH oxidase is present in a dormant state in human phagocytes and is activated when phagocytes bind and engulf opsonized microorganisms. The generation of superoxide and hydrogen peroxide by the active NADPH oxidase is essential for the killing of these phagocytized microorganisms as evidenced by severe clinical problems in patients having an inherited defect in this enzyme system. The disease associated with defective NADPH oxidase activity is called chronic granulomatous disease (CGD), characterized by recurrent severe bacterial and fungal infections. The most common pathogens encountered in CGD patients are catalase-positive organisms, because in catalase-negative organisms bacterial hydrogen peroxide may be used by the CGD neutrophils to mediate the killing process. Pivotal for the killing of engulfed microorganisms is the formation of hypochloric acid (HOCl) from hydrogen peroxide and chloride ions in a myeloperoxidase-mediated reaction. CGD is a rare, but also a very heterogeneous disorder; clinically because of several antimicrobial systems that can partially compensate for the defect in oxygen-dependent killing and biochemically because of the complicated genetic origin of CGD.[1,2] Proper activation of the NADPH oxidase requires the presence of several proteins (now called *phox* proteins for phagocyte oxidase proteins). A defect in any of these proteins will cause a partial or complete absence of enzyme activity. Four *phox* proteins have been identified through studies with CGD cells[3–9]: two membrane-bound components, gp91-*phox* and p22-*phox*, and two components, p47-*phox* and p67-*phox*, that reside in the cytosol of resting phagocytes, but translocate to the membrane upon cell activation. The two membrane-bound components are associated with each other already in resting cells, forming a complex now known as cytochrome b558. The observation by Segal[10] that in most X-linked CGD neutrophils the spectroscopic signal characteristic for this cytochrome is absent has really been the beginning of the characterization of the NADPH oxidase in human phagocytes. The reason for this absence in X-linked CGD became apparent when the cDNA encoding gp91-*phox* was cloned and the

[a]Address correspondence to: Arthur J. Verhoeven, Ph.D., Department of Experimental Immunohematology, CLB, Plesmanlaan 125, 1066 CX Amsterdam, The Netherlands. Phone, 31-20-5123317; Fax, 31-20-5123310.

gene was found to be on the X-chromosome.[3] Subsequently, deficiencies in other CGD subtypes have been correlated with the absence of p22-*phox*,[11] p47-*phox*,[7] or p67-*phox*.[9] The complete electron transfer appears to occur within an activated gp91/p22 heterodimer with the NADPH and the FAD binding site being present on gp91-*phox*,[12–14] one heme group also bound to gp91-*phox* and one heme group bound between the two subunits of cytochrome b558.[15,16]

In most CGD patients, there is complete absence of one of the *phox* proteins, explaining the absence of NADPH oxidase activity. In some CGD patients, however, all *phox* proteins are present in the neutrophils at normal or near-normal levels, but oxidase activity is absent due to critical point mutations or small deletions. These mutations or deletions will either prevent proper assembly of the NADPH oxidase from its various components or the electron transfer within the cytochrome b558 itself. This review will focus on the lessons that can be learned from the analysis of these rare cases of CGD with respect to the structure-function relationships between the *phox* proteins. First, a short description is given of the rapid detection of CGD neutrophils with normal expression of *phox* proteins.

DETECTION OF CGD NEUTROPHILS

In the past, CGD neutrophils have been detected by their inability to consume oxygen upon appropriate stimulation,[17] their inability to produce superoxide as measured by the SOD-sensitive reduction of ferricytochrome c,[18] or their inability to release hydrogen peroxide as measured by scopoletin oxidation.[19] The underlying defect was then subsequently analyzed by performing immunoblots with antibodies specific for each *phox* protein on neutrophil lysates or neutrophil fractions obtained after sonication.[5,6,20] In these experiments, great care has to be taken to prevent proteolysis of the *phox* proteins, especially of p67-*phox* (Verhoeven and colleagues, unpublished observations).

More recently, fluorescent dyes suitable for flow cytometry have been used to measure NADPH oxidase activity in human neutrophils. Bass and colleagues[21] have shown that dichlorofluorescein diacetate can be used to detect oxidase activation in a flow cytometer, whereas Emmendorfer and colleagues[22] applied dihydro-rhodamine-1,2,3 (DHR) for the same purpose. Although this method of detection has some important limitations,[23] the use of DHR offers an especially sensitive and rapid way of detecting oxidase activity in circulating neutrophils.[24] It would, therefore, also be desirable to have flow cytometric assays to detect simultaneously the presence or absence of the various *phox* proteins. In this way, the subtype of CGD[2] can rapidly be assigned. However, the very rare CGD cases, in which the lack of oxidase activity is accompanied by normal (or near-normal) expression of *phox* proteins are also easily recognized. In those cases, the absence of a positive signal in the DHR assay is accompanied by normal (or near-normal) signals in the immunofluorescence assay.

For the detection of cytochrome b558 in human neutrophils by flow cytometry, Nakamura and colleagues[25] have used a monoclonal antibody (mAb 7D5) that binds to an epitope on the outside of the cells, probably by binding to p22-*phox*. Alternatively, mAb 449 also binding to p22-*phox*[20] may be used. However, binding of mAb

449 can only be observed after digitonin permeabilization of the plasma membrane,[20] indicating that the epitope for mAb 449 is on a domain of p22-*phox* facing the cytoplasm. Binding of mAb 449 is very high with permeabilized neutrophils of normal, healthy donors and clearly decreased in CGD neutrophils lacking cytochrome b558 (FIG. 1). Although in most neutrophils lacking cytochrome b558 the defect is caused by a mutation in the gene encoding gp91-*phox*, there is a concomitant decrease in p22-*phox* signal in the flow cytometer (FIG. 1). A strong decrease in p22-*phox* expression in X-linked CGD neutrophils has previously been observed after immunoblotting of neutrophil extracts[4,20,26] and has been ascribed to a mutual dependence of both cytochrome b558 subunits for stable protein expression. The concomitant decrease in gp91-*phox* and p22-*phox* signals prevents an immediate distinction between Xb(0) and Ab(0) CGD. For this, an analysis of the neutrophils of the mother of the patient is indicated, which, in most cases of Xb(0) CGD, show heterogeneity in the classical NBT-slide test[27] or in the DHR assay referred to above.

In order to detect the cytosolic components of the NADPH oxidase by flow cytometry, the cells also need to be permeabilized, but in this case rapid fixation is required to prevent leakage of these proteins to the extracellular space. We found addition of a limiting amount of digitonin to neutrophils at 4°C, followed after 1 min by mild fixation in 1% paraformaldehyde, the most satisfactory procedure to achieve reliable immunodetection of p47- and p67-*phox* in a flow cytometer (Verhoeven and colleagues, manuscript in preparation).

With the flow cytometric methods described above, CGD neutrophils can readily

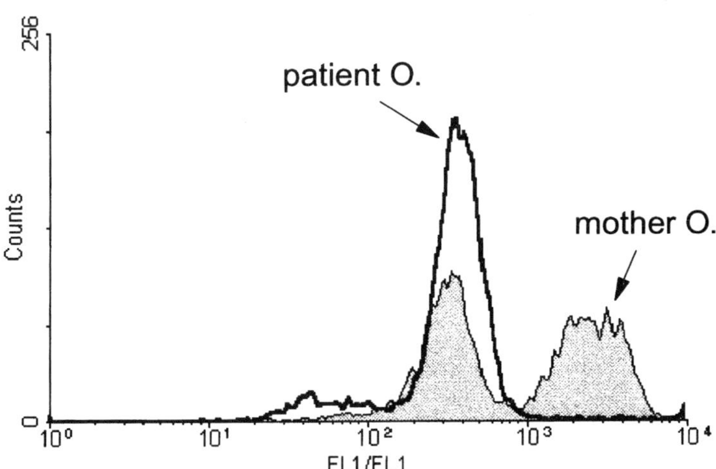

FIGURE 1. Binding of Mab 449 to the neutrophils of an Xb(0) CGD patient (*unshaded graph*) and to the neutrophils of his mother (*shaded graph*). Neutrophils were permeabilized by addition of digitonin, fixed with paraformaldedyde (1%), and incubated with Mab 449 (5 µg/ml). Subsequently, cells were washed and stained with FITC-labeled goat antimouse Ig. Binding was determined in a flow cytometer (FACSCAN, Beckton-Dickinson). The mother shows a mixture of bright- and dull-staining cells, whereas the patient only shows dull-staining cells.

be detected. When a negative DHR assay is accompanied by normal (or near-normal) levels of *phox* proteins, further analysis is required to find out which component is affected. When the neutrophils of the mother of the CGD patient show positive and negative cells in the DHR assay, one obviously has to look for a mutation in the gp91-*phox* gene. When the cells of the mother show a homogeneous pattern, the mutation can be either in the gene encoding p22-, p47-, and p67-*phox*. In order to save elaborate sequencing of all these three genes, one can obtain further information by analyzing first in a cell-free activation system[28,29] the activity of the neutrophil membranes and the neutrophil cytosol. In case of a p22-*phox* mutation, the defective activity can be corrected by the addition of control membranes. In case of a p47- or a p67-*phox* mutation, the defective activity will be restored by addition of control cytosol or, even more informative, by addition of recombinant p47- or p67-*phox*.[48] With the strategy outlined here, the mutation leading to the CGD phenotype can almost certainly be found.

MUTATIONS AFFECTING ELECTRON TRANSFER

Until now, the mutations affecting electron transfer within the NADPH oxidase have been found to be confined to the gp91-*phox* gene. This supports the notion that the electron transfer within an active oxidase complex occurs within the gp91/p22 heterodimer. Further support for this notion comes from sequence homology studies between the C-terminal half of gp91-*phox* and the ferrodoxin-NADP$^+$ reductase flavoenzyme family, indicating that both NADPH and FAD may be bound by this part of gp91-*phox*,[12–14] and from the observation that oxidase activity can be achieved with solubilized neutrophil membranes in the presence of negatively charged phospholipids in the absence of p47- and p67-*phox*.[30,31]

In FIGURE 2, a schematic diagram is given of the primary protein structure of gp91-*phox*. In this diagram, the positions of mutations leading to Xb(+) CGD have been indicated. The residues indicated by open boxes most probably affect electron transfer. In some cases, a defect in electron transfer has been deduced from a normal translocation of cytosolic oxidase components not accompanied by oxidase activity (Leusen and coworkers, manuscript in preparation),[32,33] in some others from the absence of oxidase activity in the system of Koskhin and Pick referred to above.[30,31] In the neutrophils of one patient (with the P415H mutation), direct evidence for a defect in NADPH binding has been presented.[12,32] The effect of this mutation therefore strongly supports the hypothesis that the NADPH binding site is, indeed, on gp91-*phox* and not on one of the cytosolic oxidase components, as has previously been suggested.[34] The P415H mutation does not affect the translocation of p47- and p67-*phox* to the cytochrome b558 heterodimer in the membrane.[32,35] Similarly, in the Xb(+) CGD patient, reported by Cross and colleagues,[32] carrying a R54S mutation in the N-terminal part of gp91-*phox*, translocation of the cytosolic components is normal, but in this case electron transfer appears to be disturbed beyond the flavin center. The R54S mutation leads to a subtle change in the heme absorbance spectrum, indicating a change in the heme-binding domain resulting in a failure to accept electrons from FAD.[32]

Taylor and colleagues[36] have constructed a three-dimensional model of the C-ter-

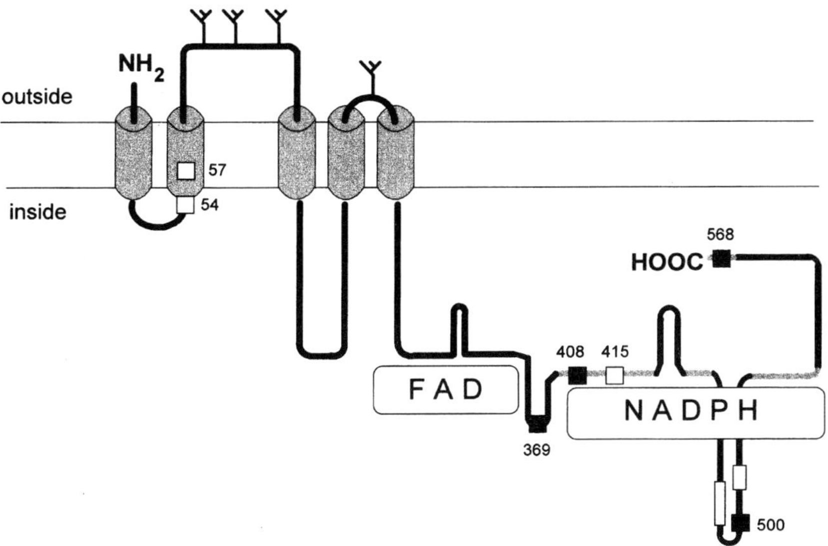

FIGURE 2. Schematic diagram of mutations in gp91-*phox* leading to Xb(+) CGD. In the primary structure of gp91-*phox*, mutations without an effect on translocation of cytosolic components are given by open boxes. Mutations disturbing translocation are depicted as shaded boxes. Grey sequences indicate regions involved in NADPH binding.

minal part of gp91-*phox* on the basis of crystallographic data of the ferrodoxin-NADP$^+$ reductase. In this model, the ^{415}Pro residue is also very near the FAD binding site and buried within the protein (Dr. N. Keep, personal communication). The G408E mutation on gp91-*phox* is on the central strand of the beta sheet region facing the NADPH molecule, probably inducing a defect in NADPH binding. This mutation prevented oxidase activity as measured in the absence of p47- and p67-*phox*,[30,31] but translocation of cytosolic components was disturbed as well (Leusen and coworkers, manuscript in preparation). Probably, the G408E leads to major alterations in the protein structure affecting both electron transfer and translocation of cytosolic components. The second patient with both a defective electron transfer and a disturbed translocation is carrying a D500G mutation.[35] In the three-dimensional model referred to above[36] residue ^{500}Asp is on top of an inserted α-helix, which has been proposed to regulate access of NADPH to the NADPH binding site.[36] Clearly, this α-helix is on the surface of the gp91-*phox* protein, because a peptide mimicking this domain is inhibitory for oxidase assembly in the cell-free system.[35]

The data reported by Azuma and colleagues[33] seem to contradict the hypothesis that the inserted α-helix comprising residues 484 to 503 is important for both the electron transfer within gp91-*phox* and the binding of cytosolic components. The aberrant gp91-*phox* gene in this Xb(+) CGD patient results in a replacement of residues 507-509 (Gly-Lys-Thr) by four amino acids (His-Ile-Trp-Ala) without apparently affecting the translocation of cytosolic oxidase components.[33] Possibly, this change only marginally affects the position of the α-helix having its major effect on NADPH binding itself.

MUTATIONS AFFECTING OXIDASE ASSEMBLY

The first step in the assembly of an active NADPH oxidase is the association of p22- and gp91-*phox* which, together with heme, form the cytochrome b558 heterodimer. Porter and coworkers[37] have demonstrated that this association occurs during the biosynthesis of both peptide chains, because conversion of the high-mannose precursor chain of gp91-*phox* into the mature complex sugar chain appears to depend on the presence of p22-*phox*. More recently, Porter and coworkers[38] reported at least three mutations in gp91-*phox* resulting in a similar blockade of sugar chain processing, indicating that also in these CGD neutrophils the association with p22-*phox* does not occur. Two of these mutations lead to amino acid substitutions (P56L and C244S), one results in the deletion of exon 3, comprising residues 48-84. Interestingly, the P56L mutation and the 48-84 deletion are near the R54S mutation that has been shown to influence the spectral properties of one of the heme groups.[32] The effects of these mutations are therefore in line with the proposal that at least one of the heme groups is coordinated by amino acid residues from both p22- and gp91-*phox*.[15]

Once the cytochrome b558 heterodimer is formed, it is transported to the specific granules and secretory vesicles of the maturing neutrophils. The targeting to specific granules and secretory vesicles is probably determined by the timing of gene expression,[39] that of p22- and gp91-*phox* being in tune with other proteins ending up in these organelles. As mentioned above, the cytochrome b558 heterodimer requires the association with cytosolic components to become active in electron transfer. With an artificial stimulus of neutrophils (the phorbol ester PMA), this activation already occurs at the membrane of the intracellular compartments containing the cytochrome,[40] with phagocytic stimulation of neutrophils this activation mainly takes place at the phagosomal membrane after fusion of specific granules with the phagosomal membrane. Several mutations leading to CGD have been found that disturb the association of cytosolic components with the cytochrome b558 heterodimer in the membrane. The first one is the D500G mutation in gp91-*phox* mentioned above,[35] that resides in a domain exposed to the cytosol and probably controls the binding of NADPH.[36] Other mutations in gp91-*phox* affecting oxidase assembly are C369R, G408E, and E568K (Leusen and colleagues, manuscript in preparation). According to the three-dimensional model constructed by Taylor and coworkers,[36] the C369R mutation also resides in a loop exposed to the cytosol. The G408E mutation would be expected to be buried within the protein and probably results in a significant change in tertiary structure affecting the normal position of the domains important for binding. The importance of the C-terminus of gp91-*phox*, in which the E568K mutation is located, for the binding of cytosolic oxidase components has previously been deduced from inhibition of oxidase assembly by a synthetic peptide mimicking this region.[41,42] Clearly, the negative effect of these mutations demonstrates that at least three different domains of the C-terminal part of gp91-*phox* are involved in the binding of p47- and/or p67-*phox*.

Another mutation disturbing the assembly of an active oxidase concerns a mutation in the gene encoding p22-*phox*. The resulting amino acid replacement (P156Q) is in a proline-rich region of p22-*phox*, disrupting a counter structure for a SH3 domain.[43] Most probably, the SH3 domain normally interacting with this domain of p22-*phox* resides in p47-*phox*.[44] Careful analysis of the separate effects of p47- and p67-*phox* on the electron transfer within cytochrome b558 has indicated a distinctive role of these proteins in facilitating electron transfer.[45,46] The reduction of the FAD bound to the C-terminus of gp91-*phox* seems to be influenced by p67-*phox*, whereas p47-*phox* facilitates the subsequent reduction of the heme group. Taken together, these observations lend support for a model, predicting binding of p67-*phox* to the C-terminal part of gp91-*phox* and binding of p47-*phox* primarily to p22-*phox* being in close contact with the N-terminal part of gp91-*phox*. However, the binding of each cytosolic component is clearly influenced by binding of the other component.[47]

CONCLUDING REMARKS

Activation of the NADPH oxidase of human phagocytes involves the association of cytosolic proteins with the membrane-bound cytochrome b558 to induce electron transfer within the latter protein. For a stable association, several protein-protein interactions are required as indicated by the fact that different mutations, as detected in the neutrophils of some rare CGD patients, all result in a defect in oxidase activity. Several methods are now available to detect these rare cases of CGD and to analyze in detail the cause of defective oxidase activity.

REFERENCES

1. SMITH, R. M. & J. T. CURNUTTE. 1991. Blood **77:** 673–686.
2. ROOS, D., M. DE BOER, F. KURIBAYASHI, C. MEISCHL, R. S. WEENING, A. W. SEGAL, A. AHLIN, K. NEMET, J. P. HOSSLE, E. BERNATOWSKA-MATUSZKIEWICZ & H. MIDDLETON-PRICE. 1996. Blood **87:** 1663–1681.
3. ROYER-POKORA, B., L. M. KUNKEL, A. P. MONACO, S. C. GOFF, P. E. NEWBURGER, R. L. BAEHNER, F. S. COLE, J. T. CURNUTTE & S. H. ORKIN. 1986. Nature **322:** 32–38.
4. PARKOS, C. A., R. A. ALLEN, C. G. COCHRANE & A. J. JESAITIS. 1987. J. Clin. Invest. **80:** 732–742.
5. VOLPP, B. D., W. M. NAUSEEF & R. A. CLARK. 1988. Science **242:** 1295–1297.
6. NUNOI, H., D. ROTROSEN, J. I. GALLIN & H. L. MALECH. 1988. Science **242:** 1298–1301.
7. LOMAX, K. J., T. L. LETO, H. NUNOI, J. I. GALLIN & H. L. MALECH. 1989. Science **245:** 409–412.
8. VOLPP, B. D., W. M. NAUSEEF, J. E. DONELSON, D. R. MOSER & R. A. CLARK. 1990. Proc. Natl. Acad. Sci. USA **86:** 7195–7199.
9. LETO, T. L., K. J. LOMAX, B. D. VOLPP, H. NUNOI, J. M. SECHLER, W. M. NAUSEEF, R. A. CLARK, J. I. GALLIN & H. L. MALECH. 1990. Science **248:** 727–730.
10. SEGAL, A. W. 1978. Nature **276:** 515–517.
11. DINAUER, M. C., E. A. PIERCE, G. A. BRUNS, J. T. CURNUTTE & S. H. ORKIN. 1990. J. Clin. Invest. **86:** 1729–1737.
12. SEGAL, A. W., I. WEST, F. WIENTJES, J. H. NUGENT, A. J. CHAVAN, B. HALEY, R. C. GARCIA, H. ROSEN & G. SCRACE. 1992. Biochem. J. **284:** 781–788.
13. ROTROSEN, D., C. L. YEUNG, T. L. LETO, H. L. MALECH & C. H. KWONG. 1992. Science **256:** 1459–1462.
14. SUMIMOTO, H., N. SAKAMOTO, M. NOZAKI, Y. SAKAKI, K. TAKESHIGE & S. MINAKAMI. 1992. Biochem. Biophys. Res. Commun. **186:** 1368–1375.

15. QUINN, M. T., M. L. MULLEN & A. J. JESAITIS. 1992. J. Biol. Chem. **267:** 7303–7309.
16. CROSS, A. R., J. RAE & J. T. CURNUTTE. 1995. J. Biol. Chem. **270:** 17075–17077.
17. WEENING, R. S., D. ROOS & J. A. LOOS. 1974. J. Lab. Clin. Med. **83:** 570–576.
18. BABIOR, B. M. 1978. N. Engl. J. Med. **298:** 659–668.
19. DE LA HARPE, J. & C. F. NATHAN. 1985. J. Immunol. Methods **78:** 323–336.
20. VERHOEVEN, A. J., B. G. J. M. BOLSCHER, L. J. MEERHOF, R. VAN ZWIETEN, J. KEIJER, R. S. WEENING & D. ROOS. 1989. Blood **73:** 1686–1694.
21. BASS, D. A., J. W. PARCE, L. R. DECHATELET, P. SZEJDA, M. C. SEEDS & M. THOMAS. 1983. J. Immunol. **130:** 1910–1917.
22. EMMENDORFFER, A., M. HECHT, M. L. LOHMANN MATTHES & J. ROESLER. 1990. J. Immunol. Methods **131:** 269–275.
23. VAN PELT, L. J., R. VAN ZWIETEN, R. S. WEENING, D. ROOS, A. J. VERHOEVEN & B. G. J. M. BOLSCHER. 1996. J. Immunol. Methods **191:** 187–196.
24. VOWELLS, S. J., T. A. FLEISHER, S. SEKHSARIA, D. W. ALLING, T. E. MAGUIRE & H. L. MALECH. 1996. J. Pediatr. **128:** 104–107.
25. NAKAMURA, M., S. SENDO, R. VAN ZWIETEN, T. KOGA, D. ROOS & S. KANEGASAKI. 1988. Blood **72:** 1550–1552.
26. SEGAL, A. W. 1987. Nature **326:** 88–92.
27. MEERHOF, L. J. & D. ROOS. 1986. J. Leukoc. Biol. **39:** 699–711.
28. HEYNEMAN, R. A. & R. E. VERCAUTEREN. 1984. J. Leukocyte Biol. **36:** 751–759.
29. BROMBERG, Y. & E. PICK. 1985. J. Biol. Chem. **260:** 13539–13545.
30. KOSHKIN, V. & E. PICK. 1993. FEBS Lett. **327:** 57–62.
31. KOSHKIN, V. & E. PICK. 1994. FEBS Lett. **338:** 285–289.
32. CROSS, A. R., P. G. HEYWORTH, J. RAE & J. T. CURNUTTE. 1995. J. Biol. Chem. **270:** 8194–8200.
33. AZUMA, H., H. OOMI, K. SASAKI, I. KAWABATA, T. SAKAINO, S. KOYANO, T. SUZUTANI, H. NUNOI & A. OKUNO. 1995. Blood **85:** 3274–3277.
34. SMITH, R. M., J. T. CURNUTTE & B. M. BABIOR. 1989. J. Biol. Chem. **264:** 1958–1962.
35. LEUSEN, J. H. W., M. DE BOER, B. G. J. M. BOLSCHER, P. M. HILARIUS, R. S. WEENING, H. D. OCHS, D. ROOS & A. J. VERHOEVEN. 1994. J. Clin. Invest. **93:** 2120–2126.
36. TAYLOR, W. R., D. T. JONES & A. W. SEGAL. 1993. Protein Sci. **2:** 1675–1685.
37. PORTER, C. D., M. H. PARKAR, A. J. VERHOEVEN, R. J. LEVINSKY, M. K. COLLINS & C. KINNON. 1994. Blood **84:** 2767–2775.
38. PORTER, C. D., F. KURIBAYASHI, M. H. PARKAR, D. ROOS & C. KINNON. 1996. Biochem. J. **315:** 571–575.
39. BORREGAARD, N. 1996. Curr. Opin. Hematology **1:** 11–18.
40. LUNDQVIST, H., P. FOLLIN, L. KHALFAN & C. DAHLGREN. 1996. J. Leuk. Biol. **59:** 270–279.
41. ROTROSEN, D., M. E. KLEINBERG, H. NUNOI, T. LETO, J. I. GALLIN & H. L. MALECH. 1990. J. Biol. Chem. **265:** 8745–8750.
42. KLEINBERG, M. E., D. MITAL, D. ROTROSEN & H. L. MALECH. 1992. Biochemistry **31:** 2686–2690.
43. LEUSEN, J. H. W., B. G. J. M. BOLSCHER, P. M. HILARIUS, R. S. WEENING, W. KAULFERSCH, R. A. SEGER, D. ROOS & A. J. VERHOEVEN. 1994. J. Exp. Med. **180:** 2329–2334.
44. SUMIMOTO, H., Y. KAGE, H. NUNOI, H. SASAKI, T. NOSE, Y. FUKUMAKI, M. OHNO, S. MINAKAMI & K. TAKESHIGE. 1994. Proc. Natl. Acad. Sci. USA **91:** 5345–5349.
45. CROSS, A. R., J. L. YARCHOVER & J. T. CURNUTTE. 1994. J. Biol. Chem. **269:** 21448–21454.
46. CROSS, A. R. & J. T. CURNUTTE. 1995. J. Biol. Chem. **270:** 6543–6548.
47. UHLINGER, D. J., K. L. TAYLOR & J. D. LAMBETH. 1994. J. Biol. Chem. **269:** 22095–22098.
48. LEUSEN, J. H. W., A. DE KLEIN, P. M. HILARIUS, A. AHLIN, C. I. E. SMITH, D. DIEKMANN, A. HALL, A. J. VERHOEVEN & D. ROOS. 1996. J. Exp. Med. **184:** 1243–1249.

Endothelial Activation by Cytokines[a]

ALBERTO MANTOVANI,[b,c,d] SILVANO SOZZANI,[c]
AND MARTINO INTRONA[c]

*[c]Istituto di Ricerche Farmacologiche "Mario Negri"
via Eritrea 62
20157 Milan, Italy*

*[d]Section of General Pathology
Department of Biotechnology
Università di Brescia*

INTRODUCTION

Endothelial cells (EC) have long been considered a "layer of nucleated cellophane," endowed with negative properties, the most important one being that of representing a non-thrombogenic substrate for blood. As such, EC were seen to participate in tissue reactions essentially as targets for injurious agents. This view has changed radically. It is now evident that hemostasis, inflammatory reactions, and immunity involve close interactions between immunocompetent cells and vascular endothelium.

EC are strategically located at the interface between blood and tissues. In addition to responding rapidly (seconds to minutes) to agonists such as histamine and thrombin, vascular cells, upon exposure to cytokines, undergo profound alterations of function that involve gene expression and protein synthesis, require hours to develop, and are relatively long-lasting.

Vascular cells are both a target for and a source of cytokines. These soluble polypeptide mediators serve as communication signals with leukocytes as well as with diverse tissues and organs. The spectrum of responses elicited in endothelial cells by different cytokines is extremely vast and varied. Different cytokines activate distinct, largely non-overlapping, sets of functions that can be grouped into programs of activation/differentiation. The phenomenology of endothelial cell activation by cytokines was reviewed in detail previously.[1–4] Here we will update these previous descriptions, emphasize production and action of relatively novel mediators (e.g., chemokines) as well as the molecular basis for EC activation, and analyze emerging clinical implications of EC activation.

[a]This work supported by special project AIDS from Istituto Superiore della Sanità and by the Italian Association for Cancer Research

[b]Address correspondence to: Prof. Alberto Mantovani, Istituto di Ricerche Farmacologiche "Mario Negri," via Eritrea 62, 20157 Milano, Italy. Phone, (02)39014.1; Fax, (02)3546277; E-mail, MANTOVANI@IRFMN.MNEGRI.IT.

FUNCTIONAL PROGRAMS

IL-1 and TNF

As previously described in detail, IL-1 and TNF induce the expression of a functional program related to thrombosis and inflammation. Briefly, these cytokines facilitate thrombus formation by inducing procoagulant activity, inhibiting the thrombomodulin/protein C anticoagulation pathway, and blocking fibrin dissolution via stimulation of the type I inhibitor of plasminogen activator.

Cytokines and autocoids constitute interlaced systems of soluble mediators that participate in microvascular homeostasis during host defense. A well-established example is the production of platelet activating factor (PAF) or prostanoids by EC stimulated with TNF or IL-1. The PAF synthesis requires the neo-synthesis of an elastase like protease,[5] which is the final effector of the synthesis of PAF. PAF expressed on EC surface cooperates with adhesion molecules (E-selectin) in the transmigration of leukocytes. A small amount of PAF is also secreted and can prime or activate circulating cells or EC, and triggers a vicious circle of activation leading to recruitment of more inflammatory cells (reviewed in Bussolino and Camussi[6]). Furthermore, PAF produced by ECs is a secondary mediator of angiogenesis induced by inflammatory cytokine.[7] Prostanoids synthesis is strictly dependent on the induction of the pivotal enzymes phospholipase A2 and cyclooxygenase 1 and 2.[8,9] Furthermore, IL-1 induces the transcription of prostaglandin G/H synthase 2, and in combination with aspirin, increases the synthesis of a new class of lipoxins during endothelial cell–leukocyte interaction, having an inhibitory effect on neutrophil adhesion.[10]

NO is a representative of a new class of autocoids serving a variety of functions in several different tissues including vasculature, and acting through an independent receptor mechanism (reviewed in Nathan and Xie[11]). Nitric oxide synthase (NOS) type II (inducible, Ca^{2+}-independent isoform) and type III (constitutive, endothelial cell isoform) are present in ECs and catalyze the conversion of arginine into citrulline and NO. The former continuously produces "quanta" of NO, which especially participates in the regulation of vascular tone.[11] In man, experiments done on ECs from large vessels demonstrate that inflammatory cytokines increase the activity of NOS III and the synthesis of NO.[12,13] The effect of inflammatory cytokines on metabolic pathways leading to NO formation is characterized by a decrease of stability of NOS III mRNA,[12] by an increase of GTP cyclohydrolase I, the rate-limiting enzyme of tetrahydrobiopterin synthesis, and of tetrahydrobiopterin, a cofactor for full activity of NOS III.[12,13] However, the increase of tetrahydrobiopterin is compensated for by a decrease in stability of NOS III mRNA,[14] necessary to counteract the toxic effect of NO and its metabolite peroxynitrite on EC themselves.

Results obtained in several laboratories have demonstrated that the enhancement of NO production in murine, rat, porcine, and bovine ECs observed upon cytokine challenge is mediated by transcription of NOS II gene.[15–18] Interestingly, the promoter of this gene contains cis-acting DNA elements that are targets of cytokine-activated transcriptions factors NF-kB/Rel and IRF,[19,20] while recent data point to a role of Sp1 and GATA factors for the endothelial, basal transcriptions of the NOS III gene.[21] At present, unequivocal information on the role of this NOS isoform in human ECs is lacking, since experiments have only been done on EC from large vessels. However, we can speculate that NOS II is operative in human microvasculature after induction by inflammatory cytokines because it has been detected in EC lining the vessels localized in synovia of patients with rheumatoid arthritis[22] and in brain tumors.[23]

The ability of different cytokines alone or in combination to induce NO production is in dispute. In human EC, the combination of at least three cytokines (IL-1, TNF, and INF) is required to enhance NO synthesis.[12] In other animal species only one cytokine is sufficient to elicit NO synthesis.[15,18] The analysis of these data could indicate that in humans a complex and refined mechanism for NO synthesis in EC has been developed during evolution.

The complexity of this phenomenon is also stressed by the opposite effect of one cytokine in different animal species or on different NOS isoforms. For instance IFN-γ is required for NO synthesis in human EC,[12] but is an inhibitor in bovine EC stimulated with TNF.[15] Furthermore, TGFβ inhibits NOS II,[24] but upregulates NOS III.[25]

NO produced by EC acts in both an autocrine and paracrine manner. For example, alteration of NO levels in ECs has as the primary target EC themselves and modifies their biological properties. The inhibition of basal production of NO by competitive analogues of arginine increase the adhesion of leukocytes to EC surface, by a mechanism in part dependent on the upregulation of VCAM-1 and PAF synthesis.[26,27] Furthermore, the treatment of EC with NO donors reduces the expression of VCAM-1 induced by IL-1, IL-4, TNF, or LPS.[27] NO also decreases the expression of other adhesion molecules (ICAM-1 and E-selectin) and secretable cytokines (IL-6, MCP-1, IL-8, and M-CSF).[27–29] These effects of NO do not appear to involve stimulation of guanylate cyclase, the classical intracellular target of NO, but are mediated by an inhibition of NF-kB through the induction and stabilization of NF-kB inhibitor.[27,30] The finding that inhibition of endogenous, cytokine-independent NO production by arginine analogues could activate NF-kB suggests that constitutively produced NO may play an important physiologic role in tonically inhibiting the expression of NF-kB–dependent pro-inflammatory genes.[26,27,30] Moreover, NO produced by cytokine stimulation attenuates the inflammatory effects of these molecules.

However, NO is not only an intracellular regulator of EC function, but is instrumental in EC response. For example, a NO-dependent killing of *Schistosoma mansoni* has been described in murine EC stimulated with IFN-γ, IL-1, or TNF.[31] NO participates in long-term morphogenetic activities of vasculature, as in delayed hypersensitivity response, chronic inflammation, or in atherogenesis. It enhances the motility of EC, inhibits the proliferations of vascular smooth cells, is angiogenic *in vivo*, and reduces neointima formation.[32–34] Finally, in septic shock, NO produced by EC cooperates in the pathogenesis of the depression in contractile function of myocardium.[35,36]

Inflammatory cytokines promote leukocyte extravasation by altering the rheology of microcirculation and, by induction of adhesion molecules [E selectin, vascular cell adhesion molecule-1 (VCAM-1), and intercellular adhesion molecule-1 (ICAM-1)] and chemotactic cytokines. The regulated expression of adhesion molecules in the multistep process of recruitment has been the object of recent extensive reviews and chemokine production is discussed below. TNF and IFNγ cause redistribution of CD31 on the EC surface[37] and this could be important given the role of this molecule in transmigration. IL-1 and TNF cause production of PAF in EC.[4] A serine protease is involved in the synthesis of PAF in activated EC.[5,38] PAF can act on leukocytes as well as on EC themselves.[39] PAF is not important for leukocyte adhesion, but primes leukocytes and facilitates transmigration.[40]

The membrane attack complex of complement augments TNF-induced expression of adhesion molecules[41] and induces tissue factors by inducing IL-1α.[42] Interestingly, in turn, IL-1 augments production of C3 and factor B by EC.[43]

Endothelial cells have been the object of several efforts aimed at cloning IL-1 or TNF-inducible genes. New genes have been characterized including: a novel zinc finger transcription factor, A20, which subsequently was shown to be able to protect against TNF-induced cytotoxicity in a variety of cell types[44]; B12, a novel gene differentially expressed in the heart and liver during mouse embryogenesis and rapidly degraded[45]; C-193, which localizes to the nucleus; C-28 and B94, which are expressed in a complex modulated way during vasculogenesis, hematopoietic differentiation, and spermatogenesis.[46] The secreted B61 protein[47] was shown to be a chemoattractant *in vitro* for endothelial cells and an angiogenetic factor *in vivo*.[48] Its proposed function as the ligand for the Eck receptor may provide a clue for one circuit of angiogenesis during inflammation. The first long pentraxin PTX3, also known as TSG14,[49] was cloned as an IL-1–inducible gene in EC.[50,51] It is a secreted molecule consisting of a C terminal domain, encoded by the third exon, with sequence and structural similarity to classical pentraxins (e.g., CRP), coupled with an unrelated N terminal portion. PTX3 is produced by various cell types *in vitro*, prominently by EC and mononuclear phagocytes. Intriguingly, after LPS administration in mice, PTX3 is expressed predominantly by heart and skeletal muscle EC.[51] Recent results suggest that PTX3 binds C1q and activates C and thus may represent a mechanism of amplification of innate immunity (Bottazzi and colleagues, unpublished work).

IL-1 and TNF induce production of various cytokines in EC, including chemokines, CSF, IL-6, and IL-1 itself.[2,4] *In vitro* passage of EC results in spontaneous expression of IL-1α and refractoriness to exogenous IL-1.[52,53] Endogenous IL-1 may represent a mediator limiting the lifespan of EC in culture. EC produce IL-1, but efforts to demonstrate expression of the IL-1 receptor antagonist (IL-1ra) in umbilical vein cells yielded negative results.[54] IL-1ra blocks the action of IL-1 on EC, and these cells may represent a major target for the therapeutic activity of this molecule *in vivo*.

EC express both the p55 and the p75 TNF receptor, the latter being the most abundant on the cell membrane.[55] The p55 receptor is expressed at much lower levels in the membrane but is more abundant overall and it is detectable mainly in the Golgi apparatus and in cytoplasmic vacuoles.[55]

TNF activates EC predominantly via the p55 receptors.[56–58] The contribution of the p75 receptor is best observed at low TNF concentrations, consistent with the "ligand passing" model of function of this molecule.[59] The transmembrane form of TNF is the prime ligand of p75 and it may play an important role in juxtacrine interactions between EC and monocytes.[60–62]

EC express only the type I IL-1 receptor.[63] Under resting conditions or upon exposure to inducers (e.g., IL-4) active on myelomonocytic cells, EC do not express the type II decoy receptor,[63] a molecule without a demonstrable role in signaling, capable of blocking IL-1.[64]

IL-6

Various stimuli induce production of copious amounts of IL-6 in EC.[65] Production of IL-6 is elicited by diverse agents and stimuli, including, most prominently, IL-1, TNF, IL-4, IL-13, oncostantin M, IL-17 (S. Lebege, personal communication) infectious agents and their products, and hypoxia.[66] NF IL-6 is involved in the latter response.[66] EC also produce the functionally related cytokine LIF,[67] but not IL-11.[68] Original studies on IL-6 production by human umbilical vein EC (HUVEC) concluded that this cytokine did not affect several EC functions,[69] a conclusion repeatedly confirmed, though there are indications of involvement of this molecule in angiogenesis and vascular tumor formation. Observations in IL-6 KO mice (M. Romano and colleagues, unpublished data) prompted us to reexamine the interaction of IL-6 with EC. HUVEC express the signal-transducing gp130 chain but not the IL-6R chain. Soluble IL-6R and IL-6 alone did not affect EC function, but the two together activated EC. Interestingly, soluble IL-6 receptor, at physiological levels, in concert with IL-6, induced chemokine production in EC, with no other measurable response. Hence, recent *in vitro* and *in vivo* data suggest that IL-6 plays an unsuspected role as a pathway of amplification of leukocyte recruitment and that IL-6, in concert with its soluble receptor, activates a unique functional program in EC.

Hematopoietic Growth Factors

EC are an important source of CSFs. Hematopoietic growth factors produced by EC include stem cell factor,[70] G-CSF, GM-CSF, and M-CSF. CSF production is induced or augmented by a variety of stimuli including LPS, IL-1, and TNF[1-3] and minimally modified low-density lipoproteins (MM-LDL).[71]

The hematopoietic growth factors GM-CSF, G-CSF, IL-3, and erythropoietin were shown to affect EC (see Bussolino and colleagues[72] for recent review). By and large, these factors are relatively weak agonists, which affect migration and proliferation and amplify EC responsiveness to other signals.[72] In the same studies M-CSF was inactive, though, in one study M-CSF induced expression of monocyte chemotactic protein-1 (MCP-1) in endothelial cells.[73] Analysis of receptor expression revealed that EC express c-kit, the β chain common to the GM-CSF, IL-3, and IL-5 receptors, the α chain for IL-3 and GM, but not that for IL-5, and the M-CSF receptor c-fms. Endothelial cells express the IL-3Rα chain and TNF and IFNγ augment expression of IL-3Ra chain.[74] Accordingly IL-3 and TNF synergize in terms of induction of IL-8 and adhesion molecules and the same occurs with IFNγ in terms of class II MHC. It has been speculated that the ability of various hemopoietic cytokines to affect EC is a memoir of common ancestors, i.e., a reflection of the common ontogenetic origin of hematopoietic and endothelial elements in blood islands.[72]

IL-10, IL-4, and IL-13

Information on the interaction of IL-10 with vascular endothelium is scanty and fragmentary. This cytokine was a weak stimulus for expression of chemokines and

IL-6 in mouse Polyoma middle T (PmT) immortalized EC lines and amplified the action of IL-1 and TNF.[75] This effect was associated with prolongation of mRNA half life. Stimulation of HUVEC was variable and not reproducible. The effect of IL-10 on IL-8 production has been the object of conflicting reports.[76,77] IL-10 was reported to inhibit antigen presentation by human dermal microvascular EC,[78] induction of tetrahydrobiopterine in HUVEC,[79] amplification by LPS of irradiation-induced apoptosis,[80] and IL-1α induction of adhesion molecules.[81]

IL-4 has growth factor activity and induces uPA in microvascular EC, but not in macrovascular EC (see Mantovani and colleagues[4] and Wogta and colleagues[82] for review). It is intriguing that IL-4 and IL-13, but not IL-10, inhibited induction of RANTES expression in EC stimulated by IFNγ and TNF.[83] IL-4 selectively induces VCAM-1 and inhibits ICAM-1 and E-selectin expression. IL-4 is a weak inducer of IL-6 and MCP-1 in EC and amplifies production of these mediators in concert with other stimuli.[4] Recently it was shown that IL-13 has similar activities on EC.[84] Sharing of receptor components may underlie the similarity of action of IL-4 and IL-13 in EC.[85] EC do not express the common γ chain.[85] It is intriguing that these cytokines have divergent effects on monocytes (where they inhibit), and EC (where they amplify production of certain cytokines). Stimulation of certain EC functions may be important in the induction and local expression of TH2 type responses, by, for instance, inducing recruitment of eosinophils and basophils and favoring the transition to the late phase reaction.

Interferons and IL-12

Interferonγ (IFNγ) was the first molecularly identified cytokine shown to affect EC.[2] IFNγ induces EC expression of MHC class II antigens and of the invariant chain and augments class I. It also amplifies responses to TNF, slowly stimulates ICAM-1 expression, and augments LPs-induced production of IL-1. EC express CD40 and IFNγ, and IFNβ, IL-1, and TNF, augment its expression.[86–88] Engagement of CD40 amplifies induction of adhesion molecules.[88] Thus, ping-pong reciprocal stimulation may occur when CD40L expressing cells interact with EC.

IL-12 is a heterodimeric cytokine active on T cells and NK cells with antitumor activity against a variety of murine tumors. Recently IL-12 was shown to have potent anti-angiogenic activity *in vivo*.[89] In a murine opportunistic vascular tumor, IL-12 is the most effective single agent studied to date (Vecchi and colleagues, unpublished data). Circumstantial evidence suggests that IL-12 does not act per se on EC, but rather via induction of IFNγ.[89] IFNs have long been known to have anti-angiogenic activity and IFNα is used in the treatment of human hemangiomas.[90] IFNγ, in turn, may act on EC via induction of the C-X-C chemokine IP-10 (see below). Thus, IL-12 may set in motion a cytokine cascade involving IFNγ and IP10, which eventually results in inhibition of angiogenesis.

Chemokines

Chemokines are a key element in the multistep process of leukocyte recruitment and are produced by EC in response to molecules involved in inflammatory reactions, immunity, and thrombosis.[91] The chemokine repertoire of EC includes members of both the C-X-C (IL-8, IP10, and groα) and C-C (MCP-1, MCP-3, RANTES) family of chemokines, with most studies focused on the prototypic molecules IL-8 and MCP-1. Inducers include the proinflammatory cytokines IL-1 and TNF, bacterial products, IL-4 and IL-13[92] (which are less potent), IL-17 (S. Lebege, personal communication), minimally modified low density lipoproteins,[93] thrombin,[94] fibrin,[95] histamine,[96] and hypoxia.[97–99] M-CSF was reported to induce MCP-1 expression in EC[73] (and see above for critical discussion). One interesting pathway of chemokine induction is represented by monocytes and platelets,[100,101] which can activate EC via juxtacrine pathways involving adhesion molecules IL-1 and TNF. The C-X-C chemokine IP10, which unlike other members of the family acts on T cells and monocytes, but not on neutrophils, is expressed by certain endothelia of mice exposed *in vivo* to IFNγ or LPS,[102,103] but there is no data on *in vitro* expression in EC. RANTES is induced *in vitro* in EC exposed to IFNγ and TNF[69] and *in vivo* at sites of delayed type hypersensitivity and kidney allograft rejection.[104–105]

Given the different spectrum of action of chemokines, one would expect expression of molecules such as MCP-1 and IL-8 to be independently regulated. However there are few examples of selective regulation of different chemokines. It was found that IFNγ selectively induces MCP-1 in microvascular EC[106] as found also in monocytes, where this molecule stimulates MCP-1 and inhibits IL-8.

By and large, the spectrum of action of chemokines is restricted to leukocytes, but recent evidence suggests that some members of this superfamily of inflammatory mediators may affect EC function. IL-8, groα, and other C-X-C chemokines were reported to induce EC migration and proliferation *in vitro* and to be angiogenic *in vivo*.[107–109] The expression of high affinity receptors and responsiveness to IL-8 of EC has however been the object of conflicting results.[110,111]

Platelet factor 4, a C-X-C chemokine contained in the α granules of platelets, inhibits growth factor–induced proliferation of EC and angiogenesis.[112] Also, IP10 was shown to have angiostatic properties *in vivo*, though conflicting results have been obtained as to its capacity to inhibit bFGF-induced proliferation of HUVEC *in vitro*.[113,114] IP-10 induced via IFNγ may represent the ultimate mediator of the anti-angiogenic activity of IL-12.[89] A three amino-acid motif (Glu-Leu-Arg) (ELR), is highly conserved in all members of the C-X-C family that activate neutrophils. Recent results, including the action of ELR⁺ versus ELR⁻ molecules and the activity of IL-8 muteins, suggest that the presence or absence of an ELR motif dictates whether C-X-C chemokines induce or inhibit angiogenesis.[115] However, the observation that groβ inhibits angiogenesis is not consistent with this model of function.[116]

Three types of chemokine binding sites have been identified. Chemokines activate leukocytes via seven transmembrane domain, G protein-coupled, receptors. A promiscuous chemokine receptor identical to the Duffy blood group antigen (DARC) has been identified on erythrocytes where it may act as a sink for chemokines leaking from inflamed tissues. This promiscuous receptor is expressed by EC at postcapillary venules *in vivo*, but not by endothelial cells *in vitro*.[117] The structure of the promiscuous chemokine receptor is that of a seven-transmembrane–type molecule, but there is no clear evidence of signaling activity. Finally, chemokines bind heparin and heparin-like proteoglycans[118] and these molecules on endothelial cells present at least certain chemokines to leukocytes in the multistep process of recruitment.

In conclusion, EC cells, strategically located at the tissue/blood interface, produce chemokines and present at least some of these molecules to circulating leukocytes. EC-produced and presented chemokines, when produced in massive amounts, as in cancer or chronic inflammation, could contribute to systemic antiinflammation[119] by inducing, for instance, rapid release of the TNF p75R and the IL-1 type II decoy R.[120] Recent evidence also suggests that at least certain chemokines act on EC exerting pro- or anti-angiogenic activity. It will be important to define unequivocally the structural basis and receptors involved in the divergent action of chemokines on EC.

MOLECULAR BASIS FOR ENDOTHELIAL CELL ACTIVATION BY CYTOKINES

In this section we will focus on recent observations on the molecular mechanisms involved in the cytokine-regulated expression of several genes. In particular, we will review available information on genes studied in the context of the endothelial cells, even for genes (e.g., VCAM-1) whose expression is not restricted to these cells, in an effort to summarize molecular information that could provide hints to the largely unresolved issue of endothelial specificity.

Following binding to specific receptors (see above), phosphorylation has been frequently observed along with endothelial activation, although its direct role in the modification of transcription factors involved in controlling the expression of genes in endothelial cells can only be a matter of speculation. For example, the ATF2 factor is clearly involved in the regulation of the activity of the E-selectin promoter,[121,122] and it can be the target of JNK 1/2 phosphorylation (JNK = c-jun NH_2-terminal protein kinase).[123] Previous studies had shown that pharmacological elevations of cAMP in EC perturb E-selectin expression[124] and a role for PKA-mediated phosphorylation was suggested in studies of forskolin-mediated activation of EC.[125] Nonetheless, no direct evidence for this mechanism in endothelial cells is so far available.

It is well established that NF-kB elements are tightly controlled by several inhibitors belonging to the I-kB family.[126] In endothelial cells, it has been demonstrated that TNF exposure induces phosphorylation and subsequently proteolytic degradation of I-kB α.[127] Similarly, several serine-protease inhibitors have been shown able to inhibit the I-kB α degradation and, consequently, to block the TNF-induced upregulation of adhesion molecules.[128] Following cell activation, while I-kB α protein levels fall rapidly[127,129] RNA levels are dramatically upregulated[130] because the I-kB α gene is itself under NF-kB control. This circuit may provide a model for the transient induction of many cytokine-inducible genes. More recently, the regulated expression of NF-kB and I-kB α system has been demonstrated *in vivo* in an animal model of arterial injury.[131]

Interestingly, many data suggest a role for reactive oxygen intermediates (ROI) as a common and critical denominator for various activating signals leading to NF-kB activation. In particular, many different antioxidants [such as N-acetyl-L-cysteine (NAC), dithiocarbamates, vitamin E derivates, metal chelators, and pyrrolidine dithiocarbamate (PDTC)] have been shown to effectively block the NF-kB activation and subsequent gene induction. This issue has been scarcely explored so far in endothelial cells: α-tocopherol was shown to inhibit the cytokine-induced expression of E-selectin, but the authors failed to detect any change in NF-kB activity on the promoter.[132] Other agents like PDTC and NAC were shown, on the contrary, to inhibit the expression of VCAM-1, possibly through a reduction in the binding of NF-kB proteins to promoter elements, but interestingly in the same study no effect was reported with respect to E-selectin or ICAM.[133] PDTC has been shown able to abrogate TF expression following activation.[134]

The best characterized promoter in endothelial cells, so far, is from the E-selectin gene. Canonical p50/p65 NF-kB heterodimers (NF-kB = nuclear factor kB) are able to bind to three distinct sites,[121,135,136] now identified as PDI (PD = positive regulatory domain), PDII, and PDIV, respectively.[137] PDI and III are simultaneously occupied while PDIV is not, but the occupancy of these sites is largely dependent upon cell activation.[137] An additional element is a CRE/ATF-like binding site (CRE = cyclic AMP responsive element; ATF = activating transcription factor, previously known as CRE binding protein), now identifed as PDII, which is mainly occupied by ATF2 dimers (a factor of the basic leucine zipper family), which plays a major role in cytokine inducibility.[122,138] Finally, the HMGI (Y) protein binds to a region within PDII[139] as well as to the AT-rich regions in the kB sites contained in PDI, PDIII, and PDIV, possibly facilitating the binding of the NF-kB and ATF factors. All in all, the overall organization of the promoter is very reminiscent of the IFNβ promoter and a similar stereospecific model has been therefore hypothesized.[137]

The characterization of the VCAM-1 promoter has shown the presence of a tandem of NF-kB elements, both necessary for the cytokine-mediated expression, bound by classical heterodimers p65/ p50 or p65 homodimers.[137,140–142] More recently, other elements have been described, including one interferon-regulatory factor-1 (IRF-1) and one Sp-1 binding sites.[143]

Finally, and similarly to what has been observed for the E-selectin promoter, the HMGI (Y) protein (HMGI = high mobility group protein I) appears to facilitate the NF-kB and IRF-1 binding and seems to be a crucial element for the cytokine-inducibility of the gene.[144]

The ICAM-1 promoter shows three functionally relevant elements: one atypical NF-kB site, which mediates binding of p50/p65 heterodimers as well as c-Rel/p65 and p65 homodimers[145,146]; one γ-activated sequence (GAS) element, which mediates binding to p91 (STAT1 = signal transducer and activator of transcription 1) in response to IFNγ[147]—the functional role of this element has been highlighted in epithelial cells, while the modest induction of ICAM-1 in endothelial cells by IFNγ seems to imply the presence of tissue-specific negative regulatory factors[148]; and one c/EPB element (c/EBP = CCAAT / enhancer binding protein), which mediates binding to a mixture of factors (C/EBP α and β).[137] Interactions between different factors (as in the case of NF-kB and C/EBP) are being explored for the possibility of additional elements implicated in the ICAM-1 inducibility by different signals (i.e., one AP-1 element and the ets transcription factor when the gene is activated by exposure to H_2O_2.[149]

Recently, the tissue factor (TF) promoter has been characterized. The TNF inducibility seems to require a cooperation between two AP-1 binding sites and one NF-kB element[134,150,151] and possibly also Sp-1[152] factor. As for the ICAM-1, this NF-kB element is a variant sequence that is able to mediate c-Rel/p65 binding.[146] So far, monocytes and endothelial cells show the same usage of transcription factors on the TF promoter, following activation by LPS and cytokines.[151]

These results show the basis for a new level of comprehension of EC activation. Still, the central issue of specificity of the expression of certain genes to endothelium remains unresolved.[137] Recently, observations on the VCAM-1 promoter indicate that an equilibrium between different members of the NF-kB family acting on the tandem element (see above) may in part explain the endothelial expression of the gene.[153] The difficulty in transfecting primary EC and the lack of appropriate EC lines may have hampered solving this critical question.

PATHOLOGY

Diseases involving a wide range of cellular and organ systems involve EC as targets or active participants. Here we will focus on selected disorders in which the interplay between EC and cytokines plays a primary role.

Infectious Diseases

Viral, bacterial, or protozoan infections directly or indirectly involve EC. Viruses infect or interact with EC and induce or modify cytokine production. For instance, Epstein-Barr virus and cytomegalovirus (CMV) infect EC. These agents as well as EBV cell lines induce IL-6 production.[154,155] We recently found high levels of MCP-1 in the cerebrospinal fluid of patients with HIV infection, specifically associated with CMV encephalitis (Bernasconi and colleagues, unpublished observation), and immunoreactive MCP-1 was detected in brain EC (L. Vago, unpublished observation).

EC cytokine networks have assumed an increased relevance in HIV-1 infection and associated clinical disorders, including Kaposi's sarcoma, bacillary angiomatosis, vasculitis, psoriasis, and localization of non-Hodgkin's lymphomas in the central nervous system. The interaction between infected monocytes with EC increases the virus replication. This response appears to be via both cell contact and EC-derived cytokines (IL-6, GM-CSF, and IL-1).[156] Furthermore, an imbalance of inflammatory cytokine production has been described in AIDS patients and precedes the appearance of Kaposi's sarcoma.[157] A combination of inflammatory cytokines (IFNγ, IL-1, and TNF) induce EC *in vitro* to acquire phenotypic and functional features closely resembling cultured and *in situ* Kaposi's sarcoma spindle cells. These include spindle morphology, the responsiveness to HIV-Tat protein, and the neo-expression or upregulation of adhesion molecules, such as ICAM-1, VCAM, and E-selectin. Finally these ECs become angiogenic in nude mice.[158,159] These data suggest that *in vivo* hyperplasia of EC observed in Kaposi's sarcoma and angiogenesis may be due to a chronic exposure to inflammatory cytokines.

Rickettsia rickettsiae and *R. conorii* cause spotted fevers characterized by prominent, generalized vascular inflammation. Rickettsiae enter and proliferate in EC. EC functions affected include permeability, expression of adhesion molecules, and release of von Willebrandt factor. *R. conorii* was shown to induce IL-1α in EC and cell associated IL-1α was, in turn, responsible for induction of IL-8 and IL-6.[160] Therefore a cytokine cascade initiated by rickettsial infection of EC may play an important role in spotted fever–associated vasculitis.

Gram-positive and gram-negative bacteria and their products interact with EC and induce cytokine production. This interaction accounts for some of the systemic manifestations of sepsis as well as for localized reactions. *S. aureus*, a gram-positive bacterium, interacts with EC and, after internalization, induces IL-1 and IL-6 production.[161] EC are a major determinant of systemic inflammatory response syndrome (SIRS)/toxic shock. Hypotension and coagulation abnormalities are likely primarily dependent upon EC activation by LPS or LPS-induced IL-1 and TNF (see Bradley and colleagues[162] for review). Bacterial lipopolysaccharides (LPS) elicit a spectrum of EC responses similar to that of IL-1 and TNF.[4] It has recently been shown that EC, which are CD14⁻, interact with soluble CD14 and LPS-binding protein, both present in plasma.[163–167] While direct activation of EC by LPS does occur, the indirect pathway involving mononuclear phagocyte activation and production of inflammatory cytokines is more effective in stimulation of EC by this bacterial product.[168]

Among parasitic disorders vascular involvement is a prominent feature of cerebral malaria, a fatal complication of *Plasmodium falciparum* infection in man. Circumstantial evidence in human and murine models suggests that cytokines, TNF in particular, and alterations of endothelial cells play pivotal roles in the arrest of erythrocytes in the brain and subsequent vascular damage.[169,170] The mechanisms responsible for selective involvement of the brain vascular bed remain undefined. Hemolytic uremic syndrome (HUS), the most common cause of acute renal failure in infants and small children, is caused by infection with verotoxin (VT, or Shiga-like toxin)–producing *E. coli*.[171] VT is toxic for EC, activates them in a pro-inflammatory/prothrombotic sense, and synergizes with IL-1 and TNF.[65,172] These cytokines enhance galactosyltransferase and consequent surface expression of globotriaosylceramide (Gb3).[65] The VT receptor is expressed in greater amounts on EC of certain vascular beds, such as the kidney. Therefore, augmentation of Gb3 underlies synergism between inflammatory cytokines and VT and explains the selective organ involvement in HUS.

Neoplasia

Formation of new blood vessels is a limiting determinant of tumor growth and progression. An analysis of pro- and anti-angiogenic factors is beyond the scope of this review. IFNs, IL-12, and chemokines were discussed above and here selected aspects of IL-1 and TNF, mainly related to hemorrhagic necrosis and promotion of metastasis, will be discussed.[170]

IL-1 and TNF regulate the lifespan of EC and angiogenesis with seemingly contradictory actions. Endogenous IL-1α has been suggested to reduce the lifespan of EC by acting intracellularly and localizing to the nucleus.[52] IL-1 and TNF are not growth factors for EC, but TNF induces EC migration *in vivo* and angiogenesis *in vivo*.[4] These functions may be indirect. TNF (and IL-1) induce production of the secreted protein B.61, which functions as an EC chemoattractant and angiogenic factor by acting as the ligand for the eck tyrosin receptor.[47]

Other molecules cloned as IL-1/TNF–inducible genes in EC may be relevant to vasculogenesis or angiogenesis. A20 is a zincfinger transcription factor that may be important in protection of EC and other cell types against TNF toxicity. B24 is a gene of unknown function expressed in a complex way during vasculogenesis.[173] Finally,

IL-1 and TNF induce chemokines in EC, which act as pro- or anti-angiogenic factors (see above).

At least certain tumors utilize the same molecular pathways as leukocytes for interacting with endothelial cells and seeding at distant anatomical sites. Cytokines expressed constitutively by cancer cells or produced locally augment expression of adhesion molecules recognized by tumor cell counter-receptors (e.g., VLA4-VCAM-1 in melanoma) (see Chirivi and colleagues[170] for review). In the same vein, EC-derived chemokines may play a role in cancer seeding at specific sites.[174]

The eponymous function of TNF shared by other inflammatory cytokines is to cause hemorrhagic necrosis of neoplastic as well as of appropriately conditioned normal tissues (Schwartzman reaction). Involvement and damage of the vascular bed is a prominent feature of hemorrhagic necrosis.[4] TNF is not cytotoxic for confluent EC. The mechanism responsible for the capacity of TNF to selectively damage the vasculature of murine and human[175] tumors remains unclear.

Atherosclerosis and Cardiovascular Pathology

Monocyte recruitment is the first recognizable event in the natural history of atherosclerosis.[3] EC and smooth muscle cells produce chemokines, MCP-1 in particular, in response to pathophysiologically relevant stimuli (see above). Various studies have shown expression of MCP-1 in atherosclerotic lesions.[4] In particular, EC staining for MCP-1 was prominent in the early lesions constituted by diffuse intimal thickening and fatty streaks.[176] IL-1α was also detected in atherosclerosis.[177]

Cardiovascular disorders, such as myocardial infarction, are late consequences of atherosclerosis, associated with increased levels of inflammatory cytokines (e.g., TNF). The levels of the acute phase pentraxin C reactive protein have prognostic significance in ischemic heart disease.[178] We recently found that the long pentraxin PTX3 is preferentially expressed by heart EC[51] and is elevated in myocardial infarction (G. Peri, unpublished observation). Its significance as a direct indicator of myocardial EC function remains to be established.

Transplantation and Autoimmunity

EC are a major target for immune reactions directed against allo or xenogeneic transplanted organs[179] or self antigens. Circulating anti-endothelial cell antibodies (AECA) have been detected in a variety of autoimmune diseases with vascular involvement.

AECA are a common occurrence in a variety of autoimmune diseases, including scleroderma, SLE, and Wegener granulomatosis. Antigens recognized include proteins (e.g., protease 3), phospholipids, and protein-PL complexes. The presence of AECA is frequently associated with severe clinical symptoms, most notably thrombosis. AECA are generally not cytotoxic for EC, except for those found in Kawasaki disease. AECA activate expression of adhesion molecules, procoagulant activity, and cytokine production. Endogenous IL-1 is the ultimate mediator of at least some of these actions.[180–182] Thus, EC activation is likely a major pathogenetic factor of clinical manifestations associated with AECA.

CONCLUDING REMARKS

EC, long considered little more than a layer of nucleated cellophane, play an important, active role in the onset and regulation of inflammatory and immune reactions. The varied spectrum of responses elicited by cytokines is a dramatic demonstration of EC plasticity. The vast phenomenology of EC responses can be rationalized and represented in terms of cytokine-induced activation/differentiation programs. Recent work summarized here has begun to unravel the molecular basis of EC activation by cytokines by identifying transcription factors and regulatory elements involved in the induction or inhibition of gene expression and its time-course. However, the central issue of specificity to endothelium of expression of certain genes remains unsolved. For instance, E-selectin is exclusively expressed in cytokine-activated EC and considerable progress has been made in defining the molecular basis of induction and ensuing inhibition (see above). Yet no genetic clues as to the endothelial specificity of E-selectin are available. The difficulty in transfecting primary EC and the lack of appropriate EC lines may have hampered finding the solution to this critical question. Ultimately, *in vivo* studies in transgenic mice may be required.

A second related unsolved issue is represented by EC heterogeneity. Vascular endothelia are remarkable heterogeneous in terms of morphology, marker expression (e.g., von Willebrandt factor), and function. Heterogeneity is evident at multiple levels and emerges from analysis of macrovascular versus microvascular EC, of the vascular bed from different organs, and of EC obtained from different compartments in the same organ. EC heterogeneity includes the response to and production of cytokines, though data are scanty and fragmentary.[51,79,106] The phenomenology of EC heterogeneity is increasingly complex. Its molecular and cellular basis, as well as the formulation of a conceptual framework for this descriptive phenomenology, remains elusive.

The production and action of cytokines at the level of EC is a major determinant of a variety of human pathologies. The measure of molecules produced by EC and released in the circulation, such as adhesion molecules,[183] needs to be evaluated in carefully designed clinical studies. The identification of selective expression in different vascular districts of recently identified EC products (see, for example, Introna and colleagues[51]) provides potential molecular targets for therapy and diagnostic tools hopefully more representative of organ EC. The recognition of the primary role of EC in diverse human disorders provides a conceptual framework for investigation of new diagnostic tools and development of therapeutic strategies.

REFERENCES

1. MANTOVANI, A. & E. DEJANA. 1989. Cytokines as communication signals between leukocytes and endothelial cells. Immunol. Today. **10:** 370–375.
2. POBER, J. & R.S. COTRAN. 1990. Cytokines and endothelial cell biology. Physiol. Rev. **70:** 427–451.
3. LIBBY, P. & G.K. HANSSON. 1991. Biology of disease. Involvement of the immune system in human atherogenesis: current knowledge and unanswered questions. Lab. Invest. **64:** 5–15.
4. MANTOVANI, A., F. BUSSOLINO & E. DEJANA. 1992. Cytokine regulation of endothelial cell function. FASEB. J. **6:** 2591–2599.

5. BUSSOLINO, F., M. ARESE, L. SILVESTRO *et al.* 1994. Involvement of a serine protease in the synthesis of platelet-activating factor by endothelial cells stimulated by tumor necrosis factor-alpha or interleukin-1 alpha. Eur. J. Immunol. **24:** 3131–3139.

6. BUSSOLINO, F. & G. CAMUSSI. 1995. Platelet-activating factor produced by endothelial cells. A molecule with autocrine and paracrine properties. Eur. J. Biochem. **229:** 327–337.

7. MONTRUCCHIO, G., E. LUPIA, E. BATTAGLIA *et al.* 1994. Tumor necrosis factor alpha-induced angiogenesis depends on in situ platelet-activating factor biosynthesis. J. Exp. Med. **180:** 377–382.

8. JACKSON, B.A., R.H. GOLDSTEIN, R. ROY, M. COZZANI, L. TAYLOR & P. POLGAR. 1993. Effects of transforming growth factor beta and interleukin-1 beta on expression of cyclooxygenase 1 and 2 and phospholipase A2 mRNA in lung fibroblasts and endothelial cells in culture. Biochem. Biophys. Res. Commun. **197:** 1465–1474.

9. CAMACHO, M., N. GODESSART, R. ANTON, M. GARCIA & L. VILA. 1995. Interleukin-1 enhances the ability of cultured human umbilical vein endothelial cells to oxidize linoleic acid. J. Biol. Chem. **270:** 17279–17286.

10. CLARIA, J. & C.N. SERHAN. 1995. Aspirin triggers previously undescribed bioactive eicosanoids by human endothelial cell-leukocyte interactions. Proc. Natl. Acad. Sci. USA **92:** 9475–9479.

11. NATHAN, C. & Q.W. XIE. 1994. Nitric oxide synthases: roles, tolls, and controls. Cell **78:** 915–918.

12. ROSENKRANZ WEISS, P., W.C. SESSA, S. MILSTIEN, S. KAUFMAN, C.A. WATSON & J.S. POBER. 1994. Regulation of nitric oxide synthesis by proinflammatory cytokines in human umbilical vein endothelial cells. Elevations in tetrahydrobiopterin levels enhance endothelial nitric oxide synthase specific activity. J. Clin. Invest. **93:** 2236–2243.

13. WERNER FELMAYER, G., E.R. WERNER, D. FUCHS *et al.* 1993. Pteridine biosynthesis in human endothelial cells. Impact on nitric oxide-mediated formation of cyclic GMP. J. Biol. Chem. **268:** 1842–1846.

14. YOSHIZUMI, M., M.A. PERRELLA, J.C. BURNETT, JR. & M.E. LEE. 1993. Tumor necrosis factor downregulates an endothelial nitric oxide synthase mRNA by shortening its half-life. Circ. Res. **73:** 205–209.

15. LAMAS, S., T. MICHEL, T. COLLINS, B.M. BRENNER & P.A. MARSDEN. 1992. Effects of interferon-gamma on nitric oxide synthase activity and endothelin-1 production by vascular endothelial cells. J. Clin. Invest. **90:** 879–887.

16. RADOMSKI, M.W., R.M. PALMER & S. MONCADA. 1990. Glucocorticoids inhibit the expression of an inducible, but not the constitutive, nitric oxide synthase in vascular endothelial cells. Proc. Natl. Acad. Sci. USA **87:** 10043–10047.

17. SUSCHEK, C., H. ROTHE, K. FEHSEL, J. ENCZMANN & V. KOLB BACHOFEN. 1993. Induction of a macrophage-like nitric oxide synthase in cultured rat aortic endothelial cells. IL-1 beta-mediated induction regulated by tumor necrosis factor-alpha and IFN-gamma. J. Immunol. **151:** 3283–3291.

18. BALLIGAND, J.L., D. UNGUREANU LONGROIS, W.W. SIMMONS *et al.* 1995. Induction of NO synthase in rat cardiac microvascular endothelial cells by IL-1 beta and IFN-gamma. Am. J. Physiol. **268:** H1293–H1303.

19. MARTIN, E., C. NATHAN & Q.W. XIE. 1994. Role of interferon regulatory factor 1 in induction of nitric oxide synthase. J. Exp. Med. **180:** 977–984.

20. KAMIJO, R., H. HARADA, T. MATSUYAMA *et al.* 1994. Requirement for transcription factor IRF-1 in NO synthase induction in macrophages. Science **263:** 1612–1615.

21. ZHANG, R., W. MIN & W.C. SESSA. 1995. Functional analysis of the human endothelial nitric oxide synthase promoter. Sp1 and GATA factors are necessary for basal transcription in endothelial cells. J. Biol. Chem. **270:** 15320–15326.

22. SAKURAI, H., H. KOHSAKA, M.F. LIU *et al.* 1995. Nitric oxide production and inducible nitric oxide synthase expression in inflammatory arthritides. J. Clin. Invest. **96:** 2357–2363.

23. COBBS, C.S., J.E. BRENMAN, K.D. ALDAPE, D.S. BREDT & M.A. ISRAEL. 1995. Expression of nitric oxide synthase in human central nervous system tumors. Cancer Res. **55:** 727–730.

24. MURATA, J., S.B. CORRADIN, E. FELLEY BOSCO & L. JUILLERAT JEANNERET. 1995. Involvement of a transforming-growth-factor-beta-like molecule in tumor-cell-derived inhibition of nitric-oxide synthesis in cerebral endothelial cells. Int. J. Cancer **62:** 743–748.

25. INOUE, N., R.C. VENEMA, H.S. SAYEGH, Y. OHARA, T.J. MURPHY & D.G. HARRISON. 1995. Molecular regulation of the bovine endothelial cell nitric oxide synthase by transforming growth factor-beta 1. Arterioscler. Thromb. Vasc. Biol. **15:** 1255–1261.

26. NIU, X.F., C.W. SMITH & P. KUBES. 1994. Intracellular oxidative stress induced by nitric oxide synthesis inhibition increases endothelial cell adhesion to neutrophils. Circ. Res. **74:** 1133–1140.

27. DE CATERINA, R., P. LIBBY, H.B. PENG *et al.* 1995. Nitric oxide decreases cytokine-induced endothelial activation. Nitric oxide selectively reduces endothelial expression of adhesion molecules and proinflammatory cytokines. J. Clin. Invest. **96:** 60–68.

28. PENG, H.B., T.B. RAJAVASHISTH, P. LIBBY & J.K. LIAO. 1995. Nitric oxide inhibits macrophage-colony stimulating factor gene transcription in vascular endothelial cells. J. Biol. Chem. **270:** 17050–17055.

29. ZEIHER, A.M., B. FISSLTHALER, B. SCHRAY UTZ & R. BUSSE. 1995. Nitric oxide modulates the expression of monocyte chemoattractant protein 1 in cultured human endothelial cells. Circ. Res. **76:** 980–986.

30. PENG, H.B., P. LIBBY & J.K. LIAO. 1995. Induction and stabilization of I kappa B alpha by nitric oxide mediates inhibition of NF-kappa B.J. Biol. Chem. **270:** 14214–14219.

31. OSWALD, I.P., I. ELTOUM, T.A. WYNN *et al.* 1994. Endothelial cells are activated by cytokine treatment to kill an intravascular parasite, Schistosoma mansoni, through the production of nitric oxide. Proc. Natl. Acad. Sci. USA **91:** 999–1003.

32. ZICHE, M., L. MORBIDELLI, E. MASINI *et al.* 1994. Nitric oxide mediates angiogenesis in vivo and endothelial cell growth and migration in vitro promoted by substance P. J. Clin. Invest. **94:** 2036–2044.

33. FUKUO, K., T. INOUE, S. MORIMOTO *et al.* 1995. Nitric oxide mediates cytotoxicity and basic fibroblast growth factor release in cultured vascular smooth muscle cells. A possible mechanism of neovascularization in atherosclerotic plaques. J. Clin. Invest. **95:** 669–676.

34. VON DER LEYEN, H.E., G.H. GIBBONS, R. MORISHITA *et al.* 1995. Gene therapy inhibiting neointimal vascular lesion: in vivo transfer of endothelial cell nitric oxide synthase gene. Proc. Natl. Acad. Sci. USA **92:** 1137–1141.

35. SCHULZ, R., D.L. PANAS, R. CATENA, S. MONCADA, P.M. OLLEY & G.D. LOPASCHUK. 1995. The role of nitric oxide in cardiac depression induced by interleukin-1 beta and tumour necrosis factor-alpha. Br. J. Pharmacol. **114:** 27–34.

36. SATO, K., K. MIYAKAWA, M. TAKEYA *et al.* 1995. Immunohistochemical expression of inducible nitric oxide synthase (iNOS) in reversible endotoxic shock studied by a novel monoclonal antibody against rat iNOS. J. Leukoc. Biol. **57:** 36–44.

37. ROMER, L.H., N.V. MCLEAN, H.C. YAN, M. DAISE, J. SUN & H.M. DELISSER. 1995. IFN-gamma and TNF-alpha induce redistribution of PECAM-1 (CD31) on human endothelial cells. J. Immunol. **154:** 6582–6592.

38. HELLER, R., F. BUSSOLINO, D. GHIGO *et al.* 1992. Human endothelial cells are target for platelet-activating factor. II. Platelet-activating factor induces platelet-activating factor synthesis in human umbilical vein endothelial cells. J. Immunol. **149:** 3682–3688.

39. BUSSOLINO, F., F. SILVAGNO, G. GARBARINO *et al.* 1994. Human endothelial cells are tar-

gets for platelet-activating factor (PAF). Activation of alpha and beta protein kinase C isozymes in endothelial cells stimulated by PAF. J. Biol. Chem. **269:** 2877–2886.

40. HILL, M.E., I.N. BIRD, R.H. DANIELS, M.A. ELMORE & M.J. FINNEN. 1994. Endothelial cell-associated platelet-activating factor primes neutrophils for enhanced superoxide production and arachidonic acid release during adhesion to but not transmigration across IL-1 beta-treated endothelial monolayers. J. Immunol. **153:** 3673–3683.

41. KILGORE, K.S., J.P. SHEN, B.F. MILLER, P.A. WARD & J.S. WARREN. 1995. Enhancement by the complement membrane attack complex of tumor necrosis factor-alpha-induced endothelial cell expression of E-selectin and ICAM-1. J. Immunol. **155:** 1434–1441.

42. SAADI, S., R.A. HOLZKNECHT, C. PATTE, D.M. STERN & J.L. PLATT. 1995. Complement-mediated regulation of tissue factor activity in endothelium. J. Exp. Med. **182:** 1807–1814.

43. COULPIER, M., S. ANDREEV, C. LEMERCIER *et al.* 1995. Activation of the endothelium by IL-1 alpha and glucocorticoids results in major increase of complement C3 and factor B production and generation of C3a. Clin. Exp. Immunol. **101:** 142–149.

44. OPIPARI, A.W.J., H.M. HU, R. YABKOWITZ & V.M. DIXIT. 1992. The A20 zinc finger protein protects cells from tumor necrosis factor cytotoxicity. J. Biol. Chem. **267:** 12424–12427.

45. WOLF, F.W., R.M. MARKS, V. SARMA *et al.* 1992. Characterization of a novel tumor necrosis factor-alpha-induced endothelial primary response gene. J. Biol. Chem. **267:** 1317–1326.

46. WOLF, F.W., V. SARMA, M. SELDIN *et al.* 1994. B94, a primary response gene inducible by tumor necrosis factor-alpha, is expressed in developing hematopoietic tissues and the sperm acrosome. J. Biol. Chem. **269:** 3633–3640.

47. HOLZMAN, L.B., R.M. MARKS & V.M. DIXIT. 1990. A novel immediate-early response gene of endothelium is induced by cytokines and encodes a secreted protein. Mol. Cell Biol. **10:** 5830–5838.

48. PANDEY, A., H. SHAO, R.M. MARKS, P.J. POLVERINI & V.M. DIXIT. 1995. Role of B61, the ligand for the Eck receptor tyrosine kinase, in TNF-alpha-induced angiogenesis. Science **268:** 567–569.

49. LEE, T.H., G.W. LEE, E.B. ZIFF & J. VILCEK. 1990. Isolation and characterization of eight tumor necrosis factor-induced gene sequences from human fibroblasts. Mol. Cell Biol. **10:** 1982–1988.

50. BREVIARIO, F., E.M. D'ANIELLO, J. GOLAY *et al.* 1992. Interleukin-1-inducible genes in endothelial cells. Cloning of a new gene related to C-reactive protein and serum amyloid P component. J. Biol. Chem. **267:** 22190–22197.

51. INTRONA, M., V. VIDAL ALLES, M. CASTELLANO *et al.* 1996. Cloning of mouse PTX3, a new member of the pentraxin gene family expressed at extrahepatic sites. Blood **87:** 1862–1872.

52. MAIER, J.A., P. VOULALAS, D. ROEDER & T. MACIAG. 1990. Extension of the life-span of human endothelial cells by an interleukin-1 alpha antisense oligomer. Science **249:** 1570–1574.

53. MAIER, J.A., M. STATUTO & G. RAGNOTTI. 1994. Endogenous interleukin 1 alpha must be transported to the nucleus to exert its activity in human endothelial cells. Mol. Cell Biol. **14:** 1845–1851.

54. BERTINI, R., M. SIRONI, I. MARTIN PADURA *et al.* 1992. Inhibitory effect of recombinant intracellular interleukin 1 receptor antagonist on endothelial cell activation. Cytokine **4:** 44–47.

55. BRADLEY, J.R., S. THIRU & J.S. POBER. 1995. Disparate localization of 55-kd and 75-kd tumor necrosis factor receptors in human endothelial cells. Am. J. Pathol. **146:** 27–32.

56. MACKAY, F., H. LOETSCHER, D. STUEBER, G. GEHR & W. LESSLAUER. 1993. Tumor necrosis factor alpha (TNF-alpha)-induced cell adhesion to human endothelial cells is under dominant control of one TNF receptor type, TNF-R55. J. Exp. Med. **177:** 1277–1286.

57. PALEOLOG, E.M., S.A. DELASALLE, W.A. BUURMAN & M. FELDMANN. 1994. Functional activities of receptors for tumor necrosis factor-alpha on human vascular endothelial cells. Blood **84:** 2578–2590.

58. SLOWIK, M.R., L.G. DE LUCA, W. FIERS & J.S. POBER. 1993. Tumor necrosis factor activates human endothelial cells through the p55 tumor necrosis factor receptor but the p75 receptor contributes to activation at low tumor necrosis factor concentration. Am. J. Pathol. **143:** 1724–1730.

59. TARTAGLIA, L.A., D. PENNICA & D.V. GOEDDEL. 1993. Ligand passing: the 75-kDa tumor necrosis factor (TNF) receptor recruits TNF for signaling by the 55-kDa TNF receptor. J. Biol. Chem. **268:** 18542–18548.

60. GRELL, M., E. DOUNI, H. WAJANT *et al.* 1995. The transmembrane form of tumor necrosis factor is the prime activating ligand of the 80 kDa tumor necrosis factor receptor. Cell **83:** 793–802.

61. SCHMID, E.F., K. BINDER, M. GRELL, P. SCHEURICH & K. PFIZENMAIER. 1995. Both tumor necrosis factor receptors, TNFR60 and TNFR80, are involved in signaling endothelial tissue factor expression by juxtacrine tumor necrosis factor alpha. Blood **86:** 1836–1841.

62. LUKACS, N.W., R.M. STRIETER, V. ELNER, H.L. EVANOFF, M.D. BURDICK & S.L. KUNKEL. 1995. Production of chemokines, interleukin-8 and monocyte chemoattractant protein-1, during monocyte endothelial cell interactions. Blood **86:** 2767–2773.

63. COLOTTA, F., M. SIRONI, A. BORRE *et al.* 1993. Type II interleukin-1 receptor is not expressed in cultured endothelial cells and is not involved in endothelial cell activation. Blood **81:** 1347–1351.

64. COLOTTA, F., F. RE, M. MUZIO *et al.* 1993. Interleukin-1 type II receptor: a decoy target for IL-1 that is regulated by IL-4. Science **261:** 472–475.

65. VAN DE KAR, N.C., T. KOOISTRA, M. VERMEER, W. LESSLAUER, L.A. MONNENS & V.W. VAN HINSBERGH. 1995. Tumor necrosis factor alpha induces endothelial galactosyl transferase activity and verocytotoxin receptors. Role of specific tumor necrosis factor receptors and protein kinase C. Blood **85:** 734–743.

66. YAN, S.F., I. TRITTO, D. PINSKY *et al.* 1995. Induction of interleukin 6 (IL-6) by hypoxia in vascular cells. Central role of the binding site for nuclear factor-IL-6. J. Biol. Chem. **270:** 11463–11471.

67. GROSSET, C., B. JAZWIEC, J.L. TAUPIN *et al.* 1995. In vitro biosynthesis of leukemia inhibitory factor/human interleukin for DA cells by human endothelial cells: differential regulation by interleukin-1 alpha and glucocorticoids. Blood **86:** 3763–3770.

68. SUEN, Y., M. CHANG, S.M. LEE, J.S. BUZBY & M.S. CAIRO. 1994. Regulation of interleukin-11 protein and mRNA expression in neonatal and adult fibroblasts and endothelial cells. Blood **84:** 4125–4134.

69. SIRONI, M., F. BREVIARIO, P. PROSERPIO *et al.* 1989. IL-1 stimulates IL-6 production in endothelial cells. J. Immunol. 142: 549–553.

70. MEININGER, C.J., S.E. BRIGHTMAN, K.A. KELLY & B.R. ZETTER. 1995. Increased stem cell factor release by hemangioma-derived endothelial cells. Lab. Invest. **72:** 166–173.

71. RAJAVASHISTH, T.B., A. ANDALIBI, M.C. TERRITO *et al.* 1990. Induction of endothelial cell expression of granulocyte and macrophage colony-stimulating factors by modified low-density lipoproteins. Nature **344:** 254–257.

72. BUSSOLINO, F., E. BOCCHIETTO, F. SILVAGNO, R. SOLDI, M. ARESE & A. MANTOVANI. 1994. Actions of molecules which regulate hemopoiesis on endothelial cells: memoirs of common ancestors? Path. Res. Pract. **190:** 834–839.

73. SHYY, Y.J., L.L. WICKHAM, J.P. HAGAN *et al.* 1993. Human monocyte colony-stimulating factor stimulates the gene expression of monocyte chemotactic protein-1 and increases the adhesion of monocytes to endothelial monolayers. J. Clin. Invest. **92:** 1745–1751.

74. KORPELAINEN, E.I., J.R. GAMBLE, W.B. SMITH, M. BOTTORE, M.A. VADAS & A.F. LOPEZ. 1995. Interferon-gamma upregulates interleukin-3 (IL-3) receptor expression in human

endothelial cells and synergizes with IL-3 in stimulating major histocompatibility complex class II expression and cytokine production. Blood **86:** 176–182.

75. SIRONI, M., C. MUNOZ, T. POLLICINO *et al.* 1993. Divergent effects of interleukin-10 on cytokine production by mononuclear phagocytes and endothelial cells. Eur. J. Immunol. **23:** 2692–2695.

76. CHEN, C.C. & A.M. MANNING. 1996. TGF-beta1, IL-10 and IL-4 differentially modulate the cytokine-induced expression of the IL-6 and IL-8 in human endothelial cells. Cytokine **8:** 58–65.

77. DEBEAUX, A.C., J.P. MAINGAY, J.A. ROSS, K.C.H. FEARON & D.C. CARTER. 1995. Interleukin-4 and interleukin-10 increase endotoxin-stimulated human umbilical vein endothelial cell interleukin-8 release. J. Interferon Cytokine Res. **15:** 441–445.

78. VORA, M., H. YSSEL, J.E. DE VRIES & M.A. KARASEK. 1994. Antigen presentation by human dermal microvascular endothelial cells. Immunoregulatory effect of IFN-gamma and IL-10. J. Immunol. **152:** 5734–5741.

79. SCHOEDON, G., M. SCHNEEMANN, N. BLAU, C.J. EDGELL & A. SCHAFFNER. 1993. Modulation of human endothelial cell tetrahydrobiopterin synthesis by activating and deactivating cytokines: new perspectives on endothelium-derived relaxing factor. Biochem. Biophys. Res. Commun. **196:** 1343–1348.

80. EISSNER, G., F. KOHLHUBER, M. GRELL *et al.* 1995. Critical involvement of transmembrane tumor necrosis factor-alpha in endothelial programmed cell death mediated by ionizing radiation and bacterial endotoxin. Blood **86:** 4184–4193.

81. KRAKAUER, T. 1995. IL-10 inhibits the adhesion of leukocytic cells to IL-1-activated human endothelial cells. Immunol. Lett. **45:** 61–65.

82. WOJTA, J., M. GALLICCHIO, H. ZOELLNER, E.L. FILONZI, J.A. HAMILTON & K. MCGRATH. 1993. Interleukin-4 stimulates expression of urokinase-type-plasminogen activator in cultured human foreskin microvascular endothelial cells. Blood **81:** 3285–3292.

83. MARFAINGKOKA, A., O. DEVERGNE, G. GORGONE *et al.* 1995. Regulation of the production of the RANTES chemokine by endothelial cells—Synergistic induction by IFN-gamma plus TNF-alpha and inhibition by IL-4 and IL-13. J. Immunol. **154:** 1870–1878.

84. SIRONI, M., F.L. SCIACCA, C. MATTEUCCI *et al.* 1994. Regulation of endothelial and mesothelial cell function by interleukin-13: selective induction of vascular cell adhesion molecule-1 and amplification of interleukin-6 production. Blood **84:** 1913–1921.

85. GARCIA DE FRUTOS, P., Y. HARDIG & B. DAHLBACK. 1995. Serum amyloid P component binding to C4b-binding protein. J. Biol. Chem. **270:** 26950–26955.

86. HOLLENBAUGH, D., N. MISCHEL PETTY, C.P. EDWARDS *et al.* 1995. Expression of functional CD40 by vascular endothelial cells. J. Exp. Med. **182:** 33–40.

87. YELLIN, M.J., J. BRETT, D. BAUM *et al.* 1995. Functional interactions of T cells with endothelial cells: the role of CD40L-CD40-mediated signals. J. Exp. Med. **182:** 1857–1864.

88. KARMANN, K., C.C. HUGHES, J. SCHECHNER, W.C. FANSLOW & J.S. POBER. 1995. CD40 on human endothelial cells: inducibility by cytokines and functional regulation of adhesion molecule expression. Proc. Natl. Acad. Sci. USA **92:** 4342–4346.

89. VOEST, E.E., B.M. KENYON, M.S. O'REILLY, G. TRUITT, R.J. D'AMATO & J. FOLKMAN. 1995. Inhibition of angiogenesis in vivo by interleukin-12. J. Natl. Cancer Inst. **87:** 581–586.

90. EZEKOWITZ, R.A., J.B. MULLIKEN & J. GOLKMAN. 1992. Interferon alfa-2a therapy for life-threatening hemangiomas of infancy [see comments] [published errata appear in N Engl J Med 1994 Jan 27;330(4):300 and 1995 Aug 31;333(9):595-6]. N. Engl. J. Med. **326:** 1456–1463.

91. GYETKO, M.R., S.B. SHOLLENBERGER & R.G. SITRIN. 1992. Urokinase expression in mononuclear phagocytes: cytokine-specific modulation by interferon-gamma and tumor necrosis factor-alpha. J. Leukoc. Biol. **51:** 256–263.

92. GALEA, P., G. THIBAULT, M. LACORD, P. BARDOS & Y. LEBRANCHU. 1993. IL-4, but not tumor necrosis factor-alpha, increases endothelial cell adhesiveness for lymphocytes by activating a cAMP-dependent pathway. J. Immunol. **151:** 588–596.

93. CUSHING, S.D., J.A. BERLINES, A.J. VALENTE *et al.* 1990. Minimally modified low density lipoprotein induces monocyte chemotactic protein 1 in human endothelial cells and smooth muscle cells. Proc. Natl. Acad. Sci. USA **87:** 5134–5138.

94. COLOTTA, F., F.L. SCIACCA, M. SIRONI, W. LUINI, M.J. RABIET & A. MANTOVANI. 1994. Expression of monocyte chemotactic protein-1 by monocytes and endothelial cells exposed to thrombin. Am. J. Pathol. **144:** 975–985.

95. QI, J.F. & D.L. KREUTZER. 1995. Fibrin activation of vascular endothelial cells—Induction of IL-8 expression. J. Immunol. **155:** 867–876.

96. KORPELAINEN, E.I., J.R. GAMBLE, W.B. SMITH *et al.* 1993. The receptor for interleukin 3 is selectively induced in human endothelial cells by tumor necrosis factor alpha and potentiates interleukin 8 secretion and neutrophil transmigration. Proc. Natl. Acad. Sci. USA **90:** 11137–11141.

97. JEANNIN, P., Y. DELNESTE, P. GOSSET *et al.* 1994. Histamine induces interleukin-8 secretion by endothelial cells. Blood **84:** 2229–2233.

98. KAPLANSKI, G., R. PORAT, K. AIURA, J.K. ERBAN, J.A. GELFAND & C.A. DINARELLO. 1993. Activated platelets induce endothelial secretion of interleukin-8 in vitro via an interleukin-1 mediated event. Blood **81:** 2492–2495.

99. KARAKURUM, M., R. SHREENIWAS, J. CHEN *et al.* 1994. Hypoxic induction of interleukin-8 gene expression in human endothelial cells. J. Clin. Invest. **93:** 1564–1570.

100. KAPLANSKI, G., R. PORAT, K. AIURA, J.K. ERBAN, J.A. GELFAND & C.A. DINARELLO. 1993. Activated platelets induce endothelial secretion of interleukin-8 in vitro via an interleukin-1-mediated event. Blood **81:** 2492–2495.

101. KAPLANSKI, G., C. FARNARIER, S. KAPLANSKI *et al.* 1994. Interleukin-1 induces interleukin-8 secretion from endothelial cells by a juxtacrine mechanism. Blood **84:** 4242–4248.

102. NARUMI, S., L.M. WYNER, M.H. STOLER, C.S. TANNENBAUM & T.A. HAMILTON. 1992. Tissue-specific expression of murine IP-10 mRNA following systemic treatment with interferon-gamma. J. Leukoc. Biol. **52:** 27–33.

103. GÓMEZ-CHIARRI, M., T.A. HAMILTON, J. EGIDO & S.N. EMANCIPATOR. 1993. Expression of IP-10, a lipopolysaccharide- and interferon-gamma-inducible protein, in murine mesangial cells in culture. Am. J. Pathol. **142:** 433–439.

104. DEVERGNE, O., A. MARFAING-KOKA, T.J. SCHALL *et al.* 1994. Production of the RANTES chemokine in delayed-type hypersensitivity reactions: Involvement of macrophages and endothelial cells. J. Exp. Med. **179:** 1689–1694.

105. PATTISON, J., P.J. NELSON, P. HUIE *et al.* 1994. RANTES chemokine expression in cell-mediated transplant rejection of the kidney. Lancet **343:** 209–211.

106. BROWN, Z., M.E. GERRITSEN, W.W. CARLEY, R.M. STRIETER, S.L. KUNKEL & J. WESTWICK. 1994. Chemokine gene expression and secretion by cytokine-activated human microvascular endothelial cells—Differential regulation of monocyte chemoattractant protein-1 and interleukin-8 in response to interferon-gamma. Am. J. Pathol. **145:** 913–921.

107. KOCH, A.E., P.J. POLVERINI, S.L. KUNKEL *et al.* 1992. Interleukin-8 as a macrophage-derived mediator of angiogenesis. Science **258:** 1798–1801.

108. STRIETER, R.M., S.L. KUNKEL, V.M. ELNER *et al.* 1992. Interleukin-8. A corneal factor that induces neovascularization. Am. J. Pathol. **141:** 1279–1284.

109. WEN, D., A. ROWLAND & R. DERYNCK. 1989. Expression and secretion of *gro*/MGSA by stimulated human endothelial cells. EMBO J. **8:** 1761–1766.

110. SCHONBECK, U., E. BRANDT, F. PETERSEN, H.D. FLAD & H. LOPPNOW. 1995. IL-8 specifically binds to endothelial but not to smooth muscle cells. J. Immunol. **154:** 2375–2383.

111. PETZELBAUER, P., C.A. WATSON, S.E. PFAU & J.S. POBER. 1995. IL-8 and angiogenesis:

Evidence that human endothelial cells lack receptors and do not respond to IL-8 in vitro. Cytokine **7:** 267–272.

112. MAIONE, T.E., G.S. GRAY, J. PETRO *et al.* 1990. Inhibition of angiogenesis by recombinant human platelet factor-4 and related peptides. Science **247:** 77–79.

113. LUSTER, A.D., S.M. GREENBERG & P. LEDER. 1995. The IP-10 chemokine binds to a specific cell surface heparan sulfate site shared with platelet factor 4 and inhibits endothelial cell proliferation. J. Exp. Med. **182:** 219–231.

114. ANGIOLILLO, A.L., C. SGADARI, D.D. TAUB *et al.* 1995. Human interferon-inducible protein 10 is a potent inhibitor of angiogenesis in vivo. J. Exp. Med. **182:** 155–162.

115. STRIETER, R.M., P.J. POLVERINI, S.L. KUNKEL *et al.* 1995. The functional role of the ELR motif in CXC chemokine-mediated angiogenesis. J. Biol. Chem. **270:** 27348–27357.

116. CAO, Y.H., C. CHEN, J.A. WEATHERBEE, M. TSANG & J. FOLKMAN. 1995. Gro-beta, a -C-X-C- chemokine, is an angiogenesis inhibitor that suppresses the growth of Lewis lung carcinoma in mice. J. Exp. Med. **182:** 2069–2077.

117. PEIPER, S.C., Z.X. WANG, K. NEOTE *et al.* 1995. The Duffy antigen receptor for chemokines (DARC) is expressed in endothelial cells of Duffy negative individuals who lack the erythrocyte receptor. J. Exp. Med. **181:** 1311–1317.

118. ROT, A. 1992. Endothelial cell binding of NAP-1/IL-8: role in neutrophil emigration. Immunol. Today **13:** 291–294.

119. LEY, K., J.B. BAKER, M.I. CYBULSKY, M.A. GIMBRONE & F.W. LUSCINSKAS. 1993. Intravenous interleukin-8 inhibits granulocyte emigration from rabbit mesenteric venules without altering L-selectin expression or leukocyte rolling. J. Immunol. **151:** 6347–6357.

120. COLOTTA, F., S. ORLANDO, E.J. FADLON, S. SOZZANI, C. MATTEUCCI & A. MANTOVANI. 1995. Chemoattractants induce rapid release of the interleukin 1 type II decoy receptor in human polymorphonuclear cells. J. Exp. Med. **181:** 2181–2188.

121. WHITLEY, M.Z., D. THANOS, M.A. READ, T. MANIATIS & T. COLLINS. 1994. A striking similarity in the organization of the E-selectin and beta interferon gene promoters. Mol. Cell Biol. **14:** 6464–6475.

122. KASZUBSKA, W., R.H. VAN HUIJSDUIJNEN, P. GHERSA *et al.* 1993. Cyclic AMP-independent ATF family members interact with NF-kappa B and function in the activation of the E-selectin promoter in response to cytokines. Mol. Cell Biol. **13:** 7180–7190.

123. GUPTA, S., D. CAMPBELL, B. DERIJARD & R.J. DAVIS. 1995. Transcription factor ATF2 regulation by the JNK signal transduction pathway. Science **267:** 389–393.

124. POBER, J.S., M.R. SLOWIK, L.G. DE LUCA & A.J. RITCHIE. 1993. Elevated cyclic AMP inhibits endothelial cell synthesis and expression of TNF-induced endothelial leukocyte adhesion molecule-1, and vascular cell adhesion molecule-1, but not intercellular adhesion molecule-1. J. Immunol. **150:** 5114–5123.

125. GHERSA, P., R. HOOFT VAN HUIJSDUIJNEN, J. WHELAN, Y. CAMBET, R. PESCINI & J.F. DELAMARTER. 1994. Inhibition of E-selectin gene transcription through a cAMP-dependent protein kinase pathway. J. Biol. Chem. **269:** 29129–29137.

126. MIYALOTO, S., M. MAKI, M.J. SCHMITT, M. HATANAKA & I.M. VERNA. 1994. Tumor necrosis factor alpha-induced phosphorylation of IkBalpha is signal for its degradation but not dissociation from NF-kB. Proc. Natl. Acad. Sci. USA **91:** 12740–12744.

127. READ, M.A., M.Z. WHITLEY, A.J. WILLIAMS & T. COLLINS. 1994. NF-kappa B and I kappa B alpha: an inducible regulatory system in endothelial activation. J. Exp. Med. **179:** 503–512.

128. CHEN, C.C., C.L. ROSENBLOOM, D.C. ANDERSON & A.M. MANNING. 1995. Selective inhibition of E-selectin, vascular cell adhesion molecule-1, and intercellular adhesion molecule-1 expression by inhibitors of I kappa B-alpha phosphorylation. J. Immunol. **155:** 3538–3545.

129. DE MARTIN, R., B. VANHOVE, Q. CHENG *et al.* 1993. Cytokine-inducible expression in en-

dothelial cells of an I kappa B alpha-like gene is regulated by NF kappa B. EMBO J. 12: 2773–2779.

130. D'ANIELLO, E.M., F. BREVIARIO, I. MARTIN PADURA *et al.* 1993. Interleukin-1 and tumor necrosis factor induce transient expression of an inhibitor of nuclear factor kB in endothelial cells. Endothelium **1:** 161–165.

131. LINDNER, V. & T. COLLINS. 1996. Expression of NF-kB and IkB-alpha by aortic endothelium in an arterial injury model. Am. J. Pathol. **148:** 427–438.

132. FARUQI, R., C. DE LA MOTTE & P.E. DICORLETO. 1994. Alpha-tocopherol inhibits agonist-induced monocytic cell adhesion to cultured human endothelial cells. J. Clin. Invest. **94:** 592–600.

133. MARUI, N., M.K. OFFERMANN, R. SWERLICK *et al.* 1993. Vascular cell adhesion molecule-1 (VCAM-1) gene transcription and expression are regulated through an antioxidant-sensitive mechanism in human vascular endothelial cells. J. Clin. Invest. **92:** 1866–1874.

134. ORTHNER, C.L., G.M. RODGERS & L.A. FITZGERALD. 1995. Pyrrolidine dithiocarbamate abrogates tissue factor (TF) expression by endothelial cells: evidence implicating nuclear factor-kappa β in TF induction by diverse agonists. Blood. **86:** 436–443.

135. SCHINDLER, U. & V.R. BAICHWAL. 1994. Three NF-kappa B binding sites in the human E-selectin gene required for maximal tumor necrosis factor alpha-induced expression. Mol. Cell Biol. **14:** 5820–5831.

136. HOOFT VAN HUIJSDUIJNEN, R., R. PESCINI & J.F. DELAMARTER. 1993. Two distinct NF-kappa B complexes differing in their larger subunit bind the E-selectin promoter kappa B element. Nucleic Acids Res. **21:** 3711–3717.

137. COLLINS, T., M.A. READ, A.S. NEISH, M.Z. WHITLEY, D. THANOS & T. MANIATIS. 1995. Transcriptional regulation of endothelial cell adhesion molecules: NF-kappa B and cytokine-inducible enhancers. FASEB J. **9:** 899–909.

138. PESCINI, R., W. KASZUBSKA, J. WHELAN, J.F. DELAMARTER & R. HOOFT VAN HUIJSDUIJNEN. 1994. ATF-aO, a novel variant of the ATF/CREB transcription factor family, forms a dominant transcription inhibitor in ATF-a heterodimers. J. Biol. Chem. **269:** 1159–1165.

139. LEWIS, H., W. KASZUBSKA, J.F. DELAMARTER & J. WHELAN. 1994. Cooperativity between two NF-kappa B complexes, mediated by high-mobility-group protein I(Y), is essential for cytokine-induced expression of the E-selectin promoter. Mol. Cell Biol. **14:** 5701–5709.

140. NEISH, A.S., A.J. WILLIAMS, H.J. PALMER, M.Z. WHITLEY & T. COLLINS. 1992. Functional analysis of the human vascular cell adhesion molecule 1 promoter. J. Exp. Med. **176:** 1583–1593.

141. IADEMARCO, M.F., J.J. McQUILLAN, G.D. ROSEN & D.C. DEAN. 1992. Characterization of the promoter for vascular cell adhesion molecule-1 (VCAM-1). J. Biol. Chem. **267:** 16323–16329.

142. SHU, H.B., A.B. AGRANOFF, E.G. NABEL *et al.* 1993. Differential regulation of vascular cell adhesion molecule 1 gene expression by specific NF-kappa B subunits in endothelial and epithelial cells. Mol. Cell Biol. **13:** 6283–6289.

143. NEISH, A.S., L.M. KHACHIGIAN, A. PARK, V.R. BAICHWAL & T. COLLINS. 1995. Sp1 is a component of the cytokine-inducible enhancer in the promoter of vascular cell adhesion molecule-1. J. Biol. Chem. **270:** 28903–28909.

144. NEISH, A.S., M.A. READ, D. THANOS, R. PINE, T. MANIATIS & T. COLLINS. 1995. Endothelial interferon regulatory factor 1 cooperates with NF-kB as a transcriptional activator of vascular cell adhesion molecule 1. Mol. Cell Biol. **15:** 2558–2569.

145. LEDEBUR, H.C. & T.P. PARKS. 1995. Transcriptional regulation of the intercellular adhesion molecule-1 gene by inflammatory cytokines in human endothelial cells—Essential roles of a variant NF-kappa B site and p65 homodimers. J. Biol. Chem. **270:** 933–943.

146. PARRY, G.C. & N. MACKMAN. 1994. A set of inducible genes expressed by activated hu-

man monocytic and endothelial cells contain kappa B-like sites that specifically bind c-Rel-p65 heterodimers. J. Biol. Chem. **269:** 20823–20825.

147. HOU, J., V. BAICHWAL & Z. CAO. 1994. Regulatory elements and transcription factors controlling basal and cytokine-induced expression of the gene encoding intercellular adhesion molecule 1. Proc. Natl. Acad. Sci. USA **91:** 11641–11645.

148. LOOK, D.C., M.R. PELLETIER & M.J. HOLTZMAN. 1994. Selective interaction of a subset of interferon-gamma response element-binding proteins with the intercellular adhesion molecule-1 (ICAM-1) gene promoter controls the pattern of expression on epithelial cells. J. Biol. Chem. **269:** 8952–8958.

149. ROEBUCK, K.A., A. RAHMAN, V. LAKSHMINARAYANAN, K. JANAKIDEVI & A.B. MALIK. 1995. H_2O_2 and tumor necrosis factor-alpha activate intercellular adhesion molecule 1 (ICAM-1) gene transcription through distinct cis-regulatory elements within the ICAM-1 promoter. J. Biol. Chem. **270:** 18966–18974.

150. BIERHAUS, A., Y. ZHANG, Y. BENG et al. 1995. Mechanism of the tumor necrosis factor alpha-mediated induction of endothelial tissue factor. J. Biol. Chem. **270:** 26419–26432.

151. MACKMAN, N. 1995. Regulation of the tissue factor gene. FASEB J. **9:** 883–889.

152. MOLL, T., M. CZYZ, H. HOLZMULLER et al. 1995. Regulation of the tissue factor promoter in endothelial cells. Binding of NF kappa B-, AP-1-, and Sp1-like transcription factors. J. Biol. Chem. **270:** 3849–3857.

153. AHMAD, M., N. MARUI, R.W. ALEXANDER & R.M. MEDFORD. 1995. Cell type-specific transactivation of the VCAM-1 promoter through an NF-kappa B enhancer motif. J. Biol. Chem. **270:** 8976–8983.

154. JONES, K., C. RIVERA, C. SGADARI et al. 1995. Infection of human endothelial cells with Epstein-Barr virus. J. Exp. Med. **182:** 1213–1221.

155. ALMEIDA, G.D., C.D. PORADA, S. ST JEOR & J.L. ASCENSAO. 1994. Human cytomegalovirus alters interleukin-6 production by endothelial cells. Blood **83:** 370–376.

156. FAN, S.T., K. HSIA & T.S. EDGINGTON. 1994. Upregulation of human immunodeficiency virus-1 in chronically infected monocytic cell line by both contact with endothelial cells and cytokines. Blood **84:** 1567–1572.

157. FAN, J., H.Z. BASS & J.L. FAHEY. 1993. Elevated IFN-gamma and decreased IL-2 gene expression are associated with HIV infection. J. Immunol. **151:** 5031–5040.

158. SAMANIEGO, F., P.D. MARKHAM, R.C. GALLO & B. ENSOLI. 1995. Inflammatory cytokines induce AIDS-Kaposi's sarcoma-derived spindle cells to produce and release basic fibroblast growth factor and enhance Kaposi's sarcoma-like lesion formation in nude mice. J. Immunol. **154:** 3582–3592.

159. FIORELLI, V., R. GENDELMAN, F. SAMANIEGO, P.D. MARKHAM & B. ENSOLI. 1995. Cytokines from activated T cells induce normal endothelial cells to acquire the phenotypic and functional features of AIDS-Kaposi's sarcoma spindle cells. J. Clin. Invest. **95:** 1723–1734.

160. KAPLANSKI, G., N. TEYSSEIRE, C. FARNARIER et al. 1995. IL-6 and IL-8 production from cultured human endothelial cells stimulated by infection with Rickettsia conorii a cell-associated IL-1alpha-dependent pathway. J. Clin. Invest. **96:** 2839–2844.

161. YAO, L., V. BENGUALID, F.D. LOWY, J.J. GIBBONS, V.B. HATCHER & J.W. BERMAN. 1995. Internalization of Staphylococcus aureus by endothelial cells induces cytokine gene expression. Infect. Immun. **63:** 1835–1839.

162. BRADLEY, J.R., D. WILKS & D. RUBENSTEIN. 1994. The vascular endothelium in septic shock. J. Infect. **28:** 1–10.

163. VON ASMUTH, E.J., M.A. DENTENER, V. BAZIL, M.G. BOUMA, J.F. LEEUWENBERG & W.A. BUURMAN. 1993. Anti-CD14 antibodies reduce responses of cultured human endothelial cells to endotoxin. Immunology **80:** 78–83.

164. PUGIN, J., C.C. SCHURER MALY, D. LETURCQ, A. MORIARTY, R.J. ULEVITCH & P.S. TOBIAS.

1993. Lipopolysaccharide activation of human endothelial and epithelial cells is mediated by lipopolysaccharide-binding protein and soluble CD14. Proc. Natl. Acad. Sci. USA **90:** 2744–2748.

165. HAZIOT, A., G.W. RONG, J. SILVER & S.M. GOYERT. 1993. Recombinant soluble CD14 mediates the activation of endothelial cells by lipopolysaccharide. J. Immunol. **151:** 1500–1507.

166. READ, M.A., S.R. CORDLE, R.A. VEACH, C.D. CARLISLE & J. HAWIGER. 1993. Cell-free pool of CD14 mediates activation of transcription factor NF-kappa B by lipopolysaccharide in human endothelial cells. Proc. Natl. Acad. Sci. USA **90:** 9887–9891.

167. GOLDBLUM, S.E., T.W. BRANN, X. DING, J. PUGIN & P.S. TOBIAS. 1994. Lipopolysaccharide (LPS)-binding protein and soluble CD14 function as accessory molecules for LPS-induced changes in endothelial barrier function, in vitro. J. Clin. Invest. **93:** 692–702.

168. PUGIN, J., R.J. ULEVITCH & P.S. TOBIAS. 1993. A critical role for monocytes and CD14 in endotoxin-induced endothelial cell activation. J. Exp. Med. **178:** 2193–2200.

169. WILLIMANN, K., H. MATILE, N.A. WEISS & B.A. IMHOF. 1995. In vivo sequestration of Plasmodium falciparum-infected human erythrocytes: a severe combined immunodeficiency mouse model for cerebral malaria. J. Exp. Med. **182:** 643–653.

170. CHIRIVI, R.G., M.I. NICOLETTI, A. REMUZZI & R. GIAVAZZI. 1994. Cytokines and cell adhesion molecules in tumor-endothelial cell interaction and metastasis. Cell Adhes. Commun. **2:** 219–224.

171. REMUZZI, G. & P. RUGGENENTI. 1995. The hemolytic uremic syndrome. Kidney. Int. 48: 2–19.

172. VAN DE KAR, N.C., L.A. MONNENS, M.A. KARMALI & V.W. VAN HINSBERGH. 1992. Tumor necrosis factor and interleukin-1 induce expression of the verocytotoxin receptor globotriaosylceramide on human endothelial cells: implications for the pathogenesis of the hemolytic uremic syndrome. Blood **80:** 2755–2764.

173. SARMA, V., F.W. WOLF, R.M. MARKS, T.B. SHOWS & V.M. DIXIT. 1992. Cloning of a novel tumor necrosis factor-alpha-inducible primary response gene that is differentially expressed in development and capillary tube-like formation in vitro. J. Immunol. **148:** 3302–3312.

174. WAKABAYASHI, H., P.G. CAVANAUGH & G.L. NICOLSON. 1995. Purification and identification of mouse lung microvessel endothelial cell-derived chemoattractant for lung-metastasizing murine RAW117 large-cell lymphoma cells: identification as mouse monocyte chemotactic protein 1. Cancer Res. **55:** 4458–4464.

175. LIENARD, D., P. EWALENKO, J.J. DELMOTTE, N. RENARD & F.J. LEJEUNE. 1992. High-dose recombinant tumor necrosis factor alpha in combination with interferon gamma and melphalan in isolation perfusion of the limbs for melanoma and sarcoma. J. Clin. Oncol. **10:** 52–60.

176. TAKEYA, M., T. YOSHIMURA, E.J. LEONARD & K. TAKAHASHI. 1993. Detection of monocyte chemoattractant protein-1 in human atherosclerotic lesions by an anti-monocyte chemoattractant protein-1 monoclonal antibody. Hum. Pathol. **24:** 534–539.

177. CLINTON, S.K., J.C. FLEET, H. LOPPNOW *et al.* 1991. Interleukin-1 gene expression in rabbit vascular tissue in vivo. Am. J. Pathol. **138:** 1005–1014.

178. LIUZZO, G., L.M. BIASUCCI, J.R. GALLIMORE *et al.* 1994. The prognostic value of C-reactive protein and serum amyloid a protein in severe unstable angina. N. Engl. J. Med. **331:** 417–424.

179. BACH, F.H., S.C. ROBSON, C. FERRAN *et al.* 1994. Endothelial cell activation and thromboregulation during xenograft rejection. Immunol. Rev. **141:** 5–30.

180. CARVALHO, D., C.O.S. SAVAGE, C.M. BLANCK & J.D. PEARSON. 1996. IgG antiendothelial cell autoantibodies from scleroderma patients induce leukocyte adhesion to human vascular endothelial cells in vitro. J. Clin. Invest. **97:** 111–119.

181. SIMANTOV, R., J.M. LASALA, S.K. LO, A.E. GHARAVI, L.R. SAMMARITANO & J.E. SALMON. 1995. Activation of cultured vascular endothelial cells by antiphospholipid antibodies. J. Clin. Invest. **96:** 2211–2219.

182. DEL PAPA, N., L. GUIDALI, M. SIRONI *et al.* 1996. Anti-endothelial lgG antibodies from Wegener's granulomatosis bind to human endothelial cells in vitro and induce adhesion molecule expression and cytokine secretion. Arthritis Rheum. In press.

183. GEARING, A.J. & W. NEWMAN. 1993. Circulating adhesion molecules in disease. Immunol. Today **14:** 506–512.

Evidence of Differential Mycobacterial Growth and Modulation of Mycobactericidal Property by Glucoaminylmuramyl Dipeptide in Murine Macrophages[a]

NANDAGOPAL VENKATAPRASAD[b]

Medical Research Council
Tuberculosis and Related Infections Unit
Hammersmith Hospital
London W12 0NN, United Kingdom

INTRODUCTION

Muramyl dipeptide (MDP) is widely used as an adjuvant and its minimal requirements as an adjuvant was discovered in 1974.[1,2] It is also known that several analogues of synthetic adjuvants of MDP (including glucosaminylmuramyl dipeptide) had increased nonspecific immunity to *Klebsiella pneumonia*.[3] Notably, glucosaminylmuramyl dipeptide (GMDP) has been shown to be effective as immunotherapy of postoperative complications, adjuvants for HIV gp120, or in general for viral vaccines.[4–6] Mononuclear phagocytes of monocyte-macrophage lineage are involved in the elimination of intracellular pathogens like *Mycobacterium tuberculosis*. The documented evidence indicates that mononuclear phagocytes are capable of generation of a reactive oxygen intermediates (ROI) system to eliminate the intracellular pathogens.[7,8] Johnston and colleagues have shown that human leukocytes lacking myeloperoxidase enzyme are not capable of generating O_2^- and hence develop chronic granulomatous disease (CGD).[7] Murine macrophages are also capable of generation of superoxide anion (O_2^-), which is one of the important components of the ROI system. MDP activates murine macrophages to kill *Candida albicans*[9] or chronic infection with *Mycobacterium intracellulare* in mice.[10] This study intended to evaluate GMDP as a potential immunomodulator by studying the generation of O_2^- *in vitro* and its effects on activation of mycobactericidal properties of murine macrophages.

[a]This work supported by Peptech (UK) Ltd, Gloucestershire, United Kingdom.

[b]Address correspondence to: Dr. N. Venkataprasad, MRC Tuberculosis & Related Infections Unit, Hammersmith Hospital, Du Cane Road, London, W12 0NN, United Kingdom. Telephone, (44) 181 383 3785; Fax, (44) 181 383 2064; Email, nvenkata@rpms.ac.uk.

MATERIALS AND METHODS

Animals

Female mice, 8–10 weeks old, from inbred strains of BALB/c, C57/B10, or CBA were purchased from Biological Science Unit, Royal Postgraduate Medical School, Hammersmith Hospital (London, UK).

Injection of GMDP and Preparation of Splenic, Peritoneal Adherent Cells for in Vitro *Functions*

Doses of 400 μg GMDP (Peptech, UK) or 100 μg MDP (Sigma) per mouse was given either intraperitoneally or subcutaneously. After 18 h, spleens were removed and collected in bijou bottles containing 3 ml culture medium (RPMI 1640, 2 mM L-glutamine, 5×10^{-5} M 2-mercaptoethanol). Single-cell suspensions was prepared using a syringe plunger to disrupt spleen. Peritoneal exudate cells (PEC) were harvested at 18 h after injection and collected in bijou bottles containing 3–4 ml culture medium (RPMI 1640, 100 U/ml penicillin, 2 mM L-glutamine, 5×10^{-5} M 2-mercaptoethanol). Using a 10-ml pipette, the cell suspension was transferred into 20-ml universal tubes containing 3 ml of culture medium. The cells were centrifuged at $400 \times g$ at room temperature for 5 min. The cell pellet was resuspended by tapping the universal and by adding NH_4Cl solution to cell pellets to lyse red blood cells at 37°C for 5–10 min. Ten ml of medium was added to each universal and cells were washed three times by centrifugation at $400 \times g$ for 5 min at room temperature. Fresh culture medium was added between centrifugations. The viable cells were counted using the trypan blue exclusion method and the viability of the cells were adjusted to $1–2 \times 10^6$/ml of RPMI 1640 with 10% fetal calf serum (FCS) and 100 ml per well was added to 96-well flatbottom plate. After a 90-min incubation at 37°C in 5% CO_2 the nonadherent cells were removed. A portion of cells were subsequently stimulated with GMDP for overnight.

J774 murine macrophage cell line is an actively dividing cell line. The active cell division is controlled by maintaining the cell line in RPMI medium containing 1% FCS. The cell number is adjusted by counting to 1×10^6 cells/ml of RPMI. A 100-μl aliquot of this cell suspension was added to the 96-well flatbottom plate. J774 macrophage cells were stimulated with analogues of MDP overnight, after maintaining the cell line for 48 h at 1% FCS containing RPMI 1640. The stimulated cells were washed three to four times with serum-free RPMI 1640 medium, then cells were ready for superoxide anion production and infection with mycobacteria.

Superoxide Anion Assay

This was performed following a previously described method.[9] Murine macrophages were collected either from the peritoneum or from spleen cells. After incubation at 37°C for 90 min, the nonadherent cells were removed by washing three times with media and stimulated with MDP or GMDP at various concentrations overnight. Then cells were washed three times with phenol red–free Hanks' Balanced Salt Solution (HBSS). A reagent mixture was prepared containing phorbol myristate acetate (PMA, 1 μg/ml, Sigma, UK), ferricytochrome c (1 mg/ml, Sigma, UK), without or with superoxide dismutase (SOD, 30 μg/ml, Sigma, UK) in HBSS. Cells were incubated with 100 μl of the reagent mixture at 37°C for 90 min before reading optical densities at 570 nm (Titertek plus MS212, Austria). The difference in optical density with and without SOD was converted to nanomoles per 10^5 cells using the extinction coefficient: 2.1×10^4 M^{-1} cm^{-1}.

Infection of Murine Macrophages in Vitro

After sonicating mycobacteria stock for 10 sec, an inoculum of 10^6 CFU/ml of bacteria as final concentration of bacteria in RPMI 1640 with 5% FCS serum was made without any antibiotics. Then 100 μl per well was added to the wells containing macrophages for infection and incubated at 37°C for 2 h. After the infection, the uninfected extracellular bacteria were removed by repeated washing with the media. Some of the infected cultures were further stimulated with GMDP and incubated further in some experiments. The infected macrophage cultures were harvested at various time points and the supernatants of the cultures are collected separately in cryo nunc tubes and the cells adherent to the plate were wrapped with cling film are stored at –20°C. These cells and supernatants were subsequently assessed for viability of organisms by a colony-forming unit (CFU) assay.

Colony Forming Unit Assay

The cell lysate were prepared by treating the adherent cells with 110 μl of 7H9 broth and 40 μl of 0.25% sodium dodecyl sulfate (SDS). The cell lysis solution was left for 10–15 min. Subsequently, wells containing adherent cells were scraped with pipette tips and mixed with 50 μl of 20% BSA solution in order to neutralize SDS in the cell lysate. Supernatants were thawed and diluted appropriately and plated as 30-μl droplets onto 7H11 agar plates like the cell lysates. After drying the droplet, plates were incubated at 37°C. The CFUs were counted after 3–4 weeks of incubation.

RESULTS

Superoxide Anion Levels in Murine Macrophages

The generation of superoxide anion (O_2^-) has been shown to be one of the inflammatory responses exhibited by macrophages. The effect of various doses of GMDP and MDP (0.2, 1, 5, 25, and 50 μg/ml) in *in vitro* overnight stimulation to produce O_2^- from these tissue macrophages (møs) was investigated. A modulation of O_2^- levels in these different tissue møs was revealed in this study (FIG. 1). FIGURE 1 shows data from only two concentrations of GMDP and MDP. J774 mø cell line and peritoneal mø produced similar spontaneous levels of O_2^-, whereas splenic mø produced

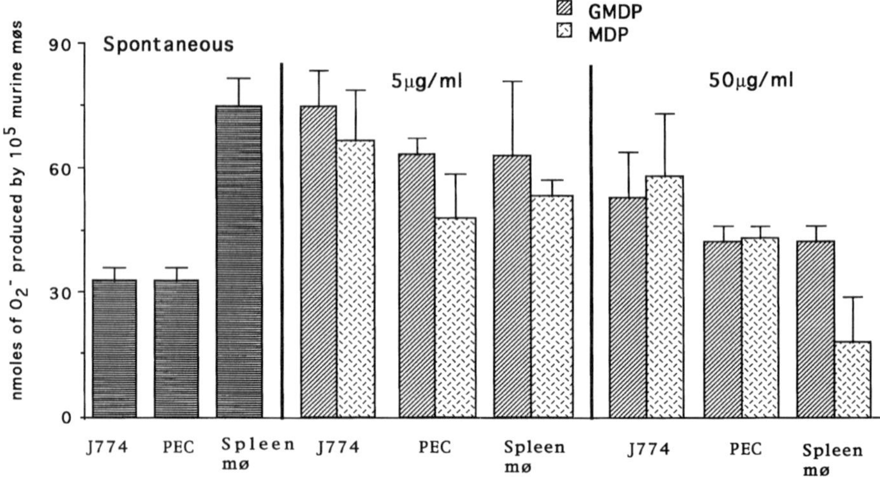

FIGURE 1. Comparison of nanomoles of superoxide anion (O_2^-) production per 10^5 J774 murine mø cell line, adherent splenic møs, and peritoneal exudate cells (PEC) per 96 well. Data shown represent mean average ± S.D. from three independent experiments from two or three BALB/c mice in each group.

higher levels of O_2^- than other types of møs. Optimal higher levels of O_2^- were produced with 5 µg/ml in J774 mø cell line and PEC, but not in splenic møs when compared with spontaneous levels. At 50 µg/ml of GMDP, there was a small effect on J774 mø cell line or peritoneal mø, but significant reduction in the O_2^- level from splenic møs in comparison with spontaneous levels.

Microbicidal Activity of Murine Macrophages

It is known that GMDP is an immunomodulatory agent and we intend to investigate the effect of GMDP *in vivo* and as well *in vitro* on microbicidal activity of mycobacteria-infected J774 mø cell line, splenic, and peritoneal møs.

J774 Murine Macrophage Cell Line

J774 mø cell line is permissive to BCG-P growth. Also there was a dose-dependent type growth inhibition of BCG-P in the J774 mø cell line, when GMDP was added to infected møs (FIG. 2). Under a similar condition, J774 mø cell line was also permissive for replication of *M. tuberculosis* (H37RV), and *M. smegmatis.* GMDP inhibited the growth of *M. tuberculosis* and *M. smegmatis* in the J774 mø cell line (FIG. 3). The microbicidal activity of the J774 mø cell line was consistent when GMDP was given *in vitro* before and after infection either at low dose of GMDP (2 µg/ml) for BCG-P and *M. smegmatis* or higher dose of GMDP (40 µg/ml) for *M. tuberculosis* (FIG. 3).

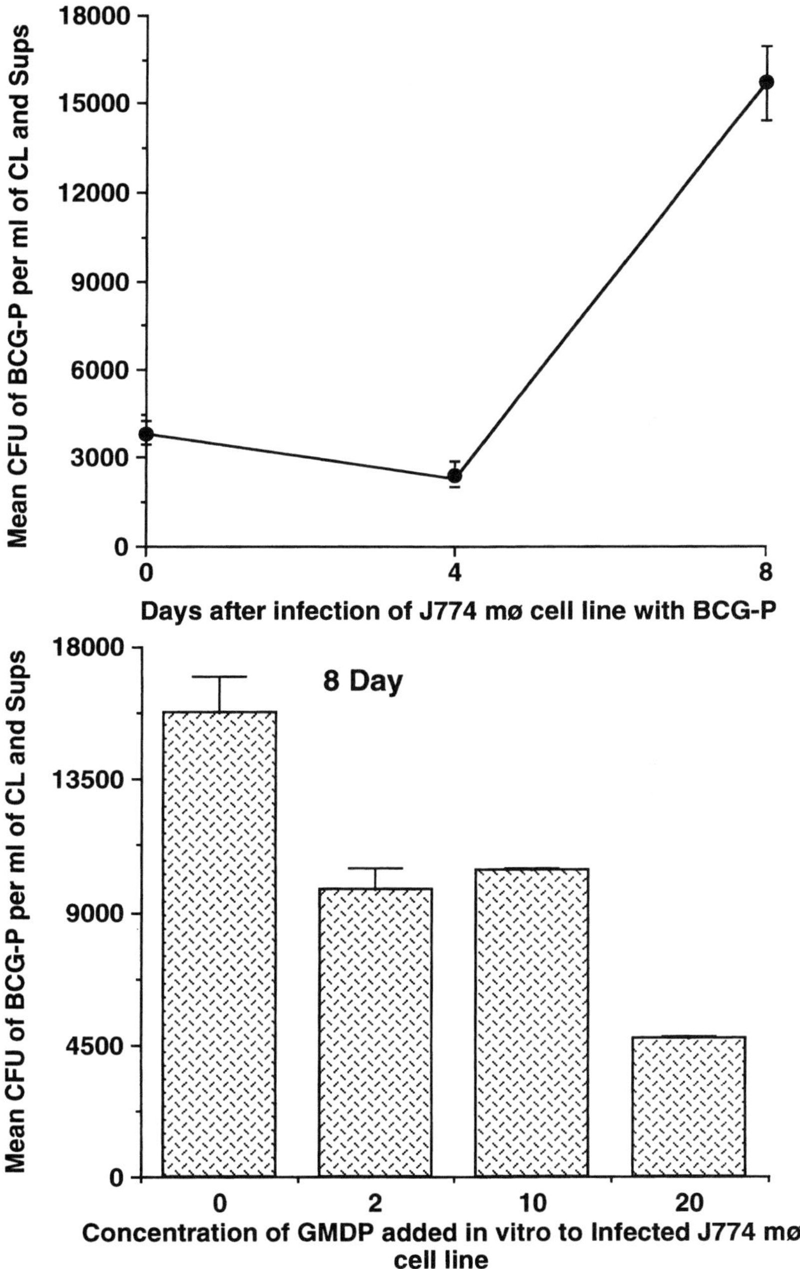

FIGURE 2. (*Top*) Growth of *M. bovis* (BCG-Pasteur strain) in J774 murine macrophage (mø) cell line. (*Bottom*) Effect of GMDP at various concentrations on growth of BCG-P in J774 mø cell line. Each value is a mean ± S.D. per ml of cell lysate and supernatants of two experiments.

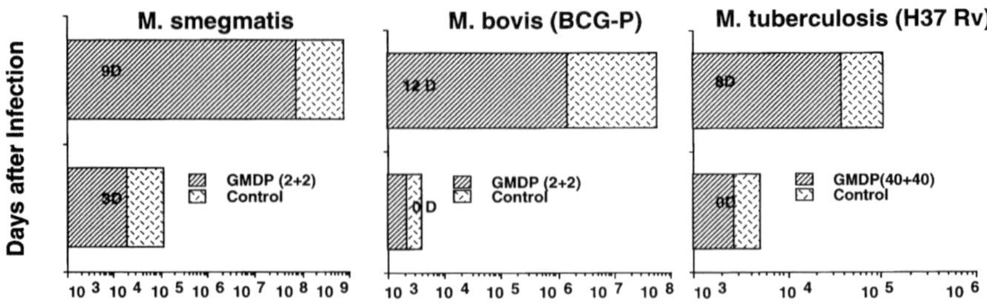

Mean CFU per ml in J774 Mø cell line CL and Sups

FIGURE 3. Growth of *M. smegmatis, M. bovis* (BCG-P), and *M. tuberculosis* in J774 murine macrophage (mø) cell line. GMDP (2 or 40 µg/ml) was given before and after infection with J774 mø cell line and indicated as GMDP (2+2 or 40+40 µg/ml) as shown in the insert. Each data point is mean per ml of cell lysate and supernatants from two to three experiments.

Splenic Macrophages

Splenic møs from *in vivo* GMDP (400 µg/mouse)– or MDP (100 µg/mouse)– treated BALB/c mice were permissive to *M. tuberculosis* growth, similar to PBS-treated mouse splenic møs (FIG. 4). This phenomenon was not identical in both BALB/c and C57/B10 strains of mice. However, growth inhibition of *M. tuberculosis* was seen in splenic mø from GMDP (400 µg/mouse) *in vivo* treated BALB/c mice, only when subsequently treated *in vitro* with 50 µg/ml of GMDP when compared with PBS-treated mice on 8-day cultures (FIG. 5). *M. tuberculosis* growth was consistently low in both *in vivo* and subsequent *in vitro* treatment of GMDP in splenic møs from C57/B10 mice.

Unlike J774 mø cell line, splenic møs were not permissive to BCG-P replication. On the other hand, when splenic møs from BALB/c, C57/B10, and CBA/ca strains were infected with BCG-P, a differential growth pattern was observed. There was also a difference in the initial infection capacity and subsequent time-dependent growth over a 6-day period. But BCG-P growth was enhanced when GMDP (2 µg/ml) was given before infection to splenic møs in 6-day culture (FIG. 6). Splenic møs were permissive to *M. smegmatis* growth as well, but did not affect the growth of *M. smegmatis* when these møs were preincubated with similar doses of GMDP over an 8-day incubation period (data not shown).

Peritoneal Exudate Macrophages

Peritoneal møs were permissive to *M. tuberculosis* and *M. avium,* but not to BCG-P growth. *In vivo* GMDP (100 µg/mouse)–treated mice peritoneal macrophages inhibited growth of *M. tuberculosis,* but did not influence the growth of *M. avium* over a 21-day culture period (FIG. 7). However, peritoneal exudate macrophages (PEC) from *in vivo* GMDP (100 µg/mouse) treated mice decreased the rate of reduction of BCG-P growth during the same length of culture (FIG. 7). Further addition of GMDP

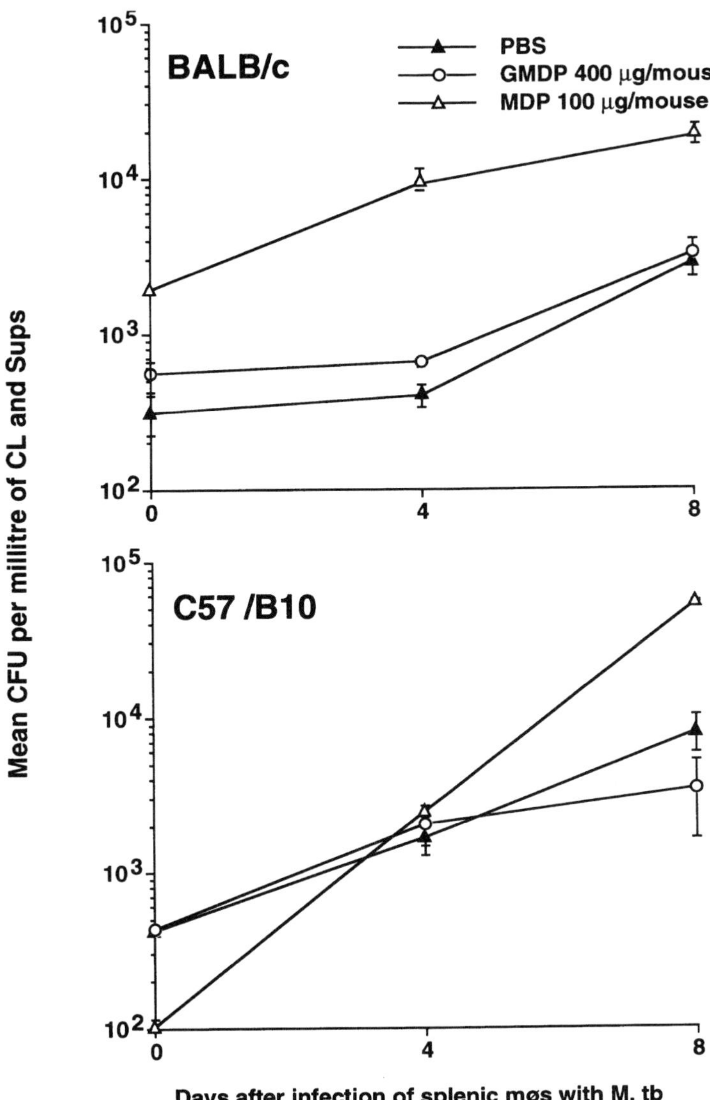

FIGURE 4. Growth of *M. tuberculosis* (H37Rv) in splenic mø from BALB/c and C57/B10 strains of mice treated with PBS or 400 or 100 µg/mouse of GMDP or MDP, respectively. Spleen cells were harvested after overnight treatment with the agents. Data shown are mean ± S.D. per ml of cell lysate and supernatants from triplicate value from a representative experiment.

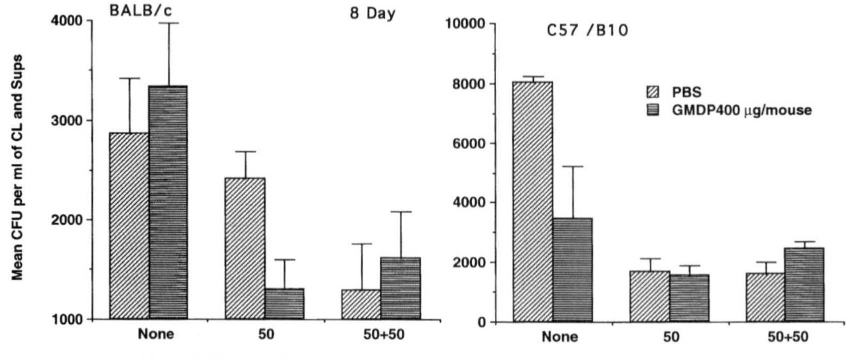

FIGURE 5. Inhibition of *M. tuberculosis* growth on Day 8 in splenic mø from BALB/c or C57/B10 strain of mice treated with PBS or 400 µg/mouse of GMDP. *In vitro* 50 µg/ml (50) of GMDP before infection and another 50 µg/ml (50+50) of GMDP after infection was given. Data shown are mean ± S.D. per ml of cell lysate and supernatants from two experiments.

(50 µg/ml) *in vitro* (before or/and after infection) did not alter *M. tuberculosis* growth in GMDP-treated groups (TABLE 1). The presence of GMDP (50 µg/ml) with *M. tuberculosis,* BCG-P, and *M. avium* (FIG. 8) or *M. smegmatis* (2 µg/ml of GMDP) (data not shown) did not influence their viability in the tissue culture medium in the absence of møs. Thus suggesting that GMDP do not possess direct mycobactericidal activity.

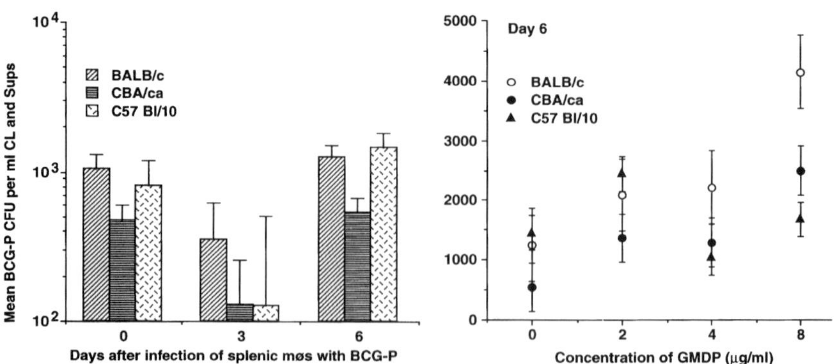

FIGURE 6. Growth of *M. bovis* (BCG-P) in splenic mø from three different strains of mice. Each data point is mean ± S.D. per ml of cell lysate and supernatants from three experiments. (*Left*) growth kinetics of BCG-P and (*Right*) growth of increment of BCG-P due to overnight (O/N) stimulation with various doses of GMDP before infection.

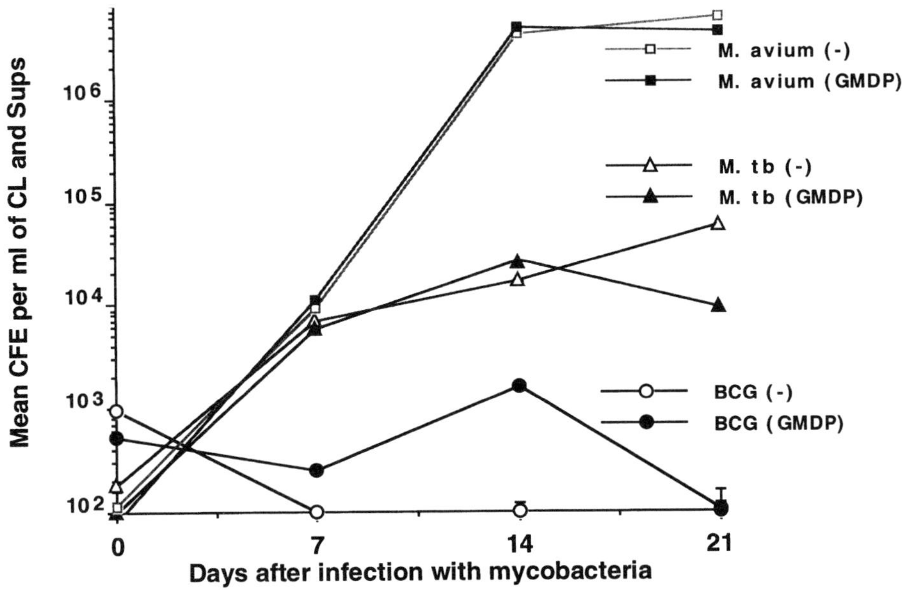

FIGURE 7. Growth kinetic of *M. tuberculosis, M. avium,* and BCG-P in peritoneal exudate cells (PEC) from BALB/c mice treated either with PBS or 100 µg/mouse of GMDP. PEC were isolated following 18 h after injection of GMDP or PBS. Each data point is mean ± S.D. per ml of cell lysate and supernatants from a triplicate value from a single experiment.

DISCUSSION

Mononuclear phagocytes (monocyte-macrophage lineage) are very important components in the pathogenesis of chronic lung diseases. These monocyte-macrophages are activated by a stimulus (like antigen or immunomodulatory agents of bacterial products) to produce inflammatory and proinflammatory response. The precise

TABLE 1. Growth of *Mycobacterium tuberculosis* in Mouse Peritoneal Macrophages at 21 Days after Infection *in Vitro*[a]

In Vivo treatment	PBS		GMDP (100 µg/mouse)	
In vitro addition before infection overnight	None	50 µg/ml	None	50 µg/ml
In vitro addition after infection				
None	5.92 ± 0.91	6.872 ± 0.42	0.932 ± 0.02	0.872 ± 0.02
50 µg/ml	13.982 ± 1.1	7.892 ± 0.45	1.162 ± 0.14	0.822 ± 0.11

[a]Values in table are mean ± S.D. × 10^4 Colony forming units per ml of cell lysate and supernatant.

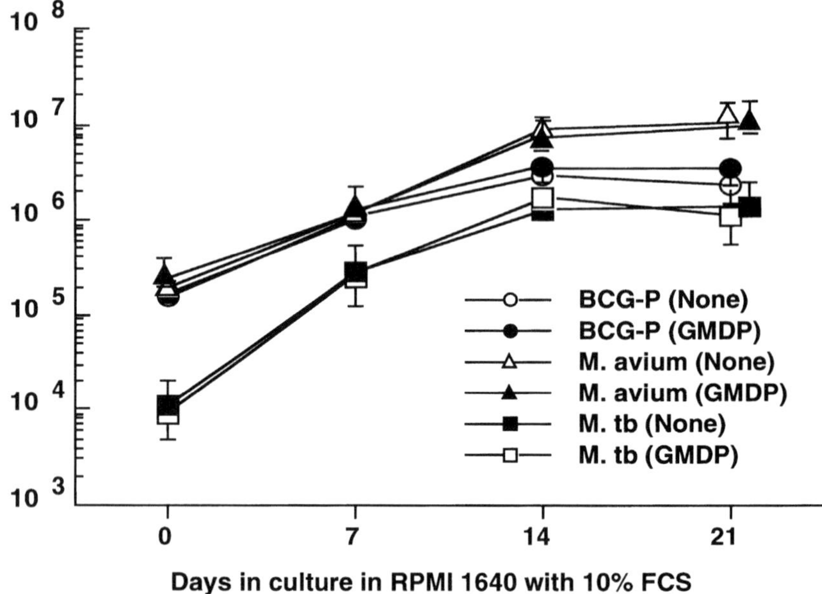

FIGURE 8. Growth of mycobacteria in the absence of macrophages. Each data is a mean ± S.D. per ml of supernatants from triplicate values from a single experiment.

role of macrophages in the pathogenesis of granulomatous lung diseases has been extensively reviewed by several investigators.[11,12] There are several reports suggesting that the activation of macrophage *in vivo* and *in vitro* to produce reactive oxygen intermediates is essential for elimination of intracellular killing for *Trypanosoma cruzi,*[13] *Toxoplasma gondii* (*T. gondii*),[14] and promastigotes of Leishmania.[15] However, Catterall and coworkers[16] demonstrated *T. gondii* was eliminated by nonoxidative pathway in human alveolar and peritoneal macrophages, unlike in the murine system.

We and others[17,18] showed similar levels of O_2^- anion production in JA4, a subclone obtained from the J774.1 cell line, composed of a heterogeneous mixture of cells. It was suggested that O_2^- anions are more crucial for intracellular killing of virulent *Listeria monocytogenes* than nitric oxide. Also, the avirulent strains of *L. monocytogenes* are eliminated by a different pathway from that of the virulent strain. Murray demonstrated a similar effect in the J774G8 clone when infected with *Leishmania donovani* (visceral etiology) and *L. tropica* (cutaneous etiology).[19] The author also suggests that the O_2^- anion played a considerable role in the intracellular killing of the promastigotes from the parasite Leishmania. It is our interest to investigate the effect of GMDP *in vivo* on mouse peritoneal macrophage similar to that which was already documented by Cummings and colleagues.[9] But to our surprise we found that in BALB/c strain of mice by using a similar concentration of GMDP (100 μg/mouse), the generation of O_2^- anion was less than in the cells from PBS-treated (control) mice. This phenomenon was consistent with two strains of mice that we have used (BALB/c and C57/B10 strains) and by both routes of administration of GMDP (intraperitoneal and subcutaneous).[20] The significant finding in the previous report[20] is the modulation of production of O_2^- anion by GMDP in resident murine macrophages when given *in vivo,* as well as modulation of activation of møs either due to priming or infection of mice with BCG-P or due to MDP administration. When administered *in vivo* at a concentration between 6 and 25 µg/mouse, GMDP produces a significant increase in the generation of O_2^- anion in the resident mouse peritoneal macrophages.[20] In this study GMDP has a similar effect on the J774 murine macrophage cell line when stimulated *in vitro.* However, mouse peritoneal and splenic macrophages stimulated with lower concentrations of GMDP used *in vitro* produced a small increase in the level of O_2^- anion, when PMA was used as restimulating agent. Proctor used a similarly high concentration (100 µg/ml) of LPS to inhibit the production of O_2^- anion, oxygen consumption, and killing of *S. aureus* and *E. coli* when preincubated with human neutrophils.[21] But we have shown that GMDP (at 100 µg/mouse) given *in vivo* not only inhibited growth of *M. tuberculosis* (in post-chemotherapy reactivation of tuberculosis); but also in general, infection of BALB/c mice with *M. tuberculosis,* where there was more reduction of CFU in the lung than in the spleen.[20]

In order to improve the clinical management of several infectious diseases, others have suggested muramyl dipeptide as an adjunctive to antimicrobial therapy to reduce the toxicity and severe side effects of those chemotherapeutic agents.[22] Although the exact mechanism of action of GMDP is not clear, Kaydalov and colleagues have proposed its mode of action in rat brain membrane,[23] while Zidek[24] showed edemagenic activity and proinflammatory activity in rats using similar analogues of MDP. But it was that found proinflammatory cytokines were inhibited by GMDP in mice presensitized with *Corynebacterium parvum* and challenged with LPS treatment.[25] A similar effect (i.e., modulation of cytokine production) by various derivatives of muramyl peptides was documented by Parant and colleagues.[26] GMDP also brought about significant changes in antitumor activity and in adenosine metabolism of murine macrophages[27] in the form of action of adenosine deaminase, which is linked to production of O_2^-. *In vitro,* in this study, we have demonstrated that GMDP activates murine macrophages to exhibit microbicidal property at a concentration that reduces O_2^- anion production in the *in vivo* system.[20] Probably GMDP, like MDP,[26] binds to brain membrane and macrophages[23] and modulates the proinflammatory cytokine response,[24,25] which results in antiinflammatory activity.

SUMMARY

These results show that given a source of mouse tissue macrophage, there is differential mycobacterial growth with different species of mycobacteria. This suggests that each species of mycobacteria generates a differential response in a given tissue macrophage within the same host for its survival. For example, BCG-P growth becomes permissive in the presence of GMDP in splenic and peritoneal macrophages. Whereas in the same tissue *M. tuberculosis* growth becomes non-permissive. From TABLE 2 it is evident that inhibition of inflammatory responses following *M. tuberculosis* infection leads to reduction of viable organisms in murine macrophages.

TABLE 2. Differential Growth of Mycobacterial Species in Murine Macrophages

	J774 MØ Cell Line		Spleen MØ		Peritoneal MØ	
	– GMDP	+ GMDP	– GMDP	+ GMDP	– GMDP	+ GMDP
M. smegmatis	↑	↓	↑	↔	N.D.	N.D.
M. bovis (BCG-P) after infection	↑	↓	↔	↑	↓	↑
M. tuberculosis	↑	↓	↑	↓	↑	↓
M. avium	N.D.	N.D.	N.D.	N.D.	↑	↔

Note: – GMDP, without GMDP treatment; + GMDP, with GMDP treatment; ↑, Increase; ↓, Decrease; ↔, No Effect; N.D., Not Done.

REFERENCES

1. ELLOUZ, F., A. ADAM, R. CIORBARU & E. LEDERER. 1974. Minimal structural requirements for adjuvant activity of bacterial peptidoglycan derivatives. Biochem. Biophys. Res. Commun. **59:** 1317–1325.
2. FLECK, J., M. MOCK, F. TYTGAT, C. NAUCIEL & R. MINCEK. 1974. Adjuvant activity in delayed hypersensitivity of the peptidic part of bacterial peptidoglycans. Nature **250:** 517–518.
3. CHEDID, L., M. PARANT, F. PARANT, P. LEFRANCIER, J. CHOAY & E. LEDERER. 1977. Enhancement of nonspecific immunity to *Klebsiella pneumoniae* infection by a synthetic immunoadjuvant (N-acetylmuamyl-L-alanyl-D-isoglutamine) and several analogs. Proc. Natl. Acad. Sci. USA **74:** 2089–2093.
4. BOMFORD, R., M. STAPLETON, S. WINSOR, A. McKNIGHT & T. ANDRONOVA. 1992. The control of the antibody isotype response to recombinant human immunodeficiency virus gp120 antigen by adjuvants. AIDS Res. Human Retroviruses **8:** 1765–1771.
5. BOMFORD, R. 1992. Adjuvants for viral vaccines. Med. Virol. **2:** 169–174.
6. KHAITOV, R. M., B. V. PINEGIN, A. A. BUTAKOV & T. M. ANDRONOVA. 1994. Immunotherapy of infectious postoperative complications with glucosaminylmuramyl dipeptide. *In* Immunotherapy of Infections. N. Masihi, Ed.: 205–211. Marcel Dekker, Inc. New York.
7. JOHNSTON, R. B., B. B. KEELE, H. P. MISHRA, J. E. LEHMEYER, L. S. WEBB, R. L. BAEHNER & K. V. RAJAGOPALAN. 1975. The role of superoxide anion generation in phagocytic bactericidal activity: Studies with normal and chronic granulomatous disease leukocytes. J. Clin. Invest. **55:** 1357–1372.
8. DRATH, D. B. & M. L. KARNVOSKY. 1975. Superoxide production by phagocytic leukocytes. J. Exp. Med. **141:** 257–262.
9. CUMMINGS, N. C., M. J. PABST & R. B. JOHNSTON. 1980. Activation of macrophages for enhanced release of superoxide anion and greater killing of *Candida albicans* by injection of muramyl dipeptide. J. Exp. Med. **152:** 1659–1669.
10. EDWARDS, C. K., H. B. HEDEGAARD, A. ZLOTNIK, P. R. GANGADHARAM, R. B. JOHNSTON & M. J. PABST. 1986. Chronic infection due to *Mycobacterium intracellulare* in mice: Association with macrophage release of prostaglandin E2 and reversal by injection of indomethacin, muramyl dipeptide or interferon-γ. J. Immunol. **136:** 1820–1827.
11. GARRETT, K. C., H. B. RICHERSON & G. W. HUNNINGHAKE. 1984. Mechanisms of granuloma formation. Am. Rev. Respir. Dis. **130:** 477–483.

12. HUNNINGHAKE, G. W., K. C. GARRETT, H. B. RICHERSON, J. C. FANTONE, P. A. WARD, S. I. RENNARD, P. B. BITTERMAN & R. G. CRYSTAL. 1984. Pathogenesis of the granulomatous lung diseases. Am. Rev. Respir. Dis. **130:** 476–477.

13. NATHAN, C., N. NOGUEIRA, C. JUANGBHANICH, J. ELLIS & Z. COHN. 1979. Activation of macrophages in vivo and in vitro: Correlation between hydrogen peroxide release and killing of *Trypanosoma cruzi*. J. Exp. Med. **149:** 1056–1068.

14. MURRAY, H. W., C. NATHAN & Z. A. COHN. 1980. Macrophage oxygen-dependent antimicrobial activity: IV. Role of endogenous scavengers of oxygen intermediates. J. Exp. Med. **152:** 1610–1624.

15. MURRAY, H. W. 1981. Susceptibility of Leishmania to oxygen intermediates and killing by normal macrophages. J. Exp. Med. **153:** 1302–1314.

16. CATTERALL, J. R., C. M. BLACK, J. P. LEVENTHAL, N. W. RIZK, J. S. WACHTEL & J. S. REMINGTON. 1987. Nonoxidative microbicidal activity in normal human alveolar and peritoneal macrophages. Infect. Immun. **55:** 1635–1640.

17. INOUE, S., S. ITAGAKI & F. AMANO. 1995. Intracellular killing of *Listeria monocytogenes* in the J774.1 macrophage-like cell line and the lipopolysaccharide (LPS)-resistant mutant LPS1916 cell line defective in the generation of reactive oxygen intermediates after LPS treatment. Infect. Immun. **63:** 1876–1886.

18. PABST, M. J. & R. B. JOHNSTON. 1980. Increased production of superoxide anion by macrophages exposed in vitro to muramyl dipeptide or lipopolysaccharide. J. Exp. Med. **151:** 101–114.

19. MURRAY, H. W. 1981. Interaction of Leishmania with a macrophage cell line: Correlation between intracellular killing and the generation of oxygen intermediates. J. Exp. Med. **153:** 1690–1695.

20. VENKATAPRASAD, N., P. LEDGER & J. IVANYI. 1997. The effect of glucosaminylmuramyl dipeptide (GMDP) injection to mice on the course of tuberculosis infection and in vitro superoxide anion production. Int. Arch. Allergy Immunol. **114:** 23–29.

21. PROCTOR, R. A. 1979. Endotoxin in vitro interactions with human neutrophils: Depression of chemiluminescence, oxygen consumption, superoxide production and killing. Infect. Immun. **25:** 912–921.

22. O'REILLY, T. & O. ZAK. 1992. Enhancement of the effectiveness of antimicrobial therapy by muramyl peptide immunomodulators. Clin. Infect. Dis. **14:** 1100–1109.

23. KAYDALOV, A. A., Y. N. UTKIN, T. M. ANDRONOVA, V. I. TSETLIN & V. T. IVANOV. 1989. Muramyl peptides bind specifically to rat brain membranes. FEBS Lett. **248:** 78–82.

24. ZIDEK, Z. 1992. Differences in proinflammatory activity of several immunomodulatory derivatives of muramyl dipeptide (MDP) with special reference to the mechanism of the MDP effects. Agents Actions **36:** 136–145.

25. ADELEYE, T. A., C. MORENO, J. IVANYI & R. ASTON. 1994. The modulation of tumor necrosis factor-α, interleukin-1α and glucose levels with GMDP and other analogues of muramyl dipeptide. APMIS **102:** 145–152.

26. PARANT, M. A., P. POUILLART, C. L. CONTEL, F. J. PARANT, L. A. CHEDID & G. M. BAHR. 1995. Selective modulation of lipopolysaccharide-induced death and cytokine production by various muramyl peptides. Infect. Immun. **63:** 110–115.

27. BALITSKY, K. P., V. Y. UMANSKY, A. M. TARAKHOVSKY, T. M. ANDRONOVA & V. T. IVANOV. 1989. Glucosaminylmuramyl dipeptide-induced changes in murine macrophage metabolism. Int. J. Immunopharmacol. **11:** 429–435.

Effects of Carbamazepine on Human PMN Function: Possible Role of Peripheral Benzodiazepine Receptors

E. CALDIROLI, A. M. FIETTA,[a] F. DE PONTI, M. COSENTINO,
F. MARINO, M. TADDEI, S. LECCHINI, AND G. M. FRIGO[b]

Department of Internal Medicine and Therapeutics
II Faculty of Medicine
[a]Department of Chemotherapy
I Faculty of Medicine
University of Pavia
21100 Varese VA, Italy

INTRODUCTION

Carbamazepine intake has been occasionally associated with the occurrence of immune adverse reactions during long-term treatment (for a review, see De Ponti and colleagues[1]). Recently, modifications of neutrophil leukocyte (PMN) migration, phagocytosis, and killing properties have been reported in chronic carbamazepine recipients,[2,3] but the mechanism(s) underlying these effects remain to be determined.

Indirect evidence suggests an interaction of carbamazepine with peripheral benzodiazepine receptors (pBZrs) both in the central nervous system[4,5] and in the periphery.[6] Several kinds of data are now available to support a role of pBZrs in modulating immune cell function. For example, Ro 5-4864, a pBZr agonist, was shown to act as a potent chemotactic agent on monocytes, its activity being antagonized by the peripheral pBZr antagonist, PK 11195,[7] while diazepam and Ro 5-4864 were reported to affect some PMN activities, an effect also antagonized by PK 11195.[8]

In the present study, we provide preliminary evidence indicating that carbamazepine affects human PMN function *in vitro* through the involvement of pBZrs.

MATERIALS AND METHODS

PMNs were isolated from heparinized venous blood (10 U/ml) from healthy adult volunteers by Ficoll-Hypaque density gradient centrifugation and by sedimentation using dextran. Contaminant erythrocytes in the PMN pellet were lysed with NH_4Cl solution. PMNs were then spin-washed with phosphate-buffered saline solution and finally suspended in Hanks' balanced salt solution to obtain a concentration of 2×10^7 PMN/ml. PMN viability, as determined by the trypan blue exclusion test, was always

[b]Address correspondence to: Prof. Gianmario Frigo, Department of Internal Medicine and Therapeutics, II Faculty of Medicine, University of Pavia, Via Ottorino Rossi, 9, 21100 Varese VA, Italy.

greater than 95%. Chemotaxis was assessed according to a previously described method[9] employing a modified Boyden Millipore system and *E. coli* lipopolysaccharide (LPS, 10 μg/ml) plus 5% normal serum or formyl-methionyl-leucyl-phenylalanine (FMLP; 10^{-7} M) as chemotactic stimuli. Zymosan-stimulated nitrobluetetrazolium (NBT) reduction frequency (number of cells with formazan deposits × 100/number of phagocytosing cells), phagocytosis index (mean number of zymosan particles/cell), and phagocytosis frequency (number of phagocytosing cells × 100/total cells) were measured according to Preisig and Hitzig[10] using 1×10^6 adherent cells incubated with 8×10^6 serum-opsonized zymosan particles. *C. albicans* lethality index was measured according to Leher and Cline[11] and expressed as [100 − (100 × survived/total microorganisms)]. Drug effects on PMN functions were tested following a 30-min preincubation period at 37°C. Controls consisted of PMN suspensions in the absence of each compound.

Stock solutions of carbamazepine (RBI, Natick, MA), 7-chloro-1,3-dihydro-1-methyl-5-(*p*-chlorophenyl)-2H-1,4-benzodiazepine-2-one (Ro 5-4864), and 1-(2-chlorophenyl)-N-methyl-N-(1-methylpropyl)-3-isoquinolinecarboxamide (PK 11195) (both from Sigma, St. Louis, MO) were prepared in methanol and stored at –20°C. Diluted fresh solutions were prepared just before assay.

Data were analyzed by Dunnett's test or Student's *t* test with Bonferroni's correction for multiple comparisons, as appropriate.

RESULTS

Carbamazepine (42–84 μM) inhibited chemotaxis induced by FMLP- or LPS-activated human serum (FIGS. 1 and 2). Inhibition of FMLP- and LPS-induced chemotaxis by 42 μM carbamazepine (a concentration within the therapeutic range) was 47.8±6.6 and 63.6±5.6% ($N = 16$), respectively ($p<0.01$). Phagocytosis index, phagocytosis frequency, NBT reduction frequency, and *C. albicans* lethality index were not affected by 84 μM carbamazepine (TABLE 1).

PK 11195 at a concentration of 1 μM (per se ineffective) reversed the inhibitory effect of carbamazepine on chemotaxis induced by FMLP (FIG. 1) or LPS (FIG. 2).

The effect of carbamazepine on chemotaxis induced by LPS or FMLP was mimicked by Ro 5-4864 (10 and 100 μM; FIGS. 1 and 2). Ro 5-4864 had no effect on the other parameters (TABLE 1).

DISCUSSION

The present study indicates that carbamazepine, at concentrations overlapping the therapeutic range (16.8–50.4 μM), affects some human PMN functions *in vitro*. Indeed, chemotaxis induced by LPS or FMLP was significantly inhibited already in the presence of 42 μM carbamazepine. This effect can probably be ascribed to an interaction with the pBZrs, as indicated by the fact that it was reversed by the selective antagonist PK 11195 and mimicked by the selective agonist Ro 5-4864. Accordingly, none of the PMN functions unaffected by carbamazepine was modified by Ro 5-

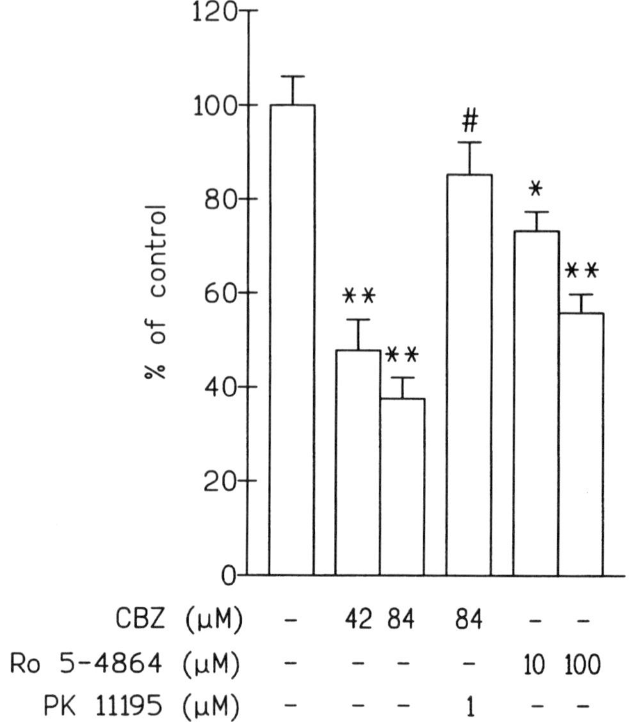

FIGURE 1. Inhibitory effect of carbamazepine (CBZ) and Ro 5-4864 on chemotaxis induced by FMLP. Note reversal by PK 11195 of the inhibitory effect of carbamazepine. Values are means ± SE (N = at least 6 experiments) and are expressed as percentage of control (48.7 ± 3.0 μm). *$p<0.05$ vs. control; **$p<0.01$ vs. control; #$p<0.001$ vs. carbamazepine alone.

4864. Thus, pBZrs seem to contribute not only to the anticonvulsant action of carbamazepine,[4,5] but also to some of the effects on immune cell function.

The fact that these effects can be observed at concentrations achieved in the clinical setting raises the question about their possible clinical relevance. Little information is available on PMN function in carbamazepine-treated patients. Epileptic patients on carbamazepine for at least two years have been reported to have increased PMN phagocytosis and killing properties,[2] while in a psychiatric setting chronic administration of this drug was associated with enhanced chemotaxis, phagocytosis, oxidative metabolism, and reduced microbicidal activity.[3] Although these clinical data are somehow difficult to reconcile and differ from the present *in vitro* data, nevertheless they clearly indicate that carbamazepine can affect human PMN function. Discrepancies may be ascribed to many factors, such as differences between acute *in vitro* and chronic *in vivo* exposure, dose and duration of treatment, and underlying disease.

Investigations on expression and role of pBZrs in PMNs in chronic carba-

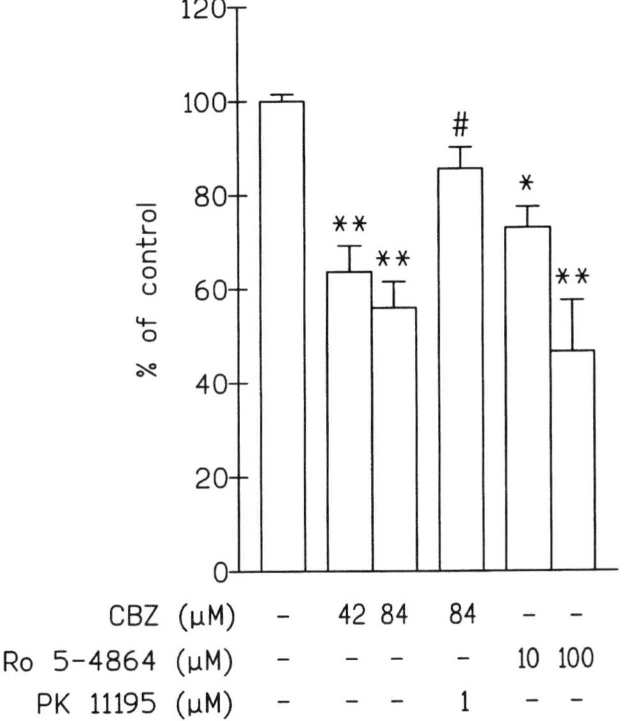

FIGURE 2. Inhibitory effect of carbamazepine (CBZ) and Ro 5-4864 on chemotaxis induced by LPS. Note reversal by PK 11195 of the inhibitory effect of carbamazepine. Values are mean±SE (N = at least 6 experiments) and are expressed as percentage of control (91.4±1.4 μM). *p<0.05 vs. control; **p<0.01 vs. control; [#]p<0.01 vs. carbamazepine alone.

TABLE 1. Effect of Carbamazepine and Ro 5-4864 on Some Human PMN Functions

	Controls	Carbamazepine (84 μM)	Ro 5-4864 (100 μM)
Phagocytosis index (N)	2.2±0.4	2.0±0.5	2.0±0.2
Phagocytosis frequency (%)	71.9±5.2	66.6±9.3	70.3±6.9
NBT reduction frequency (%)	88.9±3.2	88.3±6.0	92.1±3.7
C. albicans lethality index (%)	52.6±7.8	51.5±7.9	56.0±6.2

Values are given as mean ± SE; N = at least 3 experiments.

mazepine recipients will help to clarify the possible contribution of these receptors to the *in vivo* effects of this drug on PMN function.

ACKNOWLEDGMENTS

The authors are grateful to Marco Manstretta for his skillful technical assistance in performing the *in vitro* assays.

REFERENCES

1. DE PONTI, F., S. LECCHINI, M. COSENTINO, C. M. CASTELLETTI, A. MALESCI & G. M. FRIGO. 1993. Immunological adverse effects of anticonvulsants. What is their clinical relevance? Drug Safety **8:** 235–250.
2. PACIFICI, R., L. PARIS, S. DI CARLO, S. PICHINI & P. ZUCCARO. 1991. Immunologic aspects of carbamazepine treatment in epileptic patients. Epilepsia **32:** 122–127.
3. COSENTINO, M., A. M. FIETTA, E. CALDIROLI, F. MARINO, L. RISPOLI, M. COMELLI, S. LECCHINI & G. M. FRIGO. 1996. Assessment of lymphocyte subsets and neutrophil leucocyte function in chronic psychiatric patients on long-term drug therapy. Prog. Neuropsychopharmacol. Biol. Psychiatry **20:** 1117–1129.
4. WEISS, S. R. B., R. M. POST, J. PATEL & P. J. MARANGOS. 1985. Differential mediation of the anticonvulsant effects of carbamazepine and diazepam. Life Sci. **36:** 2413–2419.
5. WEISS, S. R. B. & R. M. POST. 1991. Contingent tolerance to carbamazepine: a peripheral-type benzodiazepine mechanism. Eur. J. Pharmacol. **193:** 159–163.
6. WEIZMAN, A., Z. TANNE, L. KARP, Y. MARTFELD, S. TYANO & M. GAVISH. 1987. Carbamazepine up-regulates the binding of [^{3}H]PK 11195 to platelets of epileptic patients. Eur. J. Pharmacol. **141:** 471–474.
7. RUFF, M. R., C. B. PERT, R. J. WEBER, L. M. WAHL, S. M. WAHL & S. M. PAUL. 1985. Benzodiazepine receptor-mediated chemotaxis of human monocytes. Science **229:** 1281–1283.
8. FINNERTY, M., T. J. MARCZYNSKI, H. J. AMIRAULT, M. URBANCIC & B. R. ANDERSEN. 1991. Benzodiazepines inhibit neutrophil chemotaxis and superoxide production in a stimulus dependent manner; PK-11195 antagonizes these effects. Immunopharmacology **22:** 185–194.
9. WILKINSON, P. C. 1977. Neutrophil leukocyte function test. Techniques. *In* Clinical Immunology. R. A. Thompson, Ed.: 201–204. Blackwell Scientific Publication. Oxford.
10. PREISIG, E. & W. H. HITZIG. 1971. Nitroblue-tetrazolium test for the detection of chronic granulomatous disease—Technical modification. Eur. J. Clin. Invest. **1:** 409–412.
11. LEHRER, R. I. & M. J. CLINE. 1969. Leukocyte myeloperoxidase deficiency and disseminated candidiasis: The role of myeloperoxidase in resistance to Candida infection. J. Clin. Invest. **48:** 1478–1488.

Human and Bovine Endothelial Cell Monolayers Are Differentially Activated for Neutrophil Transmigration by Human Plasma[a]

CHRISTIAN J. WIEDERMANN,[b] PETER SCHRATZBERGER,
STEFAN DUNZENDORFER, STEFAN KIECHL,[c]
NORBERT REINISCH, CHRISTIAN M. KÄHLER,
AND JOHANN WILLEIT[c]

Department of Internal Medicine
[c]Department of Neurology
University of Innsbruck
6020 Innsbruck, Austria

INTRODUCTION

The migration of leukocytes across the endothelial lining of blood vessels and into the interstitium can be divided experimentally into several stages.[1] The first steps comprising the initial attachment to and rolling on the endothelial cells (EC) have been demonstrated to be mediated in most cases by the selectins and their carbohydrate-rich ligands, the mucins.[1] As the leukocytes roll, they may become activated, thereby entering into the next phase of tight adhesion, in which leukocytes stop rolling, attach firmly to the EC, and spread out. These steps are mediated by the integrin family of cell adhesion molecules and result in a temperature- and divalent cation–dependent binding of leukocytes to their EC ligands, which, where they have been identified, are members of the immunoglobulin superfamily.[2]

Activation of integrins can be induced by a variety of factors. Endotoxin (LPS) or chemoattractants (e.g., FMLP) and cytokines/factors produced by host EC or leukocytes already present in the tissue (such as TNF, platelet-activating factor, and IL-8), can have this effect.[3–5] Integrin activation can also occur via an adhesion cascade, in which adhesion via one adhesion molecule pair activates another adhesion molecule on the cell surface.[6]

The transmigration step occurring subsequently has been the least investigated. Several groups have developed *in vitro* assays to study this phenomenon.[7–11] Initially, monolayers of EC were grown on connective tissue derived from amniotic membrane and used to examine the transendothelial migration (TEM) of leukocytes.[12] Later, EC monolayers were cultured on collagen matrices or microporous membranes to create transmigration assays that were more physiologic.[7–11,13] Most of the available assays

[a]This work supported by Austrian Science Funds grant number 09977 to C. J. W.

[b]Address correspondence to: Christian J. Wiedermann, M.D., Department of Internal Medicine, University of Innsbruck, Anichstrasse 35, 6020 Innsbruck, Austria.

135

enable investigation of mechanisms of transmigration under static conditions.[7–13] With the development of parallel flow chamber techniques,[14] however, studies can be also performed under dynamic conditions. Assay modifications also allow investigation of leukocyte-specific mechanisms of transendothelial passage of neutrophils[4–6,9–14] as well as of monocytes[7,8,15] and lymphocytes.[16]

Normally, EC grow to growth-arrested cobblestone monolayers. In most of the abovementioned assay systems, resting monolayers do not express the known cytokine-inducible endothelial adhesion molecules and do not bind neutrophils or lymphocytes but can be activated to do so by appropriate stimulation.[13,15,17] Thus, priming of EC led to a significant increase in incomplete layer passage of leukocytes occurring in the absence of an external chemotactic gradient.[15] Using the assays, it was found that tight binding of leukocytes to the apical surface of the monolayer could be dissected from the subsequent step of TEM. One molecule that appears to be critical specifically for TEM of neutrophils and monocytes is platelet/endothelial cell adhesion molecule 1 (PECAM-1, CD31), as actual transmigration of leukocytes between the EC junctions into the subendothelial matrix can be stopped by anti-PECAM reagents both *in vitro* and *in vivo*.[18]

EC used in TEM assays have been derived from several different sources including human umbilical vein (HUV), adult artery, and saphenous vein,[13] as well as bovine pulmonary artery[19] and microvasculature.[12] Assays with the various EC gave congruent results.[13] Assaying of neutrophils with either human and bovine EC[12,19] was considered acceptable because adhesion and transmigration studies showed that specific interactions occur between the two cell types[20,21] including the binding between bovine P-selectin and human mucin.[21]

Recently, a transmigration assay that employs HUVEC-covered Transwell™ (Costar, Cambridge, MA) cell culture chamber inserts for *in vitro* studies of leukocyte TEM has been used for screening potential sources of human lymphocyte chemoattractant activities in the supernatants of stimulated peripheral blood mononuclear cells.[16] Plasma may also be a potential source of TEM-inducing agents. Plasma-induced activation of EC for enhanced transmigration of leukocytes may be pathophysiologically relevant in several clinical situations, e.g., systemic inflammatory response syndrome, reperfusion injury, or arteriosclerosis. In order to identify possible species differences with regard to transmigration of neutrophils, we compared the effects of human plasma on HUVEC with that on calf pulmonary artery (CPA) EC.

MATERIALS AND METHODS

Assay of Transendothelial Neutrophil Migration

Materials

Materials used in this study include the recombinant human cytokine tumor necrosis factor-alpha (TNF) (specific activity 4×10^7 U/mg protein; Genentech Inc., South San Francisco, CA), secretoneurin (Neosystems; Strasbourg, France), polymyxin B, gelatin, dextran 485,000, heparin, and Percoll (all from Sigma Chemical Co., St. Louis, MO), 0.05% trypsin/EDTA, RPMI-1640, Medium-199, Trypan blue, and heat-inactivated fetal calf serum (FCS) (all from Biological Industries, Beth Heamek, Israel), EC growth supplement (ECGS; Collaborative Research, Bedford, MA), penicillin-streptomycin, gentamycin, and glutamine (Gibco Laboratories, Grand Island, NY). Plasma samples were stored undiluted at –80°C.

Purification of Human Neutrophils

From the peripheral blood (anticoagulated with EDTA) of healthy volunteers donating blood at the Blood Bank of the University Hospital of Innsbruck, neutrophils were obtained after discontinuous density gradient centrifugation of whole blood on Percoll or from buffy coat residues (mixed with normal saline in a ratio of 3:1) by dextran sedimentation and centrifugation through a layer of Ficoll-Hypaque as described,[19] followed by hypotonic lysis of contaminating erythrocytes and washing in HBSS. The cell preparations (>95% PMNs by morphology in Giemsa stains, >99% viable by Trypan blue dye exclusion) were resuspended in RPMI-1640/0.5% BSA for migration experiments.

Growth of Endothelial Cells

HUVEC from fresh placental cords were isolated by previously described methods[22] and grown until confluence at 37°C in 5% CO_2. The growth medium consisted of Medium-199 supplemented with 20% fetal calf serum, 200 μg/ml ECGS, 100 U/ml penicillin-streptomycin, 50 μg/ml gentamycin, 2 mM glutamine, and 50 μg/ml sodium heparin. Cells used for experiments were from passage 4 to 8.

CPAEC (ATCC, Rockville, MD), which were previously shown to interact with human neutrophils in a manner comparable to human EC,[21] were cultured in 25-cm^2 culture flasks (Falcon, Becton-Dickinson) in the medium described above for HUVEC.

At confluence, EC were detached using 0.05% trypsin/EDTA and seeded out on PVP-free polycarbonate filters bearing 5 μm pores in Transwell™ culture plate inserts (6.5 mm diameter, Transwell 3421; Costar, Cambridge, MA). The filters were prepared by coating with 30 μl of 0.2% gelatin for 30 min followed by removal of excess fluid and air drying. EC at 1.0×10^5 cells/culture plate insert were added to the cups above the filter in 0.1 ml Medium-199 containing 10% FCS, and 0.6 ml of the same medium was added to the lower compartment beneath the filter. The EC formed a tight permeability barrier in 5–7 days. Medium was exchanged for fresh medium 2 days before (usually day 4 or 5) the monolayers were used for migration studies on day 6 or 7.

Test of Endothelial Monolayer Permeability

To evaluate the functional integrity of the EC monolayer, medium was removed and 100 μl of undiluted Trypan blue was added to the upper compartment above the endothelial cell monolayers on the filters. One to 60 minutes later, 50 μl samples were taken from the upper compartment and the lower chamber beneath the filter for colorimetric determination with an ELISA reader at 600 nm wave length (Labsystems, Helsinki, Finland). Passage of Trypan blue across gelatin-coated filter alone resulted in a total equilibrium between the upper and lower compartments within less than 2 minutes. When endothelial cell monolayers were grown to confluency, the passage of Trypan blue into the lower chamber was less than 3% of equilibrium after 5 minutes and between 5% and 10% of equilibrium after 10 to 60 minutes (data not shown).

Neutrophil Transendothelial Migration

For assays, EC monolayers on the filters in the upper compartment and the lower compartment were washed twice with HBSS. EC were then stimulated for 60 minutes by addition of 10 ng/ml of TNF or of 1:10 dilutions of plasma to the upper compartment in fresh RPMI-1640/0.05% BSA. Pretreatment of EC monolayers for 60 minutes allows for submaximal stimulation of neutrophil transmigration by TNF.[13] Additional plasma-derived agents with potential EC-activating properties (e.g., proinflammatory neuropeptides, such as secretoneurin) may reach maximal stimulatory action earlier (TABLE 1). After pretreatment of CPAEC for 60 minutes, optimal activation of TEM of neutrophils by plasma was seen at a dilution of 1:10 (TABLE 2). Therefore, in all further experiments plasma was used at a 1:10 dilution for 60 minutes. Furthermore, TEM experiments using aliquots from blood sampling tubes filled with LPS-free medium with and without 10 μg/ml of polymyxin B revealed that blood sampling did not lead to LPS contamination of plasma probes (data not shown).

Following incubation with the plasma samples, the upper and lower surfaces of the filter cup were washed with HBSS and the cup was transferred to a new, clean well (lower compartment). To this well 0.6 ml of RPMI-1640/0.05% BSA was added. Before immersion of the filter cup, 0.1 ml of neutrophils suspended in the same medium was added to the upper compartment (cup). After 90 minutes of incubation, migration was stopped by vigorously washing the upper compartment twice with 0.1 ml of HBSS to remove non-adherent neutrophils. In order to remove neutrophils adherent to the upper surface of the filter, cups were filled with ice-cold phosphate-buffered saline/0.05% EDTA and kept at 4°C for 30 minutes. Then buffer was aspirated and cups were centrifuged at 2,000 rpm for 10 minutes in a Beckman GPR centrifuge to detach cells adhering to the lower surface of the filter. Cells at the bottom of the lower compartments were finally counted in three microscopic fields/cup at 100-fold magnification using an inverted microscope.[19]

Results are given as transmigration index, which is the number of cells per microscopic field that migrated through an endothelial cell monolayer and a micropore filter membrane after pretreatment of endothelium with plasma, divided by the number of cells per microscopic field that migrated after pretreatment of endothelium with medium.

Plasma Samples

Study Population

Population recruitment, baseline examination, and collection of plasma specimens were performed as part of the Bruneck Study from July to November, 1990.[23] The

TABLE 1. Time-Dependent Activation of CPAEC Monolayers for Neutrophil Transmigration by the Proinflammatory Neuropeptide, Secretoneurin ($N = 6$)

Time (min)	TEM Index[a] Mean	SEM
0	1.000	—
15	1.031	0.045
30	1.218	0.056
45	1.464	0.064
60	1.876	0.104
120	2.207	0.052
180	2.199	0.114
240	2.199	0.050

CPAEC monolayers were pretreated with 10 nM secretoneurin for various times before washing of EC and adding neutrophils for TEM.

[a]TEM index is the ratio of cells per microscopic field (magnification = 100×) that migrated through monolayers after pretreatment with secretoneurin to cells that migrated after pretreatment with medium.

study population comprises an age- and sex-stratified random sample of all inhabitants of Bruneck (Province of Bolzano, Italy) aged 40 to 79 years (125 men and 125 women per decade). The current evaluation focused on the age group of 50 to 69 years because of the nearly equal proportions of subjects with (48%) and without (52%) atherosclerotic diseases in this subgroup. Of 469 participants who satisfied the above age criteria (participation rate, 93.8%), 9 were regarded ineligible due to incomplete data or missing ultrasound records. In the remaining male population, frozen plasma samples were available from a random sample of 152 men.

TABLE 2. Dose-Dependent Activation of CPAEC Monolayers for Neutrophil Transmigration by Normal Human Pool Plasma ($N = 6$)

Plasma Dilution	TEM Index[a] Mean	SEM
1:1	1.940	0.167
1:10	2.062	0.133
1:100	1.706	0.179
1:1000	1.040	0.028
Medium	1.000	—

CPAEC monolayers were pretreated with plasma for 60 min before washing of EC and adding neutrophils for TEM.

[a]TEM index is the ratio of cells per microscopic field (magnification = 100×) that migrated through monolayers after pretreatment with plasma to cells that migrated after pretreatment with medium.

Examination of Subjects

All individuals underwent detailed general examination with cardiological and neurological priority and were given a standardized questionnaire for evaluation of risk factors for atherosclerosis.[23]

Laboratory Methods

Venous blood specimens were taken between 07:30 and 09:30 a.m. after 12 h of fasting and abstinence from smoking. In the case of a known acute infection, the definitive samples were drawn up to 6 weeks later. Commercially available test kits (Merck, Darmstadt, Germany) were used for determination of cholesterol and triglycerides. High density lipoprotein (HDL) cholesterol was measured in supernatants after precipitation of apolipoprotein B containing lipoproteins with phosphotungstic acid and Mg^{2+}. Apolipoproteins A-I and B were determined by an immunonephelometric fixed-time method (Behring AG, Marburg, Germany). Plasma levels of soluble adhesion molecules VCAM-1, ICAM-1, E-selectin, and P-selectin were measured using the test kit from R&D Systems (Wiesbaden-Nordenstadt, Germany).

Assessment of Carotid Arteriosclerosis

Quantification of carotid arteriosclerosis was carried out using a duplex ultrasound system (ATL UM8 Advanced Technology Laboratories, Bothel, WA) with a 10 MHz imaging probe (B-mode) and a 5 MHz Doppler. All subjects were examined in the supine position by the same experienced sonographer, and images were recorded on videotape. Stenosis exceeding 50% was defined by a peak systolic velocity of more than 1.3 m/sec or, when no hemodynamic disturbances were detectable, by a percentage diameter reduction of more than 50%. Nonstenotic atherosclerotic plaques were visualized and quantified on the near or far wall of proximal and distal segments in the internal and common carotid arteries (atherosclerotic score), as described in detail and validated previously.[23]

Statistical Methods

Data were processed with the BMDP and SPSS software. The relation of plasma-induced neutrophil transmigration to vascular risk attributes and soluble adhesion molecules was assessed by Pearson correlation coefficients (continuous variables) and the unpaired t-test (dichotomized variables). To account for slight deviations from an assumed normal distribution, these analyses were supplemented and confirmed by corresponding nonparametric procedures (Spearman rank-correlation test, Mann-Whitney U test; data not presented). Limits of agreement were estimated according to Altman and Bland.[24]

RESULTS AND DISCUSSION

Using 10 ng/ml of TNF as positive control for activating EC monolayers to enhance TEM of neutrophils, the inter-assay coefficients of variation were 14.0 ($N =$

113; mean $\pm$ SD of transmigration index, 2.09 ± 0.294) for CPAEC and 19.1 ($N = 28$; mean $\pm$ SD of transmigration index, 3.06 ± 0.585) for HUVEC. The number of neutrophils with complete passage of CPAEC layers was 118 ± 2.0 per microscopic field in the absence of stimulants and 245 ± 5.0 after activation of CPAEC with 10 ng/ml of TNF (mean $\pm$ SD, $N = 113$). The number of neutrophils with complete passage of HUVEC layers was 63 ± 15.1 per microscopic field in the absence of stimulants and 188 ± 24.4 after activation of HUVEC with 10 ng/ml of TNF (mean $\pm$ SD, $N = 28$). Spontaneous TEM of neutrophils was higher when CPAEC were used for monolayer formation as compared to HUVEC ($p < 0.0001$, two-tailed Student t-test). Human recombinant TNF was more powerful in activating TEM in HUVEC as compared to CPAEC ($p < 0.0001$, two-tailed Student t-test). Inter-assay coefficients of variation were similar in both HUVEC and CPAEC.

Plasma-mediated activation of EC for enhanced TEM of neutrophils was tested by pretreatment of EC monolayers with human plasma at a 1:10 dilution for 60 min, followed by washing of the cells. Thereafter neutrophils were added and evaluated for complete TEM. Indices of plasma-mediated TEM or CPAEC and HUVEC monolayers were 1.148 ± 0.283 and 1.660 ± 0.625 (mean $\pm$ SD, $N = 152$), respectively. Indices of TEM are significantly higher in HUVEC assays than in CPAEC assays ($p < 0.001$, two-tailed Student t-test paired samples). FIGURE 1 illustrates that, as compared to CPAEC assays, the variability of TEM indices is higher in assays using HUVEC. For 79% of tested plasma samples, TEM indices were higher in HUVEC assays than in CPAEC assays. Correspondingly, in 21% of cases TEM indices were higher in CPAEC assays. The mean ratio of TEM indices for HUVEC/CPAEC obtained with the two different test systems is 1.520 (range 0.2–2.7); limits of agreement of 0.856 and 2.184 indicate that the two assay types cannot replace each other.

As a measure of the strength of a relation, the correlation coefficient between the two methods was calculated. For the total population ($N = 152$), no significant correlation was observed (r $= 0.0555$; $p > 0.1$). Since plasma samples were obtained from a heterogeneous population of subjects with and without carotid arteriosclerosis, possibly affecting species-specific activation or EC for TEM of neutrophils, the strength of a relation between the TEM assays with HUVEC and CPAEC was calculated separately for the two groups. In patients with carotid arteriosclerosis ($N = 79$), again no significant correlation was seen (r $= 0.0730$; $p > 0.1$). Stimulation of HUVEC and CPAEC monolayers for TEM of neutrophils, however, occurred in a related manner (r $= 0.2612$; $p < 0.05$) when plasma samples from subjects without evidence of carotid arteriosclerosis ($N = 73$) were used for analysis (FIG. 2).

Interactions of neutrophils with EC *in vivo* may be reflected by circulating levels of soluble adhesion proteins, some of which are known to exhibit species-specific effects.[2,25] Consequently, the presence of soluble adhesion molecules in plasma samples used for activating TEM in this study may be responsible for the differential results. Levels of soluble ICAM-1, VCAM-1, E-selectin, and P-selectin have therefore been determined in a random sample, and their relation to TEM indices of HUVEC and CPAEC studies was calculated (TABLE 3). Results demonstrated that plasma levels of soluble adhesion protein P-selectin are inversely related to plasma-mediated activation of endothelium for neutrophil transmigration only in HUVEC but not in CPAEC. No association was found with E-selectin, ICAM-1, and VCAM-1. As plasma levels of soluble adhesion proteins are reported to be elevated in arteriosclerosis,[26] and CPAEC and HUVEC appear to support human plasma-mediated TEM of

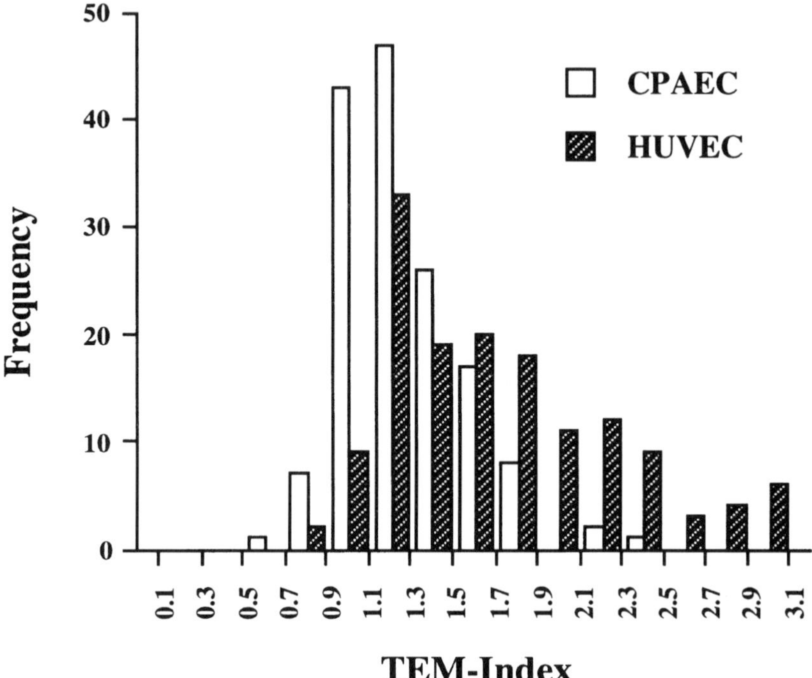

FIGURE 1. Frequency histograms of indices of neutrophil transmigration through CPAEC and HUVEC monolayers stimulated by human plasma. Monolayers were pretreated for 60 min with plasma samples (dil. 1:10) from 152 men 50 to 69 years old. TEM index is the ratio of cells per microscopic field (magnification = 100 ×) that migrated through monolayers after pretreatment with plasma to cells that migrated after pretreatment with medium.

neutrophils in a comparable manner only in the absence of arteriosclerosis (FIG. 2), data suggest that the elevated plasma levels of soluble adhesion proteins are responsible for the species differences in TEM of neutrophils. Elevated plasma levels of soluble P-selectin are associated with reduced activation of HUVEC for TEM (TABLE 3).

The lack of correlation between plasma levels of soluble P-selectin and activation for TEM in CPAEC assays may allow the detection of other factors. An association of Apo-AI levels in plasma and plasma-induced TEM of neutrophils, for instance, was observed only in CPAEC but not in HUVEC (TABLE 1).

Comparing the use of CPAEC and HUVEC in micropore filter assays of TEM for human neutrophils, both systems appear to support TEM. However, lower spontaneous and higher cytokine-activated TEM rates can be achieved with the use of HUVEC monolayers. Human recombinant TNF stimulated TEM stronger in human than in bovine EC. There was also a difference between the two as far as plasma-activated TEM is concerned. Again, higher transmigration indices and higher rates of variability are seen with the use of HUVEC monolayers. Thus, in plasma-mediated EC activation for TEM of human neutrophils, the use of EC from two different species led to differential results.

Human plasma probably contains both kinds of EC-activating agents, those without any species specificity, such as endotoxin and arachidonic acid metabolites,[27] and those with activities restricted to certain species, such as cytokines. Therefore one would expect that human plasma samples can activate human EC more powerfully than bovine EC. Interestingly, CPAEC- and HUVEC-derived TEM data were significantly related only when plasma samples from subjects without carotid arteriosclerosis were used for EC activation, but not when plasma samples from all subjects were used for analysis. This finding suggests that EC priming activity is present in plasma of patients with carotid arteriosclerosis and acts in a species-specific manner. The observed association of plasma-induced HUVEC activation with levels of soluble P-selectin may implicate soluble adhesion proteins in the regulation of EC function in arteriosclerosis.

SUMMARY

Endothelial cells used in transendothelial migration assays have been derived from different sources including human umbilical vein and bovine pulmonary artery. As

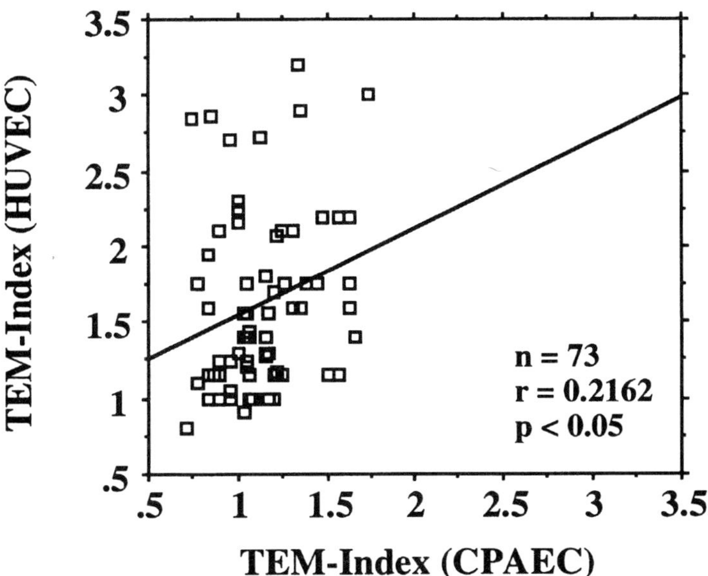

FIGURE 2. TEM of neutrophils measured after pretreatment of CPAEC and HUVEC monolayers with plasma samples (dil. 1:10) from 73 men 50 to 69 years old without evidence of carotid arteriosclerosis. TEM index is the ratio of cells per microscopic field (magnification = 100×) that migrated through monolayers after pretreatment with plasma to cells that migrated after pretreatment with medium.

TABLE 3. Correlation between Plasma-Induced Activation of CPAEC and HUVEC Monolayers for Neutrophil Transmigration and Plasma Levels of Lipoproteins, Triglyceride, and Soluble Adhesion Proteins

Variable (N)	CPAEC		HUVEC	
	r	p Value	r	p Value
Apo B (152)	−0.0407	0.619	−0.0892	0.275
Apo A-I (152)	−0.1634	0.044[a]	0.1040	0.202
HDL (152)	−0.0743	0.363	0.0553	0.499
Triglyceride (152)	−0.0019	0.982	0.0125	0.878
Soluble P-Selectin (65)	0.0167	0.895	−0.2543	0.041[a]
Soluble E-Selectin (71)	0.0078	0.949	−0.0332	0.784
Soluble ICAM-1 (71)	0.1010	0.402	0.0298	0.805
Soluble VCAM-1 (71)	−0.1211	0.314	0.0645	0.593

Apo, apolipoprotein; HDL, high-density lipoprotein; r, Pearson correlation coefficients
[a]Statistically significant, $p < 0.05$.

plasma-induced activation of endothelial cells for enhanced transmigration of leukocytes may be pathophysiologically relevant, the role of species differences between plasma and endothelial cells was studied. The effects of human plasma on human umbilical vein and bovine pulmonary artery endothelial cells with regard to transmigration of neutrophils were compared. Transendothelial migration of neutrophils was tested employing endothelial cell–covered Transwell™ cell culture chamber inserts with micropore filters of 5 μm pore size. Results showed that human plasma induces neutrophil transmigration of both human umbilical vein and bovine pulmonary artery endothelial cell monolayers. Plasma samples from 50 to 69 year old men with and without carotid arteriosclerosis ($N = 152$) stimulated endothelial cells of human origin significantly stronger for transmigration of neutrophils than endothelial cells of bovine origin. Analyses of limits of agreement and of correlation of the two methods indicated that bovine pulmonary artery and human umbilical vein endothelial cells cannot replace each other in assays of plasma-induced activation of transmigration. Plasma levels of soluble adhesion molecule P-selectin, which are elevated in patients with arteriosclerotic diseases, are inversely related to plasma-induced activation of neutrophil transmigration of endothelial monolayers of human origin but not of bovine origin ($N = 65$). As rates of transmigration that were induced by plasma from subjects without carotid arteriosclerosis ($N = 73$) were significantly related between human and bovine endothelium, elevated plasma levels of soluble P-selectin may thus affect results of assays for plasma-induced activation of neutrophil transmigration of endothelial monolayers in a species-specific manner.

REFERENCES

1. SPRINGER, T. A. 1994. Traffic signals for lymphocyte recirculation and leukocyte emigration: the multistep paradigm. Cell **76:** 301–314.

2. CARLOS, T. M. & J. M. HARLAN. 1994. Leukocyte-endothelial cell adhesion molecules. Blood **84:** 2068–2101.

3. WRIGHT, S. D., R. RAMOS, A. HERMANOWSKI-VOSATKA, P. ROCKWELL & P. A. DETMERS. 1991. Activation of the adhesive capacity of CR3 on neutrophils by endotoxin: dependence on lipopolysaccharide binding protein and CD14. J. Exp. Med. **173:** 1281–1286.

4. SMITH, C. W., S. D. MARLIN, R. ROTHLEIN, C. TOMAN & D. C. ANDERSON. 1989. Cooperative interactions of LFA-1 and Mac-1 with intercellular adhesion molecule-1 in facilitating adherence and transendothelial migration of human neutrophils in vitro. J. Clin. Invest. **83:** 2006–2017.

5. DETMERS, P. A., D. E. POWELL, A. WALZ, I. CLARK-LEWIS, M. BAGGIOLINI & Z. A. COHN. 1991. Differential effects of neutrophil-activating peptide 1/IL-8 and its homologues on leukocyte adhesion and phagocytosis. J. Immunol. **147:** 4211–4217.

6. BERMAN, M. E. & W. A. MULLER. 1995. Ligation of platelet/endothelial cell adhesion molecule 1 (PECAM-1/CD31) on monocytes and neutrophils increases binding capacity of leukocyte CR3 (CD11b/CD18). J. Immunol. **154:** 299–307.

7. PAWLOWSKI, N. A., G. KAPLAN, E. ABRAHAM & Z. A. COHN. 1988. The selective binding and transmigration of monocytes through the junctional complexes of human endothelium. J. Exp. Med. **168:** 1865–1882.

8. NAVAB, M., G. P. HOUGH, L. W. STEVENSON, D. C. DRINKWATER, H. LAKS & A. M. FOGELMAN. 1988. Monocyte migration into the subendothelial space of a coculture of adult human aortic endothelial and smooth muscle cells. J. Clin. Invest. **82:** 1853–1863.

9. HUBER, A. R. & S. J. WEISS. 1989. Disruption of subendothelial basement membrane during neutrophil diapedesis in an in vitro construct of a blood vessel. J. Clin. Invest. **83:** 1122–1136.

10. LUSKINSKAS, F. W., M. I. CYBULSKY, J. M. KIELY, C. S. PECKINS, V. M. DAVIS & M. R. GIMBRONE, JR. 1991. Cytokine-activated human endothelial monolayers support enhanced neutrophil transmigration via a mechanism involving both endothelial-leukocyte adhesion molecule-1 and intercellular adhesion molecule-1. J. Immunol. **146:** 1617–1625.

11. HAKKERT, B. C., J. M. RENTENAAR, W. G. VAN AKEN, D. ROSS & J. A. VAN MOURIK. 1990. A three-dimensional model system to study the interactions between human leukocytes and endothelial cells. Eur. J. Immunol. **20:** 2775–2781.

12. FURIE, M. B., B. L. NAPRSTEK & S. C. SILVERSTEIN. 1987. Migration of neutrophils across monolayers of cultured microvascular endothelial cells. J. Cell Sci. **88:** 161–175.

13. MOSER, R., B. SCHLEIFFENBAUM, P. GROSCURTH & J. FEHR. 1989. Interleukin 1 and tumor necrosis factor stimulate human vascular endothelial cells to promote transendothelial neutrophils passage. J. Clin. Invest. **83:** 444–455.

14. PIERCE, J. W., M. A. READ, H. DING, F. W. LUSCINSKAS & T. COLLINS. 1996. Salicylates inhibit $I_\kappa B_\alpha$ phosphorylation, endothelial-leukocyte adhesion molecule expression, and neutrophil transmigration. J. Immunol. **156:** 3961–3969.

15. MULLER, W. A. & S. A. WEIGL. 1992. Monocyte-selective transendothelial migration: dissection of the binding and transmigration phases by an in vitro assay. J. Exp. Med. **176:** 819–828.

16. ROTH, S. J., M. W. CARR, S. S. ROSE & T. A. SPRINGER. 1995. Characterization of transendothelial chemotaxis of T lymphocytes. J. Immunol. Meth. **188:** 97–116.

17. KUIJPERS, T. W., B. C. HAKKERT, M. H. L. HART & D. ROSS. 1992. Neutrophil migration across monolayers of cytokine-prestimulated endothelial cells: a role for platelet-activating factor and IL-8. J. Cell Biol. **117:** 565–572.

18. MULLER, W. A. 1995. The role of PECAM-1 (CD31) in leukocyte emigration: studies in vitro and in vivo. J. Leukocyte Biol. **57:** 523–528.

19. WIEDERMANN, C. J., P. SCHRATZBERGER & C. M. KÄHLER. 1994. Migration of neutrophils

across endothelial monolayers is stimulated by treatment of the monolayers with beta-endorphin. Brain Behav. Immun. **8:** 261–269.

20. GUDEWICZ, P. W., L. E. ODEKON, P. J. DEL VECCHIO & T. M. SABA. 1988. Generation of neutrophil chemotactic activity by phorbol ester stimulated calf pulmonary artery endothelial cells. J. Leukocyte Biol. **44:** 1–7.

21. STRUBEL, N. A., M. NGUYEN, G. F. KANSAS, T. F. TEDDER & J. BISCHOFF. 1993. Isolation and characterization of a bovine cDNA encoding a functional homologue of human P-selectin. Biochem. Biophys. Res. Commun. **192:** 338–344.

22. WIEDERMANN, C. J., B. AUER, B. SITTE, N. REINISCH, P. SCHRATZBERGER & C. M. KÄHLER. 1996. Induction of endothelial cell differentiation into capillary-like structures by substance P. Eur. J. Pharmacol. **298:** 335–338.

23. WILLEIT, J. & S. KIECHL. 1993. Prevalence and risk factors of asymptomatic extracranial carotid artery atherosclerosis: a population-based study. Atheroscl. Thromb. **13:** 661–668.

24. ALTMAN, D. G. & J. M. BLAND. 1983. Measurement in medicine: the analysis of method comparison studies. Statistician **32:** 307–317.

25. GEARING, A. J. H. & W. NEWMAN. 1993. Circulating adhesion molecules in disease. Immunol. Today **14:** 506–512.

26. BLANN, A. D., C. N. McCOLLUM, M. STEINER & M. I. V. JAYSON. 1995. Circulating adhesion molecules in inflammatory and atherosclerotic vascular disease. Immunol. Today **16:** 251–252.

27. CASALE, T. B. & M. K. ABBAS. 1990. Comparison of leukotriene B_4-induced neutrophil migration through different cellular barriers. Am. J. Physiol. **258:** C639–C647.

The Cathelicidin Family of Antimicrobial Peptide Precursors: A Component of the Oxygen-Independent Defense Mechanisms of Neutrophils[a]

MARGHERITA ZANETTI,[b] RENATO GENNARO, AND DOMENICO ROMEO[c]

Dipartimento di Scienze e Tecnologie Biomediche
Università di Udine
Via Gervasutta 48
I-33100 Udine, Italy

[b]*Laboratorio Nazionale Consorzio Interuniversitario Biotecnologie*
AREA Science Park
Padriciano 99
I-34012 Trieste, Italy

[c]*Dipartimento di Biochimica*
Biofisica e Chimica delle Macromolecole
Università di Trieste
Via Giorgieri 1
I-34127 Trieste, Italy

This review will focus on a recently identified heterogeneous group of myeloid antimicrobial peptides derived from precursors showing a highly conserved preprosequence. Members of this family, named cathelicidins, have been identified by the use of conventional protein biochemistry approaches and recombinant DNA techniques.

ANTIMICROBIAL PEPTIDES: A CONSERVED COMPONENT OF INNATE IMMUNITY

Host protection from invading pathogens involves cellular and humoral effectors and results from the concerted action of both non-adaptive (innate) and adaptive (acquired) immunity. The latter is based on specific immunological recognition mediated by clonally distributed receptors, is a recent acquisition of the immune system, and is present only in vertebrates. The former evolved well before the development of adaptive immunity and consists of a variety of cells and molecules distributed

[a]This work was supported by grants from the National Research Council (CNR) and from the Italian Ministry for the University and Research (MURST 40% and 60% grants).
[b]Address correspondence to: M. Zanetti, Dipartimento di Scienze e Tecnologie Biomediche, Università di Udine, Via Gervasutta 48, I-33100 Udine, Italy.

throughout the organism with the task of keeping potential pathogens under control, before they can cause an overt infection.

As opposed to adaptive immunity, which is characterized by a highly specific but relatively slow response, innate immunity is based on effector mechanisms that are triggered by differences in the structure of microbial components relative to the host. These mechanisms can mount a fairly rapid initial response, often sustained by amplification/recruitment of effector systems, which may lead to neutralization of the noxious agents. Reactions of innate immunity are the only defense strategy of the lower phyla and have been retained in vertebrates as a first line of defense before the adaptive system is mobilized.

In mammals, the primary effector cells of innate immunity are neutrophils, macrophages, and natural killer cells, whereas the humoral components in this pathway are the complement cascade, a variety of lectins, and binding proteins (such as the mannose-binding protein, C-reactive protein, and lipopolysaccharide-binding protein).

An important and powerful component of innate immunity is a rich variety of peptides of fewer than one hundred amino acid residues, that are able to kill microbes.[1] In the last 15 years more than 100 different antimicrobial peptides have been isolated from a variety of organisms, ranging from insects to mammals, which points to a widespread distribution of these molecules in nature.[1,2] In addition to these peptides, several larger antimicrobial polypeptides have also been identified, although, in general, these are not as common as peptides in nature. The animal antimicrobial proteins in particular include some important components of the mammalian antimicrobial arsenal, such as the BPI protein[3] and the serprocidins[4] (TABLE 1).

Antimicrobial peptides are also produced by bacteria as antagonistic substances

TABLE 1. Antimicrobial Peptides and Proteins of Mammalian Neutrophils

	MW (kD)	Species	Activity
Peptides			
Defensins	4	Human, rabbit, guinea pig, cow, rat	G+, G–, F, EV, P, M
Cathelicidin-derived peptides:			
α-helical	3–5	Human, pig, rabbit, cow, sheep, mouse	G+, G–, F, P, M
Pro and Arg-rich	4.5–9	Cow, pig, sheep	G–, G+, EV
Trp-rich	2	Cow	G+, G–, F, M
One disulfide	1.6	Cow, sheep	G+, G–, M
Two disulfide	2	Pig	G+, G–, F
Proteins			
Lactoferrin	78	Human, rabbit, cow	G+, G–, F
BPI protein	60	Human, rabbit, cow	G–
Serprocidins	30	Human, cow	G+, G–, F, P, M
Lysozyme	14.5	Human, horse	G+

G, bacteria (+ and – refer to Gram staining); F, fungi; EV, enveloped viruses; P, parasites; M, mammalian cells.

against competing organisms.[5] These may derive from gene-encoded precursors, as the animal antimicrobial peptides, or may be products of the microbial secondary metabolism and synthesized stepwise by different enzymes.

A Historical Overview

The history of peptides with antibiotic activity began with the discovery of these metabolites in prokaryotes and traces back to the early 1940s, when Hotchkiss and Dubos purified two bactericidal compounds from *Bacillus brevis* cultures. These turned out to be peptides composed of both L- and D-amino acids and were named tyrocidin and gramicidin.

The first appreciation that endogenous antimicrobial (poly)peptides are also present in animals came from the studies of Hirsch in the 1950s. He showed that a crude acid extract from rabbit polymorphonuclear leukocytes, containing a mixture of cationic polypeptides, killed both Gram-positive and Gram-negative bacteria *in vitro*.[6] The active components of this fraction were found to be associated with the cytoplasmic granules of neutrophils.[7] Subsequent investigations by Zeya and Spitznagel[8] indicated that the main antimicrobial components of rabbit and guinea pig leukocyte extracts are several cationic peptides with a mass less than 8 kD. These pioneering observations were extended some 15 years later when fractionation technologies allowed a better resolution of the active components of granular extracts. Lehrer and coworkers purified several low molecular weight (*ca.* 4 kD) antibacterial peptides from extracts of rabbit macrophages and granulocytes.[9] These peptides were the first to be characterized in mammals and were named defensins, on the basis of their putative role in host defense.

In the same years, Boman and coworkers were investigating the immune response in insects by using pupae of the *Hyalophora cecropia* moth. Their studies led to the discovery that the major bactericidal factors induced in pupae challenged with bacteria were a family of peptides named cecropins.[10] These seminal investigations disclosed the world of the diverse antibiotic peptides produced by insects.

Occasionally, the presence of antimicrobial peptides in the skin secretions of amphibian species was also observed during the 1960s.[11] This source of antibacterial peptides became prominent when the magainins from *Xenopus laevis* were first described by Zasloff.[12] A number of other peptides were subsequently isolated both from skin and gastrointestinal epithelia of various frogs.[11]

In the last few years, investigations carried out in a number of laboratories have greatly expanded our knowledge of these key components of animal immunity. Readers interested in this subject will find excellent reviews on animal and plant antimicrobial peptides in the proceedings of a recent Ciba Foundation Symposium.[13]

General Features of Animal Antimicrobial Peptides

Antimicrobial peptides are produced to meet the requirements for a rapid response to microbial challenge, and for this reason they are expressed in strategic settings. In fact, they are found at those anatomical sites most exposed to microbial invasion, are secreted into internal body fluids in response to a microbial challenge, or are stored in the cytoplasmic granules of professional phagocytes.

Skin and mucosal surfaces are critical biological boundaries. They work as an effective barrier to most infectious agents, but may become an easy access point for microbial invasion after breaching. To withstand this emergency, several antimicrobial agents, including peptides, are secreted at epithelial surfaces (e.g., the sex-specific antibacterial peptides that are expressed in the epithelial cells of both the male and female reproductive tracts of insects[1]). In insects, antimicrobial peptides can also be induced in cuticular epithelial cells, when the epicuticle is lightly abraded in the presence of live bacteria or bacterial cell-wall components.[14] A variety of antimicrobial agents have also been found strategically located at critical boundaries in amphibian and mammalian species. In the frog, they are produced and stored in specialized dermal structures called granular glands, which release their contents into the external surface upon injury or adrenergic stimulation.[15] Similar antimicrobial peptides are also produced in the gastric mucosa of frogs by large multicellular structures closely resembling the granular glands of the skin, from which they are likely secreted into the lumen of the stomach.[15] Several antimicrobial peptides have also been found in mammalian mucosal surfaces.[15–17] In mammals, they also provide an important tool for the non-oxidative killing activity of the professional phagocytes of mammals.[18,19] Other potential sites of action of these molecules, which can be secreted upon cellular stimulation,[20] are extracellular fluids (such as wound[21] and ascitic fluids[22]).

Based on sequence similarity, the antimicrobial peptides isolated so far have been grouped into several families. When compared, members of different families show a significant diversity in size, sequence, and structure, although they show some common features that appear to be required for their activity. These features include a high content of positively charged residues and a general tendency to adopt an amphipathic conformation. Both features seem mandatory for their functioning as membrane-active agents.

A useful way of classifying known antimicrobial peptides relies on the absence or presence of disulfide bonds in their sequence. The two classes comprise several groups, each containing peptide families and/or individual peptides.

Among the peptides without disulfide bridges, one group consists of linear, mostly α-helical peptides with or without a hinge. Well-characterized peptide families, such as the frog magainins, which can be configured as single, amphipathic α-helices, and the insect cecropins, which are made of two α-helices joined by a central hinge region, belong to this group.[1] Another group in this class includes linear peptides characterized by a high content of specific residues such as proline and arginine (i.e., Bac5, Bac7[23], PR-39[24], and prophenin[25]) or tryptophan-rich peptides (such as indolicidin[26]) expressed in mammalian myeloid cells.

The cysteine-containing class can be subdivided into groups according to the number of disulfide bonds present in the sequences. The first group includes peptides with a single disulfide bridge, such as the cyclic dodecapeptide from bovine[27] and ovine[28] granulocytes. Two disulfide bridges are present in peptides such as protegrins from porcine neutrophils.[29] A third group comprises a number of peptides with three disulfide bridges. This includes the α-defensins, found in neutrophils and macrophages of several mammals and in the small intestine of mouse and man,[30] and β-defensins, found in bovine granulocytes and lingual and tracheal epithelial cells, in avian and turkey heterophils,[30] and, more recently, in human plasma and kidney and vaginal tissues.[31]

The spectrum of organisms susceptible to the antimicrobial peptides is broad, including various bacteria, protozoa, fungi, and in some cases, virally infected cells and tumor cells. Their antimicrobial and cytotoxic effects are in most cases mediated by the ability to bind and permeabilize the surface membrane of the target cells.[1] The initial binding is thought to depend on electrostatic interactions between the positively charged residues of the peptides and the negatively charged molecules exposed at the target cell surface. They may then float with their hydrophobic face buried in the lipid bilayer, or form transmembrane channels in a voltage-dependent manner. These interactions lead to alteration of membrane permeability, with leakage of metabolites.

Mammalian Antimicrobial Peptides

A variety of antimicrobial peptides appears to contribute to host defense in mammals. In general, each species is equipped with a different array of these peptides that likely represents the outcome of an evolutionary selection dictated by the preferential association of a specific set of microbes with a given species. Consistent with a defense function, antimicrobial peptides are present in various tissues, where they are thought to play a role in protecting anatomical compartments, such as the oral cavity, the respiratory, urogenital and digestive tracts, from bacterial invasion and colonization. In fact, they have been found to be expressed in bovine respiratory and lingual epithelial cells,[15,16,32] where their expression is induced by the bacterial lipopolysaccharide, tumor necrosis factor, and injury;[16,17,32] in human and murine Paneth cells of the small intestine,[15] which have long been known to synthesize lysozyme; and in various human tissues.[31,33] In addition, numerous antimicrobial peptides have been identified in professional phagocytes of several mammalian species. The neutrophil granules in particular store a rich variety of these peptides (TABLE 1) that are utilized, in addition to the oxygen-dependent mechanisms, to kill engulfed microorganisms. Several important and well-characterized antimicrobial proteins are also included in this nonoxidative arsenal (TABLE 1), and are likely to act in synergy with these peptides.[22]

In spite of relatively wide structural variety, all the known mammalian antimicrobial peptides fall into one of two major groups, that is, the cysteine- and arginine-rich α- and β-defensins, and the heterogeneous group of the cathelicidin-derived antimicrobial peptides. We will focus here on the latter group of peptides, while referring in particular to the work of Lehrer and coworkers,[9] Martin and coworkers,[30] and Selsted and Ouellette[34] for α- and β-defensins.

MYELOID CATHELICIDINS ARE PRECURSORS OF NUMEROUS AND STRUCTURALLY VARIED ANTIMICROBIAL PEPTIDES

The cathelicidin-derived antimicrobial peptides are a group of structurally diverse myeloid peptides that have been identified in several mammalian species. They are made as precursors in which highly identical N-terminal preprosequences are followed by highly varied C-terminal sequences that correspond to antimicrobial peptides after removal of the prosequence at specific cleavage sites[35] (FIG. 1). The prosequence of all these congeners is highly identical to the sequence of a protein named cathelin. This protein was isolated from porcine leukocytes,[36] and is likely the proregion of a processed precursor of this type, from which the C-terminal antimicrobial peptide has been cleaved off. Based on the presence of a conserved cathelin-like domain, these precursors have been grouped into a family named the cathelicidin family.[35]

Structural Features

Cathelicidins have molecular masses of 16–26 kD and have been identified in bovine,[37–40] ovine,[28,41] porcine,[42–48] rabbit,[49,50] and human[33,51,52] myeloid cells. In addition, several myeloid mouse cathelicidins have appeared in the EMBL/GenBank database, and a related phosphoprotein has been isolated from bovine bone.[22] Most of these congeners have been identified through molecular biological approaches that are based on the high conservation of their prosequence.[35]

Analysis of their cDNAs indicates that cathelicidins do not originate by post-transcriptional processing. As shown for several porcine,[53–55] one human,[56] and several bovine (M. Scocchi *et al.,* unpublished observation) congeners, the cathelicidin genes contain four exons. The three first exons specify the preproregion, while the cleavage site and the varied antimicrobial domain are in the fourth exon. Several potential regulatory motifs, including the consensus sites for nuclear factors (NF) involved in hematopoiesis, inflammation, and acute phase reaction (such as NF-IL6, NF-κB, acute phase-response factor (APRF), and γ-interferon response element (γIRE)) have been identified in the 5′ flanking sequences of these genes. The predicted preproregion is 128–143 amino acid residues long, and includes a putative 29–30 residue signal peptide and a propiece of 99–114 residues. The C-terminal domain is 12–100 residues long (FIG. 1). The preproregions share a high similarity, with an intra-species identity ranging from 75% for bovine, to complete identity for some of the porcine congeners. Four invariant cysteines clustered in the C-terminal region of the cathelin-like propiece are arranged to form two intramolecular disulfide bonds,[57] which may impose structural constraints on the molecule. When the prosequence is compared with other known proteins, the best alignment scores are with members of the cathelicidin family, immediately followed by members of the cystatin superfamily, proteins known to inhibit cysteine proteinases.[58] The most significant alignments are with the cystatin-like domains of kininogens.[35] The presence of a cystatin-like prosequence suggests a common evolutionary origin of these molecules and places the cathelicidin family within the cystatin superfamily. This is further supported by the moderate inhibitory effects exerted by several bovine cathelicidins on the activity of the cysteine proteinase cathepsin L.[57,59] Like other members of the cystatin superfamily, the cathelicidins are precursors of biologically active peptides and their prosequence in particular may be considered a modular unit or cassette associated with a number of different and rapidly evolving C-terminal domains. Although a specific function for this prosequence has not been established yet, the evolutionary pressure exerted towards its conservation suggests it may play an important biological function, such as targeting of the antimicrobial peptides to the granules or aiding their correct proteolytic maturation.

The structural organization of cathelicidins poses interesting questions concerning the genetic mechanisms by which they have been generated. Some indications have come from cDNA sequence analysis of the protegrin gene, which appears to have arisen from insertion of a protegrin coding region into a pre-existing prophenin gene.[47] Similar insertional events may have generated bovine Bac7 and porcine PR-39 from a common ancestor gene,[40] although these mechanisms cannot fully explain the high diversity shown by this family.

Biosynthesis and Maturation

Cathelicidins are expressed early in myeloid differentiation, and their mRNAs are not detected in mature neutrophils.[60] Their biosynthesis and intracellular processing have been studied in detail with the precursors of the bovine Bac5 and Bac7, the most extensively characterized antimicrobial peptides of this group. These are synthesized in bone marrow myeloid cells as prepropeptides and processed to propeptides by the removal of the signal peptide. ProBac5 and proBac7 are stored in the large granules of bovine neutrophils,[60] whereas the specific granules are the storage compartment of the proforms of human FALL-39/human CAP18[52] and of a murine congener (nucleotide sequence accession number L37297), as well as of rabbit p15s.[22] Processing of the proforms to mature antimicrobial peptides occurs by proteolytic removal of the propiece upon degranulation of activated neutrophils.[20,21] In particular, studies on the maturation of the bovine Bac5 and Bac7 have shown that the propiece is cleaved off by the azurophilic elastase under conditions that favor concomitant release of the contents of the large granules and the azurophils (i.e., granule discharge into phagocytic vacuoles).[20,61] This enzyme liberates the mature antimicrobial peptide at a specific valyl residue of the precursor. Most cathelicidins have cleavage sites for elastase at corresponding positions and may undergo a similar processing. However, processing to an active C-terminal peptide is not required for the rabbit congener p15 in order to exert antimicrobial activity.[22]

As shown for bovine proBac5 and proBac7,[20] and human FALL-39/CAP18,[21] cathelicidins can be released extracellularly as uncleaved proforms. Interestingly, purified proBac5 and proBac7 do not display antimicrobial activity,[61] most likely because the cationic C-terminal peptide is shielded by the anionic propiece. The propiece may thus be a means to protect the host from potential detrimental effects of the peptides.

A brief account of the characteristic features of the peptides derived from cathelicidins is given below. They have been grouped according to the abovementioned classification of antimicrobial peptides and include α-helical peptides, linear peptides with abundance of certain residues (Pro and Arg-rich, Trp-rich peptides), and peptides with one or two disulfide bonds.

Proline- and Arginine-rich Peptides

These include the bovine Bac5 and Bac7, the ovine Bac7.5, and the porcine PR-39 and prophenin-1 and -2.

Bac5 and Bac7 were first isolated from bovine neutrophil leukocytes as mature peptides.[62] Subsequent cloning of their cDNAs[38,39] indicated that both are derived from cathelicidin precursors. Investigations on these peptides were prompted by early biochemical and ultramicroscopic studies. It was observed that ruminant neutrophils, in addition to the common azurophil and specific granules, contain a third population of granules, which are denser, larger, and more numerous than the other two types.[63] These granules, designated as *large granules,* are formed at a myelocyte stage of neutrophil maturation in the bovine bone marrow.[64] They lack the typical enzymatic activities that characterize the azurophils and share lactoferrin, but not the vitamin B_{12}-binding protein, with the specific granules. Furthermore, the results of bactericidal assays indicated that the large granules are the store of oxygen-independent antimicrobial activity of bovine neutrophils.[63] This activity was found in a highly cationic protein fraction. Acid extracts of bovine neutrophil granules were thus used as starting material for the purification of antimicrobial (poly)peptides. The cyclic dodecapeptide described below was the first antibiotic to be isolated by this procedure.[27] Soon after, two other peptides were purified and shown to exert potent antibacterial effects *in vitro.*[62] The two peptides were named bactonecins and denoted as Bac5 and Bac7 from their apparent molecular masses of 5 and 7 kD, respectively.

A characteristic feature of Bac5 and Bac7 is their high content of proline and arginine (approximately 45% and 23%, respectively), the remaining amino acids being, in general, hydrophobic (isoleucine, leucine, and phenylalanine).[23] Bac5 is a C-terminally amidated peptide with 43 amino acid residues and a repeated motif of Arg-Pro-Pro triplets alternating with single apolar residues, whereas Bac7 comprises 60 amino acid residues and includes three tandem repeats of a tetradecamer characterized by several Pro-Arg-Pro triplets, also spaced by single hydrophobic amino acids (Fig. 1).

Both peptides are mainly active against enteric Gram-negative bacteria, although some Gram-positive microorganisms are also susceptible to their action. Bac5 and Bac7 efficiently kill *E. coli, S. typhimurium, K. pneumoniae, E. cloacae, S. epidermidis,* and *B. megaterium* at 0.5–20 μM. At these concentrations, Bac7 also suppresses the growth of *P. aeruginosa.*[62] Both peptides are also active against spirochetes such as *Leptospira interrogans* and *Leptospira biflexa,* while two *Borrelia burgdorferi* strains are resistant to their action.[65]

In vitro assays, using the *E. coli* ML-35 strain, showed that the lethal effects of Bac5 and Bac7 are mediated by a rapid increase in the permeability of the bacterial outer and inner membranes.[66] Conversely, they fail to lyse human erythrocytes at 50 μM, thereby suggesting a high degree of specificity for prokaryotic membranes. The mechanism of membrane perturbation has not yet been fully clarified, although preliminary studies using planar lipid bilayers seem to rule out channel formation (Gennaro and colleagues, unpublished observations). Bacterial respiration, which depends on the integrity of the inner membrane, is rapidly and significantly decreased by bactericidal concentrations of Bac5 or Bac7. This inhibitory effect is coupled to a concomitant drop in ATP levels and to a marked decrease in the transmembrane transport and subsequent incorporation of [^{3}H]uridine and [^{3}H]leucine into RNA and protein, respectively.[66] The decrease in bacterial viability thus appears to be causally related to the increase in membrane permeability and the subsequent drop in the respiration-linked proton motive force, with loss of cellular metabolites and alteration of energy-requiring, membrane-associated processes.

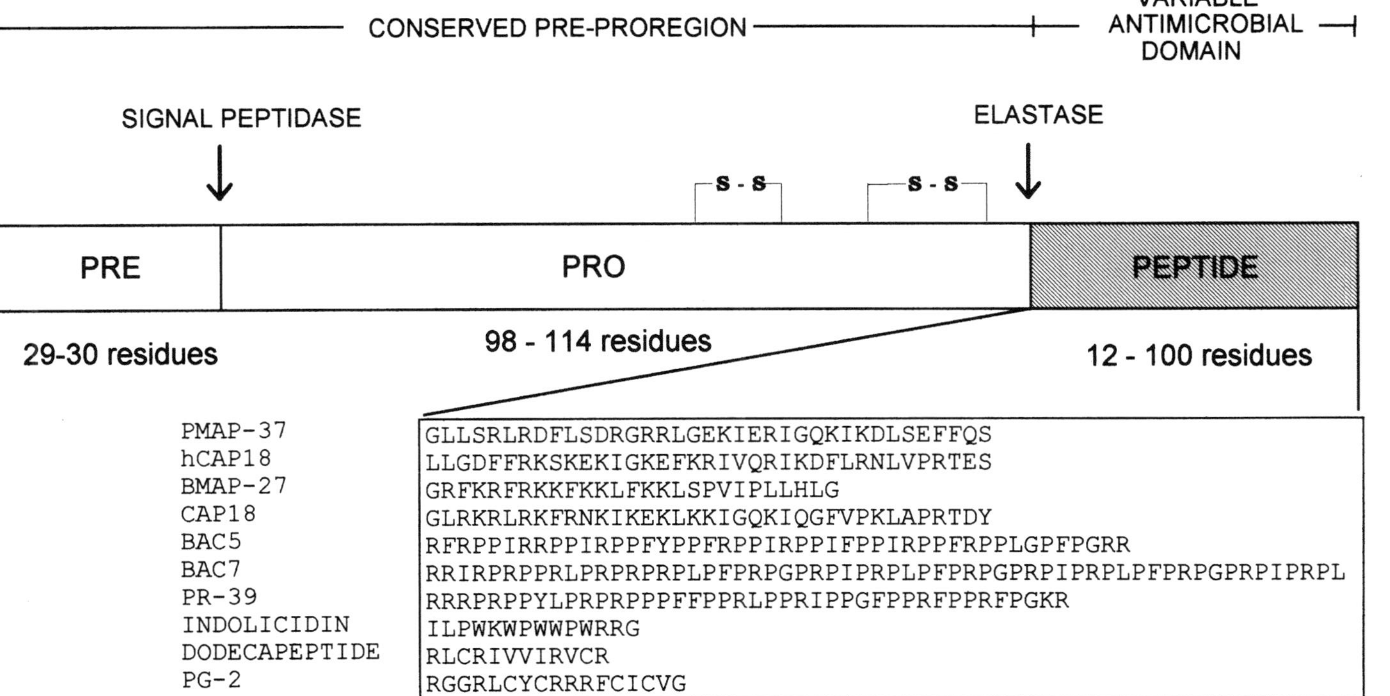

FIGURE 1. Schematic representation of propeptides of the cathelicidin family. Some of the C-terminal antimicrobial peptides are shown, representative of α-helical (PMAP-37, CAP18h, BMAP-27, CAP18r), Pro- and Arg-rich (Bac5, Bac7, PR-39), Trp-rich (indolicidin), one disulfide bridge (dodecapeptide), and two disulfide bridges (protegrin PG-2) sequences.

A 60-residue Pro- and Arg-rich peptide has more recently been deduced from ovine myeloid cDNA and not further characterized.[28] The putative peptide appears to be the ovine Bac7 homologue and has been named Bac7.5.

Two other Pro- and Arg-rich peptides have been isolated from pig and have been named PR-39 and prophenin-1. The former is a C-terminally amidated 39-residue peptide isolated from the small intestine.[24] The mRNA of this peptide has been identified in pig myeloid cells.[42] The sequence 1–14 of the antimicrobial peptide is highly similar to the stretch 2–15 of Bac7 (85% identity), while the rest is composed of the repeated module X-Pro-Pro-Y, where X is a single apolar residues and Y is frequently an arginine, in some way reminiscent of Bac5 (FIG. 1). Investigations performed by CD and Fourier-transformed infrared spectroscopy suggest a polyproline type structure for PR-39.[67]

At micromolar concentrations, this peptide is active against several strains of Gram-negative (*E. coli, S. typhimurium,* and *A. calcoaceticus*) and of Gram-positive (*B. megaterium, B. subtilis,* and *S. pyogenes*) bacteria, while others, such as *P. vulgaris, P. aeruginosa,* and *S. aureus* are resistant even at 200–300 μM.[24] Experiments with *E. coli* have suggested that PR-39 acts by a mechanism that stops protein and DNA synthesis and results in their degradation.[68] In addition to having antimicrobial activity, PR-39, as purified from wound fluid, induces the expression of cell surface heparan sulfate proteoglycans (syndecan-1 and -4), as part of the wound repair process.[69] This peptide has also been shown to inhibit the phagocyte NADPH oxidase activity by binding to Src homology 3 (SH3) domains of the cytosolic oxidase component p47, and has been suggested to limit excessive tissue damage during inflammation by regulating the production of oxygen-reactive species.[70] These findings may thus indicate that PR-39 is a multifunctional peptide involved in several functions related to injury.

Prophenin-1 is a 79-residue peptide highly rich in proline (53%) and phenylalanine (19%), which was deduced from the cDNA[44] and purified from pig leukocytes.[25] As observed with Bac7, the sequence of this peptide is characterized by the presence of several tandem repeats. In particular, the decamer FPPPNFPGPR is repeated six times between residue 2 and 61, in a near-perfect manner. This peptide has a potent antibacterial activity against *E. coli,* a weak activity against *Listeria monocytogenes,* and is inactive towards *C. albicans.*

Indolicidin: A Tryptophan-rich Peptide

Indolicidin is a tridecapeptide amide purified from the cytoplasmic granules of bovine neutrophils[26] and named after the presence of five tryptophan residues in its sequence (FIG. 1), which is the highest Trp percentage observed among known sequences.

Natural and synthetic indolicidin preparations are highly active against Gram-positive and Gram-negative bacteria, as well as against fungi (*C. albicans* and *C. neoformans*) at 0.1–1 μM.[26] At similar concentrations, the peptide rapidly permeabilizes the outer and inner membranes of a susceptible *E. coli* strain. Indolicidin also shows a considerable nonselective cytotoxicity. Interestingly, *in vivo* studies have shown that the therapeutic index is significantly improved when this peptide is administered as liposomally entrapped, as shown with *Aspergillus fumigatus*–infected mice.[71]

Peptides with Disulfide Bonds

The cyclic dodecapeptide is an arginine-rich dodecapeptide (FIG. 1) likely maintained in a cyclic structure by a disulfide bond between the two cysteines in position 3 and 11. This peptide was isolated from extracts of bovine neutrophil granules,[27] and its proform has recently been shown to be present in neutrophils as a dimer.[57] The cDNA of a homologue peptide has also been identified in ovine myeloid cells.[28,41] The dodecapeptide, to date the shortest known natural antibiotic peptide from animals, exhibits bactericidal activity against *E. coli* and *S. aureus* at micromolar concentrations.[27] It also shows a selective toxicity to neuronal and glial cells not exerted by other antibiotic peptides, such as cecropin P1, magainins, and apidaecin.[72]

Peptides with two disulfide bonds include five protegrins, denoted PG-1 to PG-5. Three such peptides have been isolated and sequenced from porcine leukocytes,[29] and two additional congeners have been deduced from cDNA and gene cloning, respectively.[47,54]

Sequence analysis shows that these highly similar peptides resemble the antimicrobial tachyplesins from horseshoe crab. They are small, cationic, 17–18 residue peptides (FIG. 1) with an amidated C-terminus and contain four cysteines linked to form two intramolecular disulfide bonds. However, the different placement and spacing of the cysteines in protegrins and tachyplesins indicate that these peptides belong to distinct families. Interestingly, the spacing of the first three Cys residues in protegrins is identical to that of the first three cysteines in defensins. In addition, a 10-residue stretch of PG-3 has eight amino acids identical to those found in positions 1–10 of rabbit defensin NP-3A.[29] The solution structure of PG-1 has been determined. The peptide has two parallel disulfide bridges stabilizing a rod-shaped, β-sheet structure with two antiparallel strands linked by a β-turn. The central region is hydrophobic, while the two ends are hydrophilic.[73] Protegrins bind LPS with an affinity comparable to that of polymyxin B.[15]

The spectrum of activity of protegrins is broad. Various Gram-negative bacteria including *Chlamydia trachomatis*,[74] Gram-positive bacteria, *Mycobacterium tuberculosis*,[75] fungi, and certain enveloped viruses,[29] are susceptible to these peptides. Electrophysiological studies using *Xenopus laevis* oocytes indicate that protegrins induce membrane permeabilization by forming weakly selective ion channels. Moreover, the presence of the disulfide bonds is a prerequisite for membrane permeabilization, but not for the antimicrobial activity.[76]

α-Helical Peptides

Cathelicidin-derived α-helical peptides include pig PMAP-23, PMAP-36, and PMAP-37 (standing for "porcine myeloid antimicrobial peptides" of 23, 36, and 37 residues)[45,46,48]; rabbit CAP18(106–142)[49]; human FALL-39/hCAP18(104–140)[33,51]; SMAP-29 from sheep[28,41]; and the bovine BMAP-27 and BMAP-28 (unpublished).

These peptides have been deduced from the sequence of myeloid cathelicidin cDNAs.

The sequences corresponding to the antimicrobial peptides are 26–39 amino acids in length, are highly cationic, due to the presence of a number of Lys and Arg residues (FIG. 1), and, when arranged according to the Edmundson plot, form an amphipathic α-helix.

The rabbit congener CAP18(106–142) has been purified from rabbit peritoneal granulocytes,[77] while BMAP-27, BMAP-28, SMAP-29, PMAP-23, PMAP-37, FALL-39/human CAP18(104–140), and a highly cationic fragment of PMAP-36 comprising residues 1–20, have been chemically synthesized.

The results obtained by CD and NMR spectroscopy confirm that these peptides can assume the predicted helical conformation in an apolar environment.

In general, all these peptides are active against both Gram-positive and Gram-negative bacteria, although their spectra of activity show some differences. For instance, at micromolar concentrations, PMAP-36(1–20) is more active against Gram-positive (*S. aureus* and *B. megaterium*) than Gram-negative (*E. coli* and *S. typhimurium*) microorganisms, while the opposite has been observed with PMAP-37.[35] Others, i.e., the two BMAPs and SMAP, are equally active against Gram-negative and Gram-positive bacteria, and are also active against fungi. As expected from their structure, all these peptides exert their activity by interacting with the membranes of susceptible bacteria. They have been shown to rapidly permeabilize the inner membrane of a susceptible *E. coli* strain in a dose-dependent manner at concentrations comparable to those found to be antibacterial.

In addition to killing bacteria, rabbit CAP18(106–142) and human CAP18(104–140) bind LPS, neutralize some of its effects *in vitro,* and protect mice from LPS lethality.[78,51] These findings suggest a therapeutic potential for these peptides in the treatment of the septic shock.

PERSPECTIVES

Many gene-encoded antimicrobial peptides have been identified in recent years in a variety of animals. As only a small fraction of the existing biodiversity has been explored as yet, it is expected that many more will be found in the future. In fact, antimicrobial peptides have virtually been found in all the species where they have been looked for, indicating that they constitute an important mechanism of the innate immunity.

One future goal is the clarification of still open questions, such as the precise mechanism of action of these peptides and its relationship to structure, as well as the basis of the high degree of specificity towards microbial membranes shown by most of them. Further studies are also required to increase our limited knowledge of the gene structure of several families of these peptides and, most important, to identify the regulatory elements that control their expression, also in view of the possible induction of these antibiotic peptides in the site of infection where they are needed.

In addition to shedding light on the mechanisms of innate immunity, these investigations also provide molecules that have the potential to be used in the control of pathogens under various contexts. For these purposes, the antimicrobial peptides might either be used as such, or as lead compounds for rational drug design, as suggested by a number of structure/activity relationship studies that have been successfully performed to improve their activity while maintaining their specificity.[79] The biotechnical potential of these peptides has induced several established biotechnology companies (e.g., Calgene Inc. and Ingene Inc.) to set up programs for their development as antiinfective agents, while new companies have been founded to pursue this goal (e.g., Magainin Pharmaceuticals, Inc. and IntraBiotics, Inc.). The applications of natural antibiotic peptides, or of their synthetic analogues, that are currently under investigation, include: (*1*) the development of transgenic plants, by the transfer of genes encoding animal antibiotic peptides into the plant genome to increase resistance to various plant pathogens; (*2*) the use of antibiotic peptides as food preservatives, in place of current chemical agents with potentially adverse effects, and (*3*) the use of these peptides, topically or systemically administered, for the treatment of various infectious diseases. The latter development in particular is urged by the emergence of bacterial strains that are resistant to most of the classical antibiotics currently in use. Hopefully, these efforts will result in a novel generation of successful therapeutic agents capable of overcoming the spread of bacterial resistance. Finally, since at least some of these peptides have been shown to bind LPS, to stimulate wound healing, and to kill a variety of tumor cells *in vitro,* investigations are also carried out to exploit the above properties.

ACKNOWLEDGMENT

We thank Dr. A. Tossi for critically reading the manuscript.

REFERENCES

1. BOMAN, H. G. 1995. Annu. Rev. Immunol. **13:** 61–92.
2. BOMAN, H. G. 1994. *In* Antimicrobial Peptides. Ciba Foundation Symposium. J. Marsh & J. A. Goode, Eds. **186:** 1–4. John Wiley & Sons. Chichester.
3. ELSBACH, P. 1994. *In* Antimicrobial Peptides. Ciba Foundation Symposium. J. Marsh & J. A. Goode, Eds. **186:** 176–189. John Wiley & Sons. Chichester.
4. GABAY, J. E. 1994. *In* Antimicrobial Peptides. Ciba Foundation Symposium. J. Marsh & J. A. Goode, Eds. **186:** 237–249. John Wiley & Sons. Chichester.
5. SAHL, H. G. 1994 *In* Antimicrobial Peptides. Ciba Foundation Symposium. J. Marsh & J. A. Goode, Eds. **186:** 27–53. John Wiley & Sons. Chichester.
6. HIRSCH, J. G. 1956. J. Exp. Med. **103:** 589–611.
7. COHN, Z. A. & J. G. HIRSCH. 1960. J. Exp. Med. **112:** 983–994.
8. ZEYA, H. I. & J. K. SPITZNAGEL. 1968. J. Exp. Med. **127:** 927–941.
9. LEHRER, R., A. K. LICHTENSTEIN & T. GANZ. 1993. Annu. Rev. Immunol. **11:** 105–128.
10. HULTMARK, D., H. STEINER, T. RASMUSON & H. G. BOMAN. 1980. Eur. J. Biochem. **106:** 7–16.
11. KREIL, G. 1994. *In* Antimicrobial Peptides. Ciba Foundation Symposium. J. Marsh & J. A. Goode, Eds. **186:** 77–90. John Wiley & Sons. Chichester.
12. ZASLOFF, M. 1987. Proc. Natl. Acad. Sci. USA **84:** 5449–5453.
13. MARSH, J. & J. A. GOODE, Eds. 1994. Antimicrobial Peptides. Ciba Foundation Symposium. Vol. 186. John Wiley & Sons. Chichester.

14. BREY, P. T., W.-J. LEE, M. YAMAKAWA, Y. KOIZUMI, S. PERROT, M. FRANCOIS & M. ASHIDA. 1993. Proc. Natl. Acad. Sci. USA **90:** 6275–6279.

15. BEVINS, C. L. 1994. *In* Antimicrobial Peptides. Ciba Foundation Symposium. J. Marsh & J. A. Goode, Eds. **186:** 250–260. John Wiley & Sons. Chichester.

16. SCHONWETTER, B. S., E. D. STOLZENBERG & M. A. ZASLOFF. 1995. Science **267:** 1645–1648.

17. RUSSEL, J. P., G. DIAMOND, A. P. TARVER, T. F. SCANLIN & C. L. BEVINS. 1996. Infect. Immun. **64:** 1565–1568.

18. GENNARO, R., D. ROMEO, B. SKERLAVAJ & M. ZANETTI. 1991. *In* Blood Cell Biochemistry. J. R. Harris, Ed. **3:** 335–368. Plenum Publishing. New York.

19. WEISS, J. 1994. Curr. Opin. Hematol. **1:** 78–84.

20. ZANETTI, M., L. LITTERI, G. GRIFFITHS, R. GENNARO & D. ROMEO. 1991. J. Immunol. **146:** 4295–4300.

21. FROHM, M., H. GUNNE, A.-C. BERGMAN, B. AGERBERTH, T. BERGMAN, A. BOMAN, S. LIDEN, H. JORNVALL & H. G. BOMAN. 1996. Eur. J. Biochem. **273:** 86–92.

22. LEVY, O. 1996. Eur. J. Haematol. **56:** 263–277.

23. FRANK, R., R. GENNARO, K. SCHNEIDER, M. PRZYBLYLSKI & D. ROMEO. 1990. J. Biol. Chem. **265:** 18871–18874.

24. AGERBERTH, B., J.-Y. LEE, T. BERGMAN, M. CARLQUIST, H. G. BOMAN, V. MUTT & H. JORNVALL. 1991. Eur. J. Biochem. **202:** 849–854.

25. HARWIG, S. L., V. N. KOKRYAKOV, K. M. SWIDEREK, G. M. ALESHINA, C. ZHAO & R. I. LEHRER. 1995. FEBS Lett. **362:** 65–69.

26. SELSTED, M. E., M. J. NOVOTNY, W. L. MORRIS, Y.-Q. TANG, W. SMITH & J. S. CULLOR. 1992. J. Biol. Chem. **267:** 4292–4295.

27. ROMEO, D., B. SKERLAVAJ, M. BOLOGNESI & R. GENNARO. 1988. J. Biol. Chem. **263:** 9573–9575.

28. BAGELLA, L., M. SCOCCHI & M. ZANETTI. 1995. FEBS Lett. **376:** 225–228.

29. KOKRYAKOV, V. N., S. S. L. HARWIG, E. A. PANYUTICH, A. A. SHEVCHENKO, G. M. ALESHINA, O. V. SHAMOVA, H. A. KORNEVA & R. I. LEHRER. 1993. FEBS Lett. **327:** 231–236.

30. MARTIN, E., T. GANZ & R. I. LEHRER. 1995. J. Leukocyte Biol. **58:** 128–136.

31. BENSCH, K. W., M. RAIDA, H. J. MAGERT, P. SCHULZ-KNAPPE & W.-G. FORSSMANN. 1995. FEBS Lett. **368:** 331–335.

32. DIAMOND, G., J. P. RUSSEL & C. L. BEVINS. 1996. Proc. Natl. Acad. Sci. USA **93:** 5156–5160.

33. AGERBERTH, B., H. GUNNE, J. ODEBERG, P. KOGNER, H. G. BOMAN & G. H. GUDMUNDSSON. 1995. Proc. Natl. Acad. Sci. USA **92:** 195–199.

34. SELSTED, M. E. & A. J. OUELLETTE. 1995. Trends Cell Biol. **5:** 114–119.

35. ZANETTI, M., R. GENNARO & D. ROMEO. 1995. FEBS Lett. **374:** 1–5.

36. RITONJA, A., M. KOPITAR, R. JERALA & V. TURK. 1989. FEBS Lett. **255:** 211–214.

37. DEL SAL, G., P. STORICI, C. SCHNEIDER, D. ROMEO & M. ZANETTI. 1993. Biochem. Biophys. Res. Commun. **187:** 467–472.

38. STORICI, P., G. DEL SAL, C. SCHNEIDER & M. ZANETTI. 1992. FEBS Lett. **314:** 187–190.

39. ZANETTI, M., G. DEL SAL, P. STORICI, C. SCHNEIDER & D. ROMEO. 1993. J. Biol. Chem. **268:** 522–526.

40. SCOCCHI, M., D. ROMEO & M. ZANETTI. 1994. FEBS Lett. **352:** 197–200.

41. MAHONEY, M. M., A. Y. LEE, D. J. BREZINSKI-CALIGURI & K. M. HUTTNER. 1995. FEBS Lett. **377:** 519–522.

42. STORICI, P. & M. ZANETTI. 1993. Biochem. Biophys. Res. Commun. **196:** 1058–1065.

43. STORICI, P. & M. ZANETTI. 1993. Biochem. Biophys. Res. Commun. **196:** 1363–1368.

44. PUNGERCAR, J., B. STRUKELJ, G. KOPITAR, M. RENKO, B. LENARCIC, F. GUBENSEK & V. TURK. 1993. FEBS Lett. **336:** 284–288.

45. Storici, P., M. Scocchi, A. Tossi, R. Gennaro & M. Zanetti. 1994. FEBS Lett. **337:** 303–307.
46. Zanetti, M., P. Storici, A. Tossi, M. Scocchi & R. Gennaro. 1994. J. Biol. Chem. **269:** 7855–7858.
47. Zhao, C., L. Liu & R. I. Lehrer. 1994. FEBS Lett. **346:** 258–288.
48. Tossi, A., M. Scocchi, M. Zanetti, P. Storici & R. Gennaro. 1995. Eur. J. Biochem. **228:** 941–946.
49. Larrick, J. W., J. G. Morgan, I. Palings, M. Hirata & M. H. Yen. 1991. Biochem. Biophys. Res. Commun. **179:** 170–175.
50. Levy, O., J. Weiss, K. Zarember, C. E. Ooi & P. Elsbach. 1993. J. Biol. Chem. **268:** 6058–6063.
51. Larrick, J. W., M. Hirata, R. F. Balint, J. Lee, J. Zhong & S. C. Wright. 1995. Infect. Immun. **63:** 1291–1297.
52. Cowland, J. B., A. H. Johnsen & N. Borregaard. 1995. FEBS Lett. **368:** 173–176.
53. Gudmundsson, G. H., K. P. Magnusson, B. P. Chowdhary, M. Johansson, L. Andersson & H. G. Boman. 1995. Proc. Natl. Acad. Sci. USA **92:** 7085–7089.
54. Zhao, C., T. Ganz & R. I. Lehrer. 1995. FEBS Lett. **368:** 197–202.
55. Zhao, C., T. Ganz & R. I. Lehrer. 1995. FEBS Lett. **376:** 130–134.
56. Gudmundsson, G. H., B. Agerberth, J. Odeberg, T. Bergman, B. Olsson & R. Salcedo. 1996. Eur. J. Biochem. **238:** 325–332.
57. Storici, P., A. Tossi & D. Romeo. 1996. Eur. J. Biochem. **238:** 769–776.
58. Rawlings, N. D. & A. J. Barrett. 1990. J. Mol. Evol. **30:** 60–71.
59. Verbanac, D., M. Zanetti & D. Romeo. 1993. FEBS Lett. **317:** 255–258.
60. Zanetti, M., L. Litteri, R. Gennaro, H. Horstmann & D. Romeo. 1990. J. Cell Biol. **111:** 1363–1371.
61. Scocchi, M., B. Skerlavaj, D. Romeo & R. Gennaro. 1992. Eur. J. Biochem. **209:** 589–595.
62. Gennaro, R., B. Skerlavaj & D. Romeo. 1989. Infect. Immun. **57:** 3142–3146.
63. Gennaro, R., B. Dewald, U. Horisberger, H. U. Gubler & M. Gaggiolini. 1983. J. Cell Biol. **96:** 1651–1661.
64. Baggiolini, M., U. Horisberger, R. Gennaro & B. Dewald. 1985. Lab. Invest. **52:** 151–158.
65. Scocchi, M., D. Romeo & M. Cinco. 1993. Infect. Immun. **61:** 3081–3083.
66. Skerlavaj, B., D. Romeo & R. Gennaro. 1990. Infect. Immun. **58:** 3724–3730.
67. Cabiaux, V., B. Agerberth, J. Johansson, F. Homblé, E. Goormaghtigh & J.-M. Ruysschaert. 1994. Eur. J. Biochem. **224:** 1019–1027.
68. Boman, H. G., B. Agerberth & A. Boman. 1993. Infect. Immun. **61:** 2978–2984.
69. Gallo, R. L., M. Ono, T. Povsic, C. Page, E. Eriksson, M. Klagsbrun & M. Bernfield. 1994. Proc. Natl. Acad. Sci. USA **91:** 11035–11039.
70. Shi, J., C. R. Ross, T. L. Leto & F. Blecha. 1996. Proc. Natl. Acad. Sci. USA **93:** 6014–6018.
71. Ahmad, I., W. R. Perkins, D. M. Lupan, M. E. Selsted & A. S. Janoff. 1995. Biochim. Biophys. Acta **1237:** 109–114.
72. Radermacher, S. W., V. M. Schoop & H. I. Schluesener. 1993. J. Neurosci. Res. **36:** 657–662.
73. Aumelas, A., M. Mangoni, C. Roumestand, L. Chiche, E. Desaux, G. Grassy, B. Calas & A. Chavanieu. 1996. Eur. J. Biochem. **237:** 575–583.
74. Yasin, B., S. S. L. Harwig, R. I. Lehrer & E. A. Wagar. 1996. Infect. Immun. **64:** 709–713.
75. Miyakawa, Y., P. Ratnakar, A. Gururaj Rao, M. L. Costello, O. Mathieu-Costello, R. I. Lehrer & A. Catanzaro. 1996. Infect. Immun. **64:** 926–932.

76. MANGONI, M. E., A. AUMELAS, P. CHARNET, C. ROUMESTAND, L. CHICHE, E. DESAUX, G. GRASSY, B. CALAS & A. CHAVANIEU. 1996. FEBS Lett. **383:** 93–98.
77. HIRATA, M., Y. SHIMOMURA, M. YOSHIDA, J. G. MORGAN, I. PALINGS, D. WILSON, M. H. YEN, S. C. WRIGHT & J. W. LARRICK. 1994. Infect. Immun. **62:** 1421–1426.
78. LARRICK, J. W., M. HIRATA, H. ZHENG, J. ZHONG, D. BOLIN, J.-M. CAVAILLON, H. SHAW WARREN & S. C. WRIGHT. 1994. J. Immunol. **152:** 231–240.
79. MALOY, W. L. & U. PRASAD KARI. 1995. Biopolymers **37:** 105–122.

Cytokine Activation of Human Endothelial Cells Stimulates Neutrophils To Become Cytotoxic: The Role of Nitric Oxide[a]

JOHAN BRATT AND JAN PALMBLAD[b,c]

Department of Rheumatology
[b]Department of Medicine
Section for Hematology
The Center for Inflammation Research
Clinical Research Center
The Karolinska Institute at Stockholm Söder Hospital
S-118 83 Stockholm, Sweden

INTRODUCTION

One mechanism for vasculitides is when activated neutrophil polymorphonuclear (PMN) granulocytes injure endothelial cells,[1–4] a process that characterizes rheumatic diseases, reperfusion disorders, as well as the adult respiratory distress syndrome. We and others have shown that a variety of agonists for the PMN can initiate this cytotoxic process in *in vitro* systems, e.g., N-formyl-methionyl-leucyl-phenylalanine (fMLP), phorbol myristate acetate (PMA), and lipoxin A4 (LXA4).[5–7] That process is dependent on adhesion molecules and secretion of oxygen metabolites, including nitric oxide (NO), and granulae constituents.[6,7]

Cytokines, e.g., IL-1β, have been shown to activate endothelial monolayers so that PMN confer endothelial injury.[8] Several mechanisms can be assumed to be involved in this process, e.g., activation of endothelial cells to express adhesion and activation molecules for leukocytes, such as ICAM-1 and E-selectin, platelet-activating factor (PAF), the PMN activating chemokine IL-8, as well as NO.[9–14]

Against this background we sought to study the role and mechanisms of IL-1β and TNFα activation of HUVEC for neutrophil-mediated endothelial cytotoxicity. As shown here, these cytokines mediated HUVEC injury dependent on adhesion molecules and NO in the system.

[a]This study was supported by the Swedish Medical Research Council (19X-05991, 19P-8884), the Funds of the Karolinska Institute, King Gustaf V's 80-year Fund, the Funds of the Swedish Medical Association, Swedish Heart and Lung Foundation, and the Swedish Association Against Rheumatism.

[c]Address all correspondence to: Dr. Jan Palmblad, Department of Hematology, Huddinge University Hospital, S-14186 Huddinge, Sweden. Phone, 46-8-5858 2693; Fax, 46-8-7748725.

MATERIALS AND METHODS

Chemicals

These were obtained as follows: IL-1β and superoxide dismutase (SOD) from Boehringer Mannheim GmbH (Mannheim, Germany); N^G-monomethyl-L-arginine (L-NMMA) from Wellcome Research Laboratories (Beckenham, UK); α-2-macroglobulin from Calbiochem (La Jolla, CA); ^{51}Cr from Du Pont Co. (Wilmington, DE); endothelial cell growth factor from Collaborative Research, Inc. (Bedford, MA); 24-well polystyrene plates from Nunclon (Roskilde, Denmark); fetal calf serum (FCS), HEPES, penicillin, streptomycin, RPMI 1640, and Hanks' balanced salt solution (HBSS) from GIBCO (Paisley, Scotland, UK); collagenase (type 3) from Worthington (Freehold, NJ); Sephadex G25 and Percoll from Pharmacia Fine Chemicals (Uppsala, Sweden); EDTA from Merck (Darmstadt, Germany); sodium dithionite from Aldrich (Steinheim, Germany); and a monoclonal antibody to ICAM-1, Elimomab®[15] from Boehringer Ingelheim International BmgH (Ingelheim, Germany). MAb H18/7, previously shown to bind specifically to and inhibit the activity of ELAM-1,[16] was generously provided by Dr. M. Gimbrone (Department of Pathology, Brigham and Women's Hospital, Boston, MA). The control antibody D3/9 against CD45 was a kind gift from Dr. M. Patarroyo (Department of Immunology, Karolinska Institute, Stockholm, Sweden). The neutralizing monoclonal antibody against interleukin-8 (IL-8), ascites clone 6G4,[17] was generously provided by Dr. Caroline Hébert (Department of Immunology, Genentech Inch., South San Francisco, CA). All other chemicals were obtained from Sigma Chemicals Co. (St. Louis, MO).

Endothelial Cell Cultures and Preparation of Neutrophils and Oxyhemoglobin

Human umbilical vein endothelial cells (HUVEC) were obtained and grown as described[5–7,18] and utilized as primary cultures upon achieving confluence. Neutrophils were isolated by a one-step discontinuous Percoll gradient centrifugation.[19]

[51]Cr Release Cytotoxicity Assay

The assay was performed as described previously.[5] In brief, confluent HUVEC monolayers were incubated with ^{51}Cr for 24 h at 37°C. IL-1 or TNF was added to the labeled monolayer and incubated for 1–24 h at 37°C. After washes, the monolayer was covered with PMN in HBSS with 1% FCS, yielding an effector-to-target (endothelial cell) ratio of 6.25:1. Inhibitors, e.g., catalase and SOD, as well as mAbs, were added together with PMN. Dishes were incubated for 4 h at 37°C. Subsequently, supernatants were centrifuged to pellet any HUVEC that may have detached but not lysed. To each well with remaining HUVEC monolayers, 1 M NH₄OH was added to lyse the cells. The radioactivity of supernatants, pellet fractions, and the lysed HUVEC was counted. Injury of the HUVEC was expressed as percent specific ^{51}Cr release. Less than 5% of the total radioactivity lost into the media was found in the pelleted fractions in almost all our assays, indicating that only a few HUVEC were detached during the assay. All experiments were performed in duplicate.[5]

IL-8 Production

Concentrations of IL-8 in the HUVEC supernatants and cell lysates were analyzed with an ELISA technique (Medgenix Diagnostics, Fleurus, Belgium).

Statistical Evaluation

Statistical evaluation was performed with Students' two tailed t test for paired samples, when appropriate.

RESULTS

HUVEC monolayers pretreated with IL-1β or TNF-α, rinsed, and then coincubated with unstimulated PMN displayed a significantly increased ^{51}Cr release, indicating HUVEC injury compared to when PMN were coincubated with unactivated HUVEC (TABLE 1). Based on other results we exposed HUVEC to IL-1 for 4 h and to TNF for 24 h. The effects of IL-1 and TNF were dose dependent and the optimal concentrations for these cytokines were 10 IU/ml and 100 ng/ml, respectively, causing 4- and 9.5-fold increases of the injury, respectively, compared to unactivated HUVEC. IL-1 or TNF alone, i.e., in the absence of PMN, caused no cytotoxicity.

Next, we assessed whether ICAM-1 and E-selectin molecules were necessary for the cytotoxicity. Addition of mAb Enlimomab® (against ICAM-1), blocked 70% of IL-1 and 50% of the TNF induced cytotoxicity. IL-1– and TNF–induced endothelial cytolysis was inhibited in a dose-dependent manner when the E-selectin blocking mAb mAb H18/7 was present in the assays, the maximal inhibition was 65% for IL-1

TABLE 1. The Effect of the Incubation Time on Interleukin-1β, Interferon-γ, and Tumor Necrosis Factor-α Induced Neutrophil (PMN) Dependent Endothelial Cytotoxicity

Treatment	Incubation Time	% Cytolysis
PMN + HBSS	4 h	1.0 ± 0.1
	24 h	1.2 ± 0.5
PMN + IL-1β	4 h	3.8 ± 0.3^{a}
PMN + TNFα	24 h	9.5 ± 0.6^{a}

HUVEC were exposed to 10 IU/ml IL-1 or 100 ng/ml TNF for the indicated time period, washed and then unstimulated PMN were added. Mean and SE values. $^{a}p < 0001$ when compared to cytotoxicity induced by unstimulated PMN alone.

and 45% for TNF. Thus, expression of adhesion molecules on cytokine-activated HU-VEC monolayers is essential for PMNs to cause the endothelial injury.

We then studied whether the cytotoxicity might be mediated by platelet activating factor (PAF), generated and expressed by HUVEC in response to TNF. When we inhibited the binding of PAF to its PMN receptor by means of the receptor antagonist WEB-2086 no hampering effect was seen on neutrophil-mediated cytotoxicity induced by TNF-treated HUVEC. These findings suggest that PAF expression is not a critical event for cytokine-driven cytolysis.

Interleukin-8 (IL-8), a potent neutrophil chemokine produced by HUVEC,[20] might activate PMN to cytotoxicity. On exposure to TNF (100 ng/ml) for 4 h, high levels of IL-8 were produced in our system (877 pg/ml) compared to 45 pg/ml for unstimulated HUVEC. Addition of a mAb directed against IL-8 did not abrogate TNF-mediated cytotoxicity. Thus, the role of IL-8, produced by TNF-activated HUVEC, is unclear.

Based on the findings that oxygen radicals and proteases are pivotal for the cytolytic activity of fMLP- or LXA4-stimulated PMN, we added SOD, catalase, α-1-antitrypsin, or α-2-macroglobulin to the PMN suspension. None of the enzymes prevented the TNF-induced cytolysis. Thus, these released PMN granulae constituents do not seem to play a role in the PMN-mediated injury of TNF-activated HUVEC in this setting.

Finally, we assessed the role of nitric oxide (NO) in cytokine-induced neutrophil-mediated endothelial cytotoxicity. The cytotoxicity achieved by IL-1 and TNF was significantly reduced by L-NMMA, an inhibitor of the NO synthase (TABLE 2). Thus, NO appears to be of importance for the endothelial damage in this *in vitro* model of vasculitis.

DISCUSSION

This study indicates that IL-1β and TNFα are powerful promoters of cytokine-mediated, neutrophil-dependent cytotoxicity for HUVEC *in vitro,* a process dependent on expression of adhesion molecules and associated with NO produced in our system.

Many previous reports have documented that stimulated PMN can cause injury to

TABLE 2. The Effect of NO Synthase Inhibitors and the NO Scavenger Oxyhemoglobin on Neutrophil (PMN) Dependent Endothelial Cytotoxicity Induced by TNFα

Treatment	% Cytolysis
PMN + HBSS	1.2 ± 0.5
PMN + TNFα	8.5 ± 0.4
PMN + TNFα + L-NMMA	2.9 ± 0.3[a]

HUVEC were exposed to TNF for 24 h, washed and then unstimulated PMN were added. Mean and SE values. [a]$p < 0001$ when compared to cytotoxicity induced by TNF-stimulated HUVEC alone.

HUVEC.[1–7] We have shown that the chemotactic peptide fMLP or the physiologically occurring lipid product of arachidonic acid, LXA4, directly stimulate PMN to confer a significant and consistent cytotoxicity. The effect of these two stimuli is dependent on release of proteases, oxygen radicals, expression of PMN adhesion proteins, and requires Ca^{2+} and Mg^{2+} ions.[5–7] The LXA effect is also associated with endogenous PAF expression.[13] However, the cytokine-mediated process presented in this paper is an example of endothelial injury mediated by neutrophils in the absence of added neutrophil agonists. However, it is evident from the data presented here that an agonist for PMNs is produced in the system but its true nature is not yet known.

Maximal cytotoxicity here is three- to fourfold higher than observed for fMLP and LXA4, being slightly lower than what the ionophore A23187 confers.[21] Although cytotoxicity comprises less than 10% of the HUVEC in the well it is highly reproducible and consistent, with very small day-to-day variations. With other assay conditions slightly higher endothelial damage has been observed.[8] Results from different reports are not easily compared due to differences in origin and species of endothelial cells, concentrations of FCS, PMN, incubation time, etc.

Cytokine activation of the endothelium causes leukocytes to stick to the surface. IL-1 and TNF increase the expression of adhesion and activation molecules for leukocytes, such as ICAM-1 and E-selectin.[9–11,16] Here, addition of Mabs to ICAM-1 or to E-selectin consistently inhibited cytotoxicity induced by the tested cytokines. Taken together, these results demonstrate that adhesion between PMN and HUVEC is essential for the cytotoxicity and agree with a profile of activity that parallels previous findings.[5–7]

Our present experiments suggest that the injury to HUVEC was not caused by released oxygen metabolites or PMN proteases since addition of SOD, catalase, or proteinase inhibitors, such as α-2-macroglobulin and α-1-antitrypsin, failed to inhibit the TNF-mediated cytotoxicity. This is in contrast to our earlier findings that oxygen radicals and proteases are pivotal for the cytotoxic activity of fMLP- and LXA4-stimulated PMN towards HUVEC.[7]

NO appears to be a possible mediator for the cytokine-induced neutrophil-mediated injury of HUVEC. We have previously shown that NO, produced by both PMN and EC, is of importance in PMN-dependent endothelial injury induced by LXA4 and PMA.[6] In this study we were able to demonstrate that cytokine-induced PMN-dependent cytolysis is inhibited by the specific inhibitor of NO-synthase (L-NMMA).

Thus, IL-1β and TNFα act as powerful promoters of cytokine-mediated neutrophil-dependent injury to endothelial cells, an important event in the pathogenesis of different forms of vasculitis. The cytotoxic process of vascular inflammation is dependent on expression of adhesion molecules and may be associated with stimulated NO production.

ACKNOWLEDGMENT

The skillful technical assistance of Mrs. Anette Landström and Mr. Christer Forsbom is gratefully acknowledged.

REFERENCES

1. WEISS, S. J., J. YOUNG, A. F. LOBUGLIO, A. SLIVKA & N. F. NIMEH. 1981. Role of hydrogen peroxide in neutrophil-mediated destruction of cultured endothelial cells. J. Clin. Invest. **68:** 714–721.

2. WARD, P. A. & J. VARANI. 1990. Mechanisms of neutrophil-mediated killing of endothelial cells. J. Leukocyte Biol. **48:** 97–102.

3. WEISS, S. J. 1989. Tissue destruction by neutrophils. N. Engl. J. Med. **320:** 365–376.

4. VARANI, J., I. GINSBURG, L. SCHUGER, D. F. GIBBS, J. BROMBERG, K. J. JOHNSON, U. S. RYAN & P. A. WARD. 1989. Endothelial cell killing by neutrophils. Synergistic interaction of oxygen products and proteases. Am. J. Pathol. **135:** 435–438.

5. BRATT, J., R. LERNER, B. RINGERTZ & J. PALMBLAD. 1994. Lipoxin A4 induces neutrophil dependent cytotoxicity for human endothelial cells. Scand. J. Immunol. **39:** 351–354.

6. BRATT, J. & H. GYLLENHAMMAR. 1995. The role of nitric oxide in lipoxin A4-induced polymorphonuclear neutrophil-dependent cytotoxicity to human vascular endothelium in vitro. Arthritis Rheum. **38:** 768–776.

7. BRATT, J., R. LERNER, B. RINGERTZ & J. PALMBLAD. 1995. Mechanisms for lipoxin A4 induced neutrophil dependent cytotoxicity for human endothelial cells. J. Lab. Clin. Med. **126:** 36–43.

8. WESTLIN, W. F. & M. A. GIMBRONE, JR. 1993. Neutrophil-mediated damage to human vascular endothelium: Role of cytokine activation. Am. J. Pathol. **142:** 117–128.

9. BEVILACQUA, M. P., J. S. POBER, M. E. WHEELER, R. S. COTRAN & M. A. GIMBRONE, JR. 1985. Interleukin-1 activation of vascular endothelium: Effects on procoagulant activity and leukocyte adhesion. Am. J. Pathol. **121:** 393–403.

10. BEVILACQUA, M. P., S. STENGELIN, M. A. GIMBRONE, JR. & B. SEED. 1989. Endothelial leukocyte adhesion molecule 1: an inducible receptor for neutrophils related to complement regulatory proteins and lectins. Science **243:** 1160–1164.

11. DUSTIN, M. L., R. ROTHLEIN, A. F. BHAN, C. A. DINARELLO & T. A. SPRINGER. 1986. A natural adherence molecule (ICAM-1): induction by IL-1 and IFN, tissue distribution, biochemistry and function. J. Immunol. **137:** 245–254.

12. BUSSOLINO, F., M. ARESE, L. SILVESTRO, R. SOLDI, E. BENFENATI, F. SANAVIO, M. AGLIETTA, A. BOSIA & G. CAMUSSI. 1994. Involvement of a serine protease in the synthesis of platelet-activating factor by endothelial cells stimulated by tumor necrosis factor-α or interleukin-1α. Eur. J. Immunol. **24:** 3131–3139.

13. BROWN, Z., M. E. GERRITSEN, W. W. CARLEY, R. M. STREITER, S. L. KUNKEL & J. WESTWICK. 1994. Chemokine gene expression and secretion by cytokine-activated human microvascular endothelial cells. Differential regulation of monocyte chemoattractant protein-1 and interleukin-8 in response to interferon-γ. Am. J. Pathol. **145:** 913–921.

14. ROSENKRANZ-WEISS, P., W. C. SESSA, S. MILSTEIN, S. KAUFMAN, C. A. WATSON & J. S. POBER. 1994. Regulation of nitric oxide synthesis by proinflammatory cytokines in human umbilical vein endothelial cells. J. Clin. Invest. **93:** 2236–2243.

15. HAUG, C. E., R. B. COLVIN, F. L. DELMONICO, H. AUCHINCLOSS, JR., N. TOLKOFF-RUBIN, F. I. PREFFER, R. ROTHLEIN, S. NORRIS, L. SCHARSCHMIDT & A. B. COSIMI. 1993. A phase 1 trial of immunosuppression with anti-ICAM-1 (CD 54) mAb in renal allograft recipients. Transplantation **55:** 766–773.

16. LUSCINSKAS, F. W., M. I. CYBULSKY, J. M. KIELY, C. S. PECKINS, V. M. DAVIS & M. A. GIMBRONE, JR. 1991. Cytokine-activated human endothelial monolayers support enhanced neutrophil transmigration via a mechanism involving both endothelial-leukocyte adhesion molecule-1 and intercellular adhesion molecule-1. J. Immunol. **146:** 1617–1725.

17. BROADDUS, V. C., A. M. BOYLAN, J. M. HOEFFEL, K. J. KIM, M. SADICK, A. CHUNTHARAPAI & C. A. HÉBERT. 1994. Neutralization of IL-8 inhibits neutrophil influx in a rabbit model of endotoxin-induced pleurisy. J. Immunol. **152:** 2960–2967.

18. PALMBLAD, J., R. LERNER & S. H. LARSSON. 1994. Signal transduction mechanisms for leukotriene B4 induced hyperadhesiveness of endothelial cells for neutrophils. J. Immunol. **152:** 262–269.
19. RINGERTZ, B., J. PALMBLAD & J. Å LINDGREN. 1985. Stimulus-specific neutrophil aggregation: Evaluation of possible mechanisms for the stimulus-response apparatus. J. Lab. Clin. Med. **106:** 132–140.
20. BAGGIOLINI, M., A. WALZ & S. L. KUNKEL. 1989. Neutrophil activating peptide-1/interleukin-8, a novel cytokine that activates neutrophils. J. Clin. Invest. **84:** 1045–1049.
21. BRATT, J. & J. PALMBLAD. 1996. Inhibition of neutrophil dependent cytotoxicity for human endothelial cells by antirheumatic drugs. J. Lab. Clin. Med. (In press.)

Osteoclastic Bone Resorption:
Normal and Pathological

IGOR SCHEPETKIN

Department of Immunology
Research Institute of Oncology
Tomsk Scientific Centre
Siberian Branch of Russian Academy of Medical Sciences
Tomsk, 634001, Russia

INTRODUCTION

Osteoclastic resorption is an inseparable part of bone remodeling in both prenatal and postnatal periods. The ability of bone tissue to undergo reconstruction in embryonic development defined progressive evolution of surface vertebrates.[1] Specialization of cells for the resorption function became a necessary consequence of the apposition bone growth. In normal growth, there is a balance between osteogenesis by osteoblasts and bone resorption by osteoclasts. Osteosynthetic and resorption processes are regulated by systemic osteotropic hormones, local factors of microenvironment, and distribution of lines of mechanical tension. In a number of cases a balance of these processes can be broken that leads to osteoporosis and osteolysis or to osteosclerosis and hyperostosis. Molecular and genetic investigations of human subjects and experimental animals with different forms of osteopetrosis revealed a bond of disturbing functions and maturing osteoclasts with certain mutations. It is apparent that to understand the reasons of these disturbances and to develop new methods of treatment the mechanisms of the bone resorption must be understood. Additionally, the resorption of the bone tissue is a method of calcium mobilization from the bone. Regulating the osteoclastic resorption equally with calcium metabolism in the intestine (absorption and secretion) and in the kidneys (reabsorption and excretion) gives supporting physiologic calcium balance in the extracellular medium of the organism. In this review the main focus is on mechanisms of osteoclastic bone resorption, in normal and pathological conditions, and its regulation by pharmacological agents.

OSTEOCLASTS

Osteoclasts are multinucleated giant cells specializing on the resorption of mineral and organic components of the bone matrix. They are formed as a result of fusion of the postmitotic progenitor cells, which are ultimately derived from multipotential hemopoietic stem cells belonging to the monocyte-macrophage lineage.[2,3] Nevertheless, some mononucleated cells with osteoclast phenotype can perform a resorption function.[4] In normal osteogenesis, most cells are located on the surface of the endosteum covering trabecules of the spongy bone and bone marrow cavity. Osteoclasts take an active part in the bone remodeling in its growth, including forming the primitive marrow cavity (resorb and invade the calcified cartilage rudiment) in the process of the myeloid tissue development as well as in reparative osteogenesis after fracture.

Participation of osteoclasts in physiologic cartilage resorption is also discussed. The main role in this process belongs to the cells called septoclasts or chondroclasts coming, apparently, from pericytes. They have one nucleus, actively secrete cathepsins, and differ from osteoclasts, monocytes, and macrophages by antigenic determinants.[5]

The osteoclast activity is evaluated *in vitro* according to the rate of resorption lacunae formation on bone slices. Osteoclast activity depends on the method of obtaining the cells and the other experimental conditions and usually changes from 10^3 to $1-2\times10^4$ μm^2 of the digestion surface per cell in a 24-h period.[4] For histochemical identification of osteoclasts, a reaction to tartrate-resistant acid phosphatase is used. One of the early markers of osteoclast differentiation is an intercellular carbonic anhydrase II. Identifying this enzyme as well as calcitonin receptors allows us to differentiate osteoclasts from the osteoclast-like multinucleated cells forming as a result of monocyte/macrophage fusion in some pathological states.[6]

Osteoclasts are highly mobile cells that migrate and attach to the mineralized matrix with the help of their adhesive molecules. The plasma membrane under the osteoclast (an apical membrane) is gathered into folds forming the so-called ruffled border. The ends of microvilli of the ruffled border reach the bone surface. The adhesive molecules of osteoclasts are integrin transmembranous heterodimeric glycoproteins composed of two non-covalent bound subunits, a large α and a small β. They function as receptors for a greater part of ligands, including matrix proteins with an amino acid sequence of Arg-Gly-Asp (RGD). The interaction of integrins with these ligands leads to reorganization of the cytoskeleton components and to changes in the osteoclast activity. The presence of the $\alpha_v\beta_3$ for vitronectin, $\alpha_2\beta_1$ for collagen and laminin, and $\alpha_3\beta_1$ for collagen, fibronectin, and vitronectin have been detected in osteoclasts.[7,8]

COOPERATION OF OSTEOCLASTS AND OSTEOBLASTS IN THE PROCESS OF BONE RESORPTION

Bone tissue resorption is a multi-stage process that includes degradation of both mineral bone phase and the components of the organic matrix. It is believed that non-mineralized tissues, such as osteoid and non-calcified cartilage, are not able to activate osteoclasts. As the surface of quickly growing bone is covered with non-mineralized collagen, the first step of resorption is the removal of this osteoid by osteoblast's collagenase (matrix metalloproteinase-1, MMP-1), stromelysin (MMP-3), and the other Zn-dependent MMP. It is shown that the synthesis of proteinase and their tissue inhibitors by osteoblasts is regulated by the local and systemic hormones including interleukin-1 (IL-1), the tumor necrosis factor-α (TNF-α), and parathyroid hormone (PTH).[9,10] Stromelysin has broad substrate specificity and can digest proteoglycans, fibronectin, and laminin.[11] Participation of osteoblasts in the degradation of the organic matrix is similar to the function of fibroblasts in soft tissues with interstinal growth.[1]

The local MMP activity regulation is realized by tissue inhibitors of metalloproteinases (TIMPs): TIMP-1 and TIMP-2. TIMP-1 (glycoprotein) suppresses the enzymatic activity of various MMPs including stromelysin, and TIMP-2 (nonglycosylated protein) of gelatinase A. Osteoblasts support a balance between MMPs and their inhibitors, controlling the rate of degradation of not only an osteoid, but the organic bone components, in the process of its further resorption by osteoclasts as well.[12]

After removing an osteoid, the osteoclasts attach to the prepared surface of the mineralized matrix. They form a closed space under themselves where protons and cathepsins can enter. Proteolytic enzymes are secreted under fusion of vesicles of Golgi complexes with an apical membrane of the osteoclasts. An important role in this process belongs to the product of protooncogene C-src − $_{pp}60^{c\text{-src}}$, protein tyrosine kinase, phosphorylating one or several cytoskeleton proteins on tyrosine, involved in the translocation of vesicles to the apical membrane, and/or contractile proteins that activate the fusion of vesicles with a membrane and the releasing of their contents.[13] It is impossible to exclude the participation of the other src-like tyrosine kinases in this process, including the products of protooncogenes c-fyn, c-yes, and c-lyn expressed in osteoclasts.[2] In the vesicle membrane there is H^+-ATPase (vacuolar proton pump), that, after fusion of vesicles, is left in the apical membrane and excretes protons generated by carbonic anhydrase II.[14] For secretion H^+ the cells need Na^+/H^+ antiporter, which may have even greater value for osteoclasts as compared to H^+-ATPase. An important role in supporting an active state of osteoclasts is related to the formation of citrate and antiporter CI^-/HCO_3^-.[15]

Released from minerals, the collagen fibers and non-collagenic proteins are digested by acid proteases. Increasing Ca^{2+} concentration in the lacuna is conducive to increasing the collagen sensitivity to proteolysis.[16] The main enzymes taking part in collagen degradation use collagenase and cathepsins B, D, L, and N. Not long ago collagenase was found in osteoclasts.[17] However, as collagenase acts at pH 6 to 7.5, even with of its presence for developing collagenolysis in the lacunar space of osteoclasts, the pH of the lacunar medium is 4.5–4.8, indicating that the main role should belong to cathepsins. It is shown that cathepsins B, L, and D are secreted by osteoclasts into resorption lacunae.[18] Recently in osteoclasts there was found one more proteinase—cathepsin K.[19] From these lysosomic enzymes the main role in the process of degradation of collagen and bone proteoglycans should have been cathepsin L.[20] The demineralized matrix, possibly, can be considered as a "temporary glycocalyx" (compare with a glycocalyx of intestinal brush-border membrane[21]) absorbing proteases, decreasing the proteolytic load to the apical osteoclast membrane, and having the role of the "porous enzyme reactor."

The formed collagen fragments in the process of proteolysis are further subjected to hydrolysis by enzymes with gelatinase activity: gelatinase A (MMP-2) and gelatinase B (MMP-9).[22] MMP-9 keeps 50% of gelatinolytic activity at pH 5.5.[23] The possibility of pinocytosis of the formed short peptides and their further destruction in osteoclast phagolysosomes is not excluded.[17]

As a result of flowing the processes of bone mineral solubilization and organic matrix degradation there is formed a resorption pit (Howship's lacuna) under the osteoclast (Fig. 1).[24]

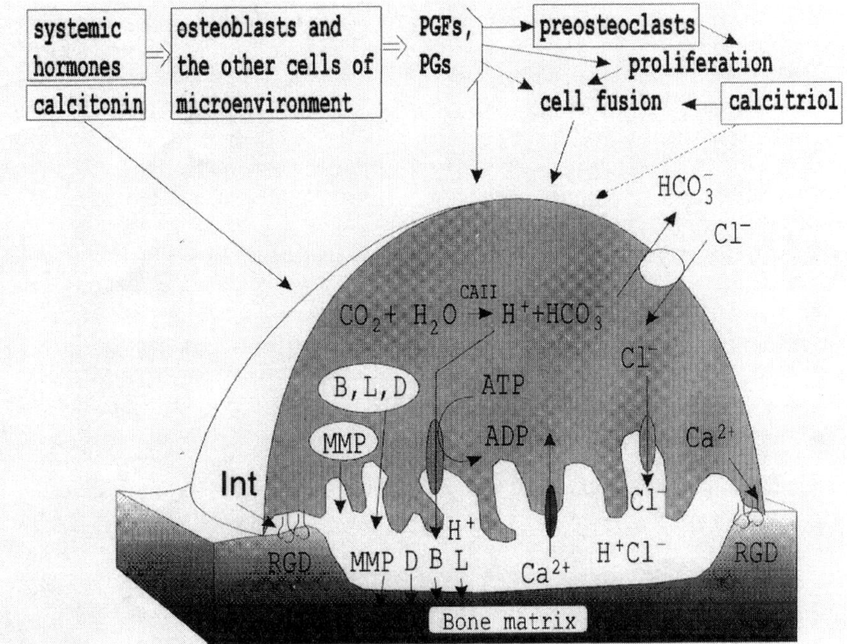

FIGURE 1. Regulating the osteoclastogenesis and osteoclastic resorption of the bone matrix. Int – integrins; RGD – amino acid sequence Arg-Gly-Asp in proteins of the bone matrix; MMPs – metalloproteinases; B, L, D – cathepsins; PGFs – polypeptide growth factors; PGs – prostaglandins; CA II – carbonic anhydrase II.

Increasing Ca^{2+} concentration in this lacuna due to hydroxyapatite dissolving in the acid medium causes Ca-receptor activation, Ca-channels opening, increases in intercellular Ca^{2+} concentration, cytoskeleton reorganization, osteoclast detachment, and movement prior to another resorption cycle.[25,26] It is reported that Ca^{2+} concentration in lacunae can reach 40 mM.[27] In high extracellular Ca^{2+} content (>20 mM) the osteoclasts become incapable of attaching to the bone slices.[28]

In microphotographs of the resorption bone surface at the osteoclast site, there is often observed demineralized collagen fibers.[29] In fact, after removing of osteoclasts, the process of proteolysis goes on, as pH of the medium in the resorption pit increases to 6.0–7.5 with a subsequent effect of collagenase secreted earlier or activated from procollagenase of the bone matrix.[17] Zymogen may be activated in a few ways (*1*) by enzymatic cascade launched by plasminogen activators (tissue activator of plasminogen and/or urokinase), (*2*) by enzymatic cascade launched by kallikrein, (*3*) by cathepsin B and, (*4*) by stromelysin.[30] The latter two variants are realized by the enzymes of the "proteolytic cocktail" of the lacunar space at the completed stage of degradation of demineralized bone matrix. On the contrary, the first two mechanisms acquire a significance at the beginning of the resorption process. In this respect the data concerning stimulating the synthesis by osteoblasts of the plasminogen tissue activator in response to 1,25-dihydroxyvitamin D_3 (calcitriol) and PTH are of great interest.[31] Owing to such cooperative action of acid and neutral proteinases, the range of pH values in which proteolysis can occur increases.

It is shown that osteoclasts are able to form superoxide anion $(O_2^{\cdot})$.[32] Addition of superoxide dismutase to isolated osteoclasts inhibits their resorption activity. Superoxide anion is secreted to the space between the ruffled border and bone surface and its concentration, probably, is regulated by 150 kD superoxide dismutase–related membrane glycoprotein that is expressed on osteoclasts in the course of their differentiation.[33] The investigators attribute two main functions to $O_2^{\cdot}$: local control of osteoclasts with participation of Ca^{2+} and nitric oxide (NO) and destruction of organic components of the bone matrix. Indeed, $O_2^{\cdot}$ also causes a degradation of osteocalcin and collagen.[32] The other short-lived regulator of the osteoclast function is NO, which can be produced both by endothelial cells in the bone marrow and the osteoclasts themselves. Nitric oxide is considered to be a strong inhibitor of the osteoclast resorption activity.[34]

Thus, the central role in physiological resorption of all the components of the bone matrix belongs to osteoclasts, while osteoblasts are promoters of this process by taking part in osteoid removal or complete destruction of a demineralized collagen. Apart from a direct participation in the bone resorption, osteoblasts and osteocytes regulate functional activity of osteoclasts. This influence is mediated by the components of the bone matrix, polypeptide cytokines, as well as short-lived mediators.

REGULATION OF OSTEOCLAST ACTIVITY BY ORGANIC COMPONENTS OF THE BONE MATRIX

The rate of degradation of the bone tissue depends on the composition of the extracellular matrix, which not only defines the enzyme-substrate correspondences but also regulates a functional activity of resorption cells.

The organic phase of the bone matrix consists of collagen I ($\approx 90\%$) and the other proteins ($\approx 10\%$): proteoglycans, glycoproteins (osteonectin, osteopontin, fibronectin, thrombospondin, and bone sialoprotein), gla-protein (osteocalcin), and polypeptide growth factors (PGFs). Most of these components are secreted by osteoblasts, the rest enter from the blood through the tissue fluid.

Osteocalcin, the peptide (5.8 kD) produced by osteoblasts and odontoblasts in the organism, diffuses through the osteoid and is bound up with mineralized bone.[35] The osteocalcin bond is realized with the help of negatively charged residue of γ-carboxyglutamic acid (gla) having a high avidity to calcium and hydroxyapatite. The gla residues are synthesized by a γ-carboxylation of glutamic acid requiring vitamin K.[36] Osteocalcin is a chemoattractant for osteoclasts and their precursors. There are no exact facts to explain the realization of this function, but, it is assumed that osteocalcin interacts with granulocyte-macrophage colony-stimulating factor (GM-CSF) accounting for its accumulation in the bone matrix.[37] Suppression of glutamic γ-carboxylation by the anticoagulant warfarin blocks ostecalcin accumulation in the bone matrix, thus increasing the bone stability to resorption by osteoclasts.[38] The osteocalcin expression in osteoblasts is modulated by calcitriol, PTH, and PGFs, and in particular, by a transforming growth factor-β (TGF-β).[39] Skeletal tissue contains 75% of osteocalcin, the remainder is in circulation in the organism and is destroyed in the liver, kidneys, and also in placenta (which, possibly, resists a significant increase in bone resorption during pregnancy).[35]

Collagen I, as well as the other components of the bone matrix (such as osteopontin, bone sialoproteins, thrombospondin, and fibronectin), have an amino acid sequence RGD serving as an adhesive "recognition site" for integrins of osteoblasts and osteoclasts. It was discovered that collagen I contains six RGD sequences, whereas fibronectin has only two RGD sequences.[40,41] The investigation of osteoclast interaction with these proteins has shown that the cells are quickly split on the substrates covered with fibronectin, bone sialoprotein II, osteopontin, and to a lesser degree, on collagen without any bond with thrombospondin. To improve the interaction of osteoclasts with collagen I its preliminary denaturation is necessary.[42] It is possible, that the RGD sequence of these proteins is required for differentiating the osteoclast precursors. Binding the osteoclast integrins with ligands leads to increasing the concentration of cytosol Ca^{2+} at the expense of its mobilization from the intracellular depot. In the bone matrix osteopontin and bone sialoprotein are present in the form of phosphoproteins. The tartrate-resistance acid phosphatase secreted by osteoclasts to the resorption region can dephosphorylate these proteins and that causes a decrease of their adhesive properties. Such a process may be one of the regulation mechanisms of osteoclast mobility on the bone surface.[43,44]

Some of PGFs have a high affinity to the components of the bone matrix. Among them one should note a GM-CSF, macrophage colony-stimulating factor (M-CSF), and TGF-β.[35,43,44] In the course of the bone resorption they are released, activated from the latent forms by a limited proteolysis (it is typical for TGF-β), and have local regulatory effects on the osteoclasts and osteoblasts. Osteoblast activation by proteins labilized from the matrix defines a change of the resorption period to an osteosynthetic one. In normal and pathological states, the rate of the remodeling cycle passage can vary to a considerable degree.

INFLUENCE OF ENDOCRINE HORMONES ON THE FUNCTION OF OSTEOCLASTS

Among osteotropic endocrine hormones one should indicate calcitonin, PTH, thyroid hormones [triiodothyronine (T_3) and thyroxin (T_4)], sex hormones (androgens and estrogens), the metabolite of vitamin D_3 (calcitriol), metabolites of vitamin A (retinoic acids), and others. Retinoids, calcitriol, thyroid, and steroid hormones are small hydrophobic molecules capable of passively passing through biological membranes. They can regulate cellular functions by interacting with specific intracellular receptors.

Calcitonin is a 32 amino-acid peptide produced by T-cells localized in thyroid, parathyroid, and thymus glands. The main physiologic role of calcitonin lies in suppressing bone resorption as a result of a direct action of a hormone to osteoclasts, which express a great number of calcitonin receptors.[47] It is assumed that calcitonin reduces the bone resorption by influencing mature osteoclasts, inhibiting differentiation, and/or in the process of fusion of mononuclear preosteoclasts.[31] Indeed, calcitonin receptors appear on the precursors long before osteoclasts become functionally competent.[48] In 2 h after binding with a receptor on the plasma membrane, calcitonin is seen in the Golgi apparatus, where it remains for 48–72 h.[48] Preprocessing osteoclasts using this hormone leads to decreasing concentrations of calcitonin receptors. In early periods it is, apparently, connected with internalization of the ligand-receptor complexes and incomplete recycling of the receptor complexes. Later, the receptor concentration decreases as a result of their reducing biosynthesis.[50] The receptors of calcitonin are present in direct contact with two types of G-proteins, one of which activates adenylate cyclase and the other activates phospholipase C. Thus, this hormone can activate two different message pathways, cAMP- and Ca^{2+}-dependent.[51] The subsequent phosphorylation by protein kinase of integrin receptors and increasing concentration of intracellular Ca^{2+} causes the loss of the ruffled border and detachment from the bone matrix. The inhibiting action to resorption activity of osteoclasts is considered transient, connected with decreasing concentration of calcitonin receptors and/or their phosphorylation after influence of this hormone.[52]

The action of PTH on the bone resorption is varied and depends on the dose and duration of the hormone.[53] Its influence on osteoclasts not having PTH receptors is mediated by cells of microenvironment.[54] In small doses PTH and its fragment 1–34 increase the bone formation; in the majority of cases PTH stimulates osteoclastogenesis. A marked proresorption action is typical for PTH-related protein (PTH-rP). At present three isoforms of PTH-rP are isolated containing 139, 141, and 173 amino acids. The first 13 amino acids in these proteins have a high homology with PTH. PTH-rP is able to bind with a receptor of PTH.[55] It is interesting that carbonyl-terminal fragments of PTH-rP (106-111 and 107-139) inhibit osteoclastic bone resorption *in vitro*. The signficance of these observations remains unclear.[56]

Thyroid hormones T_3 and T_4 are considered to be the main systemic regulators of developing and remodeling bone. It is supposed that the influence of thyroid hormones on the bone tissue is conditioned by their effect on osteoblasts, which have receptors to these ligands.[57] Increasing the osteoclast activity one should connect with stimulation by thyroid hormones of osteoblast secretion of prostaglandins or signal transmission in direct contact of these cells.[58,59] Besides, for T_3 there is the other mechanism: T_3 increases hypophyseal secretion of the growth hormone which, in its turn, stimulates production of the insulin-like growth factor-1 (IGF-1) by the liver and other organs. IGF-1 modulates the osteoblast function, including their regulation of osteoclastogenesis.[60]

Sex hormones are of great importance in controlling the speed of the osteoclastic resorption. The main biological action of estrogen-$17\beta_2$-estradiol on the bone tissue lies in decreasing the rate of its resorption as a result of a direct influence of a hormone on the osteoclast precursors and reducing osteoclastogenesis. Indeed, receptors for $17\beta_2$-estradiol on the nuclei of preosteoclasts were detected.[61] In mature osteoclasts there were no receptors to estrogens, and their action to these cells is, apparently, mediated by osteoblasts that in response to the sex hormones reduce secretion of proosteolytic PGFs. Both ovariectomy and orchidectomy lead to increasing the bone resorption due to osteoclast activation.[62] The antiosteoporotic influence of $17\beta_2$-estradiol, testosterone, dihydroxytestosterone, and androgens is explained by an inhibiting effect of the hormones upon the IL-6 formation by osteoblasts and stromal cells of the bone marrow.[63]

Biologically active retinoic acids play a vital part in regulating the growth and cell differentiation of various tissues of an organism. Retinoid hypervitaminosis leads to osteopenia, fractures, and loss of the components of the bone matrix.[64] Yet, the retinoid deficiency causes osteosclerosis. The development of diseases can be connected with a complex influence of these agents both on osteoclasts and osteoblasts. Retinoic acids promote a formation of osteoclasts in the culture of the marrow cells and activate the osteoclastic resorption.[65] On the other hand, these mediators decrease the collagen production by osteoblasts and increase the collagenase secretion.[66]

Normally, the main part of the active metabolite of vitamin D_3 (calcitriol) is formed in the kidneys. This process is regulated by the hormones supporting calcium homeostasis in the organism in the first place, PTH. An excess of vitamin D in the organism leads to the bone demineralization and their fractures even under negligible loads. Calcitriol activates the bone resorption promoting a fusion of the mature precursors of osteoclasts and a formation of multinucleated cells in such a way.[4,67] It is suggested that in addition to effects on osteoclast precursors and those mediated via osteoblasts, this mediator could exert direct effects on the active bone resorbing osteoclasts.[68–70] It is shown that calcitriol stimulates the expression of various genes in osteoclasts including carbonic anhydrase II.[71]

Often it is difficult to establish a difference between the systemic and local factors regulating osteogenesis, as one and the same mediator is secreted both out of skeletal tissue and in direct contact with bone cells. To such substances one can attribute the platelet-activating factor (PAF), a derivative of glycerophosphocholine that is synthesized and released by neutrophils, monocytes, platelets, and endothelial cells. PAF acts directly on the osteoclasts increasing their resorption activity. Osteoclasts express the high-affinity receptors on their surface to this mediator connected, like calcitonin receptors, with G-protein. PAF interaction with a receptor causes increased concentration of cytosolic Ca^{2+} at the expense of its ejection from the intracellular depot. The subsequent transient contraction of pseudopodia during 30 min is not accompanied by a loss of activity of the ruffled border, as compared to the case of calcitonin acting on osteoclasts. The half-life of PAF in plasma is less than 10 minutes, as this mediator is destroyed by PAF-acetylhydrase.[72]

LOCAL REGULATION OF OSTEOCLASTS

The investigations of the last decade have shown that osteoclastogenesis and functional activity of mature osteoclasts are under regulatory control of not only humoral factors such as hormones of thyroid and parathyroid glands, $17\beta_2$-estradiol, calcitriol, but they are also modulated by many PGFs produced in the bone microenvironment by hemopoietic and stromal cells, including osteoblasts, fibroblasts, adipocytes, macrophages, pericytes, reticular cells, and endothelial cells. Moreover, these PGFs are mediators of many systemic hormones acting on the bone tissue. Regulating the osteoclastic bone resorption of PGFs can be considered on three levels: (1) proliferation of early osteoclast precursors and their differentiation; (2) fusion of late osteoclast precursors; and (3) activation of resorption function of mature osteoclasts (FIG. 1). At present, more than 20 protein cytokines have been discovered to have an influence on the growth and differentiation of osteoclasts. Among those with a stimulating action on osteoclastogenesis and an activation of a resorption function of mature osteoclasts *in vivo* and *in vitro* were IL-1β, -1α, -3, -6, -11, TNFs (-α and -β), leukemia inhibitory factor, GM-CSF, M-CSF, osteoclast colony-stimulating factor, osteogenic protein-1, platelet-derived growth factor (PDGF), TGF-α, IGFs (-1 and -2), macrophage inflammatory protein-α, and hepatocyte growth factor.[46, 73–79] An inhibiting action was found for interferon-γ, IL-4, -8, and -18, an antagonist of a receptor to IL-1 relating to the family of interleukins.[46,80,81] For some PGFs the influence on the bone resorption can be activating or inhibiting depending on the protein concentration, the initial functional state of bone cells, and other factors of microenvironment. This is so for heterodimers of TGF-β (TGF-β_1 and TGF-β_2). The biphasic properties of these cytokines are the basis for regulating resorption in young embryonic bones by means of modulating migration and differentiation of osteoclast precursors.[82,83] Studying a detailed mechanism of PGFs influence on the bone cells has revealed that TNF-α and IL-1 stimulate secretion by IL-6 osteoblasts, which directly affects osteoclasts.[46] Thus, the local regulation of osteoclast functions is realized by a whole PGF network in reciprocal and synergistic interrelations. The biphasic properties of PGFs to osteoclasts are explained by the ability to modulate synthesis by bone cells and in their microenvironment of prostaglandins. It is known that the prostaglandins influence (reduce/increase) on the differentiation of osteoclast precursors and this effect is dependent not only on the type (E_1, E_2, $F_2\alpha$) and dose, but also on the nature of the microenvironment.[84,85] The role of the other metabolites of arachidonic acid, leukotrienes, in regulating the function of osteoclasts remains unknown.

PGFs serve as bone-resorbing mediators in rheumatoid arthritis, periodontitis, osteomyelitis, and other disease when they are actively secreted by the immunocompetent cells infiltating the bone and its surrounding tissues. In the these pathologic processes the circulating PGF level increases in the organism and their systemic action becomes more expressive.

MECHANICAL REGULATION OF OSTEOCLAST RESORPTION

At present two possible ways for mechanical signals to be transmitted to osteoclasts have been proposed: (*1*) mechanical forces directly influence mechano-receptors of osteoclasts and/or preosteoclasts and (*2*) a mechanical stress influences osteoclasts by means of osteoblasts or chondrocytes.[86] Data indicating the presence of mechanosensitive ionic channels on the osteoblasts favor the second supposition.[87] The investigations show that pressure of 13 kPa on the bone organic structure decreases the resorption of mineral bone components while pressure of 100 kPa activates this process. It is probable that transmitting a signal modulating a resorption osteoclast function is mediated by prostaglandins, which are secreted by osteoblasts in response to the increase of pressure.[86] Recently it is shown that pressure regulates M-CSF expression and osteoclast formation in the marrow culture.[88] A certain role in the bone remodeling, apparently, belongs to dynamic electric potentials appearing in the bone due to piezoeffect under mechanical deformation of the components of the extracellular matrix. Unfortunately, the mechanisms of this regulation are not being studied intensively.

DISEASES ACCOMPANIED BY INCREASING THE BONE RESORPTION

Hereditary or acquired disturbance of remodeling process accompanied by increasing bone resorption, not compensated by the formation of a new bone matrix, may be one of the reasons for osteoporosis development. A progressive destruction of bone tissue leads to disappearance of the affected bone (bones) and/or their fragments, i.e. osteolysis, which is divided into the primary idiopathic osteolysis and secondary osteolysis.

According to the international nomenclature of hereditary skeleton pathologies (1983), phalangeal, tarsocarpal, and multifocal osteolyses are related to idiopathic osteolyses. The character of the genome disturbances in these diseases remains unclear for the present. There are only isolated reports about a link of hereditary variants of osteolysis with certain genetical markers.[89]

Some authors subdivide secondary osteolyses into diseases: (*1*) of the inflammatory genesis (rheumatoid arthritis, psoriatic arthropathy, lipodermatoarthritis, juvenile chronic arthritis, sarcoidosis and disseminated granulomatosis), (*2*) of vasculopathies (scleroderma, thromboangiitis obliterans, Raynaud's disease, and massive osteolysis or Gorham's disease), (*3*) of neuropathies (lepra, syringomyelia, congenital insensitivity to pain and peripheral neuropathy), (*4*) metabolic disturbances (porphyria, hyperparathyroidism), (*5*) chronic intoxications (with vinyl chloride, trichloroethylene), and (*6*) secondary osteolyses appearing in hereditary disease (epidermolysis bullosa, pachydermoperiostosis, and some others).[90] The given classification may have osteochondropathy, osteolysis in tumor growth, and some other pathologic states added to it.

In the majority of cases of secondary osteolyses there is a degradation of the bone tissue appearing several years from the beginning of the disease manifestation, obviously, as a result of disturbing the trophicity of the bone tissue in microthrombosis, perivascular fibrosis, and calcinosis. Participation of osteoclasts in mechanisms of the bone resorption in osteolysis and osteoporosis remains poorly studied up to now. Nevertheless, it can be assumed that on the basis of the bone resorption in these diseases there are the following processes: (*1*) dilation of lumina of Haversian and Folkman canals as well as interosteocytic microcanals by means of dissolving mineral and organic components (pH decrease, activation of matrix MMPs using a limited proteolysis, and/or removal of the inhibiting activity on TIMPs, proteinases release by endotheliocytes, pericytes, and cells of the perivascular infiltrate); (*2*) invasion of capillaries to affected parts of the cartilage and bone; (*3*) resorption of the bone tissue in subchondral parts due to activation of cells by the inflammatory mediators from a synovial fluid in arthritis and osteochondropathy (the production of proteinase by chondrocytes as well as pericytes and endotheliocytes and cytokines activating osteoclasts); (*4*) sinus resorption of "devital" parts of the bone tissue as a result of extracellular dissolving of the mineral and digesting the organic components (pH decrease, activation of tissue MMPs, destruction of collagen by MMPs, and released proteinase from osteocytes) with a subsequent increase of the formed cavities due to the cell resorption. In such a consideration of the osteolysis mechanism the osteoclastic resorption takes a direct part in the third and fourth processes and it is activated in the course of the events of the first and second processes. Indeed, the experimental investigations report the increased activity of osteoclasts in neovascularization of the bone tissue. If a cause of osteolysis lies not in acute angioneurotrophic changes, then osteoporosis is preceded, as a rule by a bone loss. Let us consider the possible, mainly, osteoclastic resorbing mechanisms of osteolysis and osteoporosis development in some pathologic states.

In inflammatory diseases the main pathogenetic factor of increasing the osteoclastic resorption one can call the osteotropic cytokines, the synthesis of which increases in phagocytosis of microbes by means of macrophagal cells as well as in response to the effect of microbic lipopolysaccharides and inflammatory mediators. It is seen in infectious peridontitis, chronic osteomyelitis, and septic arthritis.[91,92] Lipopolysaccharides stimulated the osteoblasts to increasing the secretion of collagenase, plasminogen activator, and cytokines regulating osteoclastogenesis, such as GM-CSF and M-CSF.[93-95] The osteoporosis and osteolysis development in aseptic periodontitis and arthritis is also connected with the appearance of inflammatory mediators in gingival and synovial fluid, and in particular, PAF.[96,97] An important value in developing destructive processes of the bone tissue in cholesteatoma of the middle ear belongs to PDGF, TNF-α, IL-1, and IL-6.[74,98] It is possible that in sarcoidosis calcitriol has a definite pathogenetic role.[99] The level of calcitriol increases in the subject with such a disease. It should be noted that the extrarenal formation of calcitriol by macrophages is observed in some inflammatory diseases, including periodontitis and arthritis.[100] In chronic inflammation in activation of osteoclastic resorption a certain role belongs to acidosis that activates a vacuolar H^+ pump in osteoclasts.[101] In inflammatory diseases of the skeletal tissue, except osteoclasts in resorption of mineral and organic components of the matrix, the other cells of the organism, in particular, synoviocytes, chondrocytes, macrophages, and multinucleated giant cells, take an active part as well.[102,103]

The causes of disturbing coordination between the osteosynthetic and resorption processes in neuro-, vasculo-, and chondropathy can be revealed in considering the bone as an integral functional system only, the components of which, i.e., bone cells, bone marrow, microvessels, and a cartilage, have been developed from the common source (mesenchyme). In the course of ontogenesis the links between the differentiated parts of this system are not interrupted, they become more and more complex. PGFs give cooperative interrelations between the osteoblasts, osteoclasts, and cells of capillaries and bone marrow sinuses (pericytes and endotheliocytes).

The influence of endotheliocytes on the osteoclastogenesis and mature osteoclasts is considered to be versatile. It is shown that the endothelial cells can secrete both endothelin, inhibiting the bone resorption by osteoclasts, and IGF-1, which is a chemotactic factor for preosteoclasts.[73] On the contrary, in the direct contact with preosteoclasts the endotheliocytes stimulate the osteoclastogenesis. Neuroregulation of the osteoclastic resorption is, apparently, mediated by means of pericytes as it has been discovered that the nerve endings invaginate the cytoplasm of these cells.[104] Disturbance of the stated regulatory mechanisms may be one of the causes of osteolysis in neuro- and vasculopathy, including Gorham's disease. Histomorphologic structure of the affected focus in this disease is characterized by a wide net of the capillary-like vessels. The branched network of microvessels leads to the deceleration of the blood flow, local hypoxia, and pH reduction, i.e., conditions necessary for activating the hydrolytic enzymes.[105] In juvenile chondropathy the mechanism of the capillary invasion, phylogenetically worked in the course of a morphogenetic process of the enchondral ossification and forming the primitive marrow cavities, plays a pathophysiologic role.

The mechanism of developing osteoporosis and osteolysis in tumor growth is explained by activating osteoclastogenesis and mature osteoclasts by local and systemic mediators. Direct bone resorption by tumor-associated macrophages and giant cells is of importance in osteoclastomas and metastases to the bone in the late stages of a disease.[106] Multinucleated giant osteoclast-like cells of macrophage origin are discovered in osteoblastoclastoma tissue. It is considered that insensibility of these cells to the inhibiting calcitonin effect leads to the uncontrolled destruction of the bone tissue.[107] In metastatic lesions of skeletal or extraskeletal tumors, the cancer cells secrete bone-resorbing mediators that have local and generalized effects if they are produced in a large amount and/or the period of time of their existence in the organism is enough for creating the acting concentration in the remote parts of the skeleton. In multiple myeloma the main proosteolytic mediators are IL-1β, IL-6, and TNF-β; in lymphoma, IL-6; in breast cancer, renal carcinoma, and carcinoma of the skin, PTH-rP; and in ovarian cancer, PTH.[108,109] An increase of PTH-rP level, produced by the cells of bone metastases has been noted as compared to primary breast cancer. It is possible that the bone microenvironment has an activating effect on the gene expression of this protein.[109] PTH-rP, as well as fragments of PTH (1-34 and 1-84) and PTH-rP (1-34, 107-111, and 107-139) are also called the factors of hypercalcemia of tumor growth.[65,110] Increasing the level of circulating PTH-rP may be a consequence of its synthesis regulation disturbance in a malignant transformation and/or derepression of this protein gene transcription. The pathogenetic role in developing the osteolysis may have PAF found in the plasma of the oncologic patients with hypercalcemia.[111] It can be suggested that the process of neovascularization has a significant value in osteoclast activation in the tumoral growth. In Paget's disease, a slow viral infection, there is a disturbance of osteoclast functions. The osteoclasts from patients with Paget's disease mature quicker, they contain many more nuclei, they are much larger, and appear to be more metabolically active compared to the normal osteoclasts. These cells show hypersensitivity to calcitriol and hypesthesia to calcitonin.[71,112] Besides, they actively secrete IL-6, and the level of this mediator in the plasma of the bone marrow and peripheral blood increases.[112] Increasing the general activity of osteoclasts leads to the local destruction of the bone, which can be restored only partially by the formation of the inferior matrix. In osteoclasts, but not osteoblasts, isolated from the affected bone parts there were found specific inclusions representing nucleocapside proteins of *Paramyxoviridae* virus. The pathologic role of these viral inclusions is unknown. It is supposed that they play a role in tumoral transformation, i.e., the formation of giant cell tumor of bone.[112,113]

In pathogenesis of bone resorption in a total replacement of the hip joint by an endoprosthesis, the main role belongs to the microparticles formed as a result of fragmentation of the biomaterials in tribological system: bone/cement/femoral stem. The particles of a high-molecular polyethylene formed in friction of acetabular components of the endoprosthesis represent a pair: a metallic head/cap from a high-molecular polyethylene is of significant value as well. Owing to submicron dimensions (from 0.4 to 0.5 μm) the particles of polyethylene are easily transported and phagocytized. The rate of the particle formation can rise if fragments of cement or metal hit a pit between the acetabular components of head/cap as a result of abrasion by the "third body." Particle absorption by macrophages and the other cells of the surrounding tissue is accompanied by activation and a sharp increase of the secretion of a large number of cytokines and another biologically active mediators stimulating osteoclastic resorption by these cells.[114,115]

The role of osteoclasts in the mechanism of increasing bone resorption, which accompanies sarcoidosis, psoriasis, scleroderma, lepra, histiocytosis X, syringomyelia, and porphyria, is not practically investigated. Increasing the bone resorption in diabetes I and its decreasing in acute pancreatitis, probably, are partially mediated by a disturbance of forming and secreting the peptides of the pancreas, insulin and amylin. Insulin has a homology with IGF-1 and IGF-2, and amylin (a protein consisting of 37 amino acids) has a 50% homology with calcitonin gene–related protein.[116] The main osteoporotic factors in diabetes are, apparently, microangiopathy in the vascular system of the bone and myelitis.[117]

The role of osteoclastic resorption in developing a general osteoporosis may be connected with increasing the PTH and thyroid hormones levels (hyperparathyroidism, hyperthyroidism, intoxication by thyroid hormones) and the decreasing plasma levels of sex hormones and calcitonin in due to aging.[117–119] So, a postmenopausal osteoporosis is explained by a cancellation of the inhibiting effect of $17\beta_2$-estradiol on the IL-6 secretion by osteoblasts and stimulation of TGF-β synthesis.[63] The development of osteopenia in old age is defined by an increase in general activity of osteoclasts compared to osteoblasts due to decreasing a maturation of preosteoblasts, here, the proportion of the cells preosteoclast/osteoclast remains almost unchanged.[103]

DISEASES ACCOMPANIED BY DECREASING THE BONE RESORPTION

Hereditary or acquired decreases in the resorption function of osteoclasts and/or pathologic increases of bone matrix formation lead to the development of the skeleton diseases characterized by a presence of a local or generalized osteosclerosis. The local hyperostoses may be a reactive response of the regional bone tissue in osteoporosis and/or osteolysis accompanying the course of the chronic osteomyelitis, tuberculosis of bones, tumoral metastases to the bone, Paget's disease, sarcoidosis, and some other diseases.

To the osteopetrosis diseases one should attribute a group of hereditary pathologies of a skeletal tissue characterized by a generalized osteosclerosis and systemic hyperostosis, residual cartilage calcification, and pathologic fractures. In each concrete case a genome disturbance can be various. The deficiency of carbonic anhydrase II in a human leads to the syndrome accompanied by osteopetrosis, tubular acidosis, and cerebral calcification.[120] There had been described cases when in children with osteopetrosis the osteoclasts were not able to develop a ruffled border.[121] A disturbance of $O_2^{\pm}$ production neutrophils was found in patients with autosomal recessive form of osteopetrosis.[122] It is supposed that the mechanism of hyperostosis observed in craniometaphysial dysplasia is connected with a disturbance of the osteoclast function. The cells obtained in the course of osteoclastogenesis (*in vitro*) from the bone marrow cells in patients with craniometaphysial dysplasia were incapable of resorbing the bone slices due to the absence of the expression of H^+-ATPase.[123] The authors of the report believe that in patients with this disease there is also a disturbance of osteoclastogenesis that leads to the inferior osteoclast formation.

At present, biologists have a great number of lines of experimental animals with osteopetrosis mutations. Examining the animals with such mutations revealed a decrease of the osteoclast dimensions due to a disturbance of fusion of their precursors (*mi*), no ruffled borders formed (*oc*),the absence of synthesis in the organism M-CSF (*op*), the increase of calcitonin formation (*gl*) and osteoclast sensitivity to it (*mi*), deficiency of src-tyrosine kinase (*c-src-*), the absence of receptors for M-CSF (*c-fos-*), the lack of hematopoietic transcription factor PU.1, and a disturbance of osteoclastogenesis in rats due to mutation touching the microenvironment cells, probably, osteoblasts (*tl*) and also the osteocalcin deficiency in bone matrix.[121,124–128] Thus, the mutations causing certain regulatory or functional disturbances of the osteoclastic resorption can lead to the development of osteopetrosis.

MECHANISMS OF THERAPEUTIC TREATMENTS FOR DISEASES WITH BONE RESORPTION DISTURBANCE

The use of the main physiologic antiresorption hormone of calcitonin for treating the osteolytic states was not widely practiced as, in the first place, this substance is quickly decomposed in the organism and, in the second place, some days later resistance to the drug develops. Using estrogens and their analogs also has its shortcomings.[117] So, at present there is an active search for new means for treating these diseases. Bisphosphonates are related to such substances and were considered as an alternative treatment.

Bisphosponates are synthetic analogs of pyrophosphate, where phospatic groups are divided by a stable methyl group, P-CR_1R_2-P. Substitution of an oxygenous bridge P-O-P for the carbonic one P-C-P leads to a greater enzymatic stability of preparations. For treating the hypercalcemic states connected with increasing the bone resorption aledronate, pamidronate, etidronate, YM-175 and other compounds are used. Their chemical structure (groupings R_1 and R_2) as well a degree of antiresorption action are different.[129] Like pyrophosphate, bisphosphonates have a high affinity to the mineral bone phase and act as the inhibitors of growth and dissolving the calcium phosphate crystals, but compared to pyrophosphate, bisphosphonates are strong inhibitors of the bone resorption by osteoclasts.

At the present time bisphosphonates are widely used for treating diseases with a disturbance of the mineral bone metabolism including Paget's disease, tumoral hypercalcemia, and postmenopausal osteoporosis as well.[130] Apparently, for preventing the osteoporosis development in a forced hypokinesia and long space flights using these preparations may be rather promising. The effect of bisphosphonate on bone cells is considered to be versatile. It is connected with suppressing the differentiation and recruitment of the osteoclast precursors as a result of interaction with the components of the bone matrix or decreasing the resorption activity of the mature osteoclasts due to their ionic permeability disturbance.[131] Approaches for treating the hyperostosis diseases by bisphosphonates are developed to a lesser degree.

Gallium nitrate is used for treating the humoral hypercalcemia associated with tumoral growth. At present the main details of the mechanisms of the antiresorption effect of this substance have been established: due to affinity to the bone tissue gallium is included to the mineralized matrix decreasing a dissolvability of hydroxyapatite crystals and making them more stable to degradation by osteoclasts. On the other hand, gallium decreases a secretion of osteocalcin with the help of osteoblasts and its content in the bone matrix. It is assumed that the influence of gallium nitrate on the osteoclasts is conditioned by modulating the response of osteoblasts to PTH.[43,87,132,133] It is also reported that gallium suppresses the activity of enzymes in osteoclasts.[133]

Good results have been obtained in treating Paget's disease, a primary hyperparathyroidism and osteoporosis by ipriflavone, the preparation relating to the flavenoid series.[134] At the present time there is a search of the optimal variants of the antiresorptive and anabolic agents for a combined therapy of postmenopausal and age-related osteoporosis.

The approaches to treating the osteopetrosis diseases are at the developmental stage, the few publications on this subject are evidence of this fact. Injections of M-CSF preparation to mice with *op* mutation and rates with *tl* mutation increased a number of osteoclasts, restored their normal activity, and decreased osteosclerosis to a considerable degree.[121] According to the data by Key and colleagues[135] the activation of the bone resorption in patients with a hereditary osteopetrosis was achieved in an extended treatment regimen (from 1.5 to 2 years) of recombinant human interferon-γ_{1b} injections.

Thus, the effect of many preparations used for correcting a pathology of the bone resorption is directed at a decrease of the rate of the bone matrix reconstruction and a direct or mediated modulation of the osteoclast activity. Positive results of PGF treatments testify to their important role in osteoclastogenesis and a regulation of the osteoclastic bone resorption.

CONCLUSION

Compared to the other cells of the monocyte-macrophage lineage, osteoclasts realize extracellular resorption. When the extracellular mechanism of the digestion is disturbed, as in pycnodysostosis disease, osteoclastic phagocytosis of the bone mineral and collagen fragments is observed.[45] The extracellular process of resorption became possible due to the presence of rather dense substrate, i.e., bone matrix. This circumstance provides an opportunity to consider this process from a different perspective: as a corrosion of the calcium-phosphate material with organic inclusions in biological environment.[136] In this case, the bone dissolution in the hemivacuole under the osteoclast can be considered as a highly biological regulated process of "pitting corrosion." It is rather curious that multinucleated cells capable of resorbing sintered hydroxyapatite received a name of ceramoclasts.[137]

The unique peculiarity of osteoclasts lies in the fact that they can may be formed as a result of fusion both of their direct marrow precursors and monocytes of the peripheral blood.[138,139] One may say that various subpopulations of osteoclasts are evidently formed as a circulation of monocytes in the bloody channels affect their morphofunctional status. It can be assumed that the way osteoclasts are formed from monocytes is turned to be "urgent," e.g., in fractures, an inflammatory process, and some other pathologic states. There are only isolated reports devoted to a comparative characterization of osteoclasts and osteoclast-like cells in normal states and in some diseases. At the same time, the analysis of the literary data shows that there are common ways of regulating the morphogenesis, reparation, and inflammatory processes in the bone tissue. First, the presence of one and the same mediators of these processes, namely PGFs, participate in physiologic skeleton bone reparation, remodeling in embryonic and postnatal periods, and serve as local and systemic agents in the bone tissue in some pathologic states. Second, there is a similarity between the formation of multinucleated giant cells of the foreign bodies in inflammatory processes and osteoclast formation. Thus, for further explanation of mechanisms of physiologic and pathophysiologic bone resorption, the exposure of similarity and differences between the processes of osteoclastogenesis and formation of giant multinucleated cells in inflammations of granulomatous character and a comparative study of the morphofunctional peculiarities of various (by origin) osteoclasts and osteoclast-like cells can be considered as promising directions.

In conclusion, it should be noted that the observation of B. L. Alyoshin made 60 years ago[140] that "an inflammation taking part in the formation of the definite structure of an organism is turned to be a morphogenetic factor" continues to be a fundamental insight for researchers today.

ACKNOWLEDGMENTS

The manuscript was prepared with the excellent help of Tamara Ventsel and Vladimir Abrosimov.

REFERENCES

1. MAZHUGA, P. M. 1995. The mononuclear and multinuclear cell of tissue resorption and their functional characteristics. Tsitol. Genet. (Rus.) **29:** 9–108.
2. HORTON, M. A. & M. H. HELFRICH. 1992. Antigenic markers of osteoclasts. *In* Biology and Physiology of the Osteoclast. B. R. Rifkin & C. V. Gay, Eds.: 33–54. CRC Press. Boca Raton, FL.
3. TAKAHASHI, N., N. UDAGAVA, S. TANAKA, H. MURAKAMI, I. OWAN, T. TAMURA & T. SUDA. 1994. Postmitotic osteoclast precursors are mononuclear cells which express macrophage-associated phenotypes. Dev. Biol. **163:** 212–221.
4. HATTERSLEY, G. & T. J. CHAMBERS. 1989. Calcitonin receptors as markers for osteoclastic differentiation: correlation between generation of bone-resorptive cells and cells that express calcitonin receptors in mouse bone marrow cultures. Endocrinology **125:** 1606–1612.
5. LEE, E. R., L. LAMPLUGH, N. L. SHEPARD & J. S. MORT. 1995. The septoclast, a cathepsin B-rich cell involved in the resorption of growth plate cartilage. Histochem. Cytochem. **43:** 525–536.
6. LOMRI, A. & R. BARON. 1992. 1,25-Dixydroxyvitamin D_3 regulates the transcription of carbonic anhydrase II mRNA in avian myelomonocytes. Proc. Natl Acad. Sci. USA **89:** 4688–4692.

7. NESBITT, S., A. NESBIT, M. HELFRICH & M. HORTON. 1993. Biochemical characterization of human osteoclast integrins. Osteoclasts express $\alpha_v\beta_1$, $\alpha_2\beta_1$, and $\alpha_v\beta_1$ integrins. J. Biol. Chem. **268:** 16737–16745.

8. VAN DER PLUIJM, G., H. MOUTHAAN, C. BAAS, H. DE GROOT, S. PAPAPOULOS & C. LOWIK. 1994. Integrins and osteoclastic resorption in three bone organ cultures: differential sensitivity to synthetic Arg-Gly-Asp peptides during osteoclast formation. J. Bone Miner. Res. **9:** 1021–1028.

9. BERTOLINI, D. R., G. E. NEDWIN, T. S. BRINGHAM, D. D. SMITH & G. R. MUNDY. 1986. Stimulation of bone resorption and inhibitors of bone resorption in vitro by human tumor necrosis factors. Nature **319:** 516–518.

10. HEATH, J. K., S. L. ATKINSON, M. C. MEIKLE & J. J. REYNOLDS. 1984. Mouse osteoblasts synthesize collagenase in response to bone resorbing agents. Biochim. Biophys. Acta **802:** 151–154.

11. RIFAS L., A. FAUSTO, M. J. SCOTT, L. V. AVIOLI & H. G. WELGUS. 1994. Expression of metalloproteinases and tissue inhibitors of metalloproteinases in human osteoblast-like cells: differentiation is associated with repression of metalloproteinase biosynthesis. Endocrinology **134:** 213–221.

12. RIFAS, L., L. R. HALSTEAD, W. A. PECK, L. V. AVIOLI & H. G. WELGUS. 1989. Human osteoblasts in vitro secrete tissue inhibitor of metalloproteinases and gelatinase but not interstinal collagenase as major cellular products. J. Clin. Invest. **84:** 686–694.

13. HALL, T. J., M. SCHAEUBLIN & M. MISSBACH. 1994. Evidence that c-src is involved in the process of osteoclastic bone resorption. Biochem. Biophys. Res. Commun. **199:** 1237–1244.

14. BLAIR, H. C., S. L. TEITELBAUM, R. GHISELLI & S. GLUCK. 1989. Osteoclastic bone resorption by a polarized vacuolar proton pump. Science **245:** 855–857.

15. BASTANI, B., F. P. ROSS, R. P. KOPITO & S. L. GLUCK. 1996. Immunocytochemical localization of vacuolar H^+-ATPase and $Cl-HCO_3^-$ anion exchanger (erythrocyte band-3 protein) in avian osteoclasts: effect of calcium-deficient diet on polar expression of the H^+-ATPase pump. Calcif. Tiss. Int. **58:** 332–336.

16. ETHERINGTON, D. J. & H. BIRKEDAL-HANSEN. 1987. The influence of dissolved calcium salts on the degradation of hard-tissue collagens by lysosomal cathepsins. Collagen Rel. Res. **7:** 185–199.

17. DELAISSÉ, J.-M. & G. VAES. 1992. Mechanism of mineral solubilization and matrix degradation in osteoclastic bone resorption. *In* Biology and Physiology of the Osteoclast. B. R. Rifkin & C. V. Gay, Eds.: 289–314. CRC Press. Boca Raton, FL.

18. GOTO, T., T. KIYOSHIMA, R. MOROI, T. TSUKUBA, Y. NISHIMURA, M. HIMENO, K. YAMAMOTO & T. TANAKA. 1994. Localization of cathepsins B, D, and L in the rat osteoclast by immuno-light and -electron microscopy. Histochemistry **101:** 33–40.

19. INAOKA, T., G. BILBE, O. ISHIBASHI, K. TEZUKA, M. KUMEGAWA & T. KOKUBO. 1995. Molecular cloning of human cDNA for cathepsin K: novel cysteine proteinase predominantly expressed in bone. Biochem. Biophys. Res. Commun. **206:** 89–96.

20. RIFKIN, B. R., A. T. VERNILLO & A. P. KLECKNER. 1991. Cathepsin B and L activities in isolated osteoclasts. Biochem. Biophys. Res. Commun. **179:** 63–69.

21. ITO, S. 1974. Form and function of the glycocalyx of free cell surface. Phil. Trans. Roy. Soc. London. **268:** 55–66.

22. TEZUKA, K., K. NEMOTO, Y. TEZUKA, T. SATO, Y. IKEDA, M. KOBORI, H. KAWASHIMA, H. EGUCHI, Y. HAKEDA & M. KUMEGAWA. 1994. Identification of matrix metalloproteinase-9 in rabbit osteoclasts. J. Biol. Chem. **269:** 15006–15009.

23. OKADA, Y., K. NAKA, K. KAWAMURA, T. MATSUMOTO, I. NAKANISHI, N. FUJIMOTO, H. SATO & M. SEIKI. 1995. Localization of matrix metalloproteinase 9 (92-kilodalton gelatinase/type IV collagenase-gelatinase B) in osteoclasts: implications for bone resorption. Lab. Invest. **72:** 311–322.

24. BARON, R., J.-H. RAVESLOOT, L. NEFF, M. CHAKRABORTY, D. CHATTERJEE, A. LOMRI & W. HORNE. 1993. Cellular and molecular biology of the osteoclast. *In* Cellular and Molecular Biology of Bone: 445–494. Academic Press. New York.

25. ADEBANJO, O. A., V. S. SHANKAR, M. PAZIANAS, A. ZAIDI, B. SIMON, C. L. HUANG & M. ZAIDI. 1994. Modulation of the osteoclast Ca^{2+} receptor by extracellular protons: possible linkage between Ca^{2+} sensing and extracellular acidification. Biochem. Biophys. Res. Commun. **199:** 742–747.

26. ZAIDI, M. 1990. "Calcium receptors" on eukariotic cells with special reference to the osteoclast. Biosci. Rep. **10:** 493–507.

27. SILVER, I. A., R. J. MURRILLS & D. J. ETHERINGTON. 1988. Microelectrode studies on the acid microenvironment beneath adherent macrophages and osteoclasts. Exp. Cell Res. **175:** 266–276.

28. HALL, T. J. 1994. A reappraisal of the effect of extracellular calcium on osteoclastic bone resorption. Biochem. Biophys. Res. Commun. **202:** 456–462.

29. HAM, A. W. & D. H. CORMACK. 1979. Histology. J. B. Lippincott Company, PL.

30. LELOUP, G., J. M. DELAISSE & G. VAES. 1994. Relationship of the plasminogen activator/plasmin cascade to osteoclast invasion and mineral resorption in explanted fetal metatarsal bones. J. Bone Miner. Res. **9:** 891–902.

31. THOMSON, B. M., S. J. ATKINSON, A. M. MCGARRITY, R. M. HEMBRY, J. J. REYNOLDS & M. C. MEIKLE. 1989. Type I collagen degradation by mouse calvarial osteoblasts stimulated with 1,25-dihydroxyvitamin D-3: evidence for a plasminogen-plasmin-metalloproteinase activation cascade. Biochim. Biophys. Acta **1014:** 125–132.

32. KEY, L. L. JR, W. C. WOLF, C. M. GUNBERG & W. L. RIES. 1994. Superoxide and bone resorption. Bone **15:** 431–436.

33. KHALKHALI-ELLIS, Z., P. COLLIN-OSDOBY, L. LI, M. L. BRANDI & P. OSDOBY. 1997. A human homolog of the 150 kD avian osteoclast membrane antigen related to superoxide dismutase and essential for bone resorption is induced by developmental agents and opposed by estrogen in FLG 29.1 cells. Calcif. Tissue Int. **60:** 187–193.

34. DATTA, H., P. MANNING, H. RATHOD & C. J. MCNEIL. 1995. Effect of calcitonin, elevated calcium and extracellular matrices on superoxide anion production by rat osteoclasts. Exp. Physiol. **80:** 713–719.

35. EASTELL, R. 1994. Biochemical markers. Spine: State of the Art Rev. **8:** 155–170.

36. INGRAM, R. T., Y. K. PARK, B. L. CLARKE & L. A. FITZPATRICK. 1994. Age- and gender-related changes in the distribution of osteocalcin in the extracellular matrix of normal male and female bone. Possible involvement of osteocalcin in bone remodelling. J. Clin. Invest. **93:** 989–997.

37. LIGGETT, W. H., J. B. LIAN, J. S. GREENBERGER & J. GLOWACKI. 1994. Osteocalcin promotes differentiation of osteoclast progenitors from murine long-term bone marrow cultures. J. Cell. Biochem. **55:** 190–199.

38. GLOWACKI, J. & J. B. LIAN. 1987. Impaired recruitment and differentiation of osteoclast progenitors by osteocalcin-depleted bone implants. Cell Differ. **21:** 247–254.

39. STAAL, A., H. POLS, C. BUURMAN, T. VINK, G. VANDENBEMD, J. BIRKENHAGER & J. VAN-LEEUWEN. 1992. Differences in interaction between TGF-β and $1,25(OH)_2D_3$ in VDR and osteocalcin gene expression. J. Bone Miner. Res. **7:** S173.

40. GRZESIK, W. J. & P. G. ROBEY. 1994. Bone matrix RGD-glycoproteins: immunolocalization and interaction with primary cells in vitro. J. Bone Miner. Res. **9:** 487–496.

41. HELFRICH, M. H., S. A. NESBITT, E. L. DOREY & M. A. HORTON. 1992. Rat osteoclasts adhere to a wide range of RGD (arg-gly-asp) peptide-containing proteins, including the bone sialoproteins and fibronectin, via a β_3 integrin. J. Bone Mineral Res. **7:** 335–343.

42. GRANO, M., P. ZIGRINO, S. COLUCCI, G. ZAMBONIN, L. TRUSOLINO, M. SERRA, N. BALDINI, A. TETI, P. C. MARCHISIO & A. Z. ZALLONE. 1994. Adhesion properties and integrin expression of cultured human osteoclast-like cells. Exp. Cell. Res. **212:** 209–218.

43. EK-RYLANDER, B., M. FLORES, M. WENDEL, D. HEINEGARD & G. ANDERSON. 1994. Dephosphorylation of osteopontin and bone sialoprotein by osteoclastic tartrate-resistant acid phosphatase. J. Biol. Chem. **269:** 14853–14856.

44. HORNE, W. C., J. B. LEVY & R. BARON. 1993. Proto-oncogenes and osteoclast function. Ital. J. Mineral Electrolyte Metab. **7:** 185–197.

45. GLOWACKI, J. 1992. The influence of matrix components on osteoclasts. *In* Biology and Physiology of the Osteoclast. B. R. Rifkin & C. V. Gay, Eds.: 187–206. CRC Press. Boca Raton, FL.

46. MUNDY, G. R. 1992. Local factors regulating osteoclast function. *In* Biology and Physiology of the Osteoclast. B. R. Rifkin & C. V. Gay, Eds.: 171–185. CRC Press. Boca Raton, FL.

47. CHAMBERS, T. J., P. M. MCSHEEHY, B. M. THOMSON & K. FULLER. 1985. The effect of calcium-regulating hormones and prostaglandins on bone resorption by osteoclasts disaggregated from neonatal rabbit bones. Endocrinology **116:** 234–239.

48. NICHOLSON, G. C., J. M. MOSELEY, P. M. SEXTON, F. A. MENDELSON & T. J. MARTIN. 1986. Abundant calcitonin receptors in rat osteoclasts. Biochemical and autoradiographic characterization. J. Clin. Invest. **78:** 355–360.

49. IKEGAME, M., S. EJIRI & H. OZAWA. 1994. Histochemical and autoradiographic studies on elcatonin internalization and intracellular movement in osteoclasts. J. Bone Miner. Res. 9: 25–37.

50. WADA, S., T. J. MARTIN & D. M. FINDLAY. 1995. Homologous regulation of the calcitonin receptor in mouse osteoclast-like cells and human breast cancer T47D cells. Endocrinology 36: 2611–2621.

51. ZAIDI, M., H. K. DATTA, B. S. MOONGA & I. MACINTYRE. 1990. Evidence that the action of calcitonin on rat osteoclasts is mediated by two G proteins acting via separate post-receptor pathways. J. Endocrinol. **126:** 473–481.

52. DONAHUE, H. J. 1992. Signal tranduction mechanisms in osteoclasts. *In* Biology and Physiology of the Osteoclast. B. R. Rifkin & C. V. Gay, Eds.: 207–222. CRC Press. Boca Raton, FL.

53. BOIVIN, G., C. ANTHOINE-TERRIER & G. MOREL. 1994. Ultrastructural localization of endogenous hormones and receptors in bone tissue: an immunocytological approach in frozen samples. Micron **25:** 15–27.

54. MCSHEEHY, P. M. & T. J. MARTIN. 1986. Osteoblastic cells mediate osteoclastic responsiveness to parathyroid hormone. Endocrinology **118:** 824–828.

55. ORLOFF, J. J. & A. F. STEWART. 1989. Parathyroid hormone-like proteins: bichemical responses and receptor interactions. Endocr. Rev. **10:** 476–495.

56. GUISE, T. A. & G. R. MUNDY. 1996. Physiological and pathological role of parathyroid hormone-related peptide. Curr. Opinion Nephrol. Hypertension. **5:** 307–315.

57. BRITO, J. M., A. J., FENTON, W. R. HOLLOWAY & G. C. NICHOLSON. 1994. Osteoblasts mediate thyroid hormone stimulation of osteoclastic bone resorption. Endocrinology **134:** 169–176.

58. JIMI, E, I. NAKAMURA, H. AMANO, Y. TAGUCHI, T. TSURUKAI, M. TAMURA, N. TAKAHASHI & T. SUDA. 1996. Osteoclast function is activated by osteoblastic cells through a mechanism involving cell-to-cell contact. Endocrinology **137:** 2187–2190.

59. KLEIN, D. C. & L. G. RAISZ. 1970. Prostaglandins: stimulation of bone resorption in tissue culture. Endocrinology **86:** 1436–1440.

60. OHLSSON, C., J. ISGAARD, J. TORNELL, A. NILSSON, O. G. P. ISAKSSON & A. LINDAHL. 1993. Endocrine regulation of longitudinal bone growth. Acta Pediatr. Suppl. **391:** 33–40.

61. FIORELLI, G., F. GORI, M. PETILLI, A. TANINI, S. BENVENUTI, M. SERIO, P. BERNABEI & M. L. BRANDI. 1995. Functional estrogen receptors in a human preosteoclastic cell line. Proc. Natl. Acad. Sci. USA **92:** 2672–2676.

62. CLARKE, N. W., J. MCCLURE & N. J. GEORGE. 1993. The effects of orchidectomy on skeletal metabolism in metastatic prostate cancer. Scand. J. Urol. Nephrol. **27:** 475–483.

63. MANOLAGAS, S. C. & R. L. JILKA. 1992. Cytokines, hematopoiesis, osteoclastogenesis, and estrogens. Calcif. Tiss. Int. **50:** 199–202.

64. HOUGH, S., L. V. AVIOLI, H. MUIR & D. GELDERBLOM. 1988. Effects of hypervitaminosis A on the bone and mineral metabolism of the rat. Endocrinology **122:** 2933–2939.

65. KAJI, H., T. SUGIMOTO, M. KANATANI, M. FUKASE & K. CHIHARA. 1995. Retinoic acid induces osteoclast-like cell formation by directly acting on hemopoietic blast cells and stimulates osteopontin mRNA expression in isolated osteoclasts. Life Sci. **56:** 1903–1913.

66. CONNOLLY, T. J., J. C. CLOHISY, J. S. SHILT, K. D. BERGMAN, N. C. PARTRIDGE & C. O. QUINN. 1994. Retinoic acid stimulates interstinal collagenase messenger ribonucleic acid in osteosarcoma. Endocrinology **135:** 2542–2548.

67. THAVARAJAH, M., D. B. EVANS, L. BINDERUP & J. A. KANIS. 1990. $1,25(OH)_2D_3$ and calcipotriol (MC903) have similar effects on the induction of osteoclast-like cell formation in human bone marrow cultures. Biochem. Biophys. Res. Commun. **171:** 1056–1063.

68. MCSHEEHY, P. M. & T. J. CHAMBERS. 1987. Dihydroxyvitamin D_3 stimulates rat osteoblastic cells to release a soluble factor that increases osteoclastic bone resorption. J. Clin. Invest. **80:** 425–429.

69. MEE, A. P., J. A. HOYLAND, I. P. BRAIDMAN, A. J. FREEMONT, M. DAVIES & E. B. MAWER. 1996. Demonstration of vitamin D receptor transcripts in actively resorbing osteoclasts in bone sections. Bone **18:** 295–299.

70. MERKE, J., G. KLAUS, U. HUGEL, R. WALDHERR & E. RITZ. 1986. No 1,25-dihydroxyvitamin D_3 receptors on osteoclasts of calcium deficient chicken despite demonstrable receptors on circulating monocytes. J. Clin. Invest. **77:** 312–314.

71. BILLECOCQ, A., J. EMANUEL, R. LEVENSON & R. BARON. 1990. $1\alpha,25$-Dihydroxyvitamin D_3 regulates the expression of carbonic anhydrase II in nonerythroid avian bone marrow cells. Proc. Nat. Acad. Sci. USA. **87:** 6470–6474.

72. ZHENG, Z. G., D. A. WOOD, S. M. SIMS & S. J. DIXON. 1993. Platelet-activating factor stimulates resorption by rabbit osteoclasts in vitro. Am. J. Physiol. **264:** E74-81.

73. FORMIGLI, L., S. Z. ORLANDINI, S. BENVENUTI, L. MASI, A. PINTO, V. GATTEI, P. A. BERNABEI, P. G. ROBEY, P. COLLIN-OSDOBY & M. L. BRANDI. 1995. In vitro structural and functional relationships between preosteoclastic and bone endothelial cells: a juxtacrine model for migration and adhesion of osteoclast precursors. J. Cell. Physiol. **162:** 199–21.

74. FUJIOKA, O. & C.-C. HUANG. 1994. Platelet-derived growth factor in middle ear cholesteatoma. Eur. Arch. Otorhinolaryngol. **251:** 199–204.

75. GIRASOLE, G., G. PASSERI, R. L. JILKA & S. C. MANOLAGAS. 1994. Interleukin-11: a new cytokine critical for osteoclast development. J. Clin. Invest. **93:** 1516–1524.

76. KUKITA, T., H. NOMIYAMA, Y. OHMOTO, A. KUKITA, T. SHUTO, T. HOTOKEBUCHI, U. SUGIOKA, R. MIURA & T. IIJIMA. 1997. Macrophage inflammatory protein-1 α (LD78) expressed in human bone marrow: its role in regulation of hematopoiesis and osteoclast recruitment. Lab. Invest. **76:** 399–406.

77. LORENZO, J. A., S. L. SOUSA & M. CENTRELLA. 1988. Interleukin-1 in combination with transforming growth factor-α produces enhanced bone resorption in vitro. Endocrinology **123:** 2194–2200.

78. MOCHIZUKI, H., Y. HAKEDA, N. WAKATSUKI, N. USUI, S. AKASHI, T. SATO, K. TANAKA & M. KUMEGAWA. 1992. Insulin-like growth factor-1 supports formation and activation of osteoclasts. Endocrinology **131:** 1075–1080.

79. YANG, S., Y. ZHANG, R. M. RODRIGUIZ, W. L. RIES & L. L. JR. KEY. 1996. Functions of the M-CSF receptor on osteoclasts. Bone **18:** 355–360.

80. BIZZARRI, C., A. SHIOI, S. L. TEITELBAUM, J. OHARA, V. A. HARWALKAR, J. M. ERDMANN, D. L. LACEY & R. CIVITELLI. 1994. Interleukin-4 inhibits bone resorption and acutely increases cytosolic Ca^{2+} in murine osteoclasts. J. Biol. Chem. **269:** 13817–13824.

81. UDEGAWA, N., N. J. HORWOOD, J. ELLIOTT, A. MACKAY, J. OWENS, H. OKAMURA, M. KURIMOTO, T. J. CHAMBERS, T. J. MARTIN & M. T. GILLESPIE. 1997. Interleukin-18 (interferon-γ-inducing factor) is produced by osteoblasts and acts via granulocyte/macrophage colony-stimulating factor and not via interferon-γ to inhibit osteoclast formation. J. Exp. Med. **185:** 1005–1012.

82. BERGHUIS, H. M., S. C. DIEUDONNE, W. GOEI & J. P. VELDHUIJZEN. 1994. Effects of TGF-β_2 on mineral resorption in cultured embrionic mouse long bones; ^{45}Ca release and osteoclast differentiation and migration. Eur. J. Orthod. **16:** 130–137.

83. DIEDONNE, S. C., P. FOO, E. J. J. VAN ZOELEN & E. H. BURGER. 1991. Inhibiting and stimulating effects of TGF-β1 on osteoclastic bone resorption in fetal mouse bone organ cultures. J. Bone Miner. Res. **6:** 479–487.

84. QUINN, J. M. W., A. SABOKBAR, M. DENNE, M. C. DE VERNEJOUL, J. O. MCGEE & N. A. ATHANASOU. 1997. Inhibitory and stimulatory effects of prostaglandins on osteoclast differentiation. Calcif. Tissue Int. **60:** 63–70.

85. ROUX, S., F. PICHAUD, J. QUINN, A. LALANDE, C. MORIEUX, A. JULLIENNE & M. C. DE VERNEJOUL. 1997. Effects of prostaglandins on human hematopoietic osteoclastic precursors. Endocrinology **138:** 1476–1482.

86. BURGER, E. H. 1992. Mechanical effects on osteoclast function. *In* Biology and Physiology of the Osteoclast. B. R. Rifkin & C. V. Gay, Eds.: 419–432. CRC Press. Boca Raton, FL.

87. DAVIDSON, R. M., D. W. TATAKIS & A. L. AUERBACH. 1990. Multiple forms of mechanosensitive ion channels in osteoblast-like cells. Pflügers Arch. **419:** 646–651.

88. RUBIN, J., D. BISKOBING, X. FAN, C. RUBIN, K. MCLEOD & W. R. TAYLOR. 1997. Pressure regulates osteoclast formation and M-CSF expression in marrow culture. J. Cell Physiol. **170:** 81–87.

89. HUGHES, A. E., A. M. SHEARMAN, J. L. WEBER, R. J. BARR, R. G. H. WALLACE, P. H. OSTERBERG, N. C. NEVIL & R. A. B. MOLLAN. 1994. Genetic linkage of familial expansile osteolysis to chromosome 18 q. Human Mol. Genetics. **3:** 359–361.

90. TODD, G. & N. SAXE. 1994. Idiopathic phalangeal osteolysis. Arch. Dermatol. **130:** 759–762.

91. BROWN, R. A. & J. B. WEISS. 1988. Neovascularisation and its role in the osteoarthritic process. Ann. Rheum. Dis. **47:** 881–885.

92. HAUSMANN, E. 1974. Potential pathways for bone resorption in human periodontal disease. J. Periodontol. **45:** 338–343.

93. FELIX, R., P. R. ELFORD, C. STOERCKEL, M. CECCHINI, A. WETTERWALD, U. TRECHSEL, H. FLEISCH & B. M. STADLER. 1988. Production of hemopoietic growth factors by bone tissue and bone cells in culture. J. Bone Miner. Res. **3:** 27–36.

94. SISMEY-DURRANT, H. J., S. J. ATKINSON, R. M. HOPPS & J. K. HEATH. 1989. The effect of lipopolysaccharide from bacterial gingivalis and muramyl dipeptide on osteoblast collagenase release. Calcif. Tiss. Int. **44:** 361–363.

95. WEIR, E. C., K. L. INSOGNA & M. C. HOROWITZ. 1989. Osteoclastlike cells secrete granulocyte-macrophage colony-stimulating factor in response to parathyroid hormone and lipopolysaccharide. Endocrinology **124:** 899–904.

96. NOGUCHI, K., I. MORITA & S. MUROTA. 1989. The detection of platelet-activating factor in inflamed human gingival tissue. Arch. Oral Biol. **34:** 37–41.

97. PETTIPER, E. R., G. A. HIGGS & B. HENDERSON. 1987. PAF-acether in chronic arthritis. Agents Actions **21:** 98–103.

98. MARENDA, S. A. & T. B. AUFDEMORTE. 1995. Localization of cytokines in cholesteatoma tissue. Otolaryngol. Head Neck Surg. **112:** 359–368.

99. ADAMS, J. S., O. P. SHARMA, M. GACAD & F. R. SINGER. 1983. Metabolism of 25-hydroxyvitamin D_3 by cultured pulmonary alveolar macrophages in sarcoidosis. J. Clin. Invest. **72:** 1856–1860.

100. HAYES, M. E., J. Y. YUAN, A. J. FREEMONT & E. B. MAWER. 1994. Interferon-γ and eicosanoid regulation of 1,25-dihydroxyvitamin D_3 synthesis in macrophages from inflammatory arthritic joints. Int. J. Immunother. **10:** 1–9.

101. NORDSTRON, T., L. D. SHRODE, O. D. ROTSTEIN, R. ROMANEK, T. GOTO, J. N. HEERSCHE, M. F. MANOLSON, G. F. BRISSEAU & S. GRINSTEIN. 1997. Chronic extracellular acidosis induces plasmalemmal vacuolar type H^+ ATPase activity in osteoclasts. J. Biol. Chem. **272:** 6354–6360.

102. MIZEL, T. P., J.-M. DAYER, S. M. KRANE & S. E. MERGENHAGEN. 1981. Stimulation of rheumotoid synovial cell collagenase and prostaglandin production by partially purified lymphocyte-activating factor (interleukin-1). Proc. Nat. Acad. Sci. USA **78:** 2474–2477.

103. PERKINS, S. L., R. GIBBONS, S. KLING & A. J. KAHN. 1994. Age-related bone loss in mice is associated with an increased osteoclast progenitor pool. Bone **15:** 65–72.

104. MAZHUGA, P. M. 1978. Blood microvessels and reticulo-endothelial system of bone marrow. Nak. Dumk. Kiev. (Rus.).

105. PORTER, K. B., W. F. O'BRIEN & G. TOWSLEY. 1993. Pregnancy complicated by Gorham disease. Obstet. Gynecol. **81:** 808–810.

106. QUINN, J. M. W. & N. A. ATHANASOU. 1992. Tumor infiltrating macrophages are capable of bone resorption. J. Cell Sci. **101:** 681–686.

107. RATHOD, H., A. J. MALCOLM, J. I. GILLESPIE, V. BERRY, J. POOLEY, N. H. PIGGOTT & H. K. DATTA. 1994. Characterization of a subtype of primary osteoclastoma: extracellular calcium but not calcitonin inhibits aggressive HLA-DR-positive osteoclastoma possessing 'functional' calcitonin receptors. J. Pathol. **175:** 293–299.

108. TORCIA, M., M. LUCIBELLO, E. VANNIER, S. FABIANI, A. MILIANI, G. GUIDI, O. SPADA, S. K. DOWER, J. E. SIMS, A. R. SHAW, C. A. DINARELLO, E. GARACI & F. COZZOLINO. 1996. Modulation of osteoclast-activating factor activity of multiple myeloma bone marrow cells by different interleukin-1 inhibitors. Exp. Hematol. **24:** 868–874.

109. WYSOLMERSKI, J. J. & A. E. BROADUS. 1994. Hypercalcemia of malignancy: the central role of parathyroid hormone-related protein. Annu. Rev. Med. **45:** 189–200.

110. KAJI, H., T. SUGIMOTO, M. KANATANI, M. FUKASE & K. CHIHARA. 1995. Carboxyl-terminal peptides from parathyroid hormone-related protein stimulate osteoclast-like cell formation. Endocrinology **136:** 842–848.

111. NIGAM, S., S. MULER & C. BENEDETTO. 1989. Elevated plasma levels of platelet-activating factor (PAF) in breast cancer patients with hypercalcemia. J. Lipid Mediators **1:** 323–328.

112. ROODMAN, G. D. 1987. Biology of the osteoclast in Paget's disease. Sem. Arthritis Rheumatism **23:** 235–236.

113. SINGER, F. R. & B. G. MILLS. 1993. Giant cell tumor arising in Paget's disease of bone. Clin. Orthop. **293:** 293–301.

114. JACOBS, J. J., D. R. SUMNER & J. O. GALANTE. 1993. Mechanisms of bone loss associated with total hip replacement. Orthop. Clin. North Am. **24:** 583–590.

115. JIRANEK, W. A., M. MACHADO, M. JASTY, D. JEVSEVAR, H. J. WOLFE, S. R. GOLDRING & M. J. GOLDBERG. 1993. Production of cytokines around loosened cemented acetabular components. Analysis with immunohistochemical techniques and in situ hybridization. J. Bone Joint Surg. (Am.) **75:** 799–801.

116. YONEDA, T., Y. TAKAOKA, M. M. ALSINA, J. GARCIA & G. R. MUNDY. 1991. Porcine pancreas extract decreases blood-ionized calcium in mice and inhibits osteoclast formation and bone resorption in culture. FEBS Lett. **278:** 171–174.

117. FRANKE, J. & H. RUNGE. 1987. Osteoporosis. Veb Verlag Volk & Gesundheit. Berlin.

118. COINDRE, J., J. DAVID, L. RIVIEREL, J. GOUSSOT, P. ROGER, A. DE MASCAREL & P. J. MEU-

NIER. 1986. Bone loss in hypothyroidism with hormone replacement. A histomorphometric study. Arch. Intern. Med. **146:** 48–53.

119. RIZZOLI, R., C. STOERMANN, P. AMMANN & J.-P. BONJOUR. 1994. Hypercalcemia and hyperostosis in vitamin D intoxication: effects of clodronate therapy. Bone **15:** 193–198.

120. SLY, W. S., M. P. WHYTE, V. SUNDARAM, R. E. TASHIAN, D. HEWETT-EMMETT, P. GUIBAUD, M. VAINSEL, H. J. BALUARTE, A. GRUSKIN, M. AL-MOSAWI, N. SAKATI & A. OHLSSON. 1985. Carbonic anhydrase II deficiency in 12 families with the autosomal recessive syndrome of osteopetrosis with renal tubular acidosis and cerebral calcification. New Engl. J. Med. **313:** 139–145.

121. OSIER, L. K. & S. C. MARKS. 1992. Osteopetrosis. *In* Biology and Physiology of the Osteoclast. B. R. Rifkin & C. V. Gay, Eds.: 433–453. CRC Press. Boca Raton, FL.

122. BEARD, C. J., L. L. KEY, P. E. NEWBURGER, A. B. EZEKOWITZ, R. ARCECI, B. MILLER, P. PROTO, T. RYAN, C. S. ANAST & E. R. SIMONS. 1986. Neutrophil defect associated with malignant osteopetrosis. J. Lab. Clin. Med. **106:** 498–505.

123. YAMAMOTO, T., N. KURIHARA, K. YAMAOKA, K. OZONO, M. OKADA, K. YAMAMOTO, S. MATSUMOTO, T. MICHIGAMI, J. ONO & S. OKADA. 1993. Bone marrow-derived osteoclast-like cells from a patient with craniometaphyseal dysplasia lack expression of osteoclast-reactive vacuolar proton pump. J. Clin. Invest. **91:** 362–367.

124. CIELINSKI, M. J. & S. C. MARKS. 1994. Understanding bone cell biology requires an integrated approach: reliable opportunities to study osteoclast biology in vivo. J. Cell. Biochem. **56:** 315–322.

125. NAKAMURA, I., N. TAKAHASHI, N. UDAGAWA, Y. MORIYAMA, T. KUROKAWA, E. JIMI, T. SASAKI & T. SUDA. 1997. Lack of vacuolar proton ATPase association with the cytoskeleton in osteoclasts of osteosclerotic (oc/oc) mice. FEBS Lett. **401:** 207–212.

126. PEURA, S. R. & S. C. IR. MARKS. 1995. Colony-stimulating factor 1 combined with parathyroid hormone or 1,25-dihydroxyvitamin D can produce osteoclasts in cultured neonatal metatarsal from toothless (*tl*-osteopetrotic) rats. Bone **16:** 335S-340S.

127. SORIANO, P., C. MONTGOMERY, R. GESKE & A. BRADLEY. 1991. Targeted disruption of the c-src proto-oncogene leads to osteopetrosis in mice. Cell **64:** 693–702.

128. TONDRAVI, M. M., S. R. MCKERCHER, K. ANDERSON, J. M. ERDMANN, M. QUIROZ, R. MAKI & S. L. TEITELBAUM. 1997. Osteopetrosis in mice lacking haematopoietic transcription factor PU.1. Nature **385:** 81–84.

129. TOHKIN, M., S. KAKUDO, H. KASAI & H. ARITA. 1994. Comparative study of inhibitory effects by murine interferon-γ and a new bisphosphonate (aledronate) in hypercalcemic, nude mice bearing human tumor (LJC-1-JCK). Cancer Immunol. Immunother. **39:** 155–160.

130. BODY, J. J. 1993. Medical treatment of tumor-induced hypercalcemia and tumor-induced osteolysis: challenges for future research. Support Care Cancer **1:** 26–33.

131. LOWIK, C. W., G. VAN DER PLUJIM, L. J. VAN DER WEE-PALS, H. BLOYS VAN TRESLOG-DE GROOT & O. L. M. BIJVOET. 1988. Migration and phenotypic transformation of osteoclast precursors into mature osteoclasts: The effect of a bisphosphonate. J. Bone Miner. Res. **3:** 185–192.

132. GUIDON, P. T. JR., R. SALVATORI & R. S. BOCKMAN. 1993. Gallium nitrate regulates rat osteoblast expression of osteocalcin protein and mRNA levels. J. Bone Miner. Res. **8:** 103–112.

133. MERRYMAN, J. I., C. C. CAPEN & T. J. ROSOL. 1994. Effects of gallium nitrate in nude mice bearing a canine adenocarcinoma (CAC-8) model of humoral hypercalcemia of malignancy. J. Bone Miner. Res. **9:** 725–732.

134. REGINSTER, J. Y. 1993. Ipriflavone: pharmacological properties and usefulness in postmenopausal osteoporosis. Bone Miner. **23:** 223–232.

135. KEY, L. L. JR., R. M. RODRIGUIZ, S. M. WILLI, N. M. WRIGHT, H. C. HATCHER, D. R. EYRE,

J. K. CURE, P. P. GRIFFIN & W. L. RIES. 1995. Long-term treatment of osteopetrosis with recombinant human interferon gamma. New Engl. J. Med. **332:** 1594–1599.

136. SCHEPETKIN, I. 1995. Calcium-phosphate materials in biological substrates. Adv. Curr. Biol. (Rus.) **115:** 58–74.

137. DAVIES, J. B., G. SHAPIRO & B. F. LOWENBERG. 1993. Osteoclastic resorption of calcium phosphate ceramic thin films. Cell. Materials **3:** 245–256.

138. QUINN, J. M. W., J. O'D. MC GEE & N. A. ATHANASOU. 1994. Cellular and hormonal factors influencing monocyte differentiation to osteoclastic bone resorbing cells. Endocrinology **134:** 2416–2423.

139. SHIH, C. & G. W. BERNARD. 1996. Peripheral blood mononuclear cells develop into multinucleated osteoclasts in tissue culture. Anat. Rec. **245:** 41–45.

140. ALYOSHIN, B. V. 1936. Investigation of amphibian methamorphosis. 1. Resorption of larva tail as inflammation process. Arch. Anat. Histol. Embriol. (Rus.) **15:** 9–70.

Ultrastructural Changes of Neutrophils following IL-2 Treatment *in Vivo*

R. NANO,[a] E. CAPELLI,[b] S. BARNI, AND G. GERZELI

Department of Animal Biology
University of Pavia
Center of Study for Histochemistry
CNR
Pavia, Italy

[b]*Department of Genetic and Microbiology*
University of Pavia
Pavia, Italy

Interleukin-2 (IL-2) induces, directly and/or indirectly, a broad spectrum of biological effects. *In vivo* IL-2 induces changes in circulating leukocytes as: cell number (lymphopenia or rebound lymphocytosis, eosinophilia),[1–3] morphofunctional features (hand mirror shape, enzymatic activation, anergy),[4–6] and immunophenotype.[7] The discovery of circulating histiocytes with dark inclusions in patients following high doses of rIL-2 treatment, as observed in our previous study, led us to hypothesize that rIL-2 triggers apoptotic phenomena.[8] The probable morphological and functional modifications of neutrophils following IL-2 administration were not at present deeply investigated. In this study the characteristic ultrastructural changes of polymorphonucleated cells observed in cancer patients following recombinant interleukin-2 (rIL-2) treatment are described.

MATERIALS AND METHODS

Patients and Treatment

Three patients with advanced renal cell carcinoma, treated with high doses of rIL-2 (18×10^6 IU/m^2/day) by continuous intravenous administration for 5 consecutive days, were studied. Heparinized blood samples were drawn immediately before starting the first treatment cycle and 3, 6, 24, and 48 h after rIL-2 infusion.

Analysis of Peripheral Blood Smears

Blood cell smears from cancer patients obtained before and after 3, 6, 24, and 48 h of rIL-2 treatment were stained with May-Grunwald Giemsa (MGG). The leukocytic formula was determined.

[a]Address correspondence to: Prof. Rosanna Nano, Department of Animal Biology, Piazza Botta 10, University of Pavia, 27100, Pavia, Italy. Telephone, 0382-506315; Fax, 0382-506406; e-mail, nano@ipv36.unipv.it

Electron Microscopy

Freshly isolated leukocytes were examined. Pellets were fixed with 1.5% glu-taraldehyde in 0.07 M cacodylate buffer (pH 7.4) for 3 h at 4°C, washed in 0.1 M ca-codylate buffer with 7% sucrose, and post-fixed with 1% OsO_4 in the same buffer for 2 h at 4°C. After several washings the cells were pre-embedded in 2% agar in buffer, dehydrated in graded ethanols, and embedded in Epon 812. Thin silver to gold sec-tions were stained with saturated uranyl acetate in 50% acetone and with Reynold's lead citrate and were examined with a Zeiss 900 TEM operating at 50 KV.

RESULTS AND DISCUSSION

Peripheral blood cell samples obtained from the treated patients 3, 6, 24, and 48 h after rIL-2 infusion, were compared with those obtained from the blood of the same patients before the treatment. Blood cell smears stained with MGG were analyzed. According to the leukocytic formula, the basal values of peripheral blood cells were in the normal range. After rIL-2 administration, cancer patients showed a strong de-crease in lymphocytes starting from 3 h after the beginning of the treatment (18% versus 34%), while variation in the number of polymorphonucleated cells was not observed during the time of this study (0–48 h). These findings agree with our previ-ous observations that variation in the number of eosinophils, neutrophils, and ba-sophils were observed only 6 days after the beginning of the treatment. In particular a significantly increased number of eosinophils and a decrease of neutrophils was ob-served.[2]

After the rIL-2 treatment, neutrophils showed morphological changes at the nu-

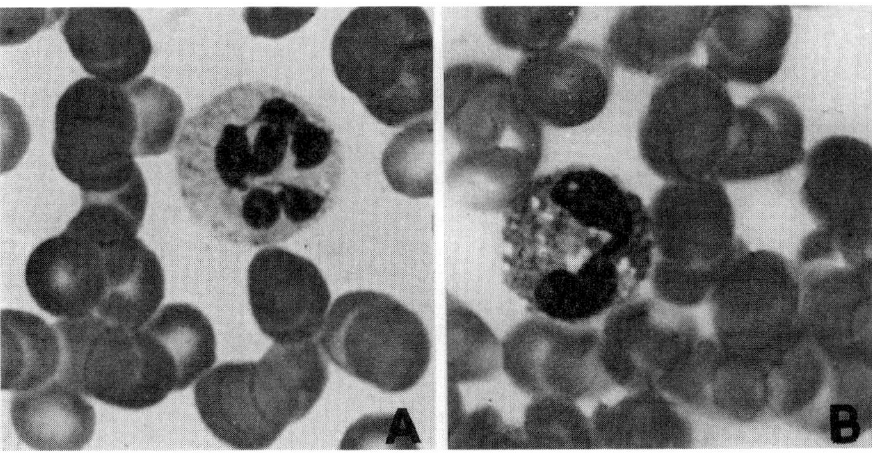

FIGURE 1. Smear of peripheral blood cells of rIL-2 treated patient showing a neutrophil with many nuclear segmentations (A) and with cytoplasmic vacuoles (B). May-Grunwald Giemsa stain (× 800).

clear and cytoplasmic levels. Nuclei showed an increased number of nuclear segmentations according to the Arneth formula (FIG. 1, A). Vacuolizations were frequently observed in the cytoplasm (FIG. 1, B).

The ultrastructural analysis revealed an increased activation of all leukocytes after rIL-2 treatment with respect to the basal situation. Morphofunctional modifications (a reduced nucleus/cytoplasm ratio, increase in cell organelles, polarization of the nucleus, hand-mirror shape), which are expression of a cell state activation, were found in the lymphocyte fraction, confirming our previous study.[8] The presence of histiocytes with vacuoles and inclusions was also observed (FIG. 2, D).

In the present work we focused our attention on polymorphonucleated cells. These cells observed 3 and 6 h after rIL-2 administration presented an increase in

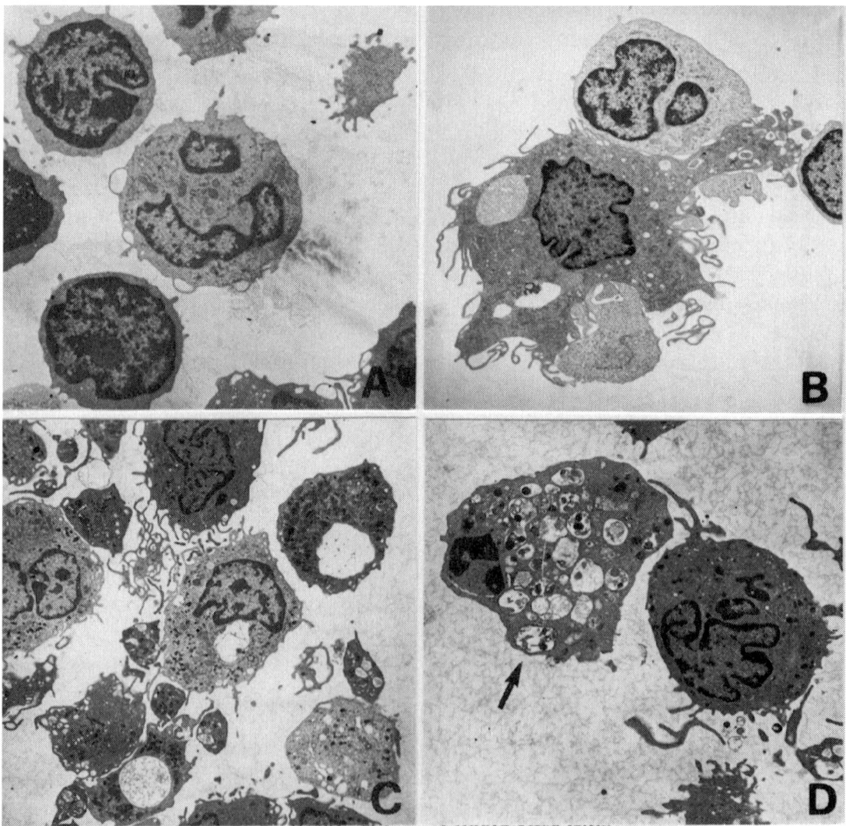

FIGURE 2. Electron micrographs of peripheral leukocytes of cancer patients after rIL-2 treatment. (A) Neutrophil with a few cytoplasmic extroflexions; (B) neutrophil exhibiting different stages of cellular internalization with presence of numerous lamellopodia; (C) neutrophils with cytoplasmic vacuoles in different stages of lytic degradation; and (D) histiocyte (*arrow*) with numerous cytoplasmic heterophagosomes (A, B, D : × 4,700; C: × 4,500).

membrane projections and cytoplasmic vacuoles with variable electron density, which indicates phagocytic activity. In FIGURES 2 and 3, the pattern of morphological changes observed in neutrophils are summarized. In the cancer patients only slight morphological features of an activation state were observed as the presence of cytoplasmic extroflexions and an increased number of cell organelles. A strong increase in membrane projections with formation of lamellopodia that trigger different stages of cellular internalization was observed in patients after rIL-2 administration. FIGURE 2(A) shows a neutrophil with some cytoplasmic extroflessions on cell membrane surface. Such a feature may be considered to be an early step in the formation of membrane projections. With the increasing time from the beginning of the treatment, membrane projections increased, forming lamellopodia. The extension of lamellopo-

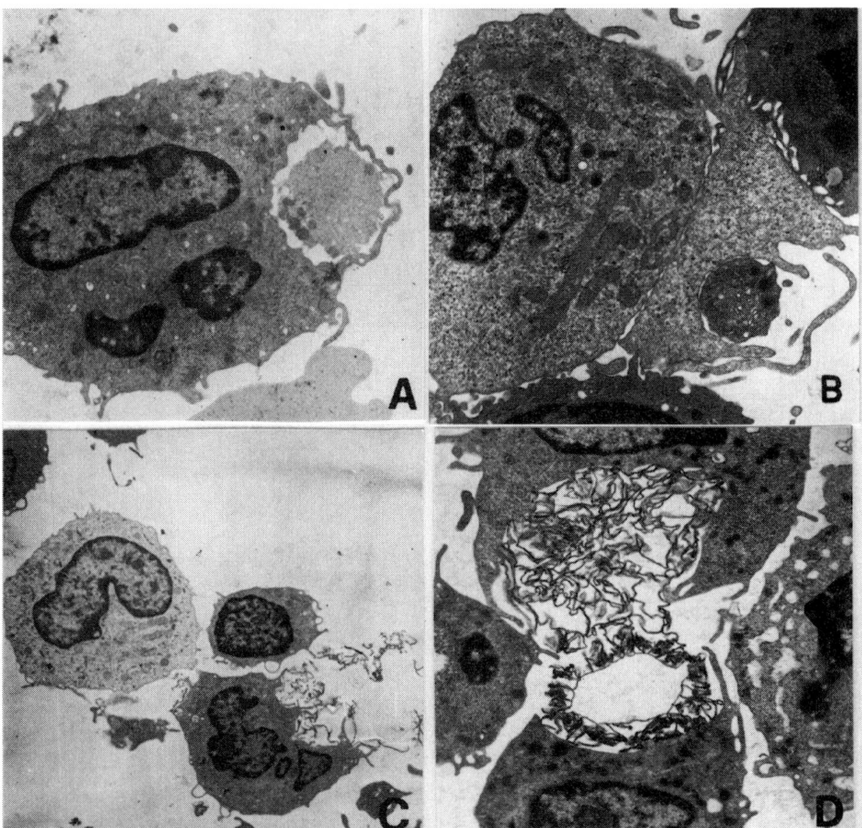

FIGURE 3. Electron micrographs of polymorphonucleated cells of rIL-2 treated patients showing particular patterns of activated state. (A) Late stage of phagocytosis in a polymorphonucleated cell; (B) a part of cell surrounded by lamellopodia; (C) late stage of lamellopodia formation in neutrophils; and (D) possible interaction between many ruffles or lamellopodia derived from two adjacent cells (A, B, D: × 5,200; C: × 4,600).

dia and ruffles caused frequently complex interactions between various types of cells (FIG. 2, B). After 24 and 48 h, quite a number of neutrophils showed cytoplasmic vacuolizations and an active phagocytic process was observed into the cytoplasm of the neutrophils that showed large vacuoles containing amorphous material (FIG. 2, B and C). In FIGURE 2(B) an early phagocytic step with electron-dense vacuoles can be seen. In FIGURE 2(C) a late phagocytic step with many large light vacuoles in the neutrophils is represented. Patterns of extreme activation of polymorphonucleated cells with lamellopodia surrounding and engulfing a part of cell (FIG. 3, A and B) or the whole cell or forming an intricate network, were sometimes observed (FIG. 3, C and D).

In conclusion, the morphofunctional modifications of neutrophils observed in peripheral blood cells of patients after rIL-2 treatment indicate an activated state of these cells. In particular the phagocytic action is so strong that the phenomena of autophagocytosis and of cell cannibalism were hypothesized (FIG. 3, B). These findings were observed early after rIL-2 administration (3 h). These data suggest a direct activation of neutrophils modulated by rIL-2 and not mediated by other cytokines produced by lymphocytes or by NK cells. Our results are in agreement with recent data that demonstrated the presence of IL-2 receptor on neutrophils.[9,10]

SUMMARY

An ultrastructural analysis of peripheral blood cells of cancer patients following recombinant interleukin-2 (rIL-2) treatment at high doses (rIL-2, 18×10^6 I.U./m^2/day) has been performed. Characteristic patterns of intense phagocytosis (neutrophils with large vacuoles containing electron-dense bodies) were observed in granulocytes of the treated patients with respect to the basal situation. These characteristics were particularly evident in the advanced stages of the therapy (24 and 48 h). The state of neutrophil activation was sometimes accompanied by the appearance of a close net of cell membranes, probably derived from lamellopodia.

REFERENCES

1. JANSSEN, R. A. J., N. H. MULDER, T. HAUW THE & LOU DE LEIJ. 1994. Cancer Immunol. Immunother. **39:** 207–216.
2. CAPELLI, E., E. MAINARDI, R. NANO, E. BOBBIO PALLAVICINI, F. TACCONI, Y. P. YANG & M. CUCCIA. 1994. *In* Proceedings of XVI International Cancer Congress Monduzzi XVI Ed. S.p.A. Bologna (Italy). 3059–3064.
3. CREMASCHI, P., E. VOLPINI, G. TERZUOLO, E. CAPELLI, R. NANO, C. NASCIMBENE, C. CATANESE & P. VITULO. 1995. Can. J. Infect. Dis. **6:** 401.
4. NANO, R., E. CAPELLI, M. CIVALLERO, L. LORUSSO, F. ARGENTINA, E. BONIZZONI & M. CERONI. 1996. Anticancer Res. **17:** 107–112.
5. LORUSSO, L., R. NANO, E. CAPELLI, K. MARINU-AKTIPI, E. BENERICETTI, G. GIARDINI & M. CERONI. 1994. Acta Neurol. **16**(4): 198–205.
6. CLEMENTI, E., E. BUCCI, G. CITTERIO, G. LANDONIO, G. CONSOGNO & C. FORTIS. 1994. Cancer Immunol. Immunother. **39:** 167–171.
7. FORTIS, C., E. FERRERO, S. HELTAI, C. BESANA, C. CORTI, G. DI LUCCA, M. FOPPOLI, G. CONSOGNO & C. RUGARLI. 1993. Eur. J. Cancer **29**(3): 474–475.

8. CAPELLI, E., S. BARNI, R. VACCARONE, C. FORTIS & R. NANO. 1996. Anticancer Res. **16:** 1775–1780.
9. GIRARD, D., J. GOSSELIN, D. HEITZ, R. PAQUIN & A. D. BEAULIEU. 1995. Blood **86**(3): 1170–1176.
10. WEI, S., D. K. BLANCHARD, J. H. LIU, W. J. LEONARD & J. Y. DJEU. 1993. J. Immunol. **150**(50): 1979–1987.

Network Analysis of Arachidonic Acid Pathophysiology in Human Phagocytes and Primary Brain Tumors[a]

H.A. LEAVER,[b] J.R. WILLIAMS, S.R. CRAIG,[c] A. GREGOR,[d]
J.W. IRONSIDE,[e] I.R. WHITTLE,[f] B.H. SU,[g] P.L. YAP[h]

*Departments of Pharmacology, [c]Surgery, [d]Clinical Oncology, [e]Pathology,
[f]Clinical Neurosciences, [g]Medical Statistics, and [h]Medicine
University of Edinburgh
Edinburgh EH8 9JZ, United Kingdom*

INTRODUCTION: ARACHIDONIC ACID IN THE RETICULOENDOTHELIAL SYSTEM

Arachidonic acid (FIG. 1) is an essential component of the leukocyte membrane. The activities of arachidonic acid have been studied in a variety of ways including dietary modification of tissue,[1–4] analysis of the *in vitro* effects of exogenous fatty acids,[5–9] and investigation of the enzymes of fatty acid metabolism.[10–19] These approaches have indicated a unique role for arachidonic acid in cell signaling in the reticuloendothelial system. Arachidonic acid has the ability to modulate cellular activities, to control the growth and development of cells, and to act as an intracellular messenger in the reticuloendothelial system.

In this paper, it will be proposed that network analysis can be applied to the study of arachidonic acid activity. Recent developments in network theory will be described that can be applied to arachidonate-mediated intracellular and intercellular events that connect elements of the reticuloendothelial system.[20–24] Three areas of arachidonic acid activity will be considered: firstly, the immediate activation of phagocyte NADPH oxidase activity; secondly, longer term homeostatic and priming activities involving arachidonic acid; and thirdly, the peroxidative pathways associated with the control of cell proliferation. In these three areas, results from our laboratory implicating arachidonic acid activity will be reviewed and compared with those of other groups. The properties of arachidonic acid activity and metabolism characteristic of connective elements in theoretical and biological networks will be discussed and the advantages of nonlinear and interactive network analysis will be considered. An advantage of network analysis is that it can determine associations and

[a]This work generously supported by a Melville Trust for the Care and Cure of Cancer Research Fellowship (J.R.W.), the Edinburgh University Cancer Research Fund, the ICRF flow cytometry facilities (Profs, Miller and Smythe), and the Edinburgh University Department of Pathology culture facilities (Profs. Wyllie and Bird).

[b]Address correspondence to: Dr. H. A. Leaver, Department of Pharmacology, 1 George Square, University of Edinburgh EH8 9JZ, Edinburgh, United Kingdom.

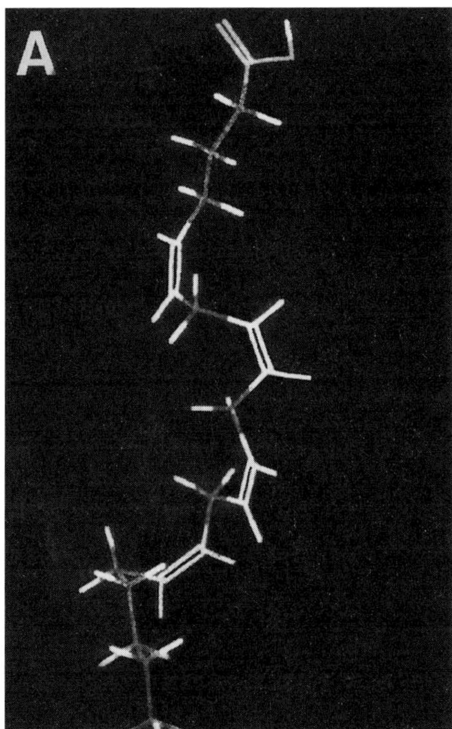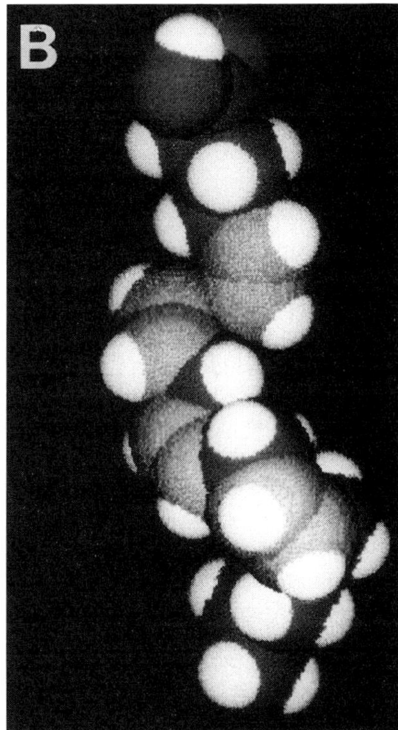

FIGURE 1. Arachidonic acid. This energy-optimized molecular configuration shows the disposition of unsaturated C=C double bonds and the helical shape of the -C-C-backbone (**A**). The molecular orbital space–filled model (**B**) shows that the helical configuration brings the methylene interrupted C=C double bonds into close apposition. This may facilitate the transfer of free radicals during peroxidation reactions. In the lipid bilayer, the proximity of unsaturated double bonds between neighboring fatty acids is increased by the parallel stacking and constant bilayer width of the helical configuration in biological membranes. The molecular configuration was modeled using the Nemesis Oxford Molecular Modelling programme, energy minimized over 400 cycles.

interactions between individual parameters. Also, using network analysis it is possible to investigate the patterns of cooperative responses and hence to define emergent or developing properties such as priming. The analysis of the effects of arachidonic acid on phagocytes of patients with lung and brain tumors will be described. In analyzing arachidonic acid effects in these cells, it was necessary to use nonlinear models of the dynamics of the oxidative response. It is proposed that network and nonlinear approaches will be useful in the analysis of multifactorial events such as trauma, cancer, and cardiovascular disease, in defining the processes and interactions in which arachidonic acid flux may play a mediatory or connective role.[1,25]

ARACHIDONIC ACID: ESSENTIAL FATTY ACID AND SIGNALING ACTIVITIES

The rapidity of arachidonic acid responses and arachidonic acid translocation indicates activity in intracellular communication. Arachidonic acid selectivity has been detected in the activation of phagocyte NADPH oxidase[26] and H^+ flux[6,8,19,27–31] and also in the mobilization of intracellular Ca^{2+}[7] and in cellular peroxidation and apoptosis.[14,29,32,33] In some pathophysiological pathways, such as Fcγ-mediated superoxide generation[5] and in tumor necrosis factor–induced cytotoxicity,[10] arachidonic acid appears to be an obligatory mediator. Arachidonic acid metabolism is closely connected with endotoxin priming of the immune system.[11,15,34] Arachidonic acid–specific pathways have also been identified in the central nervous system.[9,35,36] In these processes, arachidonic acid plays a connective role in network responses.

The oxidative burst is an important reticuloendothelial response that is sensitive to pathophysiological concentrations (100 nM–20 μM) of arachidonic acid. During this process, cytotoxic superoxide anions (O_2^-) are produced by a wide variety of immunocompetent cells in response to stimulation.[37,38] The immediate activation of phagocyte oxidative activity by arachidonic acid involves multiple sites of action. Arachidonic acid activates NADPH oxidase.[7, 26–31] This activity is a property shared by related *n*-6 essential fatty acids, such as gammalinolenic acid,[30] which however shows less activity (FIG. 2) and lower bioavailability in excitable membrane phospholipid pools.[39] Specific roles for arachidonic acid have been identified at several molecular sites associated with NADPH oxidation (FIG. 3). These include interaction of the NADPH oxidase component rap 1A with rap-GTPase activating protein.[8] The activation of rap-GTPase–activating protein by arachidonic acid causes exposure of the p47-SH3 region, crucial for oxidase assembly and the binding of cytochrome b protein p22 phox and the p67 phox protein.[18] Also, nanomolar concentrations of arachidonic acid activate GTP-binding protein.[27] Additionally, in conjunction with G proteins, arachidonic acid induces translocation of rac p21s to the membrane and the activation of NADPH oxidase.[31] Arachidonic acid also directly affects the spin state and the activity of binding site of cytochrome b_{558} with molecular oxygen.[28] The specific activation of neutrophil MAP kinase by arachidonic acid via p21[ras] and Raf1 is described in the communication of Weissman in this volume. Thus free arachidonic acid, with a range limited by the highly active enzymes of esterification and metabolism,[2,39] stimulates phagocyte NADPH oxidase over short distances.[5,8,26] The multiple sites of arachidonic acid activation of NADPH oxidase indicate that several responses may be activated by the local generation of arachidonic acid and that the resulting response of the oxidase to this arachidonic acid release would be best described by nonlinear models.

ARACHIDONIC ACID AND CONNECTIVITY IN RETICULOENDOTHELIAL NETWORKS

The analysis of network properties of biological systems has developed recently, as a result of advances in nonlinear dynamics and in immune and neural network theory.[21,40,41] These networks are not cell- or system-specific. They depend on interac-

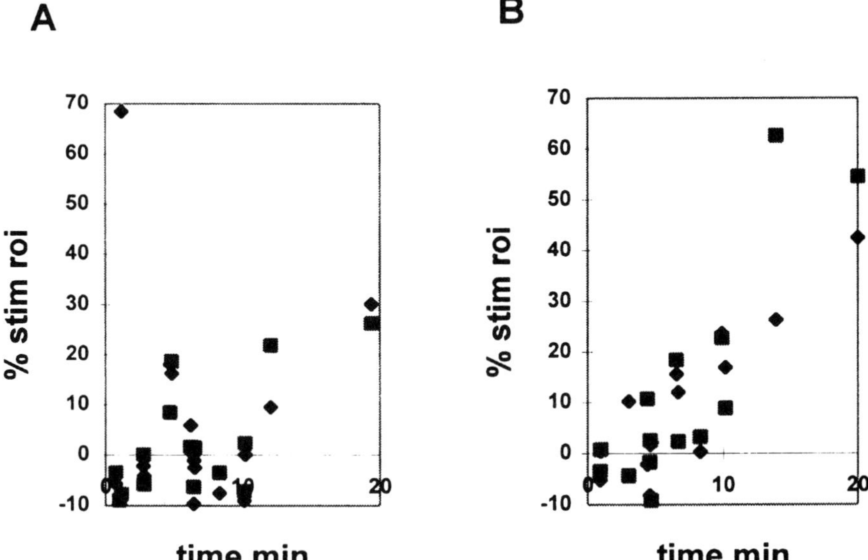

FIGURE 2. Kinetics of reactive oxygen generation in phagocytes from lung cancer patients and control subjects. Leukocyte preparations from 6 patients and from 6 paired control subjects preincubated with the oxidative probe, 2′,7′-dichlorofluorescein diacetate, 5 μM, were incubated with 8μM gammalinolenic acid from 0 minutes. The % stimulation of oxidative metabolism was derived by dividing mean cell fluorescence of phagocytes incubated in the presence of gammalinolenic acid by fluorescence of unstimulated cells from the same individual. **A** indicates the kinetics of oxidative metabolism in (■) patient and (◆) control monocytes. **B** indicates oxidative metabolism in the same (■) patients and (◆) controls. Leukocytes were taken from patients before surgery. The patient neutrophils (**B**), which showed 20% stimulation of basal oxidative activity, were significantly ($p<0.05$) less stimulated than controls in response to arachidonic acid and gammalinolenic acid.[24]

tions between connecting elements that interact via experimentally determined molecular interactions and connective factors. The properties of a network emerge from co-operativity and connectivity of participating elements. Individual elements of the network, such as cells and cytokines, are dynamically connected to each other. In this paper, it is proposed that arachidonic acid flux may mediate such dynamic connections. In network theory, each component of the network operates on the basis of its local environment but, because it is part of the network, there is overall cooperation. An important property of network analysis is that there is no necessity for a central processing unit to guide the network, nor do external influences act as the prime driving force.[21] In closely connected systems, signals may propagate very deeply into the network. These closely connected systems require control since a small perturbation could trigger the entire network or system.[22] A general principle necessary for the formation of pattern is the presence of influences that activate over short dis-

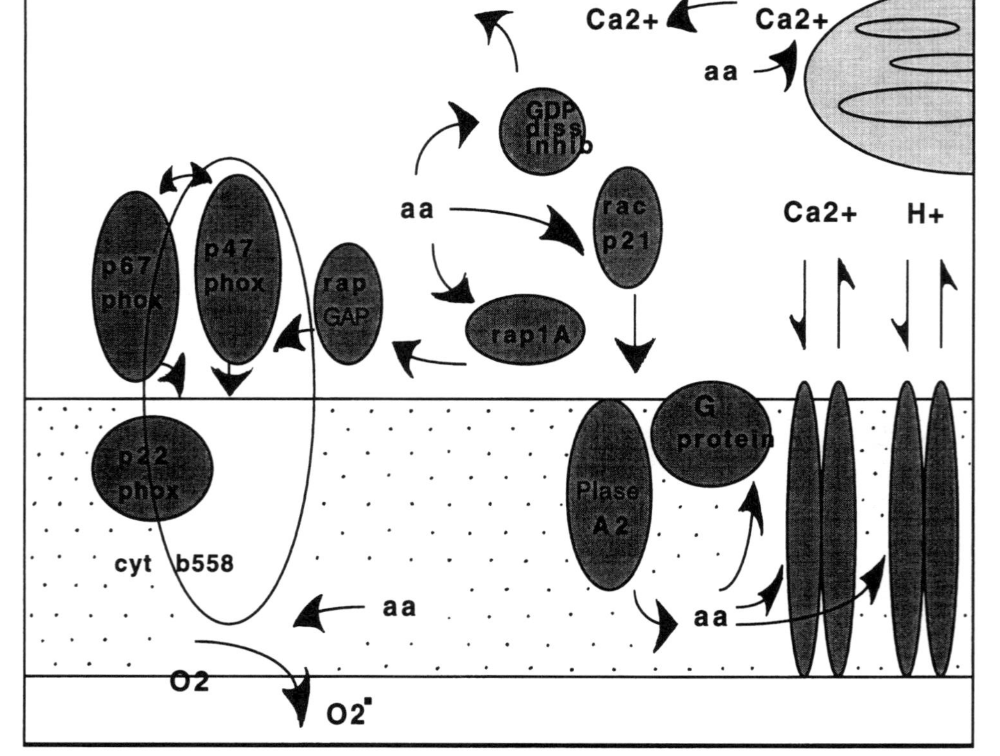

FIGURE 3. Arachidonic acid in the activation of phagocyte NADPH oxidase. This diagram indicates the multiple molecular sites at which arachidonic acid activation of components of phagocyte NADPH oxidase have been identified. Arachidonic acid (aa) interacts with rap-GTPase activating protein (rap GTPase AP) exposing a p47-SH3 region crucial for oxidase assembly and the binding of p22 phox and p67 phox. Nanomolar concentrations of arachidonic acid activate GTP-binding protein (G protein). Arachidonic acid, together with G proteins, induces translocation of rac p21s to the membrane and the dissociation of rac p21 from GDP dissociation inhibitor protein (GDP diss inhib). Arachidonic acid also directly affects the spin state and oxygen binding site of cytochrome b_{558}. Arachidonic acid interacts with both plasma membrane and intracellular ion channels to increase H^+ and Ca^{2+} flux.

tances and that inhibit over long distances.[22,23] Such properties characterize several arachidonic acid effects in the reticuloendothelial system.

A necessary property of a connective element, apart from the short range stimulation discussed above, is long range inactivation and inhibition. Both of these characteristics are typical of arachidonic acid release and metabolism. Inactivation of released arachidonic acid is partly achieved by cellular esterification into cell phospholipids and other lipids.[39] Additionally, arachidonic acid and fatty acid hydroperoxides inhibit macrophage superoxide production by depolarizing plasma and mitochondrial membranes.[6,19,36] The inhibition of NADPH oxidase activity over longer distances and times is shown by the predominant eicosanoid metabolite of arachidonic acid in leukocytes, prostaglandin E_2. Prostaglandin E_2 secreted by mononuclear phagocytes has a longer half-life and range than arachidonic acid and acts on adjacent cells to inhibit NADPH oxidase activity.[4,42] Prostaglandin E_2 also has an inhibitory effect on lymphocyte proliferation.[4,42] The dichotomy between the mediator actions of arachidonic acid in inflammation and the homeostatic antiinflammatory effects of arachidonic acid metabolites are also discussed in the contributions of Weissman and Ricevuti in this volume.

A further feature of arachidonic acid flux that makes it an appropriate network component is its extracellular action. There is evidence that arachidonic acid, released during cell stimulation, reaches adjacent endothelium, where it is converted to prostacyclin. Prostacyclin also generally acts in a homeostatic inhibitory way in target cells by increasing intracellular cyclic AMP and exerting paracrine effects similar to those of prostaglandin E_2 described above. Additionally, arachidonic acid has been shown to stimulate the efflux of calcium, which may itself play a role in intracellular activation[36] and arachidonic acid also affects the release of glutamate in the central nervous system (see following section).

IMMUNE NETWORKS, MOLECULAR MEMORY, AND ARACHIDONIC ACID DYNAMICS

The analysis of the kinetics of change in activity and development of patterns of molecular activity is important in understanding the development of reticuloendothelial responsiveness and patterns of molecular memory. For example, in the immune system it has been proposed that a central characteristic of the immune network is the definition of the individuals' molecular identity.[21] Recently, a more dynamic model of immunological memory has been advocated. Studies in autoimmunity have indicated that suppression and tolerance are dominant properties of the immune network and that suppression/tolerance reflect dynamic behavior of the network.[21,23] The emergent network properties of immunological memory have been defined in two ways[22]: A dynamic model has been proposed in which the involved cells are maintained at specific levels of activity via network interactions and autostimulation. An older, static model defines memory in terms of resting, long-lived "memory cells." There is evidence that memory may be maintained by both static and dynamic means.[22] Evidence for arachidonic acid participation in dynamic pathways of phagocyte and reticuloendothelial function has been reviewed above. The action of arachidonic acid in longer term structural and developmental processes will be discussed in this section.

An important result of network analysis in the immune system is an understanding of the endogenous dynamics of the system. Thus, it has been proposed that the function of the reticuloendothelial system is not primarily to respond to external stimuli. External influences, such as pathogens, only modify the local environment of individual components, they do not drive the system. These properties are evident in the naive immune system, which has intrinsic lymphoproliferative activity, T cell responses, immunoglobulin secretion, and phagocyte activities before any exposure to environmental antigens. However, the network properties involving the development of molecular memory have not been generally considered in relation to other activities of the reticuloendothelial system. In this paper, evidence will be presented that implicates arachidonic acid in dynamic systems involved in the acute response to surgery, in the development of neuronal synapses, in the endotoxin priming of phagocytes, and in the certain pathways leading to apoptosis.

It has been shown that the concentrations of arachidonic acid released within biological membranes are compatible with the concentrations that activate NADPH oxidase (FIG. 3), but is arachidonic acid release capable of maintaining physiologically significant phagocyte activation? The oxidative activity of phagocytes from patients undergoing pulmonary surgery indicates that arachidonic acid pathways may be involved in phagocyte activation during reactive responses to lung carcinoma and surgery.[30] In these studies, reactive oxygen production in phagocytes from lung cancer patients undergoing pulmonary resection was analyzed. Activation associated with arachidonic acid was investigated by using exogenous arachidonic acid to stimulate patient and control reactive oxygen intermediate (roi) formation. The activated phagocyte populations from these patients exhibited a decreased oxidative response to arachidonic acid and gammalinolenic acid for periods as long as seven days after surgery. The decreased stimulation of patient roi suggested that the phagocytes of patients were previously activated by arachidonic acid or that the phagocyte response via the arachidonic acid pathway was impaired by surgery.

The characteristics of arachidonic acid turnover indicate a potential role for arachidonic acid in the processes associated with memory within the reticuloendothelial system. Thus, arachidonic acid release in response to agonists (FIG. 3) is pulsatile and transitory[4] and its excitatory effects, for example on ion flux, are specific but short range.[6,7,19,20] In a more conventional model of molecular memory, short-term activation by arachidonic acid has also recently been demonstrated in the central nervous system, where $0.1–10$ μM arachidonic acid potentiated the release of glutamate[35] and activated glutamate NMDA receptor channels.[9] Such presynaptic activation may have a physiological role in developing and maintaining the synaptic links involved in memory in the central nervous system.

A characteristic reticuloendothelial emergent response is the priming of the immune system by endotoxin lipopolysaccharide. This process is crucially dependent on arachidonic acid, as evidenced by the inhibition of endotoxin effects in essential fatty acid–deficient animals.[34] There is evidence that phospholipase A_2 is upregulated by bacterial endotoxin in granulocytes.[11] The phospholipase A_2 that is induced shows arachidonyl specificity.[15] It is possible that a phospholipase A_2 metabolite, platelet-activating factor (PAF acetether) amplifies arachidonic acid release during this priming.[16] A similar pattern of phospholipase A_2 and PAF priming of granulocytes by tumor necrosis factor$_\alpha$ (TNF$_\alpha$) has been described.[17] This TNF$_\alpha$-induced phospholipase A_2 also shows arachidonic acid selectivity and has been postulated to be essential for the cytotoxic action of TNF$_\alpha$.[10] Ether phospholipids also stimulate apoptotic pathways, possibly by inhibiting arachidonate transfer into phosphatidylethanolamine, a pathway important in control of the availability of arachidonic acid in the stimulation of inflammatory cells.[39]

Arachidonic acid and eicosapentaenoic acid have recently been shown to stimulate apoptosis in premyelocytic human leukemic (HL-60) cells.[32] Analysis of population dynamics is an important consideration for agents that stimulate apoptosis. A key property of apoptosis is the rapidity of the process and the rapid removal of apoptotic bodies *in vivo*.[43] Apoptosis tends to increase where cell proliferation is occurring, for instance in deletion of self-reactive cells, in killing via Fas and in diseases of the immune system (such as deletion of CD4-positive T cells in AIDS). The dissociation of apoptosis from proliferation is thought to be important in carcinogenesis (see next section). The antiproliferative effects of arachidonic acid may be partly mediated by phagocytes but they may also arise from direct effects of arachidonic acid on the oxidative activity of tumor cells. The evidence that the anti-tumor actions of the essential fatty acids involve cellular reactive oxygen intermediates and act partly by apoptotic pathways will be reviewed.

ARACHIDONIC ACID IN THE CONTROL OF CELL TURNOVER AND APOPTOSIS

The antiproliferative effects of arachidonic acid and related essential fatty acids *in vitro* have been well characterized.[2,3,33] A pathway associated with antiproliferative activity is the generation of oxygen-derived free radicals and lipid peroxides. The polyunsaturated fatty acids of biological membranes, of which arachidonic acid is the most abundant, are highly susceptible to lipid peroxidation (FIG. 1). Under appropriate conditions, lipid peroxidation has the characteristics of a chain reaction, as lipid peroxides propagate free radical formation in adjacent polyunsaturated fatty acids.[29] Evidence for the involvement of lipid peroxidation in the control of cell proliferation includes observations that proliferating and transformed cells exhibit lower levels of lipid peroxidation and lower essential fatty acid content and that superoxide dismutase inhibits the antiproliferative effects of arachidonic acid *in vitro*.[33] It has been reported that arachidonic acid is the most potent essential fatty acid in limiting cancer cell growth *in vitro*.[2,33,44]

The rate of peroxidation in leukocytes can be stimulated by micromolar concentrations of arachidonic acid. Although the extent of peroxidation is greater in phagocytes than in many other cell types, arachidonic acid stimulation of cellular peroxidation was not limited to the phagocyte populations (see stimulation of tumor tissue peroxidation by arachidonate in FIGURE 4). In 40 primary human brain tumor preparations whose peroxidative metabolism was analyzed by flow cytometry, we detected a significant increase in the rate of peroxidation and inhibition of cell growth and also an increase in the rate of apoptosis in response to arachidonic acid (FIG. 5) and gammalinolenic acid.[14] In contrast to the effects of these *n*-6 fatty acids on phago-

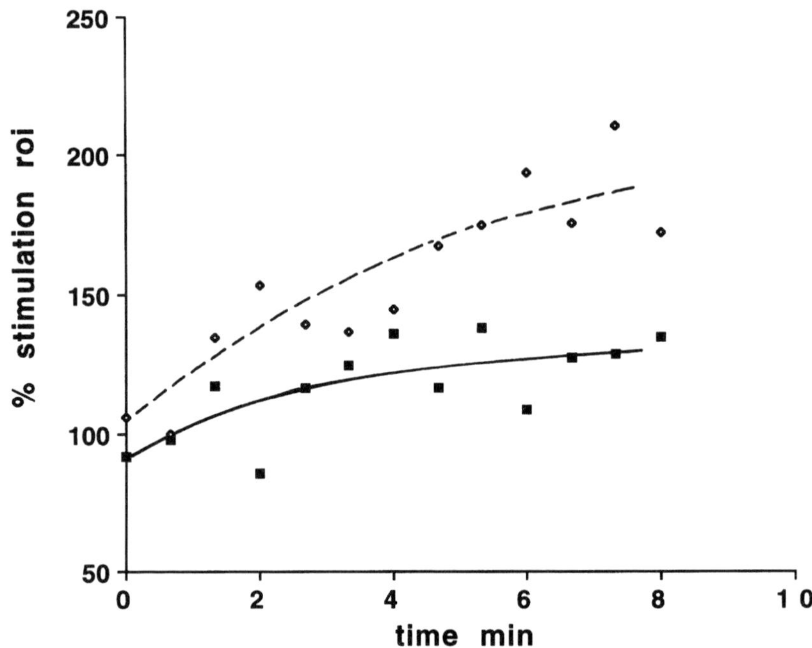

FIGURE 4. Stimulation of reactive oxygen intermediate formation in human tumor and normal unaffected brain tissue. The rate of stimulated reactive oxygen intermediate formation is shown in cells prepared from (–■–) unaffected normal brain tissue and (–◇–) oligoastrocytoma tissue from the same individual. Both preparations were incubated in the presence or absence of 18 μM arachidonic acid, reactive oxygen intermediates were detected using 2',7'-dichlorofluorescein oxidation. The rate of increase of 2',7'-dichlorofluorescein production in the total tumor and normal brain cell population was analyzed using the exponential function $y = I + \beta$ $[1 - \exp(-kt)]$, where y = the ratio of stimulated/unstimulated roi, i.e., mean 2',7'-dichlorofluorescein fluorescence in the stimulated cell preparation/mean 2',7'-dichlorofluorescein fluorescence in unstimulated cells. In each preparation, the mean cellular oxidized 2',7'-dichlorofluorescein per cell in the presence of arachidonic acid was divided by the mean unstimulated dichlorofluorescein fluorescence using cells from the same patient. The goodness of fit to the model, estimated using residual means squared (r^2) was 0.992 for tumor and 0.991 for normal tissue.

cytes, the activity of gammalinolenic acid was greater than that of arachidonic acid, indicating that peroxidative pathways may be involved. The mode of action of these antiproliferative effects are incompletely understood, but may involve the activation of apoptosis either via transcription factors such as $nF\kappa_\beta$ or other pathways. Although a stimulation of tumor phagocyte activity by exogenous n-6 fatty acids was detected, the dichlorofluorescein method also detected a significant stimulation of tumor cell peroxidation in cells characterized by glial fibrillary acidic protein expression. It is possible that these effects on apoptosis may be the result of a combination of multiple pathways, involving free arachidonic acid,[3,32] reactive oxygen intermediates,[14,23,27,46]

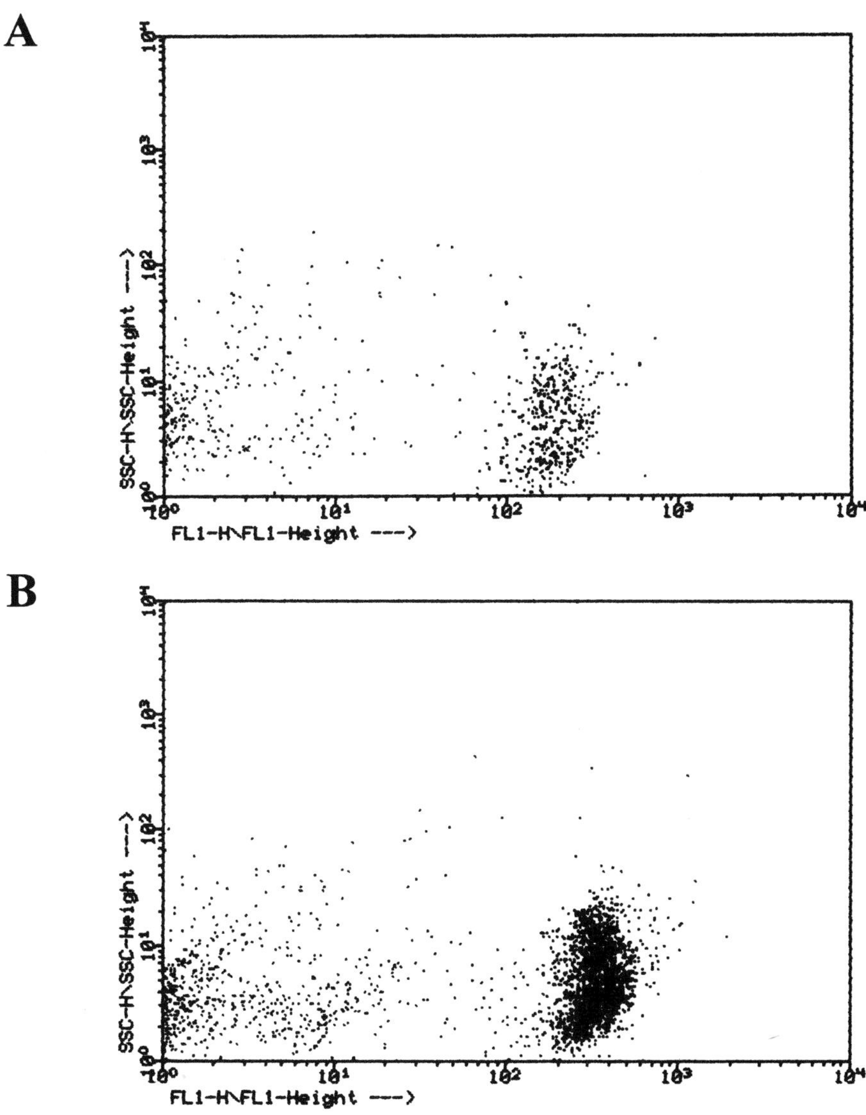

FIGURE 5. Effect of arachidonic acid on apoptosis in human brain tumor cells. Cells were prepared from a sample of cerebellar anaplastic oligodendroglioma using 200 U/ml collagenase. Isolated cells were incubated either (**A**) without arachidonic acid or (**B**) with 30 μM arachidonic acid for 15 minutes. Apoptosis in individual cells was assessed using the terminal deoxynucleotide transferase uridine nick end-labeling (TUNEL) assay analyzed by flow cytometry using a Becton-Dickinson FACScan cytometer. In each sample, 10,000 cells were analyzed and cells with fluorescence >80 were gated. TUNEL-labeled populations were characterized by high fluorescence-1 intensity (>70 FL-1 on *x* axis). The proportion of TUNEL-labeled tumor cells in **A** cells without arachidonic acid was 6.57% and in **B** the same tumor cell preparation incubated with 30 μM arachidonic acid was 20.53%.

and the pathways of arachidonyl-phospholipid metabolism.[39] Transfection experiments using Bcl-2 and Bcl-x in neuronal and myeloid cells show Bcl inhibition of sensitivity of apoptosis to peroxidation.[45] The extent and even the presence of arachidonate-associated apoptosis has shown wide variations in reported values, even for the same cell type.[32,46] The wide variation in reporting of apoptosis may partly relate to methodological deficiencies in which temporal considerations are insufficiently analyzed in defining the dynamics of apoptosis[46] and arachidonic acid flux.[39] Therefore, although the cellular pathways of the process are incompletely understood, there is increasing evidence that the endogenous release of arachidonic acid in normal cells is capable of autoregulatory activity in controlling lipid peroxidation and cell growth. It is possible that in pathological conditions involving rapid cell growth the endogenous supply of arachidonic acid is diminished and is not able to inhibit cell proliferation. Further network analysis of arachidonic acid flux and cell turnover is important to investigate this effect.

Recently, genetic evidence involving mutations in the p53 oncogene and the studies of the origin of tumor cells have supported an epigenetic network model of carcinogenesis in many solid tumors. These studies suggested that the microenvironment within a tumor can determine growth and malignancy. It was postulated that the controlling factors in these processes involved oxidative metabolism and apoptosis.[47] It was found that the selection of p53 mutations resulting in the development of tissue resistant to oxidative signals commonly occurred in solid tumors of diverse origins. A polyclonal origin of colonic adenoma has recently been identified that also indicates that multiple cells are involved in tumorigenesis.[48] Thus, the overwhelming majority of cancers present a diverse and multifactorial pathology. It has been calculated that less than 2% of tumors are related to monogenic causes and even in such cases, the final phenotype is modulated by many factors.[41] Therefore, because in at least 98% of tumors, genetic modes do not act in isolation, it is essential to analyze the interaction between pathways involving several genes responding to multiple physiological modulators. Metabolic and cellular networks, many of which are linked to arachidonic acid flux, provide the context for gene expression. In such epigenetic control systems, simple linear analysis is insufficient to provide reliable predictions. Such systems are dominated by nonlinear logic, in which environmental, developmental, and metabolic signaling play a key role in determining pathogenesis. In analysis of peroxidation in primary brain tumors, the mixed responses of the individual cell populations within the tumor made it necessary to use nonlinear modeling of the dynamics of the peroxidative response (FIG. 4). The resultant kinetic constants gave information that linked tumor peroxidative metabolism with tumor grade. This selective action of exogenous arachidonic acid (FIGS. 4 and 5) supports the hypothesis that there may be a local deficiency in arachidonic acid in rapidly growing tumors such as primary brain tumors.

NETWORK PROPERTIES OF ARACHIDONIC ACID: SUMMARY

The selective action and ubiquitous distribution of arachidonate within the cells of the reticuloendothelial and nervous systems make arachidonic acid a key candidate to act as a connective agent in intracellular communication. These properties have not been adequately defined by previous, more static, network definitions or by structural and monogenetic analysis. Network analysis is useful in determining dynamic behavior involving several pathways and responding cell types, for example, in describing metabolic flux and cell turnover in apoptosis, which involves multiple interacting pathways. In the pathways of apoptosis in phagocytes and other cells and in phagocyte NADPH oxidase activation and endotoxin priming, evidence is accumulating to suggest that arachidonic acid plays an important part in reticuloendothelial network responses. These networks describe intracellular and intercellular events during reticuloendothelial function and in the development of immunological memory.[21–23] These networks have some resemblance to neural networks in establishing spatio-temporal patterns of connectivity. Reticuloendothelial networks also resemble more fluid models of interaction between cells and mediators associated by receptor type and response pathway distribution. Network theory has the advantage of defining complex factors such as fatty acid distribution and activity in a quantitative and non-hierarchical manner. It has the disadvantage that the exact relationship between individual elements is not always easy to define. However, network analysis is already giving new insights into arachidonic acid activity in complex systems such as multiparameter flow cytometry of cell populations. Network analysis of flow cytometric data is currently being used in the analysis of phagocyte activation, in which ultrastructural changes are associated with intracellular Ca^{2+} mobilization.[49,25] The application of both specifically designed and generally available network programs will help to characterize the association between arachidonic acid flux and cell activation, transcellular signaling, and the immunomodulation associated with cell proliferation and the control of cell growth. Network and nonlinear approaches may therefore be useful in the analysis of multifactorial events such as trauma, cancer, and cardiovascular disease, conditions in which arachidonic acid has been postulated to play a mediatory role.[1,25] To discover the extent of arachidonic acid involvement in the pathophysiology of these system responses, it is important to analyze nonlinear dynamics and interactive responses.

ACKNOWLEDGMENTS

We are very grateful and to Drs. Jeanne Bell and Alastair Lammie for Pathology samples, to Dr. I. Dawson and Dr. N.H. Wilson of the Pharmacology Department for molecular modeling, to Eric Miller of the ICRF Laboratories for flow cytometry, and to Helen Bell for culture and immunocytochemistry.

REFERENCES

1. SINCLAIR, H. M. 1956. Deficiency of essential fatty acids. The Lancet: 381–383.
2. BURNS C. P. & A. A. SPECTOR. 1987. Membrane fatty acid modification in tumour cells: a potential therapeutic adjunct. Lipids **22:** 178–184.
3. TISDALE, M. J. 1993. Mechanism of lipid mobilisation associated with cancer cachexia: interaction between polyunsaturated fatty acid, eicosapentanoic acid and inhibitory guanine nucleotide regulatory protein. Prostaglandins Leukotrienes Essent. Fatty Acids **48:** 105–109.

4. JOHNSTON, P. V. 1988. Lipid modulation of immune responses. Nutrition and Immunology: 7–86. Alan R. Liss, Inc. New York.

5. SAKATA, A., E. IDA, M. TOMINAGA & K. ONOUE. 1987. Arachidonic acid acts as an intracellular activator of NADPH-oxidase in Fcγ receptor-mediated superoxide generation in macrophages. J. Immunol. **138:** 4353–4359.

6. KAPUS, A., R. ROMANEK & S. GRINSTEIN. 1994. Arachidonic acid stimulates plasma membrane H^+ conductance in macrophages. J. Biol. Chem. **269:** 4736–4745.

7. LEAVER, H. A., S. JANAH, P. L. YAP, W. B. ROSS, A. D. HILLON & L. TURNER. 1992. Pathways controlling the superoxide response during phagocyte differentiation: involvement of arachidonic acid and Ca^{2+} in response to bacterial endotoxin. FEMS Microbiol. Immunol. **105:** 261–270.

8. LIGETI, E., V. PIZON, A. WITTINGHOFER, P. GIERSCHIK & K. H. JAKOBS. 1993. GTPase activity of small GTP binding proteins in HL-60 membranes is stimulated by arachidonic acid. Eur. J. Biochem. **216:** 813–820.

9. MILLER, B., M. SARANTIS, S. F. TRAYNELIS & D. ATWELL. 1992. Potentiation of NMDA receptor currents by arachidonic acid. Nature **355:** 722–725.

10. HAYAKAWA, M., N. ISHIDA, K. TAKEUCHI, S. SHIKAMOTO, T. HORI, N. OKU, F. HO & M. TSUJIMOTO. 1993. Arachidonic acid-selective phospholipase A_2 is crucial in the cytotoxic action of tumor necrosis factor. J. Biol. Chem. **268:** 11290–11296.

11. FOREHAND, J. R., R. B. JOHNSTON & J. S. BOMALASKI. 1992. Phospholipase A_2 activity in human neutrophils: stimulation by lipopolysaccharide and possible involvement in priming for an enhanced respiratory burst. J. Immunol. **151:** 4918–4923.

12. FUJIMORI, Y., M. MURAKAMI, K. YANG, D. KIM, K. TAKAYAMA, I. KUDO & K. INOUE. 1992. Immunochemical detection of arachidonyl-preferential phospholipase A_2. J. Biochem. **111:** 54–60.

13. MACDONALD, M. L., K. F. MACK, C. N. RICHARDSON & J. A. GLOMSET. 1988. Regulation of diacylglycerol kinase in Swiss 3T3 cells. J. Biol. Chem. **268:** 1575–1583.

14. WILLIAMS J. R., H. A. LEAVER, J. W. IRONSIDE, E. P. MILLER, G. MALCOLM, I. R. WHITTLE & A. GREGOR. 1996. Antiproliferative effects of arachidonic acid on the C6 glioma cell line and human glioma tissue. J. Neuro- Oncol. (In press).

15. DOERFLER, M. E., J. WEISS, J. D. CLARK & P. ELSBACH. 1994. Bacterial lipopolysaccharide primes neutrophils for enhanced release of arachidonic acid and causes phosphorylation of a 85-kD cytosolic phospholipase A_2. J. Clin. Invest. **93:** 1583–1591.

16. GLASER, K. B., R. ASMIS & E. A. DENNIS. 1990. Bacterial lipopolysaccharide priming of P388D1 macrophage-like cells for enhanced arachidonic acid metabolism. Platelet-activating factor receptor activation and regulation of phospholipase A_2. J. Biol. Chem. **265:** 8658–8664.

17. BAULDRY, S. A., C. E. MCCALL, S. L. COUSART & D. A. BASS. 1991. Tumor necrosis Factor-α priming of phospholipase A_2 activation in human neutrophils. J. Immunol. **146:** 1277–1285.

18. SUMOMOTO, H., Y. KAGE, H. NUNOI, T. NOSE, Y. FUKUMAKI, M. OHNO, S. MINAKAMI & K. TAKESHIGE. 1994. Role of Src homology 3 domains in assembly and activation of the phagocyte NADPH oxidase. Proc. Natl. Acad. Sci. USA **91:** 5345–5349.

19. HENDERSON, L. M. & J. B. CHAPPELL. 1992. The NADPH- oxidase H^+ channel is opened by arachidonate. Biochem. J. **283:** 171–175.

20. DECOURSEY, T. E. & V. V. CHERNY. 1992. Potential, pH and arachidonate gate hydrogen ion currents in human neutrophils. Biophys. J. **65:** 1590–1598.

21. VARELA, F. J. & A. COUTINHO. 1991. Second generation immune networks. Immunol. Today **12:** 159–166.

22. PERELSON, A. S. 1989. Immune network theory. Immunol. Rev. **110:** 5–36.

23. STEWART, J. & F. J. VARELA. 1989. Exploring the meaning of connectivity in the immune network. Immunol. Rev. **110:** 37–61.

24. JERNE, N. K. 1974. Towards a network theory of the immune system. Ann. Immunol. (Paris) **125C:** 373–389.

25. VALET, G., M. VALET, D. TSCHOPE, H. GABRIEL, G. ROTHE, W. KELLERMAN & H. KAHLE. 1993. White cell and thromocyte disorders: standardised, self-learning flow cytometric list mode data classification. Ann. N.Y. Acad. Sci. **677:** 233–251.

26. HENDERSON, L. M., S. K. MOULE & J. B. CHAPPELL. 1993. The immediate activator of the NAPDH oxidase is arachidonate not phosphorylation. Eur. J. Biochem. **221:** 157–162.

27. AEBISCHER, C. P., I. PASCHE & A. JORG. 1993. Nanomolar arachidonic acid influences the respiratory burst in eosinophils and neutrophils induced by GTP-binding protein. A comparative study of the respiratory burst in bovine eosinophils and neutrophils. Eur. J. Biochem. **218:** 669–677.

28. DOUSSIERE, J., J. GAILLARD & P. V. VIGNAIS. 1996. Arachidonic acid induced transition from a low spin state of the neutrophil flavocytochrome b oxidase. Biochemistry **35:** 13400–13410.

29. LEAVER, H. A., J. R. WILLIAMS, I. DAWSON & P. L. YAP. 1995. Arachidonic acid in the reticuloendothelial system. Biochem. Soc. Trans. **23:** 279–301.

30. LEAVER, H. A., S. R. CRAIG, P. L. YAP, J. R. WILLIAMS & W. S. WALKER. 1996. Arachidonic acid metabolism and activation of monocyte and neutrophil reactive oxygen in lung cancer patients undergoing pulmonary resection. Biologicals **24**(4): 319–324.

31. SAWAI, T., M. ASADA, H. NUNOI, I. MATSUDA, S. ANDO, T. SAAKI, K. KAIBUCHI, Y. TAKAI & K. KATAYAMA. 1993. Combination of arachidonic acid and guanosine 5′-O-(3-thiotriphosphate) induce translocation of rac p21s to membrane and activation of NADPH oxidase in a cell-free system. Biochem. Biophys. Res. Commun. **195:** 264–269.

32. FINSTAD, H. S., S. O. KOLSET, J. A. HOLME, R. WIGER, A. K. FARRANTS, R. BLOMHOFF & C. A. DREVON. 1994. Effect of n-3 and n-6 fatty acids on proliferation and differentiation of premyelocytic leukemic HL-60 cells. Blood **84:** 3799–3809.

33. HORROBIN, D. F. 1990. Essential fatty acids, lipid peroxidation and cancer. *In* Omega-6 Essential Fatty Acids. D. F. Horrobin, Eds.: 351–377. Alan R. Liss, Inc. New York.

34. COOK, J. A., W. C. WISE & P. V. HALUSHKA. 1980. Elevated Thromboxane levels in the rat during endotoxic shock. Protective effects of Imidazole, 13-azaprostanoic acid or essential fatty acid deficiency. J. Clin. Invest. **65:** 227–230.

35. HERRERO, I., M. T. MIRAS-PORTUGAL & J. SANCHEZ-PRIETO. 1992. Positive feedback of glutamate exocytosis of metabotropic presynaptic receptor stimulation. Nature **360:** 163–166.

36. C. RANDRIAMAMPITA & A. TRAUTMAN. 1990. Arachidonic acid activates Ca^{2+} extrusion in macrophages. J. Biol. Chem. **265:** 18059–18062.

37. MOHAZZAB, K. M., P. M. KAMINSKI & M. S. WOLIN. 1994. NADH oxidoreductase is a major source of superoxide anion in bovine pulmonary artery endothelium. Am. J. Physiol. **226:** H2568–2572.

38. FORMAN, H. J. & E. J. KIM. 1989. Inhibition by linoleic acid hydroperoxide of alevolar macrophage superoxide production: effects on mitochondrial and plasma membrane potentials. Arch. Biochem. Biophys. **274:** 443–452.

39. SURETTE, M. E., J. D. WINKLER, A. N. FONTEH & F. H. CHILTON. 1996. Relationship between arachidonate-phospholipid remodelling and apoptosis. Biochemistry **35:** 9187–9196.

40. RATKOWSKY, D. A. 1989. *In* Handbook of Nonlinear Regression Models: 96–97. Marcel Dekker Inc. N.Y.

41. STROHMAN, R. 1994. Epigenesis: the missing beat in biotechnology? Biotechnology **12:** 156–164.

42. ROSS, W. B., H. A. LEAVER, P. L. YAP, G. M. RAAB, B. H. SU, D. C. CARTER, J. H. MAO, W. QIAN, R. J. PRESCOTT. 1993. Macrophage prostaglandin E_2 and oxidative responses to endotoxin. Prostaglandins Leukotrienes Essent. Fatty Acids **49:** 945–953.

43. MALCOMSON, R. D. G., S. H. ORAM, D. J. HARRISON. 1996. The importance of apoptosis. Biologicals **24**(4): 295–330.

44. DAS, U. N., W. K. PRASAD & D. R. REDDY. 1995. Local application of gamma-linolenic acid in the treatment of human gliomas. Cancer Lett. **94**: 147–155.

45. KANE, D. J., T. A. SARAFIAN, R. ANTON, H. HAHN, E. B. GRALLA, J. S. VALENTINE, T. ORD & D. E. BREDESEN. 1993. Bcl-2 inhibition of neural death: decreased generation of reactive oxygen species. Science **262**: 1274–1277.

46. JARVIS, W. D., R. N. KOLESNICK, F. A. FORNARI, R. S. TRAYNOR, D. A. GEWIRTZ & S. GRANT. 1994. Induction of apoptosis DNA damage and cell death by activation of the sphingomyelin pathway. Proc. Natl. Acad. Sci. USA **91**: 73–77.

47. GRAEBER, T. G., C. OSMANIAN, T. JACKS, D. E. HOUSMAN, C. J. KOCH, S. W. LOWE & A. J. GIACCIA. 1996. Hypoxia-mediated selection of cells with diminished apoptotic potential in solid tumours. Nature **379**: 88–91.

48. NOVELLI, M. R., J. A. WILLIAMSON, I. P. M. TOMLINSON, G. ELIA, S. V. HODGSON, I. C. TALBOT, W. F. BODMER & N. A. WRIGHT. 1996. Polyclonal origin of colonic adenomas in an XO/XY patient with FAP. Science **272**: 1187–1190.

49. ROTHE, G., W. KELLERMAN & G. VALET. 1990. Flow cytometric parameters of neutrophil function as early indicators of sepsis- or trauma-related pulmonary or cardiovascular organ failure. J. Lab. Clin. Med. **115**: 52–61.

The NADPH Oxidase of Phagocytic Leukocytes[a]

ANTHONY W. SEGAL AND KAROLYN P. SHATWELL

Department of Medicine
University College London
5 University Street
London WC1E 6JJ, United Kingdom

INTRODUCTION

Phagocytic leukocytes (e.g. neutrophils, monocytes, macrophages, eosinophils) are essential for immunity to infection by bacteria and fungi. These organisms are engulfed into a "phagocytic vacuole," an invagination of the plasma membrane, the neck of which fuses to form a closed compartment. Cytoplasmic granules containing an array of proteases and other antimicrobial compounds fuse with this vacuole and discharge their contents into the vacuolar lumen, in which the ingested microbe is killed and digested.

Phagocytosis, as well as a wide variety of artificial stimuli, induces a burst of oxygen consumption, known as the "respiratory burst." [1] This process involves the one electron reduction of oxygen to superoxide (O_2^-) and is essential for the efficient killing of the ingested microorganism. Defects in the superoxide-generating system are associated with the syndrome chronic granulomatous disease (CGD) in which there is a profound and often fatal predisposition to bacterial and fungal infections.[1] The various mutations in these patients leading to abnormalities in the different components of the NADPH oxidase have provided valuable tools with which to dissect out and understand the proteins and cofactors involved.[2]

THE ELECTRON TRANSPORT CHAIN OF NADPH OXIDASE

Flavocytochrome b

The electron transport chain that generates superoxide is an electrogenic membrane bound flavocytochrome b (known as b_{558} or b_{-245}), which is incorporated in the wall of the phagocytic vacuole. It takes electrons from NADPH, a product of the hexose monophosphate shunt,[3] and passes them via FAD and heme to molecular oxygen.

Flavocytochrome b_{558} is an $\alpha_1\beta_1$ heterodimer.[4] The β subunit, also known gp91^{phox} (gp for glycoprotein, 91 from a rough estimate of the molecular weight and *phox* from *ph*agocyte *ox*idase), is a heavily glycosylated protein[5] containing 569 amino acids, with a predicted molecular mass of 65 kD.[6,7] It is the main structural component of the flavocytochrome, housing all of the components of the electron

[a]This work supported by The Wellcome Trust.

transport chain. The C-terminal half comprises a hydrophilic globular domain that is exposed to the cytosol and accommodates the NADPH and FAD binding sites.[8] A degree of homology with the FNR family of reductases has enabled the nucleotide binding domains to be modeled using ferredoxin-NADP-reductase as a template[9] (FIG. 1). The N-terminal half of the β subunit has 4–6 putative hydrophobic transmembrane helices and probably carries the heme prosthetic groups.[37]

The α subunit, also called p22^{phox}, has a molecular mass of 22 kD and is believed to be anchored to the membrane by two hydrophobic transmembrane helices.[10] Its function is uncertain but the C-terminus has a proline-rich tail that appears to be important for the binding of activating cytosolic factors. These fail to translocate to the membrane if this region is mutated.[11,12] The α subunit might therefore play an essentially regulatory role. On binding the cytosolic activation complex it may transmit a conformational change to the β subunit, thereby initiating the flow of electrons across the membrane.

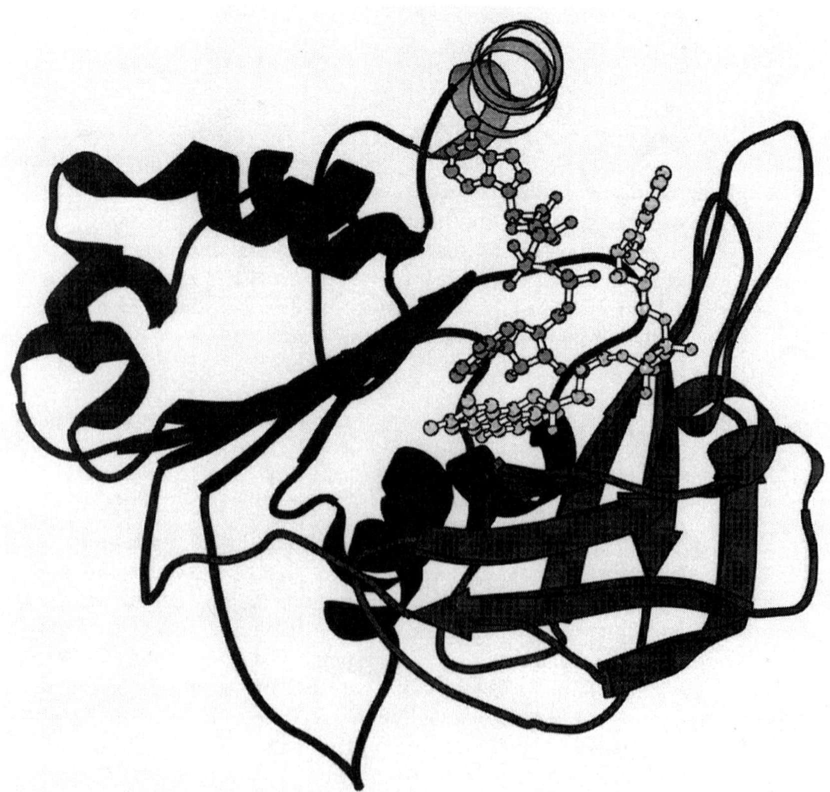

FIGURE 1. Model of the nucleotide binding domains of flavocytochrome b$_{558}$ with bound NADPH and FAD.[9]

The Flavin

Flavins are the redox cofactors usually linked to NAD(P)H and are capable of coupling a two-electron donor to a one-electron transporter, in this case heme. Compelling evidence for the involvement of a flavin group in electron transport by NADPH oxidase was provided by electron paramagnetic resonance (EPR). A FAD semiquinone free radical was detected after the addition of NADPH to membranes from activated but not unstimulated neutrophils.[13] Analysis of the flavin content of these membranes revealed almost exclusively non-covalently bound FAD.[13] Importantly, the FAD content of neutrophil membranes was shown to be depleted for the cells of patients with X-linked CGD,[8] indicating a linkage between the absence of a heme spectrum, the lack of the two subunits of what we now know to be the flavocytochrome b_{558}, and gross diminution in the amount of FAD.[8]

Binding of the flavin cofactor to the β subunit (FIG. 1) was indicated initially by

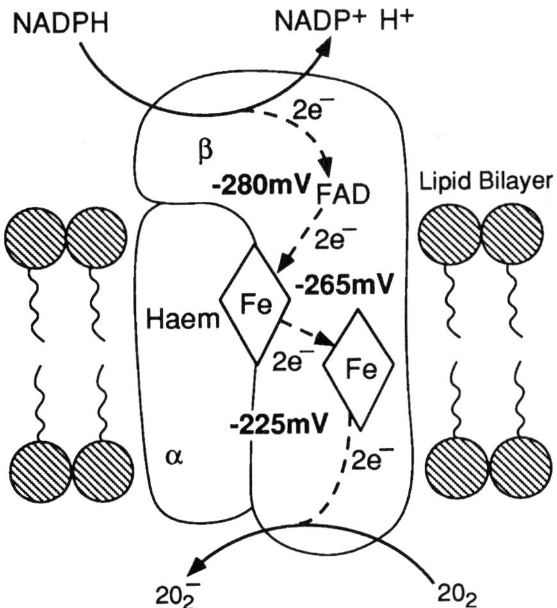

FIGURE 2. Schematic representation of flavocytochrome b_{558} in the activated NADPH oxidase. Electrons pass from NADPH in the cytoplasm, via FAD and heme, to oxygen, producing O_2^-, which is released into the phagocytic vacuole. The midpoint potentials for the different redox centers are shown in boldface.

the homology between the C-terminal half of gp91^{phox} and members of the FNR flavoenzyme family.[8] It was subsequently demonstrated directly using the photoaffinity ligand [^{3}H]NAP$_4$-FAD.[14]

The Hemes

It has long been thought that the molar ratio of heme to FAD in flavocytochrome b_{558} is 2:1.[8] However, conclusive evidence for this has only recently become available. Cross and coworkers analyzed the potentiometric titrations for flavocytochrome b_{558} from a patient with X-linked CGD attributed to an $Arg_{54}\rightarrow$Ser mutation in the β subunit. This revealed that the mutant form of the cytochrome contained two nonidentical hemes with midpoint potentials ($E_{m7.0}$) of -220 mV and -300 mV.[15] Subsequent reanalysis of earlier data for the native flavocytochrome which had, up until this point, been interpreted as a single midpoint potential of -245 mV,[16] revealed that it too contains two hemes with $E_{m7.0}$ values of -225 mV and -265 mV. This indicates that electrons flow from FAD to the hemes sequentially and then on to O_2 (FIG. 2). In the CGD patient the value of the lower potential heme was depressed to -300 mV,[15] below that of the flavin semiquinone at -280 mV, thereby blocking the flow of electrons from the flavin.

Evidence from EPR and Raman spectroscopy indicated that the hemes are low spin and six coordinate with axial imidazole or imidazolate ligands.[17] Their precise location, however, remains uncertain. Recently site-directed mutagenesis studies on the yeast ferric reductase, FRE1, a related plasma membrane cytochrome b,[18] have indicated that the hemes are coordinated between pairs of histidine residues located towards the extremities of two putative transmembrane segments in the β subunit. They are envisaged to sit between the two transmembrane α-helices, towards either edge of the membrane and perpendicular to it.[37]

Activation Mechanism

The NADPH oxidase is totally dormant until activated by phagocytosis or by a wide variety of artificial agonists. Activation requires the participation of the cytosolic *phox* proteins p47^{phox}, p67^{phox}, and p40^{phox}, as well as a small GTP binding protein p21*rac*. These proteins form a complex in the cytosol that translocates to the membrane and docks with the flavocytochrome.[19,20] The proteins interact with one another and with the flavocytochrome by virtue of SH3 and proline-rich domains.[21,22] p47^{phox},[23] and p67^{phox},[24] as well as both subunits of the flavocytochrome,[25] become phosphorylated upon activation but the precise role of phosphorylation in the activation process has still to be elucidated. p21*rac*, which attaches to p67^{phox},[26] appears to play a pivotal role, acting as a switch to activate and then subsequently inactivate the oxidase (FIG. 3).

Studies by Cross and coworkers have thrown some light on the function of the cytosolic *phox* proteins[27] p67^{phox} and p40^{phox} to which it is tightly complexed, induce the reduction of FAD without further transfer of electrons to the hemes. The latter requires the participation of p47^{phox}. p67^{phox} is thought to bind to and displace a small

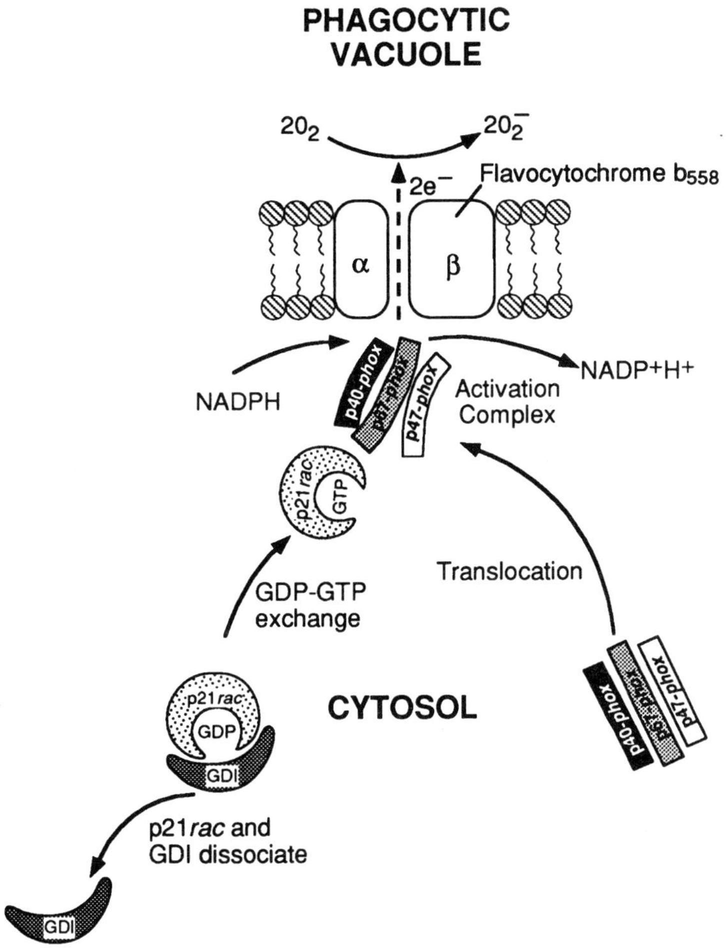

FIGURE 3. Model of the activation process of NADPH oxidase. Activation involves the translocation of a cytosolic complex of p47^{phox}, p67^{phox}, and p40^{phox} to the flavocytochrome in the membrane; p21*rac* dissociates from its complex with GDI and also translocates. The interaction of the cytosolic *phox* proteins with the cytochrome, and their interaction with the GTP form of p21*rac* causes a conformational change in the flavocytochrome subunits leading to electron transport.

α-helical region which is predicted to overly and block the NADPH binding site[9] (FIG. 1), thereby allowing access of the NADPH and the passage of electrons to FAD. Clearly this small helical region of the β-subunit is required for translocation of the cytosolic proteins to the membrane, as is the proline-rich tail of the α subunit, since mutations in both regions block movement of the activation complex to the membrane.[12,28] Binding of the cytosolic *phox* proteins together with p21*rac* in the GTP bound form probably induces the conformational changes required for the transfer of electrons to heme (FIG. 3).

THE FUNCTION OF NADPH OXIDASE

Dogma has it that the reduced oxygen species O_2^- and its derivatives, H_2O_2 and OH^-, are directly microbicidal. In addition, myeloperoxidase, which is released from the cytoplasmic granules at very high concentration into the phagocytic vacuole, is thought to use H_2O_2 as a substrate to oxidize chloride and iodide to reactive chlorine, iodine, and their hypohalous acids.[29] However, preparations of neutrophils from which the granules and nuclei have been removed, but which still phagocytose bacteria and generate superoxide, fail to kill the bacteria, indicating an absolute requirement for the granule contents.[30] Myeloperoxidase itself is unlikely to be the required factor because a deficiency of this protein, which is relatively common, does not predispose to infection.[31]

An alternative, or complementary, function of this electrogenic NADPH oxidase is to elevate the pH in the phagocytic vacuole so as to optimize conditions for microbial killing and digestion by the neutral proteinases and other enzymes released from the granules into the vacuole.[32] These proteins are maintained in the inactive state in the granules at a pH of about 5.0, whereas a pH of above 7.0 is required for their antimicrobial effect in the test tube.

The pH within the normal phagocytic vacuole has been shown to rise to 7.8–8.0 as a consequence of the NADPH oxidase pumping relatively large amounts of superoxide into this closed compartment.[32] The charged O_2^- is unlikely to easily cross the vacuolar membrane, and its dismutation to O_2^{2-} will be rapidly followed by protonation of the latter to H_2O_2. Concentrations of these molecules could theoretically reach millimolar amounts. The protons retained in the cytoplasm after the electrons have been pumped into the vacuole are exchanged for Na^+ in the extracellular medium.[33] In contrast, in CGD or anaerobic cells, although the vacuolar pH starts out the same as that of the extracellular medium, it rapidly drops to 6–6.5, well below that required for efficient killing and digestion by the granule neutral proteinases. This results in an increased risk of infection and the retention of indigestible material, which produces the granulomatous tissue response that gives CGD its name.

CHRONIC GRANULOMATOUS DISEASE

The genetic defects underlying CGD are many and varied. Defects in the *CYBB* gene, which is located on the short arm of the X chromosome at Xp21.1 and encodes the β subunit, account for about two thirds of cases.[34] The mutations have been identified in approximately 300 families with X-linked CGD and range from missense and nonsense mutations through to deletions, insertions, and splice site mutations. In the vast majority of cases, the mutation results in a complete loss of both subunits of the flavocytochrome, each being required for mutual stability.[35,36] In only about 5%

of mutations is the protein conserved and in these cases analysis of the cell biological and biochemical consequences can be very informative, as these mutations are likely to involve regulatory and catalytic rather than structural domains.

The remaining one third of cases of CGD have an autosomal recessive pattern of inheritance and can be attributed to mutations in the gene for p47^{phox} (*NCF1*) or more rarely, p67^{phox} (*NFC2*) or p22^{phox} (*CYBA*).[34] No patients have been identified in whom the primary lesion is in p40^{phox}.

At present the control of CGD is primarily aimed at prevention and aggressive treatment of infections as they occur. However, since CGD results from single-gene defects in myeloid cells, in the longer term the prospects for gene therapy look good. In principle, it should be possible to transfer the correct gene into hemopoietic stem cells, the precursors of phagocytic cells, thereby providing a complete cure.[34]

REFERENCES

1. THRASHER, A.J., N.H. KEEP, F. WIENTJES & A.W. SEGAL. 1994. Biochim. Biophys. Acta **1227:** 1–24.
2. SEGAL, A.W. & A. ABO. 1993. Trends Biochem. Sci. TIBS **18:** 43–47.
3. ZATTI, M. & F. ROSSI. 1965. Biochim. Biophys. Acta **99:** 557–561.
4. WALLACH, T.M. & A.W. SEGAL. Biochem. J. In press.
5. HARPER, A.M., M.F. CHAPLIN & A.W. SEGAL. 1985. Biochem. J. **227:** 783–788.
6. ROYER-POKORA, B., L.M. KUNKEL, A.P. MONACO, S.C. GOFF, P.E. NEWBURGER, R.L. BAEHNER, F.S. COLE, J.T. CURNUTTE & S.H. ORKIN. 1986. Nature **322:** 32–38.
7. TEAHAN, C., P. ROWE, P. PARKER, N. TOTTY & A.W. SEGAL. 1987. Nature **327:** 720–721.
8. SEGAL, A.W., I. WEST, F.B. WIENTJES, J.H.A. NUGEST, A.J. CHAVAN, B. HALEY, R.C. GARCIA, H. ROSEN & G. SCRACE. 1992. Biochem. J. **284:** 781–788.
9. TAYLOR, W.R., D.T. JONES & A.W. SEGAL. 1993. Prot. Sci. **2:** 1675–1685.
10. PARKOS, C.A., M.C. DINAUER, L.E. WALKER, R.A. ALLEN, A.J. JESAITIS & S.H. ORKIN. 1988. Proc. Natl. Acad. Sci. USA **85:** 3319–3323.
11. DINAUER, M.C., E.A. PIERCE, R.W. ERICKSON, T.J. MUHLEBACH, H. MESSNER, S.H. ORKIN, R.A. SEGER & J.T. CURNUTTE. 1991. Proc. Natl. Acad. Sci. USA **88:** 11231–11235.
12. LEUSEN, J.H., B.G. BOLSCHER, P.M. HILARIUS, R.S. WEENING, W. KAULFERSCH, R.A. SEGER, D. ROOS & A.J. VERHOEVEN. 1994. J. Exp. Med. **180:** 2329–2334.
13. KAKINUMA, K., M. KANEDA, T. CHIBA & T. OHNISHI. 1986. J. Biol. Chem. **261:** 9426–9432.
14. DOUSSIERE, J., G. BUZENET & P.V. VIGNAIS. 1995. Biochemistry **34:** 1760–1770.
15. CROSS, A.R., J. RAE & J.T. CURNUTTE. 1995. J. Biol. Chem. **270:** 17075–17077.
16. CROSS, A.R., O.T. JONES, A.M. HARPER & A.W. SEGAL. 1981. Biochem. J. **194:** 599–606.
17. HURST, J.K., T.M. LOEHR, J.T. CURNUTTE & H. ROSEN. 1991. J. Biol. Chem. **266:** 1627–1634.
18. SHATWELL, K.P., A. DANCIS, A.R. CROSS, R.D. KLAUSNER & A.W. SEGAL. 1996. J. Biol. Chem. **271:** 14240–14244.
19. HEYWORTH, P.G., J.T. CURNUTTE, W.M. NAUSEEF, B.D. VOLPP, D.W. PEARSON, H. ROSEN & R.A. CLARK. 1991. J. Clin. Invest. **87:** 352–356.
20. HEYWORTH, P.G., C.F. SHRIMPTON & A.W. SEGAL 1989. Biochem. J. **260:** 243–248.
21. LETO, T.L., A.G. ADAMS & I. DE MENDEZ. 1994. Proc. Natl. Acad. Sci. USA **91:** 10650–10654.
22. WIENTJES, F.B., G. PANAYOTO, E. REEVES & A.W. SEGAL. Biochem. J. In press.
23. Segal, A.W., P.G. Heyworth, S. Cockcroft & M.M. Barrowman. 1985. Nature **316:** 547–549.

24. Dusi, S. & F. Rossi. 1993. Biochem. J. **296:** 367–371.
25. Garcia, R.C. & A.W. Segal. 1988. Biochem. J. **252:** 901–904.
26. Diekmann, D., A. Abo, C. Johnston, A.W. Segal & A. Hall. 1994. Science **265:** 531–533.
27. Cross, A.R. & J.T. Curnutte. 1995. J. Biol. Chem. **270:** 6543–6548.
28. Leusen, J.H., M. De Boer, B.G. Bolscher, P.M. Hilarius, R.S. Weening, H.D. Ochs, D. Roos & A.J. Verhoeven. 1994. J. Clin. Invest. **93:** 2120–2126.
29. Klebanoff, S.J. 1980. Ann. Intern. Med. **93:** 480–489.
30. Odell, E.W. & A.W. Segal. 1988. Biochim. Biophys. Acta **971:** 266–274.
31. Parry, M.F., R.K. Root, J.A. Metcalf, K.K. Delaney & L.S. Kaplow. 1981. Ann. Intern. Med. **95:** 293–301.
32. Segal, A.W., M. Geisow, R. Garcia, A. Harper & R. Miller. 1981. Nature **290:** 406–409.
33. Grinstein, S. & W. Furuya. 1986. Biochim. Biophys. Acta **889:** 301–309.
34. Roos, D., M. De Boer, F. Kuribayashi, R.S. Weening, A.W. Segal, A. Ahlin, K. Nemet, J.P. Hossle, E. Bernatowska-Matuszkiewicz & H. Middleton-Price. 1996. Blood **87:** 1663–1681.
35. Parkos, C.A., R.A. Allen, C.G. Cochrane & A.J. Jesaitis. 1987. J. Clin. Invest. **80:** 732–742.
36. Segal. A.W. 1987. Nature **326:** 88–91.
37. Finegold, A. A., K. P. Shatwell, A. W. Segal, R. D. Klausner & A. Dancis. 1996. J. Biol. Chem. **271:** 31021–31024.

Influence of Interleukin-1 Receptor Antagonist on [³H]Serotonin and Histamine Release by Rat Basophilic Leukemia-2H3 Cells

PIO CONTI,[a] RENATO C. BARBACANE, MIRTO TRAKATELLIS[b],
FERNANDA C. PLACIDO, IVANA CATALDO,
AND MARCELLA REALE

Immunology Division
Institute of Experimental Medicine
University of Chieti
Via dei Vestini
66100 Chieti, Italy

[b]*Department of Biochemistry*
Aristotle University
Thessaloniki, Greece

INTRODUCTION

Mast cells located in connective tissue are unique for their metachromasia with toluidine blue and are important for their involvement in immediate and delayed hypersensitivity reactions.[1–5] Rat basophilic leukemia-2H3 cells (RBLC) are transplantable basophilic leukemia cells that are equivalent to mucosal mast cells and can differentiate in the high density stationary phase of culture by accumulating granules, histamine, and IgE receptors.[7–10]

The RBLC line is a good model system for the analysis of immunoglobulin E receptor (Fc_Σ)-mediated signal transduction and surface-engaged, Fc_Σ-induced histamine and serotonin (5HT) release.[11] The cross-linkage of the high affinity Fc_Σ receptors on mast cells and murine mast cell lines stimulate increases in messenger RNA levels and secretion of a group of cytokines classically produced by a subset of murine T cell lines, TH1 and TH2 cells.[11] Recently, it has been shown that only TH2 cells express high affinity receptors for interleukin-1 (IL-1) and require this monokine for their proliferation.[12,13] Moreover, it seems that IL-1 has no effect on the TH1 clone proliferation and in the absence of IL-1, TH2 clones proliferate less in response to antigen-presenting macrophages (IL-1-producing cells) that do not need additional IL-1.[13,14] IL-1 receptor antagonist (IL-1RA) is a new clonal protein of 22 kD (glycosylated form) and 17 kD (non-glycosylated form) that is secreted by human macrophages, is structurally similar to IL-1β, binds to the IL-1 receptor, and is a natural inhibitor of IL-1α and IL-1β.[15–27]

Since IL-1 is involved in the inflammation and hypersensitivity reactions and its

[a]Address correspondence to: Dr. Pio Conti, Associate Professor, Cattedra di Immunologia, Istituto di Medicina Sperimentale, Facoltà di Medicina, Università di Chieti, Via dei Vestini, 66100 Chieti, Italy.

role on histamine release from mast cells is still unclear,[2–29] it is pertinent to study the effect of IL-1RA on the release of histamine and 5-HT by cultured RBL cells before and after treatment with appropriate secretagogues.

MATERIALS AND METHODS

Rat Basophilic Leukemia Cells

RBL-2H3 cells, kindly provided by Dr. H. Metzger (National Institutes of Health, Bethesda, MD), were grown in S-MEM medium (GIBCO, Grand Island, NY) supplemented with 15% fetal calf serum, 100 U/ml penicillin, 0.1% streptomycin (GIBCO, Grand Island, NY) and 0.5 mM calcium chloride either in 25 cm^2 tissue culture dishes (Corning, NY) or in six-well tissue culture dishes (Costar, Cambridge, MA). Cells were plated at a density of 0.2×10^6 cells per ml taken from 3-day-old cultures grown under the same conditions. Cells were growing in an atmosphere of 5% CO_2, 95% O_2 at 37°C.

Determination of Rat Basophilic Leukemia Cell Viability

Two methods were used for determination of cell viability. Trypan blue exclusion and the ability of RBL cells to grow in fresh medium after treatment with IL-1RA. Cells either treated or not treated with IL-1RA were washed, trypsinized, and pelleted by centrifugation for 5 min at $400 \times g$. Cells were then resuspended in S-MEM medium, 0.1% trypan blue solution was added, and cells were counted under the microscope. Viability is expressed as percentage of cells that do not take up trypan blue.

Alternatively, RBL cells from 3-day-old cultures with IL-1RA were diluted to a density of 0.2×10^6/ml with fresh medium and grown without IL-1RA (these cells were totally viable). Counts were taken in triplicate from triplicated cultures.

Percent Histamine Determinations

Histamine in cells or histamine released to growth medium was estimated by a radioenzymatic method, essentially a modification of the method described by Kaplan and colleagues.[30]

RBL cells growing attached were washed, trypsinized, and harvested by centrifugation at $400 \times g$ for 5 min in 1.5 ml Eppendorf tubes. Cells were then resuspended in water (5×10^6/0.2 ml). This suspension was sonicated in Branson 1200 ultrasound device for 10 min, vortexed for 5 min, and pelleted by 10 min centrifugation at top speed in an Eppendorf microcentrifuge. Histamine in growth medium taken from growing cells or from cells treated with IgE and antigen was estimated after pelleting the cells by centrifugation at $400 \times g$ for 5 min. For each 20 μl of supernatant taken from disrupted cells or 20 μl of growth media, 2 μl 20% perchloric acid, 6 μl 1 N NaOH, and 100 μl 0.05 M sodium phosphate pH 7.4 was added. The precipitate was pelleted by 5 min centrifugation at top speed in an Eppendorf microfuge and aliquots were taken from the supernatant for further histamine assay. In 50 μl of reaction mixture for histamine assay 5–25 μl sample, 5 μl rat kidney histamine methyl transferase and S-(methyl-^{3}H) adenosyl-L-methionine (73.8 Ci/mM, Amersham) were present. Isotope and enzyme were diluted with 0.05 M sodium phosphate pH 7.4 for optimal conditions. The reaction mixture was incubated 1 h at 37°C, following which 20 μl 1.5 M perchloric acid, 20 μl 10 M NaOH, and 500 μl freshly prepared toluene-isoamylalcohol (4:1 vol/vol) was added and the mixture was shaken for 10 min. After 10 min centrifugation at 200 × g, 0.3 ml was taken from the upper phase and 4 ml of Aquasol (New England Nuclear, Boston, MA) scintillation fluid was added. Radioactivity was measured in a beta counter and the concentration of histamine was computed by using a standard curve. Samples were always performed in duplicate from duplicate cultures.

Percent of Histamine Release upon Stimulation with Anti-IgE and Antigen

Cells (1×10^6) in a six-well tissue culture dish were washed with S-MEM containing 1 mg/ml bovine serum albumin (BSA) and without Ca^{2+} to reduce spontaneous secretion. They were then sensitized in the same medium for 30 min at 37°C with 2 ml mouse monoclonal anti-DNP IgE (500 ng/ml). After sensitization the cells were washed again and treated for 30 min at 37°C with 2 ml DNP-BSA (10 ng/ml) in the same medium, but now supplemented with 0.5 mM calcium to permit secretion. Control samples without IgE were run simultaneously in the presence of 0.5 mM Ca^{2+} and these values represented nonspecific release and were subtracted from the overall histamine release. Histamine released in the medium was estimated as described earlier in *Materials and Methods.* Mouse monoclonal anti-DNP-IgE and DNP-BSA were kindly provided by Dr. Fu-Tong Liu (Scripps Clinic, La Jolla, CA).

[^{3}H]5HT Release from RBL Cells

RBL cells were loaded with [^{3}H]5HT (15–30 Ci/mmol, New England Nuclear, Boston, MA) for 1 h at 37°C, were washed twice, and were then resuspended in the indicated buffer (4×10^5/ml) in tubes (Falcon 2063) with a total sample volume of 0.5 ml/tube and preincubated for 15 min with the compound to be tested at 37°C and then adding the classic secretagogues for 10 min. At the end of the incubation, the cells were pelleted by centrifugation at 100 × g. The supernatant was removed, 2% Triton X-100 was added to the pellet to lyse the cells, and both supernatant and pellet radioactivity were quantified by a beta counter. The release was expressed as the percent of total [^{3}]5HT released, calculated as that present in the supernatant over that in the pellet and the supernatant combined. The percentage release was calculated using the formula:

$$\frac{\text{CPM supernatant}}{\text{CPM supernatant} + \text{CPM pellet (precipitate)}} \times 100 = \% \text{ release}$$

Preparation of Compounds

Compound 48/80 (C48/80) or IgE were made directly in Locke's medium. In separate tubes, in each experiment, cells were exposed to the vehicle alone, at identical concentrations, to determine non-specific release.

Interleukin-1 Receptor Antagonist

IL-1RA, a kind gift from Dr. Robert C. Thompson, Synergen, Inc. (Boulder, CO), was diluted and filter-sterilized in propylene glycol to a final concentration of 500 ng/ml.

Preparation of the Histidine Decarboxylase Probe

We used a probe made from a reverse-transcribed rat brain polyA$^+$ mRNA. Total cellular RNA was extracted from New England Deaconess Hospital rat brain. PolyA$^+$ mRNA was purified by one-step chromatography on oligodT column. A sample of 2 µg polyA$^+$ mRNA was reverse transcribed at 42°C for 40 min in a 20-µl mixture containing 4 µl 5× reverse transcriptase buffer (250 mM Tris HCl pH 8.3 at 42°C, 50 mM MgCl$_2$, 250 mM KCl, 15 mM DTT, 10 U placental RNase inhibitor, 0.5 mM each dNTP, 50 pMoles oligodT primer, and 20 U AMV reverse transcriptase. After reverse transcription, the histidine decarboxylase (HDC) cDNA was amplified by polymerase chain reaction (PCR) using two specific primers synthesized on a gene assembler plus (Pharmacia LKB): 5′ primer, 5′-ATGATGG-AGCCCAGTGAAT-ACC and 3′ primer, 5′CCAGAATTCGCATGTCTGAGG- TAG. A 4 µl single-stranded cDNA mixture was supplemented with 50 pmoles of each 5′ and 3′ primers in a volume of 50 µl, denatured for 2 min in a boiling bath, and added to a 50-µl mix prewarmed at 72°C containing 0.25 mM each dNTP, 10 µl 10× Taq polymerase buffer (500 mM KCl, 100 mM Tris-HCl pH 8.3 at 25°C, 15 mM MgCl$_2$, and 0.1% gelatin), and 1.5 U of Taq polymerase (Perkin-Elmer Cetus). The PCR program consisted of one cycle of 1 min at 55°C, and 15 min at 72°C followed by 35 cycles of 30 sec at 94°C, 30 sec at 55°C, and 4 min at 72°C, and was completed by an additional annealing at 55°C for 30 sec and a final elongation at 72°C for 15 min. PCR was performed in a Techne PHC-2 programmable heating block. Amplified products of the expected base-pair size were purified by glass-milk procedure (Geneclean BIO 101), blunt-ended with the Klenow fragment, and cut by *Eco*RI. The resulting blunt-end–*Eco*RI fragments were cloned in the p-MAL vector (Biolabs) cut by both *Stu*I and *Eco*RI restriction enzymes. The resulting recombinant plasmid was amplified in the TB1 *Escherichia coli* strain. Plasmid DNA was sequenced by the double-stranded protocol of the sequenase kit (USB Cleveland). Plasmid containing amplified HDC cDNA was prepared according to the alkaline lysis method and purified on a CL4B column.

Histidine Decarboxylase

Total RNA was isolated by guanidine hydrochloride as previously described.[44] Total RNA (10 μg/line) was fractioned by electrophoresis on a 2% agarose gel and transferred to nylon membranes (Hybond N, Amersham) and hybridized with labeled ^{32}P HDC probe (2×10^8 cpm/μg), washed at room temperature for 15 min four times in $2 \times$ SSC and 0.1% SDS, then heated to 48°C for 30 min and washed twice in $0.1 \times$ SSC and 0.1% SDS. Membranes were finally exposed to Kodak XAR5 for 3 days at –70°C. Signals were compared with ribosomal RNA to evaluate an equal quantity of RNA for each line.

Statistical Analysis

Data from different experiments were combined and reported as mean ± S.D. Student's *t* test for independent means was used to provide a statistical analysis ($p > 0.05$ was considered as not significant).

RESULTS

[³H]5HT and Histamine Release from RBLC Treated or not with IL-1RA

Basophils and/or mast cells are normal analogues of rat basophilic leukemia cells, which have histamine-containing granules and receptors for IgE. In this report we have studied RBLC and RPMC degranulation under the influence of IL-1RA, a natural and specific inhibitor of IL-1 receptor, with and without a classic specific secretagogues, anti-IgE, or a non-specific C48/80).

TABLE 1 shows, in three representative experiments, the percent release of 5HT following RBLC treatment for 48 h with or without IL-1RA (500 ng/ml). In experi-

TABLE 1. Percentage of 5HT Release by RBLC Mast Cells in Three Representative Experiments

Number of Experiments	(–IL-1RA) 500 ng/ml	(+IL-1RA) 500 ng/ml	$p <$
1　Control (untreated cells)	9.3 (*)	6.6	0.01
1a　Anti-IgE	14.5 (*)	13.9	N.S.
2　Control (untreated cells)	8.7 (*)	6.5	0.01
2a　Anti-IgE	11.9 (*)	12.3	N.S.
3　Control (untreated cells)	14.7 (*)	10.3	0.05
3a　Anti-IgE	16.8 (*)	17.0	N.S.

Note: 5HT percent release from RBLC following addition, or not, of hrIL-1RA (500 ng/ml) and treated, or not, with anti-IgE. The cells were cultured for 48 h at 37°C with 5% CO_2. *p* values (Student's *t* test) are calculated by comparing IL-1RA–untreated RBLC (*) with IL-1RA–treated cells. The values are representative of three experiments in triplicate.

ments 1–3, we report the spontaneous release of 5HT is strongly inhibited on RBLC growth in the presence of IL-1RA (500 ng/ml), compared to the untreated cells (no IL-1RA); while when IL-1RA treated and untreated cells were stimulated with a secretagogue anti-IgE, no difference was found (experiments 1a–3a). These effects were similar when the percent of histamine release was measured from cultured RBLC (FIG. 1).

Effect of hrIL-1RA on Histidine Decarboxylase mRNA in RBL-2H3

A 1,019 bp HDC cDNA probe was cloned into the p-Mal plasmid and used for Northern blot hybridization.[43] Since hrIL-1RA inhibited the spontaneous release of histamine (FIG. 1) in these studies, we cultured RBLC in the presence of IL-1RA (500 ng/ml) and Northern blot analysis was determined for HDC (FIG. 2). When IL-1RA was added, HDC mRNA was significantly inhibited compared to the controls. In FIGURE 2, we show a time-course study and steady-state levels of HDC mRNA were expressed. In Lane 1 we show the control where HDC is spontaneously activated, since these cells are immature and are spontaneously activated to proliferate. Lane 2 (30 min incubation), Lane 3 (1 h incubation), and Lane 4 (2 h incubation) gradually decreased, reaching maximum inhibition at Lane 5 (after 4 h), compared to control (Lane 1). However, the inhibitory effect of IL-1RA on HDC mRNA was

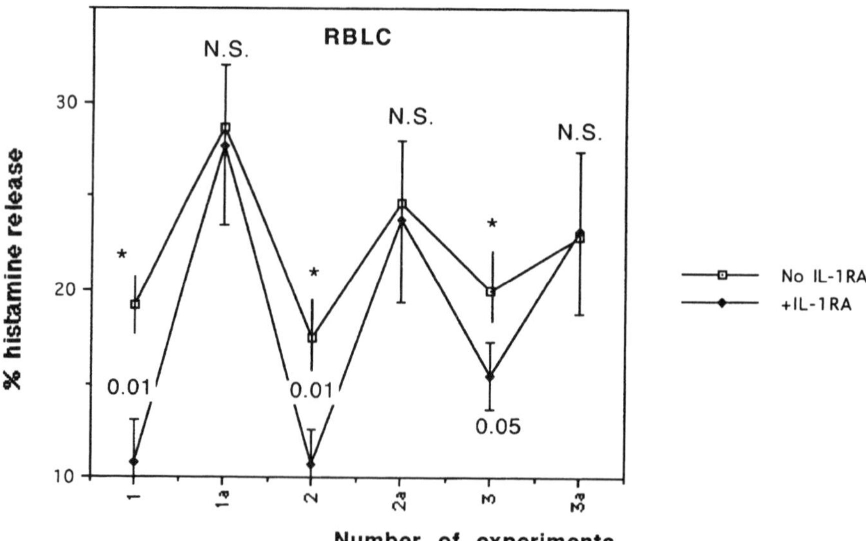

FIGURE 1. Histamine percent release from RBLC (± S.D.) following the addition (*diamond*), or not (*square*) of hrIL-1RA (500 ng/ml) (experiments 1, 2, and 3) and the corresponding samples treated with anti-IgE (experiments 1a, 2a, and 3a) plus the addition of hrIL-1RA (500 ng/ml) (*diamond*), or not (*square*). The cells were cultured for 48 h at 37°C, 5% CO_2. *p* values (Student's *t* test) are calculated by comparing IL-1RA–untreated RBLC (*) with IL-1RA–treated cell. The values ± S.D. are representative of three experiments in triplicate.

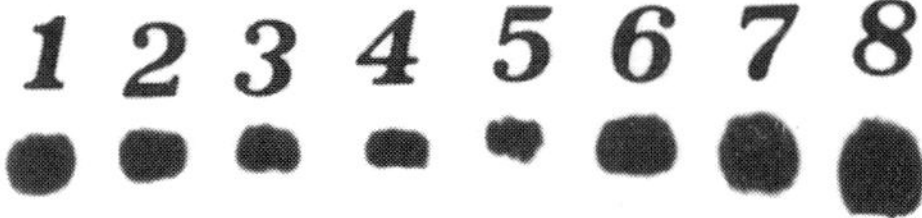

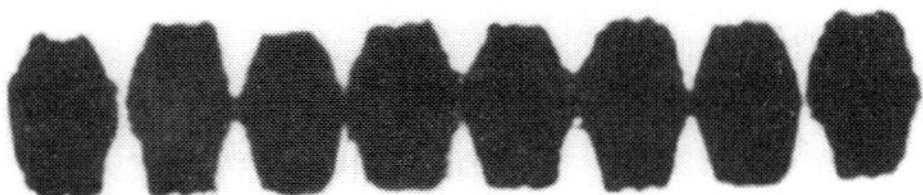

FIGURE 2. Effect of IL-1RA (500 ng/ml) on histidine decarboxylase mRNA expression in RBLC cells cultures for 30 min (Lane 2), 1 h (Lane 3), 2 h (Lane 4), 4 h (Lane 5), 18 h (Lane 6), 24 h (Lane 7), and 48 h (Lane 8). In Lane 1 (controls), the cells were not treated and received only medium at the same volume as the treated cells. This is a representative experiment of four.

completely restored when the cells were cultured for 18 h (Lane 6), 24 h (Lane 7), and 48 h (Lane 8), compared to the controls (nil).

DISCUSSION

Recently, it has been reported that mast cells generate multifunctional cytokines, including IL-1, IL-3, IL-4, IL-6, GM-CSF, and TNFα.[31–34] It is not clear if IL-1 is capable of directly inducing histamine release from basophils and/or mast cells.[29,30,35] In this report, we found that IL-1RA, a protein produced by macrophages that binds to the IL-1 receptor and is an inhibitor of transcription and translation of IL-1,[17–23] cultured for 48 h with RBLC *in vitro,* provokes a significant inhibition of spontaneous histamine and serotonin release compared to the untreated cells (control) (FIG. 1 and TABLE 1). However, when RBLC were treated after 48 h cultures with a physiologic secretagogue anti-IgE, the release of histamine or serotonin was not different between IL-1RA–treated and untreated cells. After cloning a cDNA probe into p-MAL plasmid, an HDC mRNA Northern blot hybridization was performed.[43] The addition of IL-1RA in cultures of RBLC promotes an inhibition of HDC mRNA secretion after 4 h incubation. The decrease of HDC mRNA is explained by the inhibition of the *de novo* synthesis of this enzyme, spontaneously activated in these cancer cells. This effect was abolished in the presence of cyclohexamide or actinomycin D (data not shown), compounds that inhibit protein synthesis and mRNA transcription, respectively. The inhibitory effect of IL-1RA may be low and disappear when the cells are cultured for longer periods of time (18, 24, and 48 h). This concept is supported by the fact that when cells are cultured with IL-1RA plus a strong secretagogue, the results are not significantly different from controls (non-treated cells). Therefore, it is possible that IL-1RA inhibits the intracellular formation of IL-1, which may play a pre-transcriptional and not a post-transcriptional role in histamine generation on precursor mast cells. Another hypothesis is that RBLC release low amounts of IL-1, which stimulates the autocrine loop, and IL-1RA blocks this effect through the binding of the IL-1 receptor.[28,29] Concentrations less than 500 ng/ml had little or no effect. In fact, to have a perceivable effect IL-1RA must exceed the concentration of IL-1 by 100–1,000-fold.[25] The reason IL-1RA influences non-stimulated mast cells may be linked to the fact that histamine release is more prominent in atopic individuals, but does not appear to require an interaction with IgE.[41] However, the exact mechanism of mast cell–mediated late-phase inflammatory response and IgE-dependent hypersensitivity reactions, mediated by histamine and 5HT, is unknown, but the induced release of soluble mediators, such as cytokines, is clearly important.[31,34] The concept of heterogeneity across both species and tissues is well known and there may be interspecies differences or altered cell responses seen in transformed cell lines.

Since IL-1RA has no biological effects, the inhibition of the spontaneous release of histamine and 5HT most probably involves the down-regulation of IL-1 in the RBLC cultures. The process of conversion from pre-IL-1α and pre-IL-1β to mature extracellular forms is not clear.[36] The inhibitory effect of IL-1RA on histamine and 5HT release may be exerted through the binding of this protein on IL-1 receptors, subsequently affecting the multistep peptide cleavage required for proteolytic processing of pre-IL-1 to mature IL-1, (which may have co-stimulatory properties). Moreover, since the block of IL-1 by IL-1RA does not influence the release of histamine and 5HT on RBLC challenged with secretagogues, it is possible that the mature IL-1 is not as important as is the pre-IL-1 in mast cell vasoactive amine release. Therefore, these results suggest the possible involvement of IL-1RA regulatory genes in the suppression of both pre-IL-1α and pre-IL-1β expression, and suggest that IL-1 is involved in the generation of histamine and serotonin.

SUMMARY

Mast cells located in connective tissues are a potent source of vasoactive and inflammatory mediators, such as cytokines. They accumulate in tissues in a wide variety of diseases where their function in most cases in unclear. In this report we provide evidence that rat basophilic leukemia cells (RBLC) cultured with a natural inhibitor of IL-1, interleukin-1 receptor antagonist (IL-1RA) (500 ng/ml) for 48 h, strongly inhibited the spontaneous release of serotonin (5HT) (from 25.2 to 29.9%), and histamine (from 22.50 to 43.49%), compared to untreated cells (control). When IL-IRA–treated and –untreated RBLC were stimulated with a secretagogue (anti-IgE), no difference was found in the percent of 5HT and histamine release. The present studies describe an additional biological activity of IL-1RA, inhibiting histamine and 5HT spontaneous release from RBLC cultures.

REFERENCES

1. SERAFIN, W. E. & K. E. AUSTEN. 1987. Mediators of immediate hypersensitivity reactions. N. Engl. J. Med. **317:** 87–138.

2. THEOHARIDES, T. C., P. K. BONDY, N. D. TSAKALOS & P. W. ASKENASE. 1982. Differential release of serotonin and histamine from mast cells. Nature **297**: 229.

3. PLAUT, M., J. H. PIERCE, C. J. WATSON, J. HANLEY-HYDE, R. P. NORDAN & W. E. PAUL. 1989. Mast cell lines produce lymphokines in response to cross-linkage of $Fc_{\epsilon}R1$ or to calcium ionophores. Nature **339**: 64–67.

4. SIEGHART, W., T. C. THEOHARIDES, D. S. ALPER, W. W. DOUGLAS & P. GREENGARD. 1978. Calcium-dependent protein phosphorylation during exocytotic release of mast cell secretory granules. Nature **275**: 329–331.

5. LEWIS, R. A. & K. F. AUSTEN. 1981. Mediation of local homeostasis and inflammatory by leukotrienes and other mast cell–dependent compounds. Nature **293**: 103.

6. CONTI, P., M. REALE, R. C. BARBACANE, M. R. PANARA, M. BONGRAZIO & T. C. THEO- HARIDES. 1992. Role of lipoxin A4 and B4 in the generation of arachidonic acid metabolites by rat mast cells and their effect on [^{3}H]serotonin release. Immunol. Lett. **32**: 117–124.

7. KULCZYCKI, A., C. ISERSKY & H. METZGZE. 1974. The interactions of IgE with rat basophilic leukemia cells. I. Evidence for specific binding of IgE. J. Exp. Med. **139**: 600.

8. CONRAD, D. H., I. BERCZI & A. FROESE. 1976. Characterization of the target cell receptor for IgE-I. Solubilization of IgE-receptor complexes from rat mast cells and rat basophilic leukemia cells. J. Immunol. **13**: 320–332.

9. BONIFACINO, J. S., P. PEREZ, R. D. KLAUSNER & I. V. SANDOVAL. 1986. Study of the transit of an integral membrane protein from secretory granules through the plasma membrane of secreting rat basophilic leukemia cells using a specific monoclonal antibody. J. Cell Biol. **102**: 516–522.

10. THEOHARIDES, T. C. & W. W. DOUGLAS. 1978. Secretion in mast cells induced by calcium entrapped within phospholipid vesicles. Science **201**: 1143–1145.

11. ISERSKY, C., H. METZGER & D. N. BUELL. 1975. Cell cycle-associated changes in receptors for IgE during growth and differentiation of a rat basophilic leukemia cell line. J. Exp. Med. **141**: 1147–1162.

12. WILLIAMS, M. E., T. L. CHANG, S. K. BURKE, A. H. LICHTMAN & A. K. ABBAS. 1991. Activation of functionally distinct subset of CD4+ T lymphocytes. Res. Immunol. Inst. Pasteur **142**: 23–28.

13. CHANG, T. L., C. M. SHEA, S. URIOSTE, R. C. THOMPSON, W. H. BOOM & A. K. ABBAS. 1990. Heterogeneity of helper/inducer T lymphocytes. III. Response of IL-2 and IL-4 production (TH1 and TH2) clones to antigen presented by different accessory cells. J. Immunol. **145**: 2803–2808.

14. MIZEL, S. B. 1989. The interleukins. FASEB J. **3**: 2379–2388.

15. SECKINGER, P., J. W. LOWENTHAL, K. WILLIAMSON, J.-M. DAYER & H. R. MCDONALD. 1987. A urine inhibitor of interleukin-1 activity that blocks ligand binding. J. Immunol. **139**: 1546–1549.

16. DINARELLO, C. A., L. J. ROSENWASSER & S. M. WOLF. 1982. Demonstration of a circulating thymocytes suppressor factor during endotoxin fever in humans. J. Immunol. **127**: 2517–2519.

17. HANNUM, C. H., C. J. WILCOX, W. P. AREND, F. G. JOSLIN, D. J. DRIPPS, P. L. HEIMDAL *et al.* 1990. Interleukin-1 receptor antagonist activity of a human interleukin-1 inhibitor. Nature **343**: 336–340.

18. CARTER, D. B., M. R. DEIBEL, C. J. DUNN, C. S. C. TOMICH, A. L. LABORDE, J. L. SLIGHTOM *et al.* 1990. Purification, cloning, expression and biological characterization of interleukin-1 receptor antagonist protein. Nature **344**: 633–637.

19. EISENBERG, S. P., R. J. EVANS, W. P. AREND, E. VERDERBER, M. T. BREWER, C. H. HANNUM & R. C. THOMPSON. 1990. Primary structure and functional expression from complementary DNA of a human interleukin-1 receptor antagonist. Nature **343**: 341–346.

20. AREND, W. P., H. G. WELGUS, R. C. THOMPSON & S. P. EISENBERG. 1990. Biological proper-

ties of recombinant human monocyte-derived interleukin-1 receptor antagonist. J. Clin. Invest. **85:** 1694–1697.

21. DINARELLO, C. A. 1989. Strategies for anti-interleukin-1 therapy. Int. J. Immunopathol. Pharmacol. **2:** 203–211.

22. WAKABAYASHI, G., J. A. GELFAND, W. K. JUNG, R. J. CONNOLLY, J. F. BURKE & C. A. DINARELLO. 1991. Staphylococcus epidermis induces complement activation, tumor necrosis factor and interleukin-1, a shock-like state and tissue injury in rabbits without endotoxemia. J. Clin. Invest. **87:** 1925–1935.

23. CONTI, P., C. FELICIANI, R. C. BARBACANE, M. R. PANARA, M. REALE, F. C. PLACIDO, D. N. SAUDER, R. A. DEMPSEY & P. AMERIO. 1992. Inhibition of interleukin-1β mRNA expression and interleukin-1α and β secretion by a specific human recombinant interleukin-1 receptor antagonist in human peripheral blood mononuclear cells. Immunology **77:** 245–250.

24. CONTI, P. & R. DEMPSEY. 1991. Macrophage down-regulation by interleukin-1 receptor antagonist. Am. J. Hematol. **39/4:** 310–311.

25. DINARELLO, C. A. 1989. Interleukin-1 and its biologically related cytokines. Adv. Immunol. **44:** 153.

26. CONTI, P., M. R. PANARA, R. C. BARBACANE, F. C. PLACIDO, M. BONGRAZIO, M. REALE, R. A. DEMPSEY & S. FIORE. 1992. Blocking the interleukin-1 receptor inhibits leukotriene B4 (LTB4) and prostaglandin E2 (PGE2) generation in human monocyte cultures. Cell. Immunol. **145:** 199–209.

27. CONTI, P., M. R. PANARA, S. FRIDAS, R. C. BARBACANE, M. REALE, R. A. DEMPSEY & F. C. PLACIDO. 1992. Inhibition of in vivo induced chronic inflammation by human recombinant interleukin-1 receptor antagonist (hrIL-1RA). New Adv. Cytokines **92:** 361–365.

28. HAAK-FRENDSCHO, M., C. DINARELLO & A. P. KAPLAN. 1988. Recombinant interleukin-1β causes histamine release from human basophils. J. Allergy Clin. Immunol. **82:** 218–223.

29. SUBRAMANIAN, N. & M. A. BRAY. 1987. Interleukin-1 releases histamine from human basophils and mast cells in vitro. J. Immunol. **138:** 271–275.

30. KAPLAN, A. P., M. HAAK-FRENDSCHO, A. FAUCI, C. A. DINARELLO & E. MALBERT. 1985. A histamine releasing factor from activated human mononuclear cells. J. Immunol. **135:** 2027–2032.

31. PLAUT, M., J. H. PIERCE, C. J. WATSON, J. HANLEY-HYDE, R. P. NORDON & W. E. PAUL. 1989. Mast cell lines produce lymphokines in response to cross linkage of FcΣRI or calcium ionophore. Nature **339:** 64.

32. WODNAR-FILIPOWICZ, A., C. H. HEUSSER & C. MORONI. 1989. Production of hematopoietic growth factor GM-CSF and interleukin-3 by mast cells in response to IgE receptor-mediated activation. Nature **39:** 150.

33. BURD, P. R., H. W. ROGERS, J. R. GORDON, C. A. MARTIN, S. JAYARAMAN, D. WILSON, A. M. DVORAK, S. J. GALLI & M. E. DORF. 1989. Interleukin-3-dependent and -independent mast cells stimulated with IgE and antigen express multiple cytokines. J. Exp. Med. **170:** 245.

34. ANSEL, J. C., J. R. BROWN, D. G. PAYAN & M. A. BROWN. 1993. Substance P selectively activates TNF-α gene expression in murine mast cells. J. Immunol. **150:** 4478–4485.

35. TUNG, R. & L. M. LICHTENSTEIN. 1980. In vitro histamine release from basophils of asthmatic and atopic individuals in D₂O. J. Immunol. **128:** 2067–2072.

36. KOBAYASHI, Y., K. MATSUSHIMA & J. J. OPPENHEIM. 1989. Interleukin-1, Inflammation and Disease. R. Bomford & B. Henderson, Eds.: 47–62. Elsevier. Amsterdam.

Cytokine Expression and Release by Neutrophils[a]

MARCO A. CASSATELLA,[b] SARA GASPERINI,
AND MARIA PIA RUSSO

Department of General Pathology
Strada le Grazie
University of Verona
37134 Verona, Italy

INTRODUCTION

Although it was originally thought that amongst blood cells, monocytes and lymphocytes were the predominant sources of cytokines, it is now evident that cytokines are generated by many other cell types as well. For instance, a large number of studies have established that mature polymorphonuclear leukocytes (PMN) also have the capacity to express the mRNA for, and subsequently secrete, several important inflammatory and immunoregulatory cytokines.[1,2] The fact that neutrophils clearly predominate over other cell types under various *in vivo* conditions suggests that, in some circumstances, the contribution of PMN-derived cytokines can be of foremost importance. In this review, I shall summarize the current knowledge of cytokine production by neutrophils, its molecular regulation, and other biological aspects.

GENERAL CHARACTERISTICS OF CYTOKINE PRODUCTION BY NEUTROPHILS

Most of the studies addressing neutrophil cytokine synthesis have been conducted *in vitro*, principally through the use of sensitive and specific approaches such as molecular biology techniques, *in situ* hybridization (ISH), immunohistochemistry (IH), and immunoassays. Nevertheless, numerous *in vivo* observations have confirmed the validity of the *in vitro* findings. There now remains little doubt that the release of cytokines constitutes an important aspect of neutrophil biology. FIGURE 1 lists all the cytokines that, to date, have been shown to be expressed by PMN (*in vitro* or *in vivo*), either constitutively or following appropriate stimulation. In the case of interleukin-1α/β (IL-1α/β), IL-1 receptor antagonist (IL-1ra), IL-8, IL-12, tumor necrosis factor-α (TNFα), interferon-α (IFNα), transforming growth factor-β (TGFβ), macrophage inflammatory protein-1α (MIP-1α) and MIP-1β (see Loyd & Oppenheim[1] and Cassatella[2] and references therein), MIP-2,[3,4] KC,[3] and growth-related

[a]This work was supported by grants from AIRC, M.U.R.S.T. (Fondi 40% e 60%), and ISS (VIII and IX AIDS projects #9304-33).
[b]Address correspondence to: Dr. Marco A. Cassatella, Department of General Pathology, University of Verona, Strada Le Grazie, 37134 Verona, Italy. Phone, 39-45-8098130; fax, 39-45-98127; e-mail, MCNCSS@borgoroma.univr.it.

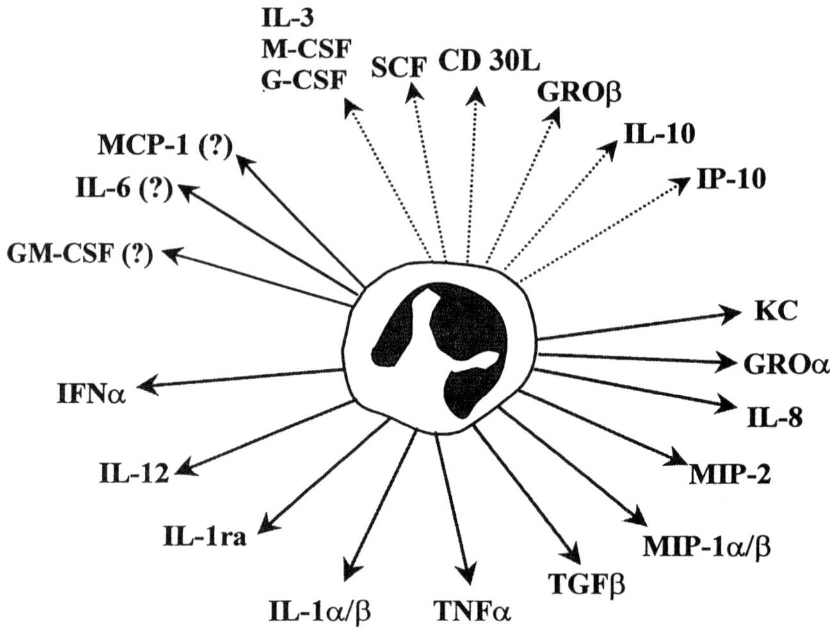

FIGURE 1. Cytokines produced by neutrophils *in vitro* or *in vivo*. The question marks in brackets indicate the fact that no general consensus exists on the ability of human neutrophils to produce IL-6, MCP-1, or GM-CSF. Production of the cytokines indicated by dashed arrows have been reported in single instances. For GROβ, CD30L, SCF, MIP-2, and KC, only mRNA expression has been reported to date.

gene product-α (GROα),[5–7] convincing evidence that PMN can release them has been generated by several groups. In contrast, mRNA expression or release of granulocyte colony-stimulating factor (G-CSF), macrophage CSF (M-CSF), IL-3,[1,2] IL-10,[8] GROβ,[9] CD30 ligand (CD30L),[10] stem cell factor (SCF)/Kit ligand (KL),[11] and interferon inducible protein-10 (IP-10)(our unpublished observations) by neutrophils have been reported in single instances, and therefore, await further confirmation. Finally, conflicting data exist in the literature concerning the issue of whether IL-6, granulocyte-macrophage colony-stimulating factor (GM-CSF), and monocyte chemotactic protein-1 (MCP-1) expression can be induced in human neutrophils. Some reports have indicated that IL-6, GM-CSF, and MCP-1[1,2,12] are expressed by human PMN, while studies from other groups, including ours, did not confirm those observations.[13–15] Whichever the case may be, the fact that neutrophils can synthesize, store, and release a wide array of cytokines should bring about a redefinition of the role of neutrophils in physiopathology.

At the molecular level, studies addressing cytokine release by neutrophils have revealed that the induction of cytokine production in PMN is usually preceded by an increased accumulation of the related mRNA transcripts. In addition, the use of Northern blotting and of related techniques have yielded important insights into the molecular mechanisms regulating cytokine gene expression in PMN. From a broad perspective, cytokine production in neutrophils can be regulated at the transcriptional, post-transcriptional, translational, and post-translational levels, as in other cell types. FIGURE 2 shows a typical Northern blot experiment, in which 10 µg of total RNA purified from PMN treated for 4.5 h with different stimuli were loaded on each gel lane. It is evident that at the selected time point, bacterial lipopolysaccharide (LPS) is the most potent inducer of IL-1β transcripts and is the only stimulus inducing IL-12p40 mRNA accumulation, while *S. Cerevisiae* opsonized with IgG (Y-IgG), formyl-methionyl-leucyl-phenylalanine (fMLP), TNFα, and LPS, differentially modulate TNFα, IL-8, and GROα mRNA steady-state levels. FIGURE 2 also shows that neutrophils do not express IL-6, a finding which, in our opinion, represents a good control of the purity of the PMN population used. Based on our studies and on re-

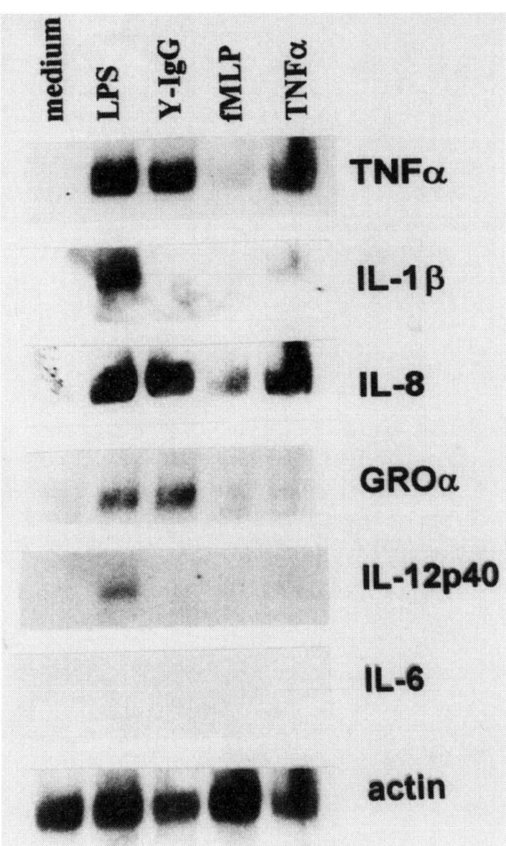

FIGURE 2. Effect of LPS, Y-IgG, TNFα, and fMLP on the steady-state levels of mRNA encoding various cytokines in human neutrophils. PMN were cultured for 4.5 h with 1 µg/ml LPS, Y-IgG at a particle/cell ratio of 2/1, 10 nM fMLP or TNFα (5ng/ml), and then subjected to Northern blot analysis. Actin mRNA expression was used to verify equal RNA loading.

ports from other laboratories,[13,16,17] the presence of IL-6 mRNA is likely to reflect the presence of contaminating monocytes in the neutrophil populations. As a result, the latter possibility should always be excluded with adequate negative controls, especially when performing Northern blot analyses (and even more so in the case of RT-PCR) or when investigating *de novo* protein synthesis.

A wide range of stimuli able to induce cytokine synthesis in PMN have been al-

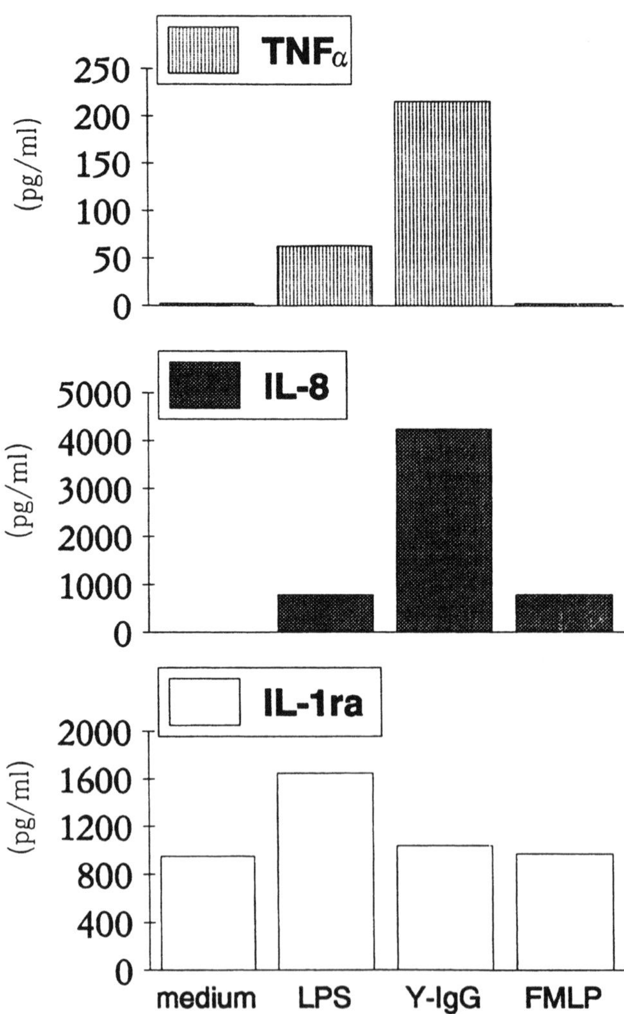

FIGURE 3. Comparison of the ability of human neutrophils to secrete various cytokines in response to different agonists. Human neutrophils were cultured for 4.5 h with LPS, Y-IgG, fMLP, or TNFα, before measuring cytokine release in their culture supernatants.

ready identified.[18] It is clear that in addition to classical agonists (such as LPS or cytokines), chemotactic factors (fMLP, leukotriene B_4, platelet-activating factor, C5a), phagocytic particles, and microorganisms (such as fungi, viruses, and bacteria) can also induce the release of cytokines by PMN. In general, not only does the magnitude and kinetics of cytokine release vary substantially depending upon the stimulus used, but the pattern of production is also influenced to a great extent by the stimulus used. For instance, FIGURE 3 shows an experiment in which TNFα, IL-8, and IL-1ra were measured in the cell-free supernatants of neutrophils cultured for 4.5 h with optimal concentrations of LPS, Y-IgG, and fMLP. It is evident that while fMLP primarily induces the production of IL-8, Y-IgG represents the most potent stimulus for IL-8 and TNFα release. In contrast, the most powerful agonist for IL-1ra secretion is LPS. The differences observed among the individual actions of the various stimuli used in the experiment in FIGURE 3 also rule out any possible contamination of fMLP or Y-IgG with trace levels of endotoxin. Since LPS can easily contaminate solutions, reagents, labware, etc.,[19] as a rule, one should carefully investigate the possibility of LPS contamination every time a given stimulus acts in a manner similar to endotoxin. This would help to avoid artifactual effects of some stimuli.

We have for a long time focused most of our investigations on the effects of Y-IgG, LPS, and fMLP, and have found different patterns of cytokine production and regulation under these experimental conditions. In the case of fMLP, or of the other chemotactic factors listed above, they seem to trigger only a transient release of IL-8[20] and GROα[5] from PMN, but apparently not that of IL-1β, TNFα, IL-12, MIP-1α/β, or IP-10. It therefore appears that chemotactic factors induce neutrophils to produce chemokines activating and recruiting more neutrophils, in a sort of positive feedback loop. In contrast, phagocytosis of Y-IgG appears to potently trigger the release of only some proinflammatory cytokines (TNFα, IL-8, and GROα), whereas LPS induces anti- and pro-inflammatory cytokines, including IL-1ra, and (in combination with interferon-γ, IFNγ) IL-12 and IP-10 as well. Thus, even though our knowledge is still incomplete and complicated by the fact that the production of cytokines by neutrophils can be also modulated by other immunoregulatory cytokines such as IL-4, IL-10, and IFNγ,[2,18] it seems that the interaction of PMN with a given agonist produces a characteristic pattern of cytokine release. Since neutrophils usually represent the first cell type encountering, and interacting with, the etiologic agent in an inflammatory context, a stimulus-specific response of neutrophils in terms of cytokine production might help in predicting the evolution of certain types of inflammatory reactions.

CHEMOKINE PRODUCTION

Convincing evidence of the ability of PMN to secrete TNFα, IL-1α/β, IL-1ra, TGFβ, and IFNα, has been reviewed elsewhere.[18] Herein, I would like to briefly expand on the production of chemokines by PMN, which provide a further means to regulate the inflammatory and immune responses. Chemokines represent a group of chemotactic cytokines whose importance in inflammatory processes is best illustrated by their ability to specifically recruit discrete leukocyte populations.[21] They have been recently classified into the subfamilies α, β, and γ, based upon their primary structure.[22] The α-subfamily includes IL-8, GRO, KC, NAP-2, IP-10, and MIP-2, which predominantly exert chemotactic and stimulatory activities towards neutrophils, except IP-10, which instead recruits lymphocytes and NK cells. The β-subfamily includes MCP-1,2,3,4,5, MIP-1α, MIP-1β and MIP-1γ, RANTES, and I-309, which predominantly have monocyte, basophil, eosinophil, and T lymphocyte-chemotactic properties. Finally, the γ-subfamily currently comprises a single member, lymphotactin,[23] which is chemotactic for lymphocytes. As mentioned above, it is now well established that neutrophils, depending upon the stimulatory conditions, can secrete IL-8, GROα, MIP-2, IP-10, MIP-1α, and MIP-1β. Therefore, it can be reasonably envisaged that neutrophils might determine the influx of different leukocyte populations to inflammatory lesions, depending upon which chemokine they produce. Should IL-8 or GROα be released, then, neutrophils will be predominantly recruited. In contrast, if MIP-1α/β or IP-10 are released, then, monocytes, eosinophils, monocytes, and lymphocyte subtypes will essentially be recruited. Obviously, these scenarios still await supporting evidence *in vivo*. However, some very recent results are reminiscent of the *in vitro* findings. In the model of experimental myocardial infarction in the rabbit, the authors demonstrated that neutrophil accumulation in myocardial tissue after ischemia and reperfusion could be explained by the sequential production of the complement fragment C5a, which recruited a certain number of neutrophils, which in turn generated IL-8, presumably in response to C5a and other stimuli.[24]

MODULATION OF CYTOKINE PRODUCTION

The *in vitro* production of chemokines (and of other cytokines) by human PMN in response to LPS appears to be regulated through a cytokine network, which involves IL-10 and IFNγ.[2] Remarkably, the fact that the release of cytokines induced by other neutrophil agonists (TNFα, fMLP, and Y-IgG)[5,25,26] is also modulated by IL-10 and IFNγ, raises the possibility that Th type 1 (Th1) and Th2 lymphocytes[27] may influence the production of cytokines by PMN. The effects of IL-10 and IFNγ can be briefly summarized as follows. IL-10 inhibits the LPS-induced extracellular release of TNFα,[16,26] IL-1α/β,[16,26] IL-8,[16,26,28] GROα,[5] IP-10, MIP-1α/β,[28] and IL-12,[29] while it potentiates that of IL-1ra.[30] By contrast, the effects of IFNγ are usually opposite to those of IL-10,[16,26] except in the case of IL-1ra (M.A. Cassatella and P.P. McDonald, unpublished observations).

The mechanisms underlying some of the modulatory actions of IL-10 and IFNγ towards cytokine mRNA accumulation in LPS-treated neutrophil have also been extensively analyzed. For instance, our nuclear run-on analyses revealed that LPS induced the transcription of the IL-8 gene in PMN stimulated for 4 h, and that this response was markedly inhibited by IFNγ and IL-10 at that selected time point.[31] Other investigators reported that the inhibitory effect of IL-10 towards LPS-induced IL-8 mRNA accumulation correlated with an enhancement of IL-8 mRNA degradation.[16,28] However, the latter two groups did not show data on the transcriptional rate of IL-8 gene. Also MIP-1α represents another cytokine gene whose modulation by IL-10 and IFNγ in PMN has been shown to be regulated at the level of both mRNA stability and transcription.[28,32] Yet, another cytokine mRNA that was found to be mainly regulated at the post-transcriptional level in neutrophils is that encoding IL-1ra. For instance, the augmented expression of IL-1ra mRNA in PMN treated with IL-13[33] and TGFβ$_1$[34] was shown to depend on a marked increase of IL-1ra transcript stability induced by both IL-13 and TGFβ$_1$. Furthermore, the half-life of IL-1ra mRNA was prolonged in PMN stimulated in the presence of IL-10 and LPS, as compared with cells stimulated with LPS alone, whereas the half-life of IL-1β mRNA was unchanged.[30] Finally, experimental evidence that IL-8 production can be modulated by IFNγ at the level of secretion was also provided.[25] Those studies revealed that the percentage of IL-8 secreted after stimulation with LPS or TNFα for up to 18 h, or with Y-IgG for 2 h, was significantly higher in PMN that were pretreated with IFNγ, relative to control cells. Thus, even though IFNγ-treated PMN synthesized less IL-8 than untreated PMN, they secreted IL-8 more efficiently after stimulation with LPS or TNFα, at all time points examined. Together, these studies indicated that the up-regulatory effect of IFNγ on LPS- and TNFα-induced secretion of IL-8 could be largely explained by a potentiating effect of IFNγ at the level of IL-8 secretion.[25]

CYTOKINE PRODUCTION BY NEUTROPHILS *IN VIVO*

Information on the production of cytokines by neutrophils *in vivo* is rapidly growing, and many different experimental animal models have been developed (TABLE 1).

TABLE 1. Cytokines Produced by Neutrophils *in Vivo*

Cytokine(s) Produced	Experimental Model	Reference
TNFα	Rats instilled intratracheally with LPS	35
IL-1α/β and TNFα	Mice injected with a colon adenocarcinoma releasing G-CSF	36
TNFα	LPS infusion of rabbits	37
TNFα, IL-1α, IL-10	Mice injected intraperitoneally with LPS	8
TNFα, IL-1β, IL-6, MIP-2	Rats instilled intratracheally with LPS	4
IL-1β	Rabbits injected intraperitoneally with casein	38
IL-1α/β and IL-1ra	Rats injected intratracheally with LPS	39
IL-1β	Rats injected intravenously with LPS	40
IL-1β	Retinal ischemia and reperfusion in rats	41
IL-1β and IL-1ra	Rabbits injected intra-articularly with IL-8	42
IL-1ra	Mice orogastrically infected with *Y. enterocolitica*	43
IL-1β, IL-8, and MIP-1β	Rabbits injected intraperitoneally with casein	44
IL-8	Dog trachea superfused with *Pseudomonas* supernatants	45
IL-8	Rabbits undergoing hyperoxia	46
IL-8	Reperfusion of ischemic myocardium in rabbits	24
MIP-2 and KC	Rats instilled intratracheally with LPS or injected intraperitoneally with thioglycollate	3
MCP-1	Rats instilled with bleomycin	47
IL-6	Mice injected intraperitoneally with LPS	48
TGFβ	New bone formation in rats	49

Using animals treated with LPS in different ways to induce specific acute inflammatory responses, it has been demonstrated by immunofluorescence of permeabilized cells, or Northern analysis, PCR and IH, that TNFα, IL-1α/β, IL-1ra, IL-6, and IL-10, can be expressed by neutrophils *in vivo*, and in some circumstances, at levels even higher than those found in mononuclear cells! However, under other experimental conditions *in vivo*, for instance after intraperitoneal injection of casein, or in sublethally irradiated mice injected with tumor cells, or even during *in vivo* infections, the genes for IL-1α/β, IL-1ra, IL-8, TNFα, TGFβ, MCP-1, MIP-1β, MIP-2 (functionally equivalent to human IL-8), and KC (functionally equivalent to GROα) were expressed in neutrophils, and in some of these situations, the production of neutrophil-derived cytokines appears to be fundamental for the evolution and/or resolution of the induced pathological process. This, therefore, not only confirms the validity of the observations made *in vitro*, but suggests that *in vivo* production of cytokines by neutrophils might have unsuspected pathogenetic consequences.

CONCLUSION

The classical role attributed to neutrophils is still based on the obsolete view that PMN are terminally differentiated, short-lived cells, with minimal, if any, transcriptional or translational activity. However, the studies that were summarized in this review clearly demonstrate the ability of neutrophils to synthesize and release various cytokines. Even though our understanding of cytokine production by PMN is far from complete, the variety of chemokines and cytokines secreted by neutrophils makes it likely that (*1*) PMN can orchestrate the infiltration of leukocytes into sites of injury, and (*2*) PMN play a pivotal role in the regulatory interactions between innate resistance (mediated by phagocytic cells and NK cells) and adaptive immunity (mediated by T and B cells). The full appreciation of cytokine synthesis by neutrophils is likely to also provide new insights into therapy of many disorders known to be influenced by PMN.

ACKNOWLEDGMENT

We would like to thank Dr. P.P. McDonald for his critical reading.

REFERENCES

1. LOYD, A.R. & J.J. OPPENHEIM. 1992. Immunol. Today **13:** 169–172.
2. CASSATELLA, M.A. 1995. Immunol. Today **16:** 21–26.
3. HUANG, S., J.D. PAULAUSKIS, J.J. GODLESKI & L. KOBZIK. 1992. Am. J. Pathol. **41:** 981–988.
4. XING, Z., M. JORDANA, H. KIRPALANI, K.E. DRISCOLL, T.J. SCHALL & J. GAULDIE. 1994. Am. J. Respir. Cell. Mol. Biol. **10:** 148–153 (erratum, Am. J. Respir. Cell. Mol. Biol. **10:** following 346.)
5. GASPERINI, S., F. CALZETTI, M.P. RUSSO, M. DE GIRONCOLI & M.A. CASSATELLA. J. Inflamm. **45:** 143–151.

6. KOCH, A.E., S.L. KUNKEL, M.R. SHAH, S. HOSAKA, M.M. HALLORAN, G.K. HAINES, M.D. BURDICK, R.M. POPE & R.M. STRIETER. 1995. J. Clin. Invest. **155:** 3660–3666.

7. HACHICHA, M., P.H. NACCACHE & S.R. McCOLL. 1995. J. Exp. Med. **182:** 2019–2025.

8. NILL, M.R., T.M. OBERYSZYN, M.S. ROSS, A.S. OBERYSZYN & F.M. ROBERTSON. 1995. J. Leuk. Biol. **58:** 563–574.

9. IIDA, N. & G. R. GROTENDORST. 1990. Mol. Cell. Biol. **10:** 5596–5599.

10. GRUSS, H.J., N. DASILVA, Z.B. HU, C.C. UPHOFF, R.G. GOODWIN & H.G. DREXLER. 1994. Leukemia **8:** 2083–2094.

11. RAMENGHI, U., L. RUGGIERI, I. DIANZANI, C. ROSSO, M.F. BRIZZI, C. CAMASCHELLO, T. PIETSCH & G. SAGLIO. 1994. Stem. Cells **12:** 521–526.

12. BURN, T.C., M.S. PETROVICK, S. HOHAUS, B.J. ROLLINS & D.G. TENEN. 1994. Blood **84:** 2776–2783.

13. BAZZONI, F., M.A. CASSATELLA, C. LAUDANNA & F. ROSSI. 1991. J. Leuk. Biol. **50:** 223–228.

14. CONTRINO, J., P.J. KRAUSE, N. SLOVER & D. KREUTZER. 1993. Pediatr. Res. **34:** 249–252.

15. STRIETER, R.M., K. KASAHARA, R. ALLEN, T.J. STANDIFORD & S.L. KUNKEL. 1990. Biochem. Biophys. Res. Commun. **173:** 725–730.

16. WANG, P., P. WU, J.C. ANTHES, M.I. SIEGEL, R.W. EGAN & M.M. BILLAH. 1994. Blood **83:** 2678–2683.

17. TAKEICHI, O., I. SAITO, T. TSURUMACHI, T. SAITO & I. MORO. 1995. Cell. Immunol. **156:** 296–309.

18. CASSATELLA, M.A. 1996. Cytokines Produced by Polymorphonuclear Neutrophils: Molecular and biological aspects. R.G. Landes Company. Austin, TX.

19. HASLETT, C., L.A. GUTHRIE, M.M. KOPANIAK, R.B. JOHNSTON, JR. & P.M. HENSON. 1985. Am. J. Pathol. **119:** 101–110.

20. CASSATELLA, M.A., F. BAZZONI, M. CESKA, I. FERRO, M. BAGGIOLINI & G. BERTON. 1992. J. Immunol. **148:** 3216–3220.

21. BAGGIOLINI, M., B. DEWALD & B. MOSER. 1994. Adv. Immunol. **55:** 97–179.

22. PRIESCHL, E. E., P. A. KULBURG & T. BAUMRUKER. 1995. Int. Arch. Allergy Immunol. **107:** 475–483.

23. KENNEDY, J., J.S. KELNER, S. KLEYENSTEUBER, T.J. SCHALL, M.C. WEISS, H.YSSEL, P.V. SCHNEIDER, B.G. COCKS, K.B. BACON & A. ZLOTNIK 1995. J. Immunol. **155:** 203–209.

24. IVEY, C.L., F.M. WILLIAMS, P.D. COLLINS, P.J. JOSE & T.J. WILLIAMS. 1995. J. Clin. Invest. **95:** 2720–2728.

25. MEDA, L., S. GASPERINI, M. CESKA & M.A. CASSATELLA. 1994. Modulation Cell. Immunol. **57:** 448–461.

26. CASSATELLA, M.A., L. MEDA, S. BONORA, M. CESKA & G. CONSTANTIN. 1993. J. Exp. Med. **178:** 2207–2211.

27. ROMAGNANI, S. 1994. Ann. Rev. Immunol. **12:** 227–257.

28. KASAMA, T., R.M. STRIETER, N.W. LUKACS, M.D. BURDICK & S.L. KUNKEL. 1994. J. Immunol. **152:** 3559–3569.

29. CASSATELLA, M.A., L. MEDA, S. GASPERINI, A. D'ANDREA, X. MA & G. TRINCHIERI. 1995. Eur. J. Immunol. **25:** 1–5.

30. CASSATELLA, M.A., L. MEDA, S. GASPERINI, F. CALZETTI & S. BONORA. 1994. J. Exp. Med. **179:** 1695–1699.

31. CASSATELLA, M.A., S. GASPERINI, F. CALZETTI, P. McDONALD & G. TRINCHIERI. 1995. Biochem. J. **310:** 751–755.

32. CASSATELLA, M.A. 1996. Immunol. Lett. **49:** 79–82.

33. MUZIO, M., F. RE, M. SIRONI, N. POLENTARUTTI, A. MINTY, D. CAPUT, P. FERRARA, A. MANTOVANI & F. COLOTTA. 1994. Blood **83:** 1738–1743.

34. Muzio, M., F. Re, M. Sironi, N. Polentarutti, A. Mantovani & F. Colotta. 1994. Eur. J. Immunol. **24:** 3194–3198.
35. Xing, Z., H. Kirpalani, D. Torry, M. Jordana & J. Gauldie. 1993. Am. J. Pathol. **143:** 1009–1015.
36. Stoppacciaro, A., C. Melani, M. Parenza, A. Mastracchio, C. Bassi, C. Baroni, G. Parmiani & M.P. Colombo. 1993. J. Exp. Med. **178:** 151–161.
37. Cirelli, R.A., L.A. Carey, J.K. Fisher, D.L. Rosolia, T.H. Elsasser, T.J. Caperna, M.H. Gee & K.H. Albertine. 1995. J. Leuk. Biol. **57:** 820–826.
38. Goto, F., K. Goto, S. Mori, S. Ohkawara & M. Yoshinaga. 1989. Br. J. Exp. Pathol. **70:** 597–606.
39. Ulich, T.R., K. Guo, S. Yin, J. Del Castillo, E.S. Yi, R.C. Thompson & S.P. Eisenberg. 1992. Am. J. Pathol. **141:** 61–68.
40. Williams, J.H., K. Patel, D. Hatakeyama, R. Arian, K.J. Guo, T.J. Hickey, S. Liao & T.R. Ulich. 1993. Am. J. Resp. Cell. Mol. Biol. **8:** 134–144.
41. Hangai, M., N. Yoshimura, M. Yoshida, K. Yabuuchi & Y. Honda. 1995. Invest. Ophthalmol. Vis. Sci. **36:** 571–578.
42. Matsukawa, A., T. Yoshimura, T. Maeda, S. Ohkawara, K. Takagi & M. Yoshinaga. 1995. J. Immunol. **154:** 5418–5425.
43. Jordan, M., I.G. Otterness, R. Ng, A. Gessner, M. Rollinghoff & H.U. Beuscher. 1995. J. Immunol. **154:** 4081–4090.
44. Mori, S., K. Goto, F. Goto, K. Murakami, S. Ohkawara & M. Yoshinaga. 1994. Int. Immunol. **6:** 149–156.
45. Inoue, H., P. Massion, I.F. Ueki, K.M. Grattan, M. Hara, L. Dohrman, B. Chan, J.A. Lausier, J.A. Golden & J.A. Nadel. 1994. Am. J. Respir. Cell. Mol. Biol. **11:** 651–663.
46. D'Angio, C.T., R.A. Sinkin, M.B. LoMonaco & J.N. Finkelstein. 1995. Am. J. Physiol. **12:** L826–L831.
47. Sakanashi, Y., M. Takeya, T. Yoshimura, L. Feng, T. Morioka & K. Takahashi. 1994. J. Leuk. Biol. **56:** 741–750.
48. Terebuth, P.D., I.G. Otterness, R.M. Strieter, P.M. Lincoln, J.M. Danforth, S.L. Kunkel & S.W. Chensue. 1992. Am. J. Pathol. **140:** 649–657.
49. Carrington, J.L., A.B. Roberts, K.C. Flanders, N.S. Roche & H. Reddi. 1988. J. Cell. Biol. **107:** 1969–1975.

Phagocytes in Ischemia Injury

KEITH A. YOUKER, HOLLY H. BIRDSALL,[a]
NIKOLAOS G. FRANGOGIANNIS, AJITH G. KUMAR,[b]
MERRY L. LINDSEY, CHRISTIE M. BALLANTYNE, C. WAYNE SMITH,[c]
ROGER D. ROSSEN,[d] AND MARK L. ENTMAN[e]

*Section of Cardiovascular Sciences
The Methodist Hospital
The DeBakey Heart Center
Department of Medicine*

[b]*Department of Medicine
University of Pennsylvania
Philadelphia, Pennsylvania*

[d]*Immunology Research Laboratory
Houston Veterans Administration Center*

[a]*Department of Otorhinolaryngology
Speros P. Martel Laboratory of Leukocyte Biology*

[c]*Department of Pediatrics
Texas Children's Hospital
Baylor College of Medicine
Houston, Texas 77030*

INTRODUCTION

In recent years, early reperfusion of the ischemic myocardium has become the mainstay of optimal therapeutic intervention in patients with evolving myocardial infarction. In clinical trials, it has become clear that early reperfusion reduces infarct size, decreases ventricular dilatation, and improves survival.[1] However, even when reperfusion occurs after a longer period of time (i.e., generally beyond that which results in reduction of myocardial necrosis) it is associated with decreased ventricular dilatation and enhanced survival.[2]

Substantial evidence has demonstrated that reperfusion of the previously ischemic myocardium is associated with the rapid onset of an intense inflammatory reaction that may extend myocardial injury.[3] In early studies, anti-inflammatory agents appeared to reduce the size of experimental myocardial infarction.[4] This led to a clinical study using methylprednisolone that resulted in an increase in ventricular rupture.[5,6] It became obvious that non-specific inhibition of the inflammatory reaction also resulted in inadequate healing and scar formation.[5] Thus, the intense inflammatory reaction ensuing upon reperfusion of the previously ischemic myocardium may be both

[e]Address correspondence to: Mark L. Entman, M.D., Department of Medicine, Cardiovascular Sciences, Baylor College of Medicine, One Baylor Plaza, Houston, Texas 77030-3498.

injurious and also an important part of ventricular healing. These observations regarding both positive and negative features associated with the inflammatory reaction to injury have led to a variety of studies designed to better understand the biological factors that control post-reperfusion injury and to attempt to differentiate those factors responsible for cellular injury from those factors critical for ventricular healing.

During the healing phase of myocardial infarction, mononuclear macrophages are found in the infarcted area regardless of whether or not reperfusion occurs.[3,7,8] Morita and colleagues demonstrated that reperfusion is associated with an increased presence of macrophages in the infarcted area when compared to non-reperfused myocardium.[9] Reperfusion has been shown to be associated with accelerated clearance of necrotic debris, which would suggest that the augmented leukocyte influx associated with reperfusion might actually accelerate the healing process.[10] Thus, reperfusion may initiate an earlier inflammatory response that accelerates recruitment of mononuclear monocytes, which may play a critical role in healing and remodeling.

In this manuscript, we will attempt to describe and quantitate the factors mediating the early influx of mononuclear macrophages that occurs after reperfusion of previously ischemic myocardium. We will identify some of the chemotactic factors that modulate mononuclear cell movement and some of the cytokinetic agents that alter mononuclear cell function. In addition to its proposed role in healing, we will present evidence that mononuclear cell function is an important modulator of the initial acute inflammatory response leading to cardiac injury. Finally, we will provide evidence that neutrophils may also perform a role generally associated with other phagocytic cells by undergoing a phenotypic transition at the site of inflammation.

METHODS

Ischemia-Reperfusion Protocols

Healthy mongrel dogs (15–25 kg) of either sex were surgically instrumented as previously described.[11,12] Anesthesia was induced intravenously with 10 mg/kg methohexital sodium (Brevital; Eli Lilly and Co., Indianapolis, IN) and maintained with the inhalational anesthetic Isoflurane (Anaquest; Madison, WI). A midline thoracotomy provided access to the heart and mediastinum, and in some experiments, the cardiac lymph duct was cannulated as previously described.[12] Subsequently, a hydraulically activated occluding device and a Doppler flow probe[11,13] were secured around the circumflex coronary artery just proximal or just distal to the first branch. The animals were allowed to recover for at least 72 h prior to occlusion. Ischemia-reperfusion protocols were performed in awake animals as previously described.[11,13–15] Coronary artery occlusion was achieved by inflating the coronary cuff occluder until mean flow in the coronary vessel was zero, as determined by the Doppler flow probe. After 50 min of occlusion, radiolabeled microspheres (for subsequent blood flow determinations) were injected into the left atrium. At the end of 1 h of occlusion the cuff was deflated and the myocardium reperfused. Reperfusion intervals ranged from 1 to 24 h. In some experiments, reperfusion was not instituted. Upon sacrifice, samples were taken systematically from the left ventricle and ischemic blood flow was quantitated. Control (no evidence of necrosis, normal blood flow) and ischemically injured myocardium (based on methods mentioned below and reductions in blood flow) were thus defined.

Myocardial Sampling and Calibration with Coronary Blood Flow

After the reperfusion periods, hearts were stopped by the infusion of saturated potassium chloride, removed from the chest, and sectioned from apex to base into four transverse rings approximately 1 cm in thickness. Transmural myocardial samples (1.0 g) were isolated from myocardial rings and labeled as control (obtained from the anterior wall) or infarcted (obtained from the posterior papillary muscle and posterior free wall) based on anatomic location within the distribution of the circumflex artery and visual inspection. Myocardial samples were then dissected into smaller pieces: first, a transmural section was taken from the middle of the sample and fixed in 2% buffered paraformaldehyde for histologic studies; then the left and right halves were cut into smaller pieces and divided in two halves. The first half was used for blood flow determinations using radiolabeled microspheres as previously described.[13,16–18] The remaining portions of each sample were immediately frozen in liquid nitrogen. Frozen tissue samples were homogenized and processed for RNA studies. Analysis of mRNA, blood flow determinations, and histopathologic examinations of samples obtained from each experiment were conducted independently (in separate laboratories) and in a blinded fashion. Once the independent analysis of the data was completed, the information was gathered and a final analysis performed.

Isolation of Mononuclear Leukocytes

Mononuclear leukocytes (MNLs) were isolated from heparinized blood of the experimental subject on the day of the occlusion-reperfusion experiment by sedimentation through Ficoll-Hypaque gradients (Organon-Teknicon, Durham, NC). Isolated MNLs were enriched for monocytes using modifications of the Recalde method reported by Fogelman and coworkers.[19]

Immunofluorescence and Flow Cytometric Evaluation[20]

Aliquots (0.1 ml) of whole blood or cardiac lymph MNLs at 0.5×10^6/ml in phosphate-buffered saline (PBS) with 30% autologous serum were placed in polypropylene tubes and all steps were carried out at 4°C. Cells were incubated with saturating concentrations of monoclonal antibodies (mAb) for 30 min and washed twice with PBS. In cases where the primary antibody was not conjugated with a fluorochrome, cells were then stained with fluorescein-conjugated, affinity-purified $F(ab')_2$ fragments of sheep anti-mouse IgG (Cappel). After a second 30 min incubation the cells were again washed twice with PBS. Red cells in whole blood samples were lysed with FACS Lysing solution (Becton Dickinson, San Jose, CA), and washed. Finally the leukocytes were fixed with 1% paraformaldehyde and analyzed by flow cytometry. At least 5,000 leukocytes were analyzed.

Histamine Assays

Histamine in lymphatic drainage was measured by competitive immunoenzymatic assay[21] (AMAC Inc., Westbrook, Maine).

TNF-α Bioassay

Lymph samples were assayed for TNF-α activity using the WEHI 164 subclone 13 fibroblast cytotoxicity assay, as previously described.[22] Units of activity were calculated using internal rTNF standards (Genzyme, Boston, MA).

Chemotaxis Assay

We polymerized 225 μl of 50% soluble collagen (Vitrogen 100, Celtrix, Santa Carlo, CA) in Millicell™ chambers (Millipore, Bedford, MA) floored with 0.45-micron filters. The chambers were placed in 24-well microtiter plates containing 450 μl of RPMI 1640 with 10% FCS (medium), freshly harvested canine cardiac lymph diluted 1:1 with medium, or chemotactic factors diluted in medium. At the same time, 225 μl containing 1×10^5 MNLs suspended in medium were added above the collagen pad in the inner chamber of each Millicell™. The 450 μl of fluid (medium + collagen) inside the Millicell™ chamber exactly balanced the 450 μl of fluid outside, effectively preventing hydrostatic forces from affecting MNL migration.

MNLs were allowed to migrate into the collagen in response to the chemotactic factors for 4 h at 37°C. Leukocytes that did not migrate into the collagen pad were removed with three 400-μl washes using Hanks Balanced saline solution (HBSS) without Ca^{2+} and Mg^{2+}. Leukocytes that had migrated into the collagen pad were recovered by digesting the collagen completely with 1 ml of 0.1% collagenase (Sigma) in HBSS with Ca^{2+}, Mg^{2+}, 1% fetal calf serum, and 0.05 M HEPES. Monocytes were positively identified by staining with phycoerythrin conjugated anti-CD14 mAb and counted by flow cytometry. To identify potential chemotaxins we added neutralizing antibodies to TGF-β (Genzyme) or MCP-1 to the cardiac lymph. We also took advantage of the observation that MNLs exposed to MCP-1 (100 ng/ml for 30 min) became insensitive to the chemotactic activity of MPC-1.

RiboProbe Generation and Selection

Riboprobes to MCP-1 and IL-6 were made (Sense and Antisense) utilizing the Genius system (Boehringer Mannheim). Briefly, T3 and T7 RNA polymerases were used (2 U/μl) on linearized template (1 μg/20 μl) to generate the sense and antisense riboprobes, respectively. The labeled RNA was then ethanol-precipitated. After two washes with 75% ethanol labeled RNA was resuspended in 50 μl of DEPC-treated water. Probe concentration was estimated by making several 10-fold serial dilutions of the probe and comparing it to a control-labeled RNA of known concentration. Probe specificity was verified by northern blot analysis following manufacturer's protocol on membranes prepared as described previously. A colorimetric reaction was detected with the antisense probe while none was seen with the sense.

Histology, Immunohistochemistry, and In Situ *Hybridization*

For histologic study, samples of cardiac tissue were calibrated for the level of coronary blood flow as previously described[13,16,17] and fixed in 2% paraformaldehyde or B*5.[23] The samples were embedded in paraffin, sectioned, and stained with hematoxylin and eosin or with hematoxylin and basic fuchsin. The latter stain was useful in identifying myocardial infarction after short periods of time.[24] The monoclonal antibody, LS27.10F7-2, to human MCP-1 was supplied by LeukoSite Corporation (Cambridge, MA) and is the same antibody used in blocking MCP-1 function (see above). Monoclonal antibodies to CD11b (MY904-ATCC), CD64 (clone #216-030, Ancell), and the neutrophil-specific antibody SG8H6 were also used to define leukocyte trafficking. Polyclonal antibody to TNF-α was provided by Genzyme$_R$. Antibody detection utilized peroxidase-based detection systems using diaminobenzidine as a substrate (Vector Laboratories$_R$).

In Situ *Hybridization in Tissue Samples*

In situ hybridization was performed on 2% paraformaldehyde embedded sections as previously described.[25] After sectioning and deparaffinization, the tissue was incubated in 2$\times$ SSC buffer once for 5 min and again for 60 min, prehybridized with 100 μl of prehybridization solution [formamide (50%) SSC (4$\times$), Denhardt's reagent (1$\times$), salmon sperm DNA (0.5 mg/ml), yeast tRNA (0.25 mg/ml), and dextran sulfate (10%)] for 1 h at room temperature. Immunologic detection utilized an antidigoxigenin antibody and nitro-blue tetrazolium staining of an alkaline phosphatase reaction as previously described[15] except that normal goat serum was substituted for sheep serum and Triton X-100 concentration was 0.2%.

In Situ *Hybridization in Cells*

The procedure for cells was identical to that for tissue with the following modifications: after fixation in 4% paraformaldehyde, cells were resuspended in 75% ethanol, placed on slides, and baked. No prehybridization step was performed and Triton X-100 was not used for immunologic detection.

RESULTS

Monocytes Rapidly Migrate into the Ischemic and Infarcted Areas

While early observations of clinical myocardial infarction suggested that mononuclear cells entered the infarct relatively late when compared to neutrophils,

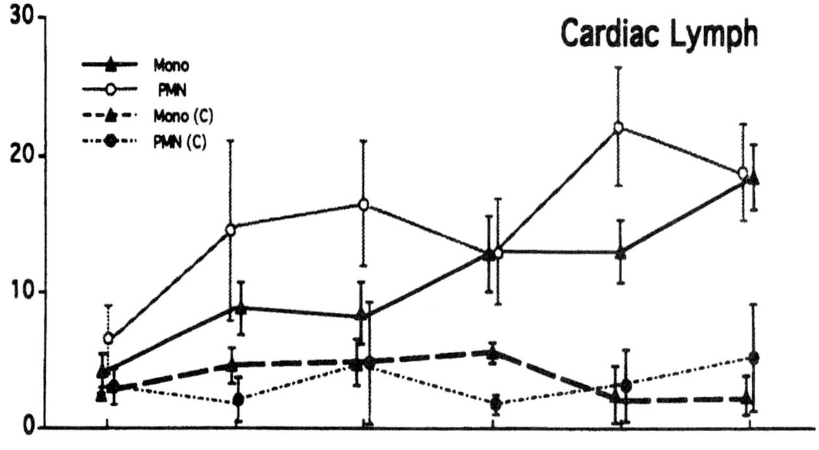

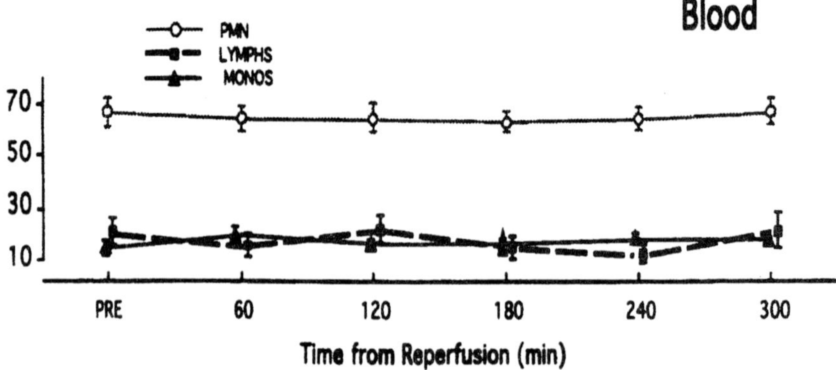

FIGURE 2. Distribution of monocytes and neutrophils in cardiac lymph during reperfusion. The top panel demonstrates the average percentage (± SEM) of monocytes (monos) and neutrophils (PMN) in canine cardiac lymph in intervals before the occlusion (PRE) and at intervals after reperfusion of the myocardium. The bottom panel summarizes the percent of neutrophils and monocytes in the blood of the same dogs at the hourly intervals after reperfusion.

dothelium of small veins. We have previously shown that these small veins mediate leukocyte endothelial transmigration.[27] Veins displaying MCP-1 mRNA are approximately 20 to 70 microns in diameter and empty into larger intravesicular veins whose endothelium does not appear to contain mRNA for MCP-1. However, MCP-1 protein could be seen in both classes of veins but not in arteries using an antibody to MCP-1 (FIG. 5B). Unlike MCP-1 mRNA, MCP-1 protein staining could not be seen until 3 h after reperfusion and increased thereafter. The induction of MCP-1 in the previously ischemic area was dependent on reperfusion and was not seen in the first 24 h in the absence of reperfusion (data not shown).

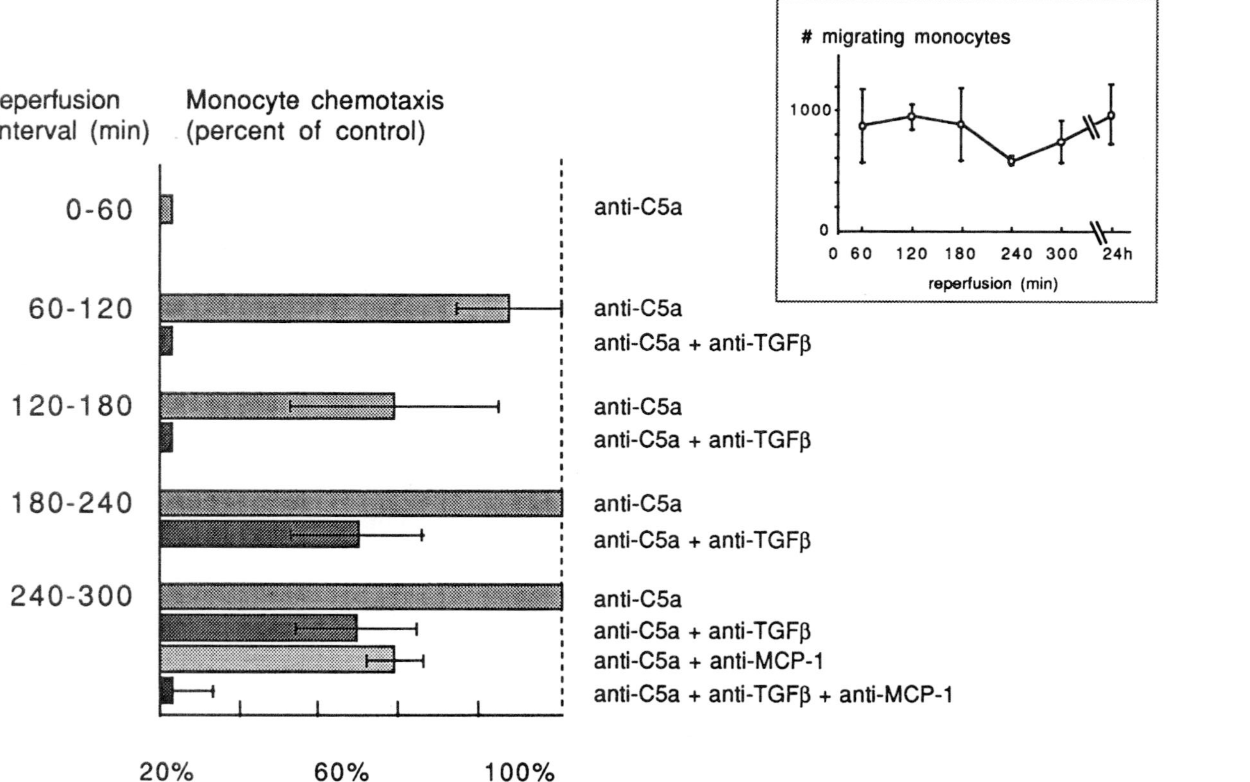

FIGURE 3. Chemotactic activity for monocytes in post-reperfusion cardiac lymph. From the first minutes of reperfusion, untreated cardiac lymph became consistently chemotactic for monocytes resulting in three- to fourfold increases in number of migratory cells (*see inset*) over pre-ischemic value (not shown). The bars in the figure describe the degree of monocyte chemotaxis using an assay described in *Methods*, remaining after treatment of cardiac lymph as described in the right portion of the figure. The results suggest that C5a provides the initial chemotactic stimulus immediately after reperfusion but that later chemotaxis is effected by TGF-β and MCP-1 (see text).

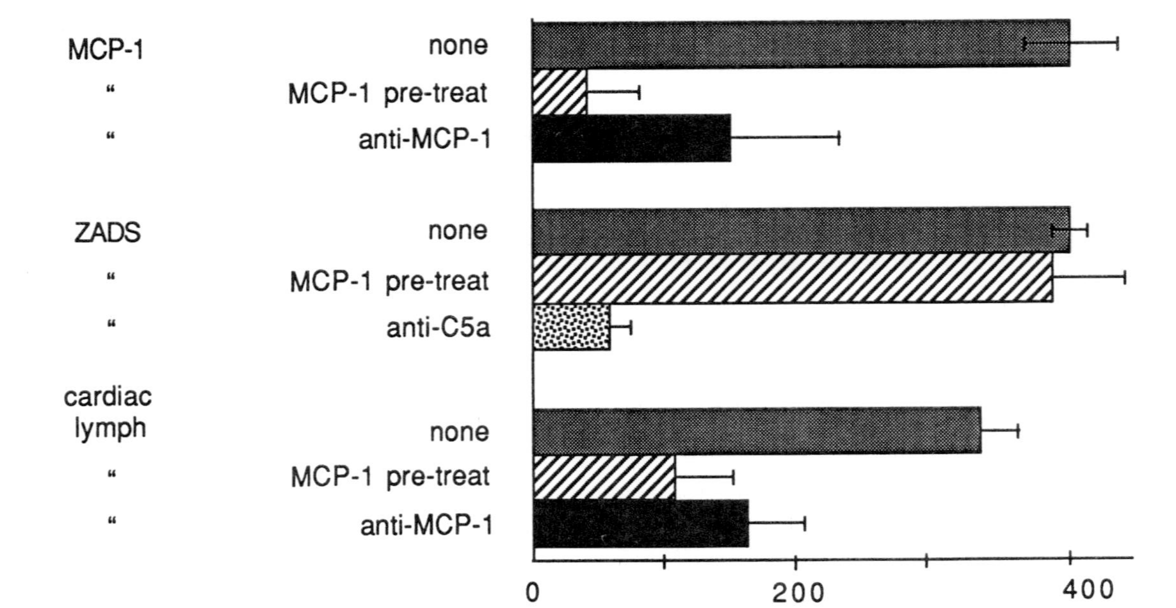

FIGURE 4. Testing cardiac lymph collected from 180–300 min of reperfusion for MCP-1 like activity. (*Top panel*) Human recombinant MCP-1 is chemotactic for monocytes and this chemotactic activity can be obviated by pretreatment of monocytes with MCP-1 to desensitize them or by the inclusion of a monoclonal antibody to MCP-1 in the reaction media. (*Middle panel*) Zymosan-activated dog serum (ZADS) provides a source of C5a. Pretreatment of monocytes with MCP-1 does not prevent chemotactic activity of ZADS. However, ZADS-induced chemotaxis is markedly inhibited by anti-C5a. (*Bottom panel*) Post-ischemic cardiac lymph selected between 180–300 min of reperfusion is strongly chemotactic for monocytes. This chemotaxis is reduced in a qualitatively and quantitatively similar way to the chemotaxis induced by MCP-1 in the top panel.

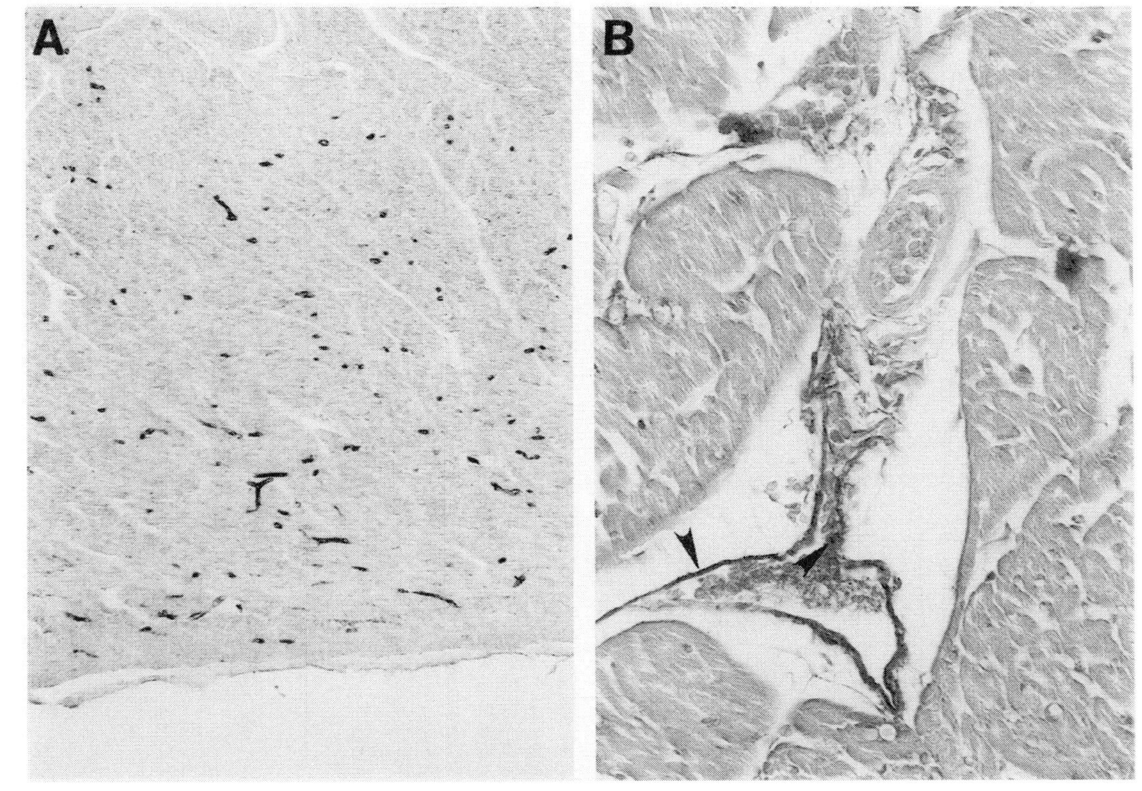

FIGURE 5. Localization of MCP-1 in ischemic myocardium. (**A**) *In situ* hybridization with riboprobe for MCP-1 mRNA showing localization in endothelium of small (20–70 micron diameter) veins. Tissue samples were taken following 1-h occlusion and 3-h reperfusion. (**B**) Immunocytochemical localization of MCP-1 on venous endothelium and leukocytes. Arrows show positive endothelial staining and positive intravascular leukocyte.

Role of Monocytes in the Acute Inflammatory Injury Associated with Early Reperfusion

In our previous work, we have presented evidence that neutrophils are capable of injuring and killing isolated cardiac myocytes through an adhesion-dependent mechanism involving activated neutrophil Mac-1 binding to ICAM-1 on stimulated cardiac myocytes. ICAM-1 is not constitutively expressed on the myocardial cells,[28,29] but can be induced by cytokine[29] and after reperfusion of infarcted myocardium.[15,16] Studies utilizing post-ischemic cardiac lymph demonstrated that IL-6 is the primary cytokine responsible for induction of myocardial cell ICAM-1 in the reperfused myocardium.[14] We have subsequently shown that both myocardial ICAM-1[28,30] and IL-6[17] are induced in the ischemic border zone surrounding a reperfused myocardial infarction and are reperfusion dependent.[17,30]

The induction of IL-6 (which precedes that of ICAM-1) is very rapid.[14,17] In FIGURE 6A, IL-6 mRNA appears in MNLs in the reperfused myocardial infarct in the first hour. IL-6 mRNA can be demonstrated in mononuclear cells appearing in the post-ischemic cardiac lymph within 15 min of reperfusion (see FIG. 6B). Thus, our data suggest that reperfusion allows mononuclear cells to enter the formerly ischemic area where they are rapidly induced to produce IL-6. IL-6 is responsible for induction of ICAM-1 on cardiac myocytes in the jeopardized border zone.[14] Thus, the mononuclear cells infiltrating the ischemic myocardium may play a critical role in generating the cytokine cascade necessary for acute inflammatory injury following reperfusion of the previously ischemic myocardium.

The rapid appearance of IL-6 suggested that the myocardium contained a preformed stimulus that can induce IL-6 production by MNLs. Post-ischemic cardiac lymph contained both histamine and TNF-α (FIG. 7). This suggested the possibility that tissue mast cells might be the source of preformed TNF-α, which was released during ischemia and washed out immediately upon reperfusion. FIGURE 8 demonstrates that cardiac tissue mast cells contain preformed TNF-α, which can be detected with polyclonal anti-TNF diluted 1:500. No other cells stain for TNF using this reagent at this dilution. In the vicinity of degranulating mast cells, TNF-α may be detected in adjacent leukocytes and endothelial cells. This suggests that the degranulating mast cell may initiate a cytokinetic signal to both endothelial and mononuclear cells. We postulate that TNF-α from mast cells (along with other factors) may be responsible for the induction of monocyte IL-6. Monocyte production of IL-6 continues throughout the first 24 h of reperfusion.[17]

Phenotypic Changes in Neutrophils That Have Migrated into Previously Ischemic Tissue

In our previous work, we demonstrated that Mac-1 is upregulated on the surface of neutrophils that have migrated through endothelium.[11] During the first hour of reperfusion, neutrophils in cardiac tissue remain primarily marginated in small veins or in the perivenular space.[27] By 3 h, however, primarily in the ischemic border zone neutrophils have migrated into the tissue (see FIG. 1B). Examination of these neutrophils, however, reveals that many of the extravascular neutrophils no longer stain

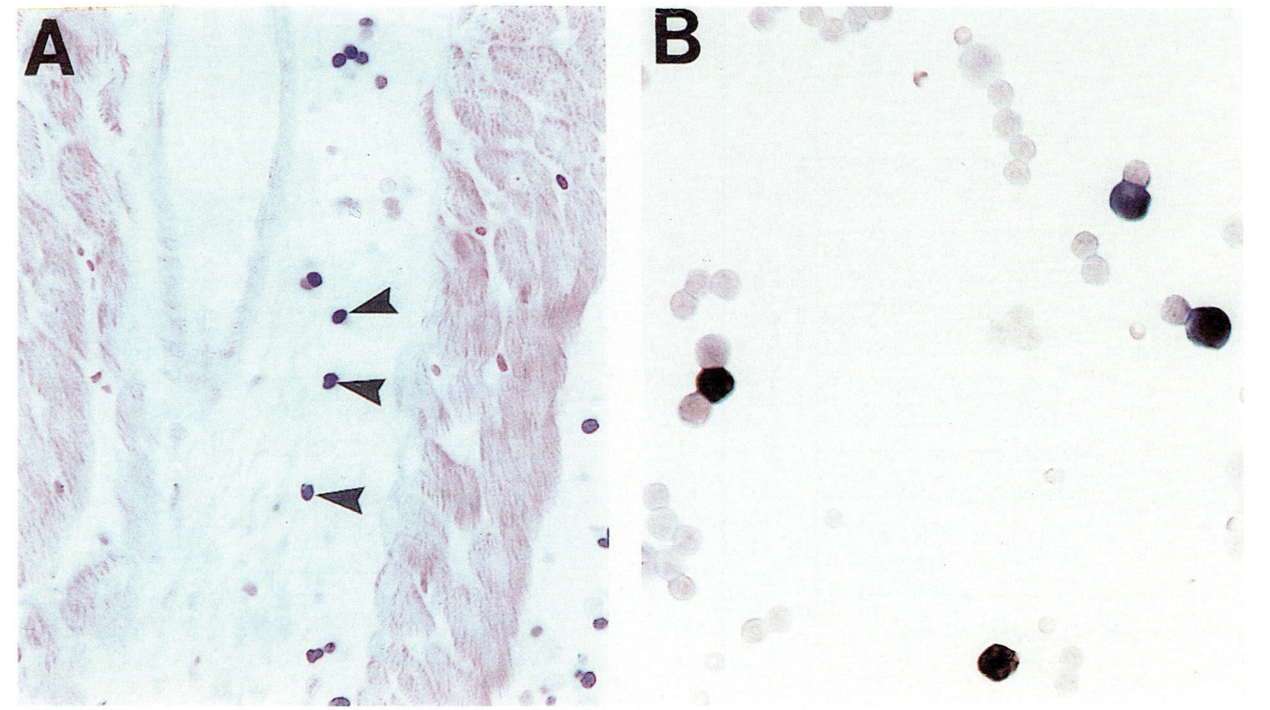

FIGURE 6. Localization of IL-6 in early reperfusion. (**A**) *In situ* hybridization of myocardium following 1-h occlusion and 3-h reperfusion demonstrates infiltrating leukocytes (identified as monocytes, not shown) as positive for IL-6 mRNA (*arrows*). (**B**) *In situ* hybridization for IL-6 mRNA of leukocytes isolated from cardiac lymph during the first 15-min of reperfusion. Only monocytes show positive staining in these samples.

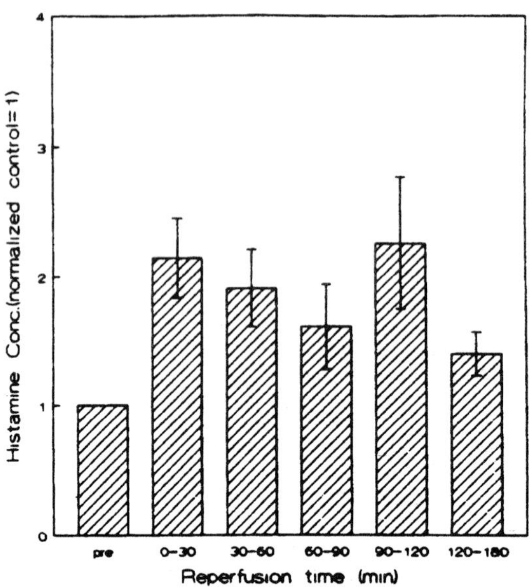

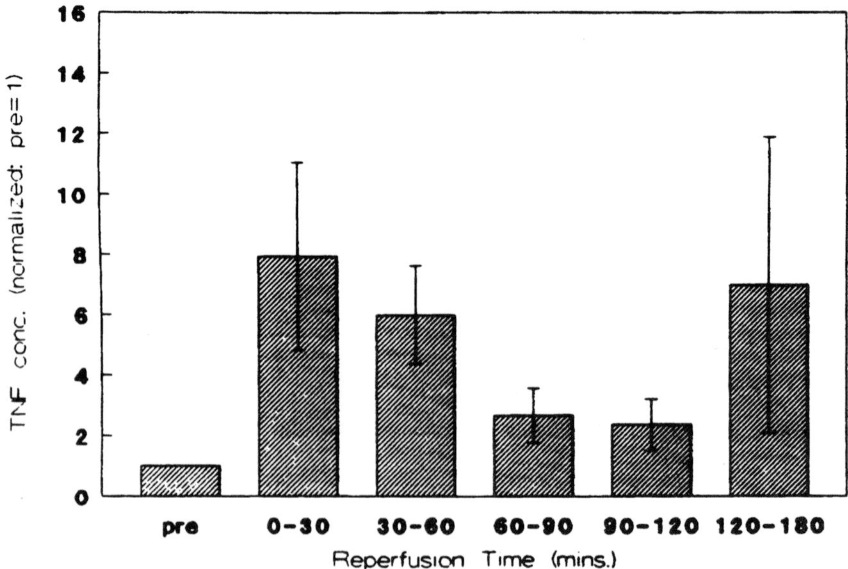

FIGURE 7. (*Top*) Kinetics of histamine release in the post-ischemic cardiac lymph. Note the early peak in histamine concentration during reperfusion ($N = 8$ for pre, 0–30 min, 30–60 min and $N = 6$ for 60–120 min and 120–180 min). (*Bottom*) Release of TNF-α bioactivity in the canine lymph following myocardial ischemia and reperfusion. The values were expressed as a percentage of the bioactivity measured in the pre-ischemic cardiac lymph (pre = 1). Note the early peak in TNF-α bioactivity ($N = 8$ for pre, 0–30 min, 30–60 min samples; $N = 6$ for 60–120 and 120–180 min samples).

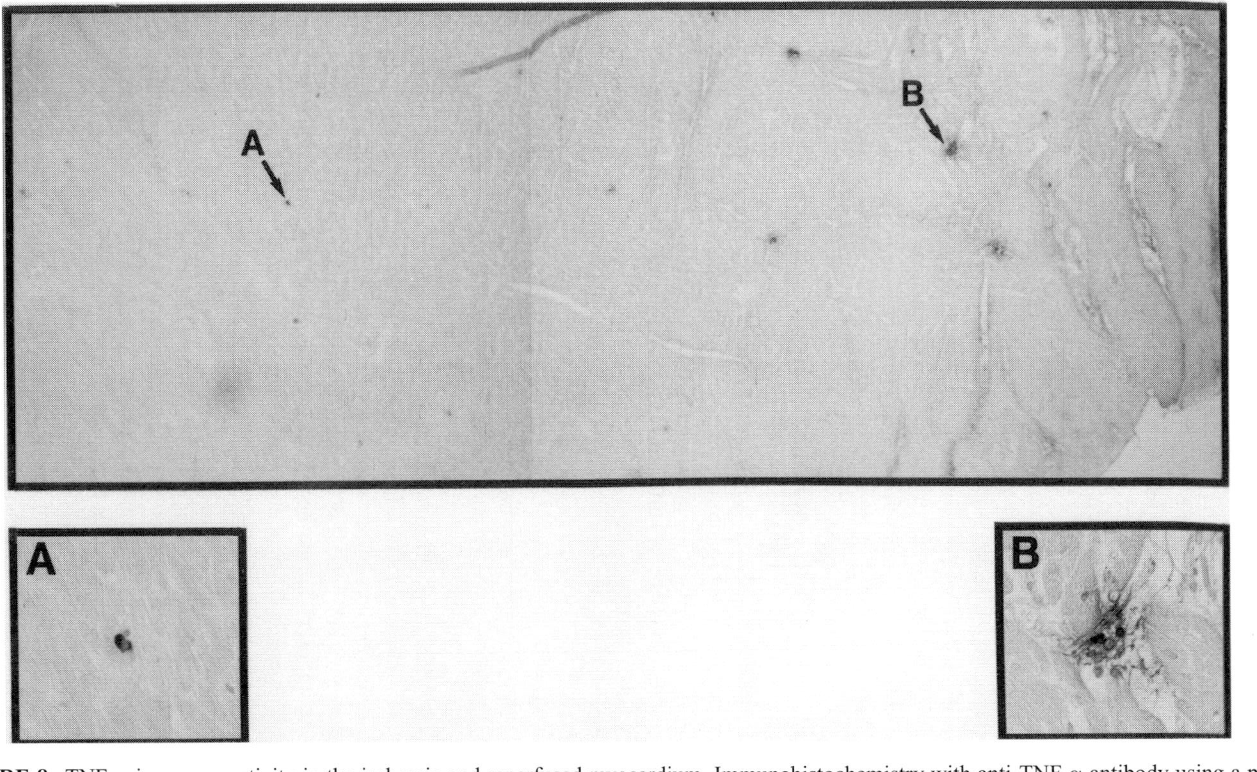

FIGURE 8. TNF-α immunoreactivity in the ischemic and reperfused myocardium. Immunohistochemistry with anti-TNF-α antibody using a peroxidase-based system and diaminobenzidine as a substrate. Sections were obtained from hearts that were ischemic for 1 h and reperfused for 3 h. A transmural 400-micron segment is demonstrated spanning from the injured subendocardial area to a normal epicardial region (100×). Note that significant mast cell degranulation is found only in cells located in the injured subendocardial area (**B**) (400×). Mast cells in the epicardial region appear fully granulated (**A**) (400×). Staining of the endothelium and the infiltrating cells is also noted in the area of mast cell degranulation.

histochemically with monoclonal antibodies to CD11b (MY904), although they all stain with antibodies to CD18 (R15.7), intravascular neutrophils continue to stain for CD11b (data not shown). By 5 h, this effect is even more striking. FIGURE 9A demonstrates that, by 5 h of reperfusion, CD11b staining is completely lost on neutrophils in the extravascular space while intravascular neutrophils retain CD11b staining. FIGURE 9B demonstrates that all neutrophils continue to stain with antibodies to CD18 (presumably because of the persistence of CD11a/CD18). Also of interest in FIGURES 9A and 9B is CD11b-positive amorphous material seen in the tissue sections at 5 h, but not before. By 24 h, neutrophils have migrated into the infarcted area (FIG. 9C) and appear to have lost Mac-1 staining except for an occasional neutrophil seen in a venule (FIG. 9D); staining of amorphous material is no longer seen. In addition to their loss of CD11b, neutrophils found in tissue sections after 5 h of reperfusion and thereafter also contain mRNA for IL-6 that is not observed earlier (FIG. 10). Thus, the neutrophil appears to undergo important phenotypic changes after transendothelial migration, substantially altering its function in the reperfused myocardium.

DISCUSSION

Inflammation is an important component of reactions to tissue injury that facilitate the healing process. Throughout the history of medicine, it has also been recognized, however, that inflammation also potentially represents a mechanism for extending tissue injury. Thus, the inflammatory reaction to injury has always represented an attractive but potentially hazardous therapeutic target. Inflammatory reaction to injury associated with myocardial infarction is a particularly good example of this conundrum. In the early 1970s, a potential for reducing injury associated with myocardial infarction with anti-inflammatory drugs was recognized based on a variety of experimental models. However, the initial clinical trial with high doses of glucocorticoids quickly exposed the hazard. Such nonspecific attacks in the inflammatory reaction impaired healing and resulted in ventricular rupture.[5,6]

Studies reporting that reperfusion of previously ischemic myocardium resulted in rapid localization and subsequent infiltration of leukocytes concentrated mainly on the neutrophil, which appears to be the primary mediator of cardiac tissue injury.[4,31] The role of monocytes has been less carefully examined; monocytes were generally considered to be important in the healing process. Only in recent years has it been recognized that reperfusion of a previously ischemic myocardium, even at later times, actually facilitates ventricular healing and is associated with an increased presence of macrophages.[1,2,9]

The present report seeks to clarify the mechanisms by which mononuclear cells are attracted to the previously ischemic and infarcted myocardium and to emphasize the rapidity with which reperfusion facilitates monocyte localization and infiltration. The data address three related issues that must be understood before we can develop treatments for reperfusion injury: (1) the chemotactic stimuli, which support monocyte tissue infiltration, (2) the role of the monocyte in the cytokine cascades promoting acute tissue injury, and (3) the evolution of the inflammatory reaction to the healing phase.

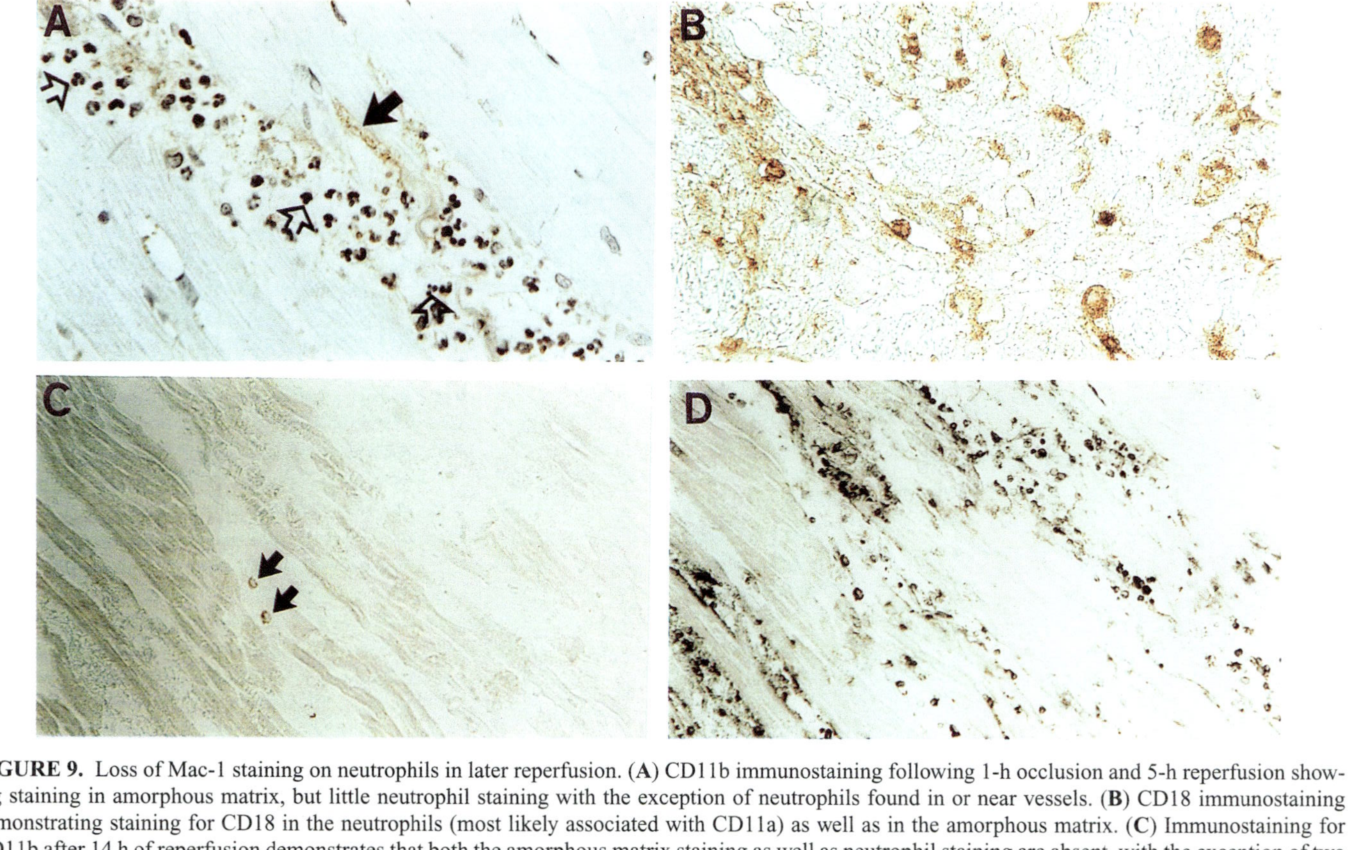

FIGURE 9. Loss of Mac-1 staining on neutrophils in later reperfusion. (**A**) CD11b immunostaining following 1-h occlusion and 5-h reperfusion showing staining in amorphous matrix, but little neutrophil staining with the exception of neutrophils found in or near vessels. (**B**) CD18 immunostaining demonstrating staining for CD18 in the neutrophils (most likely associated with CD11a) as well as in the amorphous matrix. (**C**) Immunostaining for CD11b after 14 h of reperfusion demonstrates that both the amorphous matrix staining as well as neutrophil staining are absent, with the exception of two neutrophils found within a vessel. (**D**) Dual staining of **C** with anti-neutrophil mAb indicating numerous neutrophils are found within this ischemic region.

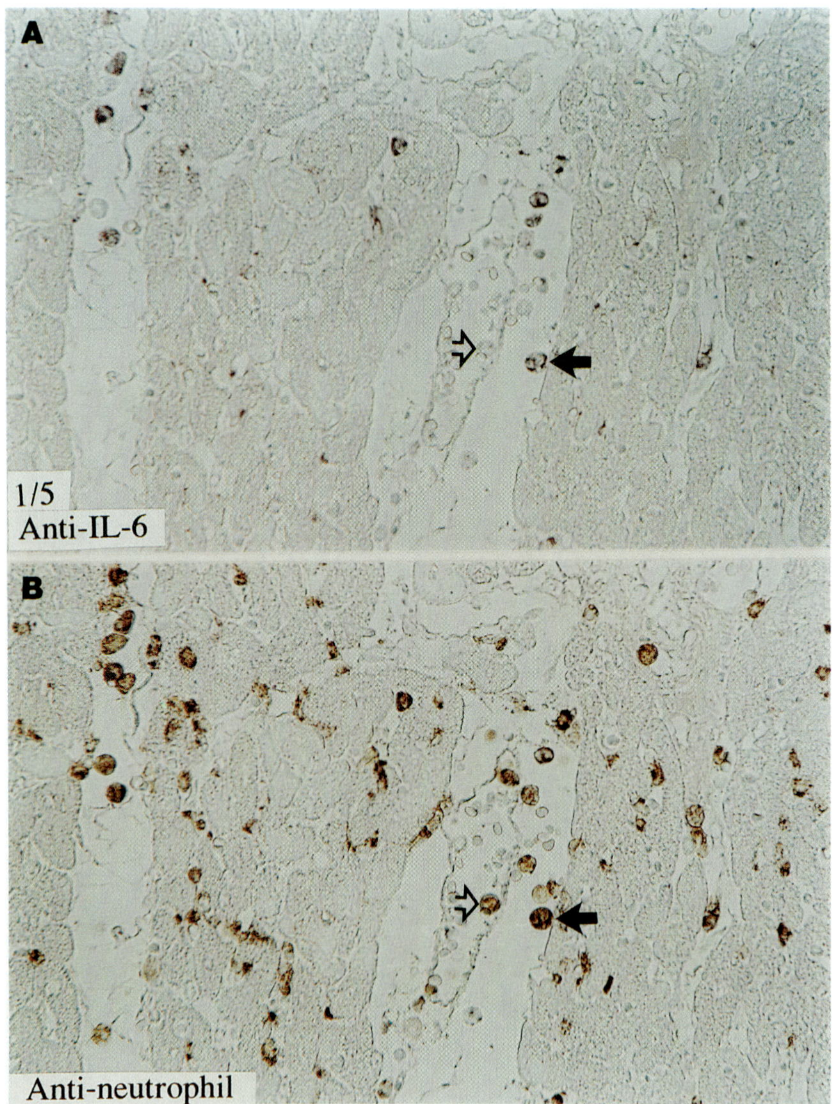

FIGURE 10. Immunostaining of IL-6 protein after 1-h occlusion and 5-h reperfusion. (**A**) Immunostaining for IL-6 protein (purple) is found in some of the extravascular leukocytes. (**B**) Dual staining with the anti-neutrophil mAb (SG8H6) of the same section shows many of the extravascular IL-6–positive cells are neutrophils. Although two intravascular neutrophils are seen, neither is positive for IL-6. In multiple samples, IL-6 protein was seen only in the extravascular neutrophils and only after 5 h of reperfusion.

Chemotactic Stimulus for Monocyte Infiltration

In our previous work we had demonstrated that C5a is a critical chemotactic attractant for neutrophils during early myocardial ischemia.[26] Clq binding proteins appear to initiate the classic complement pathway and result in the rapid appearance of C5a in the extracellular fluid within the first hour of reperfusion, as was also confirmed in the current report.[32,33] The presence of C5a in the cardiac lymph appears to be relatively short-lived while monocyte infiltration continues. The current manuscript suggests that TGF-β has an important role in the first 3 h of reperfusion. The origin of active TGF-β cannot be studied by current techniques since it is constitutively expressed in many cells (including myocardium) and exists in an inactive form subject to activation by a variety of stimuli. We would postulate TGF-β release comes from disrupted myocardial cells and that the TGF-β is subsequently washed out during reperfusion. From our data, it appears, however, that the primary control of mononuclear cell flux into the myocardium after the third hour is mediated by MCP-1. As we have previously reported,[25] MCP-1 is rapidly induced in the ischemic myocardium in a reperfusion-dependent manner. While the MCP-1 mRNA induction appears within ischemic border zone during the first hour of reperfusion, the protein cannot be stained immunohistochemically until the third hour. This observation correlates very well with the observation that MCP-1 becomes a major chemotactic factor after the third hour of reperfusion.[20] The interesting observation that MCP-1 is induced in a special class of veins[25] known to be associated with leukocyte transendothelial migration[27] speaks for the specificity of MCP-1 induction. This mode of induction is ideal for mediating monocyte transendothelial migration by a haptotactic mechanism. It is to be emphasized, however, that monocytes are not the only mononuclear cell for which MCP-1 provides chemotactic stimuli; T-lymphocytes are also attracted by MCP-1.[34] The potential role of T-lymphocytes will be discussed briefly below.

The Role of Neutrophils in Cytokine Cascade Associated with Acute Inflammatory Injury

In our earlier studies, we established that the induction of ICAM-1 on the surface of cardiac myocytes is fundamental to neutrophil-induced myocyte injury.[28,29,31] *In vitro* studies demonstrated that a compartmented transfer of reactive oxygen occurred and was mediated by the adhesion of Mac-1 on activated neutrophils to ICAM-1, induced on viable cardiac myocytes.[31] Post-ischemic cardiac lymph was found to induce ICAM-1 on cardiac myocytes via an IL-6 linked cytokinetic mechanism.[14] In contrast, endothelial ICAM-1 was not induced by IL-6.[14]

This tissue specificity led to an examination of induction of the genes for ICAM-1 and IL-6 in the jeopardized border zone following reperfusion. Initial studies demonstrated that ICAM-1 mRNA was rapidly induced in the reperfused myocardium.[16] *In situ* hybridization studies demonstrated that the induction occurred almost exclusively in viable cardiac myocytes on the border zone abutting infarcted myocardium.[35] Moreover, initial leukocyte infiltration appeared to be primarily in the border zone.[27,35] From the standpoint of *acute* inflammatory injury, however, it is important to point out that the neutrophils appear to be compartmented in the area where myocyte ICAM-1 has been induced and thus represents a potential threat to the cardiac myocytes that display ICAM-1 in their cell surface.

Studies of the induction of IL-6 demonstrated that IL-6 mRNA is very rapidly induced and appears to precede expression of ICAM-1 mRNA.[17] The IL-6 mRNA induction appears to be dependent upon reperfusion and was confined to leukocytes in the ischemic myocardium.[17] Within the first 3 h, *in situ* hybridization studies demonstrate that IL-6 mRNA is found exclusively in mononuclear cells, not in neutrophils. Induction of IL-6 mRNA is extremely rapid; studies of mononuclear cells from cardiac lymph demonstrate induction within the first 15 min of reperfusion. Thus, the mononuclear cells play an important role in the cytokine cascade through their production of IL-6, which subsequently induces myocyte ICAM-1. The rapid induction of IL-6 suggested the presence of a preformed "upstream" cytokine preexisting within the ischemic area that would allow the rapid induction of IL-6 in infiltrating monocytes. In this communication, we present evidence that mast cells contain preformed TNF-α, which has been shown *in vitro* to stimulate monocytes, and that mast cell degranulation occurs in the ischemic and reperfused myocardium. Studies of endotoxemic animals have previously demonstrated that IL-6 is upregulated only after TNF levels have risen[36–38] and that neutralization of TNF-α in sepsis prevents systemic increases in IL-6, IL-1B, and IL-8.[39]

Transition in Inflammatory Reactions That Facilitate Cardiac Healing

As reviewed above, there is substantial evidence that monocytes play important roles in myocardial healing. For the most part, it has been presumed that the monocytes function as phagocytic cells to clear cellular debris; however, monocytes are also important sources of cytokines and growth factors, which may be important in myocardial healing.

The current paper does not allow a complete discussion of the potential role of the monocyte in healing other than to identify these two factors described above. We also suggest that it is important to consider the role of other leukocytes in myocardial healing. Specifically we have provided some preliminary evidence with regard to the neutrophil. When neutrophils are activated and transmigrate in tissue their life span is markedly extended by the inhibition of normal apoptotic stimuli. Since we have identified Mac-1 (CD11b/CD18) as a critical portion of the mechanism of neutrophil-induced myocardial injury, we examined neutrophils infiltrating the myocardium and found that, after 3 h, neutrophils began to lose Mac-1 rapidly and, at least in theory, no longer had the potential to continue to injure cardiac myocytes. After the transitional time period, neutrophils begin making IL-6 mRNA and protein, neither of which is seen in neutrophils before the fifth hour of reperfusion. Since the induction of monocyte IL-6 was almost immediate, we presume this much later appearance in neutrophils is associated with significant phenotypic change in which the neutrophils begin making cytokines and perhaps other growth factors that have not yet been examined. Thus, it is possible that neutrophils may also provide cytokinetic factors for myocardial healing. Finally, it is clear that suppression of acute inflammatory mediators is a critical part of the healing process. The data suggesting MCP-1 as a chemotactic stimulus mediating mononuclear flux after the third hour of reperfusion also suggest that the T-lymphocytes may also be attracted to the ischemic and reperfused area at that time; preliminary data (not shown) suggest that this is so. As a matter of speculation, the Th_2 class of T-lymphocytes appears to be a biologically significant source of the anti-inflammatory cytokines IL-4 and IL-10; the latter is induced in response to stimulation with TNF-α. The possibility that tissue infiltrating Th_2 T-lymphocytes suppress the acute inflammatory response to myocardial injury remains for further investigation.

SUMMARY

We are now developing the means to evaluate components of this inflammatory response that may facilitate healing. A key event in the change in the inflammatory response is the development of a cytokine cascade that promotes phenotypic changes in the infiltrating leukocytes, which endow them with the ability to promote fibroblast proliferation and collagen deposition, the hallmarks of healing.

REFERENCES

1. KIM, C. B. & E. BRAUNWALD. 1993. Potential benefits of late reperfusion of infarcted myocardium. Circulation **88:** 2426–2436.
2. RICHARD, V., C. E. MURRY & K. A. REIMER. 1995. Healing of myocardial infarcts in dogs: effects of late reperfusion. Circulation **92:** 1891–1901.
3. SOMMERS, H. M. & R. B. JENNINGS. 1964. Experimental acute myocardial infarction. Histologic and histochemical studies of early myocardial infarcts induced by temporary or permanent occlusion of a coronary artery. Lab. Invest. **13:** 1491–1503.
4. ENTMAN, M. L. & C. W. SMITH. 1994. Post-reperfusion inflammation: A model of reaction to injury in cardiovascular disease. Cardiovasc. Res. **28:** 1301–1311.
5. HAMMERMAN, H., R. A. KLONER, S. HALE, F. J. SCHOEN & E. BRAUNWALD. 1983. Dose-dependent effects of short-term methylprednisolone on myocardial infarct extent, scar formation, and ventricular function. Circulation **68:** 446–452.
6. ROBERTS, R., V. DeMELLO & B. E. SOBEL. 1976. Deleterious effects of methylprednisolone in patients with myocardial infarction. Circulation **53** (suppl.I): 204–206.
7. MALLORY, G. K., P. D. WHITE & J. SALCEDO-SALGAR. 1939. The speed of healing of myocardial infarction. A study of the pathologic anatomy in seventy-two cases. Am. Heart J. **18:** 647–671.
8. KARSNER, H. T. & J. E. DWYER, JR. 1916. Studies in infarction. IV. Experimental bland infarction of the myocardium, myocardial regeneration and cicatrization. J. Med. Res. **34:** 21–41.
9. MORITA, M., S. KAWASHIMA, M. UENO, A. KUBOTA & T. IWASAKI. 1993. Effects of late reperfusion on infarct expansion and infarct healing in conscious rats. Am. J. Pathol. **143:** 419–430.
10. BOYLE, M. P. & H. F. WEISMAN. 1993. Limitation of infarct expansion and ventricular remodeling by late reperfusion. Circulation **88:** 2872–2883.
11. DREYER, W. J., C. W. SMITH, L. H. MICHAEL, R. D. ROSSEN, B. J. HUGHES *et al.* 1989. Canine neutrophil activation by cardiac lymph obtained during reperfusion of ischemic myocardium. Circ. Res. **65:** 1751–1762.

12. MICHAEL, L. H., R. M. LEWIS, T. A. BRANDON & M. L. ENTMAN. 1979. Cardiac lymph from conscious dogs. Am. J. Physiol. **237:** H311–H317.

13. KUKIELKA, G. L., C. W. SMITH, G. J. LaROSA, A. M. MANNING, L. H. MENDOZA *et al.* 1995. Interleukin-8 gene induction in the myocardium following ischemia and reperfusion *in vivo.* J. Clin. Invest. **95:** 89–103.

14. YOUKER, K. A., C. W. SMITH, D. C. ANDERSON, D. MILLER, L. H. MICHAEL *et al.* 1992. Neutrophil adherence to isolated adult cardiac myocytes: Induction by cardiac lymph collected during ischemia and reperfusion. J. Clin. Invest. **89:** 602–609.

15. YOUKER, K. A., H. K. HAWKINS, G. L. KUKIELKA, J. L. PERRARD, L. H. MICHAEL *et al.* 1994. Molecular evidence for induction of intercellular adhesion molecule-1 in the viable border zone associated with ischemia-reperfusion injury of the dog heart. Circulation **89:** 2736–2746.

16. KUKIELKA, G. L., H. K. HAWKINS, L. H. MICHAEL, A. M. MANNING, C. L. LANE *et al.* 1993. Regulation of intercellular adhesion molecule-1 (ICAM-1) in ischemic and reperfused canine myocardium. J. Clin. Invest. **92:** 1504–1516.

17. KUKIELKA, G. L., C. W. SMITH, A. M. MANNING, K. A. YOUKER, L. H. MICHAEL *et al.* 1995. Induction of Interleukin-6 synthesis in the myocardium: Potential role in post-reperfusion inflammatory injury. Circulation **92:** 1866–1875.

18. DREYER, W. J., L. H. MICHAEL, M. S. WEST, C. W. SMITH, R. ROTHLEIN *et al.* 1991. Neutrophil accumulation in ischemic canine myocardium: Insights into the time course, distribution, and mechanism of localization during early reperfusion. Circulation **84:** 400–411.

19. FOGELMAN, A. M., F. ELAHI, K. SYKES, L. B. J. VAN, M. C. TERRITO *et al.* 1988. Modification of the Recalde method for the isolation of human monocytes. J. Lipid. Res. **29:** 1243–1247.

20. BIRDSALL, H. H., D. M. GREEN, J. TRIAL *et al.* 1996. Complement C5a TGF-β1, and MCP-1, in sequence, induce migration of monocytes into ischemic myocardium within the first 1 to 5 hrs following reperfusion. Circulation (In press.)

21. McBRIDE, P., D. BRADLEY & M. KALINER. 1988. Evaluation of a radioimmunoassay for histamine measurement in biological fluids. J. Allergy Clin. Immunol. **82:** 638–646.

22. IGNATOWSHI, T. A. & R. N. SPENGLER. 1994. Tumor necrosis factor-alpha: presynaptic sensitivity is modified after antidepressant drug administration. Brain Res. **665:** 293–299.

23. BECKSTEAD, J. H. 1994. A simple technique for preservation of fixation-sensitive antigens in paraffin-embedded tissues. J. Histochem. Cytochem. **42:** 1127–1134.

24. LIE, J. T., K. E. HOLLEY & J. L. TITUS. 1972. Fuchsinorrhagia—A new histochemical indication of inapparent early myocardial ischemia. Lab. Med. **3:** 37–40.

25. KUMAR, A. G., C. M. BALLANTYNE, L. H. MICHAEL *et al.* 1996. Induction of monocyte chemoattractant protein-1 in the small veins of the ischemic and reperfused canine myocardium. Circulation (In press.)

26. DREYER, W. J., L. H. MICHAEL, T. NGUYEN, C. W. SMITH, D. C. ANDERSON *et al.* 1992. Kinetics of C5a release in cardiac lymph of dogs experiencing coronary artery ischemia-reperfusion injury. Circ. Res. **71:** 1518–1524.

27. HAWKINS, H. K., M. L. ENTMAN, J. Y. ZHU, K. A. YOUKER, K. BERENS *et al.* 1996. Acute inflammatory reaction after myocardial ischemic injury and reperfusion. Development and use of a neutrophil-specific antibody. Am. J. Pathol. **148:** 1957–1969.

28. ENTMAN, M. L., K. A. YOUKER, S. B. SHAPPELL, C. SIEGEL, R. ROTHLEIN *et al.* 1990. Neutrophil adherence to isolated adult canine myocytes: Evidence for a CD18-dependent mechanism. J. Clin. Invest. **85:** 1497–1506.

29. SMITH, C. W., M. L. ENTMAN, C. L. LANE, A. L. BEAUDET, T. I. TY *et al.* 1991. Adherence of neutrophils to canine cardiac myocytes *in vitro* is dependent on intercellular adhesion molecule-1. J. Clin. Invest. **88:** 1216–1223.

30. EISENBERG, S. P., R. J. EVANS, W. P. AREND, E. VERDERBER, M. T. BREWER *et al.* 1990. Primary structure and functional expression from complementary DNA of a human interleukin-1 receptor antagonist. Nature **343:** 341–346.

31. ENTMAN, M. L., K. A. YOUKER, T. SHOJI, G. L. KUKIELKA, S. B. SHAPPELL *et al.* 1992. Neutrophil induced oxidative injury of cardiac myocytes: A compartmented system requiring CD11b/CD18-ICAM-1 adherence. J. Clin. Invest. **90:** 1335–1345.

32. ROSSEN, R. D., J. L. SWAIN, L. H. MICHAEL, S. WEAKLEY, E. GIANNINI *et al.* 1985. Selective accumulation of the first component of complement and leukocytes in ischemic canine heart muscle: A possible initiator of an extra myocardial mechanism of ischemic injury. Circ. Res. **57:** 119–130.

33. BIRDSALL, H. H., J. TRIAL, J. A. HALLUM, A. L. DEJONG, L. K. GREEN *et al.* 1994. Phenotypic and functional activation of monocytes in HIV-1 infection; interactions with neural cells. J. Leuko. Biol. **56:** 310–317.

34. LOETSCHER, P., M. SEITZ, I. CLARK-LEWIS, M. BAGGIOLINI & B. MOSER. 1994. Monocyte chemotactic proteins MCP-1, MCP-2, and MCP-3 are major attractants for human CD4′ and CD8′ T lymphocytes. FASEB J. **8:** 1055–1060.

35. YOUKER, K. A., H. K. HAWKINS, G. L. KUKIELKA, J. L. PERRARD, L. H. MICHAEL *et al.* 1993. Molecular evidence for a border zone vulnerable to inflammatory reperfusion injury. Trans. Assoc. Amer. Physiol. **CVI:** 145–154.

36. SPINAS, G. A., D. BLOESCH, U. KELLER, W. ZIMMERLI & S. CAMMISULI. 1991. Pretreatment with ibuprofen augments circulating tumor necrosis factor-1, interleukin-6, and elastase during acute endotoxinemia. J. Infect. Dis. **163:** 89–95.

37. MARTICH, G. D., R. L. DANNER, M. CESKA & A. F. SUFFREDINI. 1991. Detection of interleukin 8 and tumor necrosis factor in normal humans after intravenous endotoxin: the effect of antiinflammatory agents. J. Exp. Med. **173:** 1021–1024.

38. HESSE, D. G., K. J. TRACEY, Y. FONG, K. R. MANOGUE, M. A. PALLADINO *et al.* 1988. Cytokine appearance in human endotoxemia and primate bacteremia. Surg. Gynecol. Obstet. **166:** 147–153.

39. VAN DEVENTER, S. J. H., M. HART, T. VAN DER POLL, C. E. HACK & L. A. AARDEN. 1993. Endotoxin and TNF-induced IL-8 release in humans. J. Infect. Dis. **167:** 461–464.

Phagocytes and Acute Lung Injury:
Dual Roles For Interleukin-1

BROOKS M. HYBERTSON, YOUNG M. LEE,
AND JOHN E. REPINE[a]

Webb-Waring Institute for Biomedical Research
University of Colorado Health Sciences Center
Denver, Colorado 80262

INTRODUCTION

Following infection, trauma, and/or numerous other disorders, certain individuals, for unknown reasons, develop a highly fatal acute edematous lung injury that is widely known as the acute respiratory distress syndrome (ARDS).[1–4] After study for many years, it is now clear that lung inflammation involving activation of resident lung alveolar macrophages (AM) along with recruitment and activation of blood neutrophils (PMN) are key features of the pathophysiology of this perplexing condition.[4,5] This impression is based largely on the multiple observations of increased numbers of inflammatory mediators and phagocytic cells in the lungs of ARDS patients. Along with other groups, our laboratory has been interested in determining the significance of the increased levels of interleukin-1 (IL-1), interleukin-8 (IL-8), and neutrophils that occur in the lungs of ARDS patients. To achieve this end, we have been investigating the acute lung injury that develops in rats that are given IL-1 intratracheally. As part of this symposium, this short paper reviews our recent laboratory findings in this model system and how these findings relate to recent promising clinical findings in a preliminary trial of ARDS patients.

RESULTS

Our initial finding was that a striking influx of neutrophils and an acute edematous leak occurred rapidly in lungs of rats given small amounts (50 ng) of IL-1 intratracheally 5 h before (FIG. 1).[6] This observation was confirmed by careful histological analysis that revealed increased lung cellularity and perivascular cuffing—an early manifestation of lung leak—in lungs of rats given IL-1 intratracheally. The dependence on IL-1 activity was further supported when treatment with the interleukin-1-receptor antagonist (IL-1ra) prevented IL-1–induced lung neutrophil accumulation and leak.[7] In addition, intratracheal administration of heated IL-1 did not cause lung inflammation or lung leak in rats.[6] Experiments were then conducted to determine the functional contribution of neutrophils to the development of lung

[a]Address all correspondence to: John E. Repine, M.D., 4200 East Ninth Avenue, Box C321, Denver, Colorado 80262. Phone, 303-315-8051 and Fax, 303-315-8541.

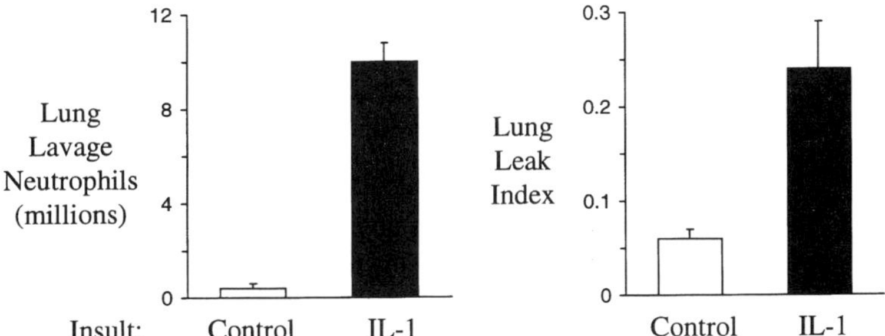

FIGURE 1. Rats given IL-1 intratracheally had increased lung lavage neutrophils and lung leak compared to control rats. (Modified from Leff *et al.*[6] with permission.)

leak. We found that rats made neutropenic by prior vinblastine treatment did not develop lung leak following IL-1 insufflation (FIG. 2).[6] This observation advanced a causative role for neutrophils in the development of IL-1–induced lung leak.

Our next objective was to determine the mechanism responsible for neutrophil recruitment. We found that cytokine-induced neutrophil chemoattractant (CINC) levels were increased in lung lavages obtained from rats given IL-1 intratracheally (FIG. 3) and that treatment with anti-CINC antibody not only decreased lung neutrophil accumulation, but also lung leak, in rats given IL-1 intratracheally (FIG. 4).[8,9] In parallel experiments, insufflating CINC at the same or concentrations exceeding 100-fold those concentrations measured in rats given IL-1 intratracheally did not cause appreciable neutrophil infiltration or lung leak.[8,9] This finding suggested that CINC was a necessary component of IL-1–induced lung inflammation, but not by itself, at the tested concentrations, sufficient to cause lung leak or lung neutrophil influx.[10] One

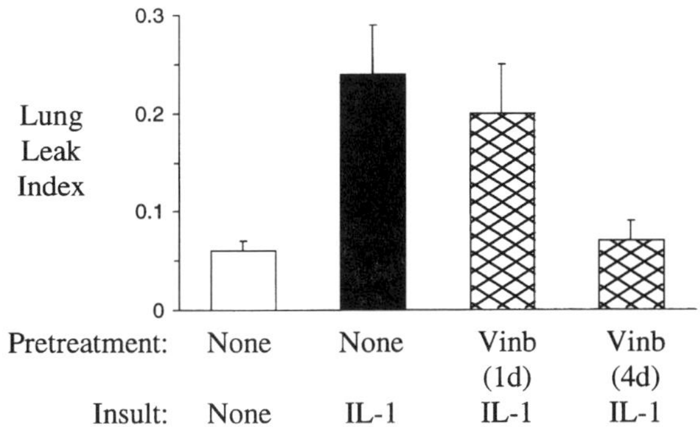

FIGURE 2. Following IL-1 instillation, rats made neutropenic by vinblastine treatment 4 days before had decreased lung leak compared to rats given vinblastine 1 day before or control rats. (Modified from Leff *et al.*[6] with permission.)

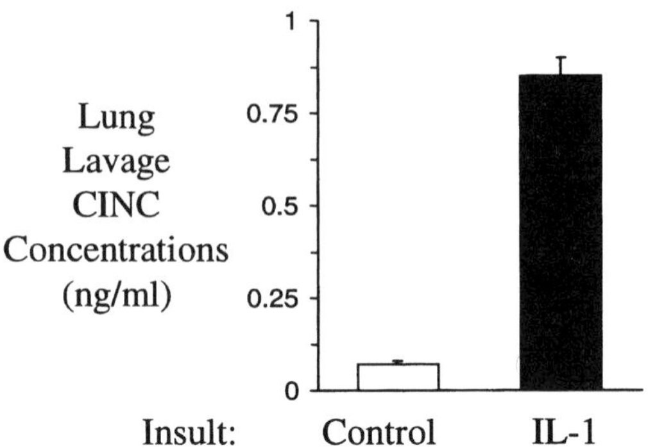

FIGURE 3. Rats given IL-1 intratracheally had increased lung lavage cytokine-induced chemoattractant (CINC) levels compared to control rats. (Modified from Koh *et al.*[9] with permission.)

possible source for CINC production *in vivo* was identified when IL-1–stimulated rat AM secreted CINC *in vitro*.[8]

Our next aim was to characterize the nature of IL-1–induced lung leak. Because of the well-appreciated ability of neutrophils to generate oxygen radicals, our hypothesis was that IL-1–induced lung leak involved an oxidative insult. We made a number of observations that supported this premise. *First*, similar to ARDS patients, rats given IL-1 intratracheally exhaled increased amounts of hydrogen peroxide (H_2O_2) compared to control rats given saline intratracheally.[6] *Second*, rats given IL-1 intratracheally had increased levels of oxidized glutathione (GSSG) compared to control rats given saline intratracheally.[6] *Third*, treatment with various oxygen-radical scavenging antioxidants, superoxide dismutase (SOD), supercritical fluid-aerosolized vitamin E,[10] or dimethylsulfoxide (DMSO), decreased lung leak in rats given IL-1 intratracheally.[6,11] SOD and DMSO treatment also reduced exhaled H_2O_2 levels and diminished GSSG increases while SOD and aerosolized vitamin E treat-

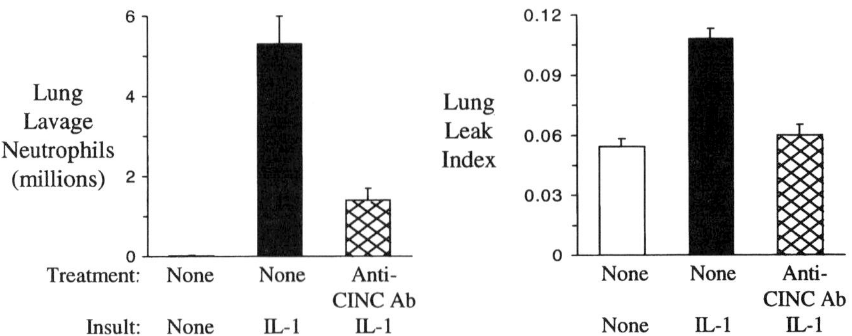

FIGURE 4. Anti-CINC antibody treatment decreased lung lavage neutrophils and lung leak in rats given IL-1 intratracheally. (Modified from Koh *et al.*[9] with permission.)

ment decreased lung leak without decreasing lung neutrophils increases in lungs of rats given IL-1 intratracheally.[6]

In 1986, a clinical study identified a positive effect of prostaglandin E_1 (PGE_1) infusion in ARDS patients,[11] but this benefit was not confirmed in a subsequent, larger and better controlled trial.[12] Afterwards, a new pharmacologic agent was discovered in which PGE_1 was associated with liposomes (TLC-C53). We found that rats given TLC-C53 at 2.5 h after IL-1 insufflation had decreased lung neutrophil influxes and lung leak compared to rats given IL-1 intratracheally (FIG. 5).[13] Subsequently, a small clinical trial was undertaken that revealed that TLC-C53 treatment dramatically reduced ventilator dependency in ARDS patients (FIG. 6).[14] A trend towards decreased mortality was also observed in this preliminary trial.[14] The exciting findings of this initial clinical study are presently being actively pursued in a large-scale, multicenter trial.

The aforementioned investigations clearly suggest that IL-1 contributes to the development of acute oxidative lung leak. However, we and others have also found that IL-1 can provide protection against oxidative insults (generally known as "tolerance").[15] For example, IL-1 pretreatment decreased not only pulmonary oxygen toxicity but also cardiac ischemia-reperfusion injury in rats.[16] To further determine the tolerance-increasing effects of IL-1, we next studied the consequences of IL-1 pretreatment in rats that would subsequently receive IL-1 intratracheally. We found that IL-1 pretreatment (given 36 h before) decreased lung leak, but not lung neutrophil increases, in rats given IL-1 intratracheally (FIG. 7).[17] In parallel investigations, lungs isolated from rats pretreated 36 h before with IL-1 intraperitoneally gained less weight following perfusion with human neutrophils and IL-1 insufflation than lungs from saline-pretreated rats. This finding suggests that lungs from IL-1–pretreated rats are intrinsically resistant to neutrophil-mediated injury. Furthermore, our recent work indicates that IL-1 pretreatment makes cultured rat lung microvascular endothelial cells resistant to injury caused by adding normal human neutrophils and phorbol myristate acetate (PMA). The mechanism responsible for the tolerance that develops following IL-1 pretreatment is unknown but does not appear to be a simple consequence of increases in traditional antioxidant enzymes. Moreover, although IL-1ra

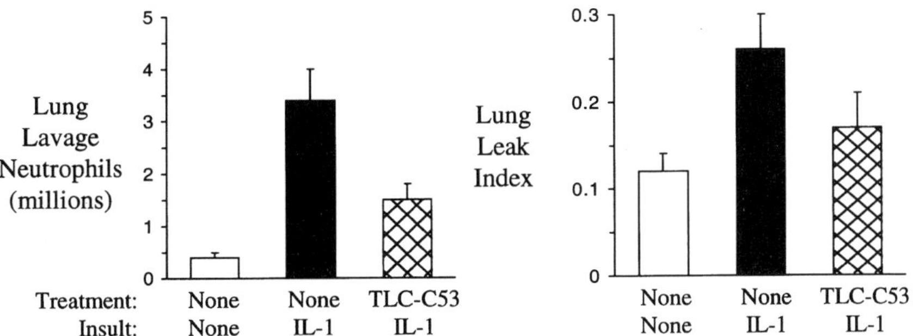

FIGURE 5. Liposomal PGE_1 (TLC-C53) treatment given 2.5 h after IL-1 administration decreased lung lavage neutrophils and lung leak in rats given IL-1 intratracheally. (Modified from Leff *et al.*[13] with permission.)

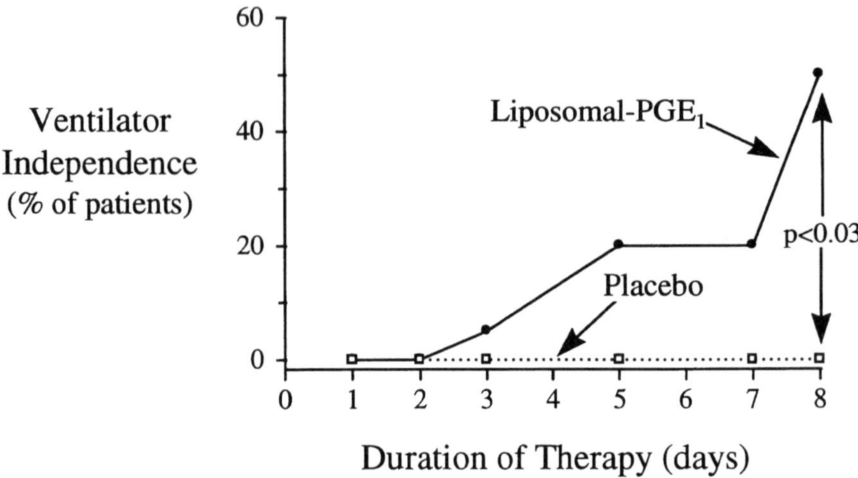

FIGURE 6. Liposomal-PGE$_1$ (TLC-C53)–treated ARDS patients had decreased ventilator dependence compared to untreated ARDS patients. (Modified from Abraham *et al.*[14] with permission.)

levels are increased in the serum of ARDS patients, it is unlikely that IL-1–induced tolerance is simply a consequence of increases in IL-1ra. This impression is based on the observation that IL-1ra treatment prevents both leak and neutrophil increases in lungs of rats given IL-1 intratracheally while IL-1–mediated tolerance involves decreases in lung leak *without* decreases in lung neutrophil accumulation.

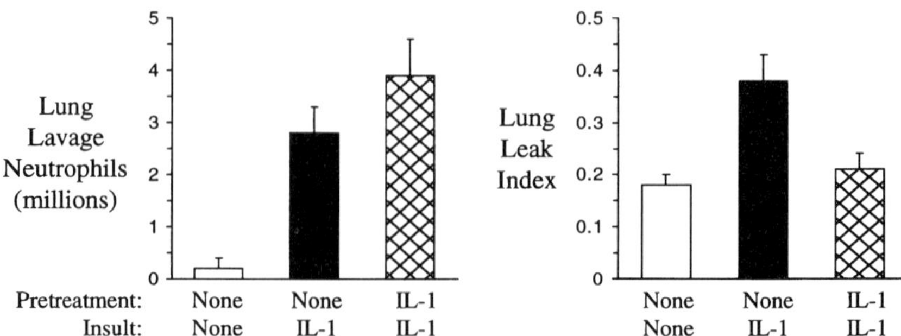

FIGURE 7. IL-1 pretreatment (given 30 ng of IL-1 intraperitoneally 36 h before) decreased lung leak, but not lung lavage neutrophils, in rats given IL-1 intratracheally. (Modified from Leff *et al.*[17] with permission.)

DISCUSSION

It is generally believed that phagocytes contribute in major ways to the development of ARDS. Release from AM of toxins and factors that recruit and activate neutrophils seems almost certain, especially when airway insults (e.g., smoke inhalation, pneumonia, and aspiration) initiate the syndrome. The massive influx of neutrophils into the lungs of ARDS patients provides *prima facie* evidence for their participation, especially when considered in conjunction with the numerous reports implicating neutrophil-mediated injury in a myriad of acute lung injury models. As more is learned about the specific mechanisms that control phagocyte-mediated lung injury, new opportunities for limiting and, hopefully, preventing this devastating condition should be forthcoming. Our enthusiasm for developing strategies to limit phagocyte responses, needless to say, must be tempered by the realization of the unquestionable value of phagocytes in combating the infections that frequently confront these patients. This duality of phagocyte function encompassing both beneficial and detrimental aspects may parallel the duality ("yin-yang") of function that relates to the influences of IL-1 as both a causative and protective force in the development of acute lung injury (FIG. 8).

SUMMARY

Interleukin-1 (IL-1) and neutrophils are increased in lungs of patients with the acute respiratory distress syndrome (ARDS). We found that rats given IL-1 intratracheally rapidly developed lung neutrophil accumulation and a neutrophil-dependent acute edematous lung leak. Lung leak was associated with increased lung lavage cytokine-induced chemoattractant (CINC) levels and increased oxidative stress that was manifested by increased exhaled H_2O_2 levels and increased lung oxidized glutathione levels. IL-1–induced lung leak was decreased by treatment with superoxide dismutase (SOD), dimethylsulfoxide (DMSO), supercritical fluid-aerosolized vitamin E,

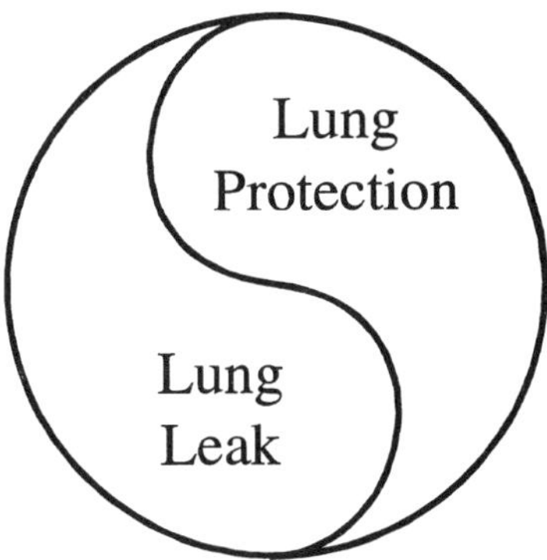

FIGURE 8. Postulated "yin-yang" dual functions of IL-1 with respect to development of lung leak and protection against lung leak.

interleukin-1–receptor antagonist (IL-1ra), or liposome-associated PGE_1 (Lip-PGE_1). Importantly, Lip-PGE_1 treatment also reduced ventilator dependence in a small clinical study of ARDS patients. Another series of investigations revealed that IL-1 pretreatment could prevent lung leak in rats given IL-1 intratracheally. These findings point to the possible dual effects of IL-1 with respect to the development of acute lung injury.

Note added in proof: Since this paper was accepted for publication, the overall clinical trial of Lip-PGE_1 was not successful. However, retrospective analysis has revealed that Lip-PGE_1 was effective in reducing ventilator dependency in ARDS patients who were treated early and did not have multiple organ failure.

Individuals who are specifically interested in this area should look for the upcoming paper reporting the results of this trial.

REFERENCES

1. ASHBAUGH, D. G., D. B. BIGELOW, T. L. PETTY & B. E. LEVINE. 1967. Acute respiratory distress in adults. Lancet **2:** 319–323.
2. DONNELLY, S. C. & C. ROBERTSON. 1993. Trauma, inflammatory cells and ARDS. [Review]. Arch. Emerg. Med. **10:** 108–111.
3. RINALDO, J. E. & R. M. ROGERS. 1982. Adult respiratory distress syndrome: Changing concepts of lung injury and repair. N. Engl. J. Med. **306:** 900–909.
4. REPINE, J. E. 1992. Scientific perspectives on adult respiratory distress syndrome. Lancet **339:** 466–469.
5. TATE, R. M. & J. E. REPINE. 1983. Neutrophils and the adult respiratory distress syndrome. Am. Rev. Respir. Dis. **128:** 552–559.
6. LEFF, J. A., J. W. BAER, M. E. BODMAN, J. M. KIRKMAN, P. F. SHANLEY, L. M. PATTON, C. J. BEEHLER, J. M. MCCORD & J. E. REPINE. 1994. Interleukin-1-induced lung neutrophil accumulation and oxygen metabolite-mediated lung leak in rats. Am. J. Physiol. **266:** 2–8.
7. LEFF, J. A., M. E. BODMAN, O. J. CHO, S. ROHRBACH, O. K. REISS, J. L. VANNICE & J. E. REPINE. 1994. Post-insult treatment with interleukin-1 receptor antagonist decreases oxidative lung injury in rats given intratracheal interleukin-1. Am. J. Respir. Crit. Care. Med. **150:** 109–112.
8. HYBERTSON, B. M., E. K. JEPSON, J. H. CLARKE, R. J. SPELTS & J. E. REPINE. 1996. Interleukin-1 stimulates rapid release of cytokine-induced neutrophil chemoattractant (CINC) in rat lungs. Inflammation **20:** 471–483.
9. KOH, Y., B. M. HYBERTSON, E. K. JEPSON, O. J. CHO & J. E. REPINE. 1995. Cytokine-induced neutrophil chemoattractant is necessary for interleukin-1–induced lung leak in rats. J. Appl. Physiol. **79:** 472–478.
10. HYBERTSON, B. M., J. A. LEFF, C. J. BEEHLER, P. C. BARRY & J. E. REPINE. 1995. Effect of vitamin E deficiency and supercritical fluid aerosolized vitamin E supplementation on interleukin-1-induced oxidative lung injury in rats. Free Radic. Biol. Med. **18:** 537–542.
11. HOLCRAFT, J. W., M. J. VASSAR & C. J. WEBER. 1986. Survival in patients with the adult respiratory distress syndrome. Ann. Surg. **203:** 371–378.
12. BONE, R. C., G. SLOTMAN, R. MAUNDER, H. SILVERMAN, T. M. HYERS, M. D. KERSTEIN, J. J. LIPSPRING & THE PROSTAGLANDIN E1 STUDY GROUP. 1989. Randomized double-blind, multicenter study of prostaglandin E1 in patients with the Adult Respiratory Distress Syndrome. Chest **96:** 114–119.
13. LEFF, J. A., J. W. BAER, J. M. KIRKMAN, M. E. BODMAN, P. F. SHANLEY, O. J. CHO, M. J. OS-

TRO & J. E. REPINE. 1994. Liposome-entrapped PGE1 posttreatment decreases IL-1 alpha-induced neutrophil accumulation and lung leak in rats. J. Appl. Physiol. **76:** 151–157.

14. ABRAHAM, E., C. PARK, P. COVINGTON, S. A. CONRAD & M. SCHWARTZ. 1996. Liposomal prostaglandin E_1 in acute respiratory distress syndrome: A placebo-controlled, randomized, double-blind, multicenter clinical trial. Crit. Care Med. **24:** 10–15.

15. REPINE, J. E. 1994. Interleukin-1-mediated acute lung injury and tolerance to oxidative injury. Env. Health Persp. **102:** 75–78.

16. BROWN, J. M., C. W. WHITE, L. S. TERADA, M. A. GROSSO, P. F. SHANLEY, D. W. MULVIN, A. BANERJEE, G. J. R. WHITMAN, A. H. HARKEN & J. E. REPINE. 1990. Interleukin 1 pretreatment decreases ischemia/reperfusion injury. Proc. Natl. Acad. Sci. USA **87:** 5026–5030.

17. LEFF, J. A., C. P. WILKE, M. J. FURMAN, M. E. BODMAN & J. E. REPINE. 1995. Interleukin-1 pretreatment prevents interleukin-1-induced lung leak in rats. Am. J. Physiol. **268:** 12–16.

Histiocytic Activation following Neutron Irradiation of Boron-Enriched Rat Liver Metastases

R. NANO,[a] S. BARNI, G. GERZELI, T. PINELLI,[b] S. ALTIERI,[b] F. FOSSATI,[b] U. PRATI,[c] L. ROVEDA,[c] AND A. ZONTA[c]

Department of Animal Biology
University of Pavia
Center of Study for Histochemistry
CNR
Pavia, Italy

[b]*Department of Nuclear and Theoretical Physics*
University of Pavia
I.N.F.N.
Pavia, Italy

[c]*Department of Surgery*
Division of General Surgery
University of Pavia
Pavia, Italy

The liver is the most common target of metastatic cells derived from colorectal and other primary tumors.[1] With the aim to realize a possible therapy to treat the unresectable diffused liver tumor, our research group has been working since 1987 to set up a methodology allowing the utilization of the boron neutron capture therapy as the intermediate phase of the liver autograft.[2,3] Various promising results have been achieved up to now and more recently the boron uptake of liver tissues has been studied using a rat model. Significant statistical results have been obtained and represent the most complete insight on this possibility.[4]

Presently, our studies are devoted to the analysis of the damage produced by alpha particles from $^{10}B(n,\alpha)^7Li$ reaction in boron-enriched liver tissues (both tumoral). In the present paper, a morphological study of rat liver metastases from colon carcinoma, before and after treatment, is reported. Our attention has been primarily focused on ultrastructural changes of neoplastic cells and on the macrophage activation.

[a]Address correspondence to: Prof. Rosanna Nano, Department of Animal Biology, Piazza Botta 10, University of Pavia, 27100, Pavia, Italy. Telephone, 0382-506315; Fax, 0382-506406; e-mail, nano@ipv36.unipv.it

MATERIALS AND METHODS

Prior to neutron irradiation, the liver metastases were obtained by intrasplenic inoculation of 2×10^7 stabilized cells from a rat colon carcinoma chemically induced in BD-IX strain rats.[5] To prevent tumor induction in two hepatic lobes, we clamped one peripheral portal vessel during the intrasplenic injection of tumor cells. We have used the healthy parenchyma as a control. Ten days later, the boron compound solution was intravenously injected into the rat (300 mg of BPA/kg). Three hours after the boron administration, the animals were sacrificed and the liver was washed by perfusion of a glucose solution. Then the liver was stored at 4°C during the irradiation (10 min) by thermal neutrons at the position inside the thermal column of the Triga Mark II Reactor of the University of Pavia. Each sample was given a neutron fluence of 10^{13} cm^{-2}. The morphological examination of the samples (H & E stain) was carried out).

Electron Microscopy

Samples of liver tissue obtained from different areas of the liver parenchyma, healthy and tumor-invaded, before and after the neutron irradiation, were processed according to the following protocol: (*1*) Fixation at 4°C for 3 h in 1.5% glutaraldehyde buffered to pH 7.4 with 0.1 M cacodylate buffer; (*2*) post-fixation in 1% osmium tetroxide in 0.1 M phosphate buffer for 1 h at 4°C; (*3*) washing in buffer and dehydration on graded ethanols; (*4*) embedding in Epon 812. Semithin sections (0.5 μm thick) were stained with 1% borated methylene blue and examined in light microscopy. Ultrathin sections were stained with saturated uranyl acetate in 50% acetone and Reynold's lead citrate solution. The specimens were examined with a Zeiss TEM 900 at 80 KV.

Acid Phosphatase Histochemistry

Small liver samples were frozen in liquid nitrogen and stored at −80°C. Cryostat sections (6 μm thick) were cut with a Reichert-Jung cryostat. The samples were incubated using an azo-coupling method: 18% PVA in 100 mM sodium acetate buffer pH 5.0; 10 mM hexarotized-p-rosanilin prepared immediately before the use from basic fuchsin (BDH, Poole, England) and 5 mM naphthol AS-BI phosphate acid (Sigma Chemical Co.). The incubation was carried out for 30 min at 37°C. The samples were washed in distilled water and mounted in glycerin-gelatin.

RESULTS AND DISCUSSION

The observations performed 10 days after the tumor induction showed two different situations of invasiveness of the liver. The first situation was the presence of free tumoral cells in the sinusoidal blood stream detectable only at the electron microscopy level (FIG. 2, A and B). The second was the aggregation of neoplastic cells

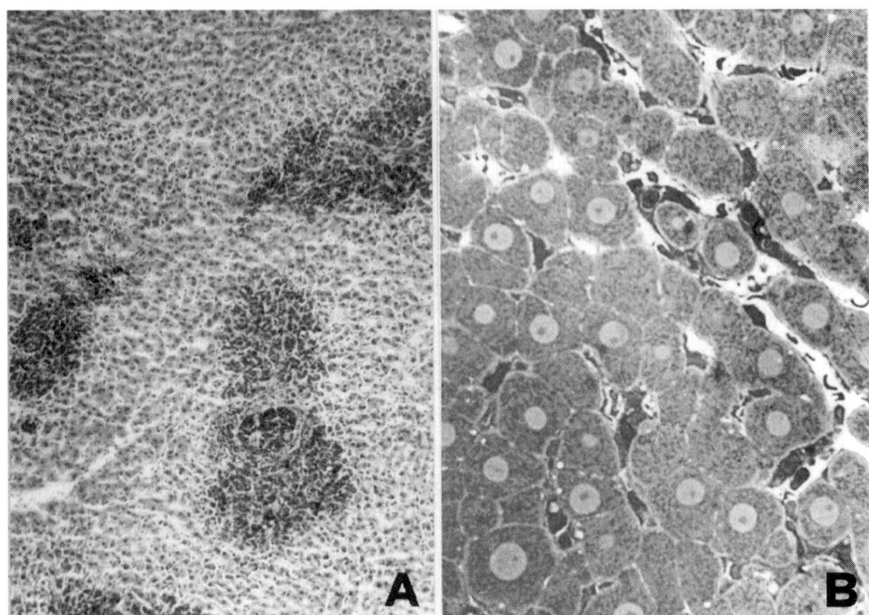

FIGURE 1. Light microscopy of (A) liver parenchyma with metastatic cells organized in nodules (H.E staining), (B) semithin section of liver parenchyma with a high incidence of Kupffer cells after the treatment (A: × 100; B: × 800).

in nodules, with different extension, scattered into the parenchyma without a preferential localization. Such structures are detectable at light microscopy (FIG. 1, A). The cell clusters appear organized in pseudoglandular formations partially showing the persistence of the "histological memory."

As regards the "free" neoplastic cells found in the sinusoids, the ultrastructural analysis shows the occasional presence of inclusions in the cytoplasm consisting of electron-dense bodies, probably containing mucous secretory material (FIG. 2, B). Such a situation is the same as that observed in the colon primary neoplastic cell in a partially differentiated stage. After the treatment with BPA and subsequent neutron irradiation, evident changes were found, in particular in the circulating neoplastic cells.

In addition to the presence of apparently undamaged neoplastic cells (FIG. 2, C), frequently debris (free nuclei, cytoplasm portions, free organelles) mixed with blood cells (FIG. 2, D) was detected in the sinusoidal lumen. This demonstrates that the ultrastructural analysis allows the evaluation of subcellular damages produced by alpha particles released in the reaction $^{10}B(n,\alpha)^{7}Li$.

Of particular interest is the observation of the liver histiocytic system after the irradiation [FIG. 1(B) and FIG. 3]. FIGURE 1(B) shows an unusual number of Kupffer

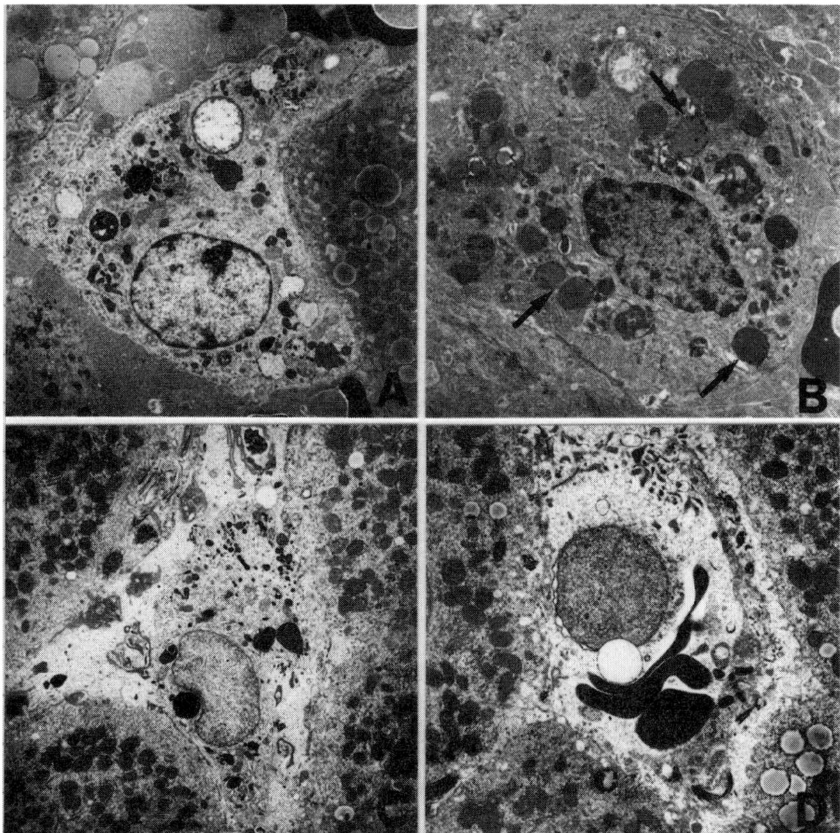

FIGURE 2. Ultrastructure of liver before (A, B) and after (C, D) treatment. Before treatment the metastatic cells circulating into the sinusoidal lumen are intact and sometimes show the presence of pseudo-secretory intracytoplasmic granules (*arrows*). After treatment the neoplastic cells show a different degree of damage (× 3,500).

cells whose morphology indicates a clear activation state (FIG. 3, A and B). At the electron microscopy level the active state of histiocytic cells is deduced by the presence of engulfing Kupffer cells (FIG. 3, A and B) with pseudopodia (FIG. 3, B) and polymorphonucleated cells with cytoplasmic phagosomes (FIG. 3, C and D). In particular, the Kupffer cells are also responsible for a strong acid phosphatase reactivity.

In conclusion, the above preliminary results give two important indications concerning the effects of the boron neutron capture therapy on liver metastases: (*1*) the subcellular details of the radioactive damage induced by the neutron irradiation in the neoplastic cells and (*2*) the increased scavenger activity of the histiocytic system present in the liver.

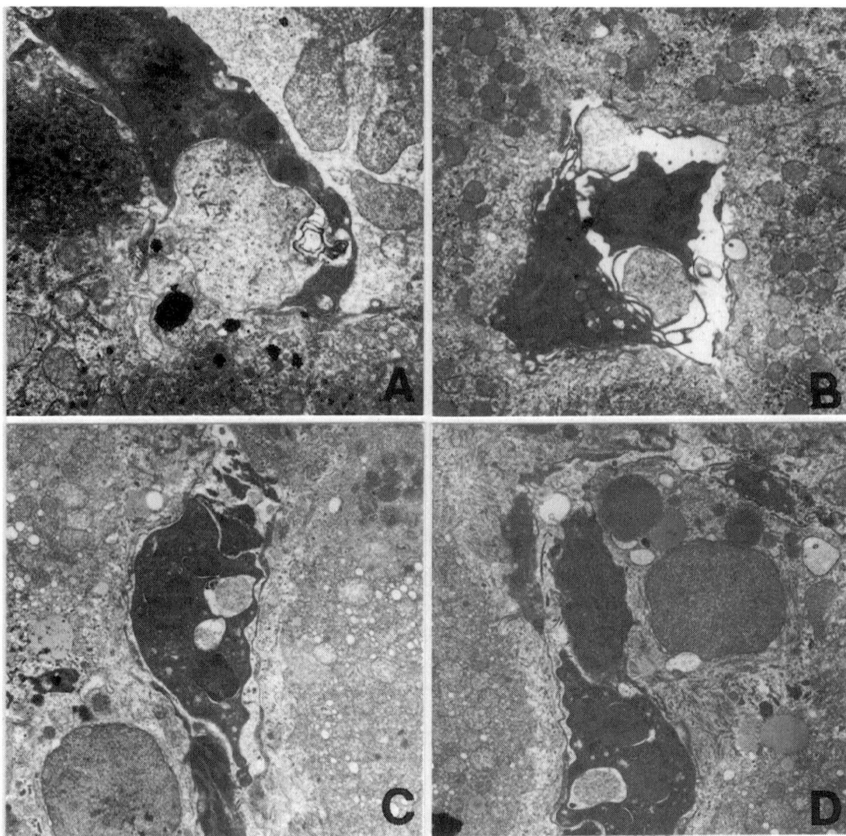

FIGURE 3. Ultrastructure of liver after treatment showing different patterns of Kupffer cells (A, B) and leukocytes (C, D) activation (phagocytosis and degradation of cellular material probably derived from the metastatic cell destruction) ($\times$ 3,500).

REFERENCES

1. VITALE, G. C. 1986. Surg. Cl. North Am. **66:** 723–725.
2. CHIARAVIGLIO, D., T. PINELLI, F. DE GRAZIA, A. ZONTA, S. ALTIERI, A. BRAGHIERI & F. FOS-SATI. 1989. Strahlenther Onkol **165:** 170–172.
3. PINELLI, T., S. ALTIERI, F. FOSSATI, A. ZONTA, D. COSSARD, U. PRATI, L. ROVEDA, G. RICEVUTI & R. NANO. 1996. *In* Cancer Neutron Capture Therapy. Mishima, Ed.: 783–796. Plenum Press. New York.
4. PINELLI, T., S. ALTIERI, F. FOSSATI, A. ZONTA, D. COSSARD, U. PRATI, C. ROVEDA, G. RICEVU-TI & R. NANO. 1996. *In* Radiation: From Theory to Multidisciplinary Applications. Piero A. Salvadori, Ed.: 23–30. Felici. Pisa.
5. CAIGNARD, A., M. S. MARTIN, M. F. MICHEL & F. MARTIN. 1985. Int. J. Cancer **36:** 273–279.

Expression of Lymphocyte Function-Associated Antigen-1 (LFA-1) in Glioblastoma Patients: A Flow Cytometric Analysis

E. CAPELLI,[a] R. NANO,[b] M. CIVALLERO,[b] K. MARINU-AKTIPI,[c] AND M. CERONI[c]

Department of Genetic and Microbiology
University of Pavia
27100 Pavia, Italy

[b]*Department of Animal Biology*
University of Pavia
Center of Study for Histochemistry
CNR
Pavia, Italy

[c]*Neurologic Institute*
Foundation "C. Mondino"
Neuropathology Laboratory
University of Pavia
Pavia, Italy

INTRODUCTION

The expression of lymphocyte function-associated antigen-1 (LFA-1, CD11a/CD18) is regulated by cytokines. These proteins are involved in the intercellular adhesion during the activation of the immune functions.[1-3] LFA-1 belongs to the family of leukocyte integrins and is detected on the membrane of many cellular lines.[4] LFA-1 expression is regulated during the differentiative stages of the cells and by exposition to inflammatory modulators.[5] Intercellular adhesion molecule-1 (ICAM-1) is a member of the immunoglobulin gene superfamily that can be expressed on non-hematopoietic cells of many lineages and on hematopoietic cells, such as tissue macrophages, mitogen-stimulated T-lymphoblasts, germinal center B-cells, and dendritic cells. ICAM-1 functions as a ligand for the LFA-1 and MAC-1 (membrane attack complex-1). ICAM-1 and its counter receptor LFA-1 act as accessory molecules in the activation of T lymphocytes. Cytokines and ICAM-1 play an important role in the recruitment of activated lymphocytes to the sites of inflammation within the central nervous system (CNS).[5] Previously we evaluated serum levels of IL-2, sIL-2R,

[a]Address correspondence to: Dott. Enrica Capelli, Department of Genetic and Microbiology, Via Abbiategrasso 207, 27100 Pavia, University of Pavia, Italy. Telephone, 0382-505528; Fax, 0382-528496.

and soluble form of ICAM-1 in patients with glioblastoma (GBL), the most anaplastic and invasive of the astrocytic tumors.[6] A significant increase of IL-2 and sIL-2R serum levels was observed in all tumor patients while soluble ICAM-1 (sICAM-1) levels were not increased.[7] In the present study, we extend the analysis of the immune system activation in GBL patients studying the expression of LFA-1. In the present study LFA-1 positive cells were detected by flow cytometric analysis using an antibody that specifically reacts with the α-L-subunit (CD11a antigen) that characterizes LFA-1 expressed on lymphocytes.[8]

MATERIALS AND METHODS

Patients and Controls

Ten patients with GBL according to the World Health Organization (WHO) classification[9,10] were examined. Blood samples of the patients were analyzed immediately before chemotherapeutic treatment. The data obtained from peripheral blood mononucleated leukocytes (PBML) of patients were compared with those obtained from the cells of 10 normal healthy donors used as controls.

Flow Cytometric Analysis

Peripheral blood mononucleated leukocytes (PBML) obtained by separation on a 1077 density gradient (Histopaque) were incubated with monoclonal antibody anti-LFA-1α labeled with FITC at the dilution of 1:20 for 30 min at room temperature. Flow cytometric measurements were performed with a FACStar Becton Dickinson (Mountain View, CA) equipped with 5 W Argon ion laser (Exc.488 nm; Em. Green 515-550 nm). For each sample 20,000 cells were analyzed. Data were stored in a list mode software program (Hewlett Packard), which allows visualization of multivariate analysis. Slide preparations were made for each sample. Slides were stained with immunofluorescent stain using the same antibody and examined with a fluorescence microscope.

Statistical Analysis

For statistical analysis all data are reported as mean $\pm$ standard deviation (SD); comparison between values were carried out using Student's *t*-test to determine the significance between groups. A level of $p < 0.05$ was accepted as statistically significant.

RESULTS AND DISCUSSION

LFA-1 expression was evaluated on PBML of GBL patients using flow cytometric measurements. TABLE 1 shows the percentage of LFA-1 positive cells obtained from

TABLE 1. Percentage of LFA-1 Positive Cells Detected on Lymphocyte Surface of GBL Patients

Cases	Mean ± SD	Range
Patients ($N = 10$)	41.9 ± 11.3	30.36–60.87
Controls ($N = 10$)	44.8 ± 7.8	33.9–55.9

Data are compared with healthy controls. The analysis was performed using a monoclonal antibody anti-LFA-1d labeled with FITC. Results are given as mean ± standard deviation.

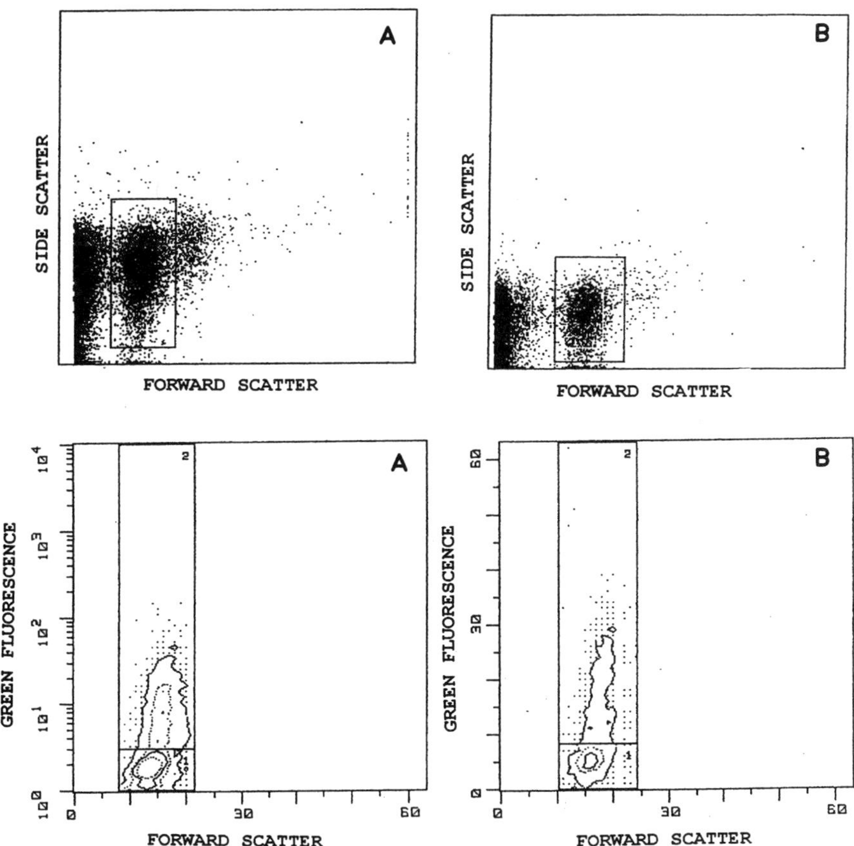

FIGURE 1. Flow cytometric measurement of PBML stained with immunofluorescence using monoclonal antibody anti-LFA-1α labeled with FITC. The forward scatter and side scatter of the cells show the cellular dimension and the percentage of the fluorescence signal, respectively. (A) healthy control blood sample and (B) GBL patient blood sample.

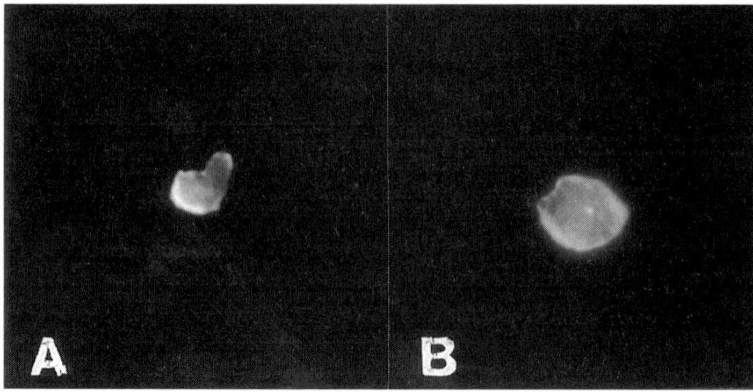

FIGURE 2. Immunofluorescence staining of GBL patient peripheral blood lymphocytes using monoclonal antibody anti-LFA-1α labeled with FITC. (A) "hand-mirror shape" lymphocyte with polar distribution of reactivity to cellular uropod and (B) round lymphocyte with intense diffuse reactivity on the cell surface (× 1,200).

patients and controls. No statistically significant differences of LFA-1 expression were found in patient lymphocytes (41.9 ± 11.3) compared with healthy control lymphocytes (44.8 ± 7.8). A wide interindividual variability of LFA-1 was observed in both groups. FIGURE 1 shows examples of flow cytometric measurements of peripheral blood cell samples from healthy controls (A) compared with those of the patients (B). Light-scattering properties of the cells are displayed as forward scatter (cell dimension) versus side scatter (green fluorescence staining of the cells). The levels of forward and side scatter of these two samples (A = control cells) (B = patient cells) presented similar regions without significant differences. FIGURE 2(A) showed a characteristic activated lymphocyte with "hand-mirror shape" and strong polarization of immunofluorescence stain. In FIGURE 2(B), a round lymphocyte is observed. The immunofluorescent staining, distributed around the cell membrane, shows intense reactivity.

An increased concentration of sICAM-1 serum levels has been repeatedly reported in patients with multiple sclerosis, viral encephalitis, and other immunological diseases.[11] These findings suggest the possibility that sICAM-1 serum levels may be considered a useful indicator of inflammatory disease in the brain.[5,11] No data on sICAM-1 serum levels in GBL patients are reported in the literature. An increased ICAM-1 expression was described on the membrane of tumor and endothelial cells of glioblastoma.[12,13] In contrast with the increased expression of ICAM-1 on tumor and endothelial cells of GBL, immunoreactivity against the brain tumor is downregulated. It could be hypothesized that the diminished immunoreactivity is due to increased sICAM-1 serum levels. Our previous data demonstrate that sICAM-1 serum levels in GBL patients are not different from those of controls.[7] Results from this study are still preliminary. Nevertheless the absence of significant difference in LFA-1 expression in GBL patients and controls suggests that the LFA-1/ICAM-1 system does not play an important role in downregulating immunoreactivity in glioblastoma.

The presence of other molecules produced by tumoral cells able to inhibit the efficacy of the immune system are probably involved.

REFERENCES

1. SANCHEZ-MADRID, F., J. A. NAGY, E. ROBBINS, P. SIMON & T. A. SPRINGEL. 1983. J. Exp. Med. **158:** 1785–1803.
2. SPRINGER, T. A., M. L. DUSTIN, T. K. KISHIMOTO & S. D. MARLIN. 1985. Ann. Rev. Immunol. **5:** 223–252.
3. ANDERSON, D. C. & T. A. SPRINGER. 1987. Annu. Rev. Med. **38:** 175–194.
4. KISHIMOTO, T. K., R. S. LARSON, A. L. CORBI, M. L. DUSTIN, D. E. STAUNION & T. A. SPRINGER. 1989. Adv. Immunol. **46:** 149–182.
5. RIECKMANN, P., U. MICHEL, M. ALBRECHT, W. BRUCK, L. WÖCKEL & K. FELGENHAUER. 1995. J. Neuroimmunol. **60:** 9–15.
6. KLEIHUES, P., F. SOYLEMEZOGLU, B. SCHAUBLE, B. W. SCHEITHAUER & P. C. BIURGER. 1995. Glia **15:** 211–221.
7. CAPELLI, E., R. NANO, F. ARGENTINA, M. CIVALLERO, K. MARINU-AKTIPI, L. LORUSSO & M. CERONI. 1996. Clin. Neuropathol. **15**(3): 166.
8. SPRINGER, T. A. & D. C. ANDERSON. 1986. *In* Human Myeloid and Hematopoietic Cells. E. L. Reinherz, B. F. Haynes, L. M. Nadler & I. D. Bernstein, Eds. Vol. 3. Springer-Verlag. New York.
9. KLEIHUES, P., P. C. BURGER & B. W. SCHEITHAUER. 1993. Brain Pathol. **3:** 255–268.
10. MICHOTTE, A. 1996. Acta Neurol. Belg. **96:** 85–88.
11. HARTUNG, H. P., M. MICHELS, K. REINERS, P. SEELDRAYERS, J. J. ARCHELOS & K. V. TOYKA. 1993. Neurology **43:** 2331–2335.
12. GINGRAS, M. C., E. ROUSSEL, J. M. BRUNER, C. D. BRANCH & R. P. MOSER. 1995. J. Neuroimmunol. **57:** 143–153.
13. LOSSINSKY, A. S., M. J. MOSSAKOWSKI, R. PLUTA & H. M. WISNIEWSKI. 1995. Brain Pathol. **5:** 339–344.

Interaction *in Vivo* between Tumor Cells and Phagocytes

ANTONIA NOTARIO, IOLANDA MAZZUCCHELLI,
GIANLUCA FOSSATI, ANDREA BALDI, AND MARIA LAURA ROLANDI

Department of Internal Medicine and Medical Therapy
Institute of Medical Therapy
University of Pavia
I-27100 Pavia, Italy

What role do phagocytes play in malignant neoplastic growth? Are the phagocytes an obstacle to tumor expansion or do they contribute directly or indirectly to tumor growth and metastatization? The answer to both questions is most likely yes; in fact a consistent number of observations outline the ambivalence of the macrophage-granulocyte system in dependence of the particular moment of the neoplastic growth and of the multifactorial activity of the cells.

The antitumoral activity of phagocytes seems to be confirmed by several different studies, but their properties are so vast that they may also have an opposite effect on the tumor progression. It is sufficient to mention the complex activities performed by cytokines produced by phagocytes and correlated cells (lymphocytes and endothelial cells) subsequent to tumor growth and the concomitant infections often present. On this basis we can understand the possible double role played by phagocytes, in function of the moment and modality of their action. The antineoplastic activity of granulocytes, monocytes, and macrophages has been documented by numerous observations of which we will mention only a few of the most significant. (*1*) Without doubt, the granulo-monocyte and macrophage (GMM) system has a fundamental role in the defense of the organism against various pathological agents, including neoplastic cells.[1–8] A possible example is given by the hepatic macrophage system, which acts as a filter against most circulating neoplastic cells that pass through the liver. It is believed that almost 100% of these cells are destroyed in this site. Only in certain conditions are some neoplastic cells capable of passing through the filter and colonizing the liver or other organs.[8] (*2*) Monocytes and granulocytes produce cytotoxic molecules (free radicals, NO, monokines, IL-1, IL-6, IL-8, TNFα, etc.), hydrogen peroxide superoxide anions, lytic enzymes (lysozyme and others), PGs, LTs, thromboxans), which have an inhibiting action on tumor growth and may determine the lysis of neoplastic cells.[9] (*3*) IL-1, IL-2, IL-4, CRP, LPS, picolinic acid, and amino acid catabolites, GM-CSF, INF, and other substances inhibiting neoplastic growth seem to work by activating the GMM system, with an increase in phagocytosis, in the production of lytic enzymes, peroxides, TNFα, and the tumoricide effect and in an exaltation of chemotaxis.[10–27] (*4*) In experimental conditions, the BCG vaccine determines an infiltrate of macrophages within the tumor and in this way inhibits the growth of the tumor.[28] (*5*) Certain bacterial extracts (streptococcal) and some viruses determine *in vitro* and *in vivo,* even in man, a regression and an involution of some tumors. This phenomenon is determined by a granulocyte-macrophage infiltrate within the tumor's microambience.[29–31]

However there are certain observations that tend to favor the other role played by phagocytes and that lead us to think, that thanks to the activity of GMM system, in particular conditions neoplastic growth may be favored. (*1*) In chronic inflammatory processes affecting different sites (lungs, kidneys, gastrointestinal tract, etc.) and caused by different pathogens (bacterial, viral, traumatic, foreign body) the GMM system reacts by liberating substances that act on the metabolism of the surrounding cells determining alterations, some of which are irreversible and transmittable, if the damaged cells are able to maintain their capacity of proliferating.[30,31] (*2*) Tumor growth depends on the possibility of developing a sufficient vascular system that is able to guarantee cellular respiration and maintain an equilibrium with the angiogenetic and angiostatic factors. Neoplastic cells participate in this process. They are responsible for the degeneration of the extracellular matrix and for stimulating the proliferation and migration of surrounding capillary endothelial cells.[32] Granulocytes and macrophages, which are the highest producers of cytokines, including growth and angiogenic factors, without doubt favor neoplastic growth.[33] (*3*) Mononucleated phagocytes present in the lymphoreticular infiltrate of malignant tumors produce procoagulating substances, which condition tumor cell formation of fibrin. This factor, under different points of view, may favor tumor progression. On the other hand, even the opposite phenomenon, the production of plasminogen activators capable of degrading the fibrin that forms around the neoplasm, may favor neoplastic growth.[34–37] (*4*) Phagocytes have an inhibitory action of the activity of the lymphocytic system and on lymphocyte response to mitogens and to DNCB.[38,40] (*5*) Experimental antigranulocyte antibodies administered to mice with ultraviolet-induced carcinoma determine the arrest of tumor growth. Also, researchers have seen that the removal of granulocytes by means of granulocyto-apheresis from the peripheral blood of patients with advanced-stage carcinoma caused an improvement of the entire clinical picture, sometimes associated with a reduction of the tumor mass.[41,42] (*6*) It has been demonstrated that metalloproteinase, liberated by monocytes present in human carcinomas of the colon and rectum, is able to degrade the matrix of the perineoplastic tissue, thus favoring the expansion of the tumor.[43] (*7*) Generally, phagocytes seem to have a negative action, not only on the tumor expansion, but on the economy of the entire organism, in that IL-6 produced by monocytes under the action of activated IL-1r seems to be responsible for the cachexia that accompanies tumors.[44,45]

It is important to remember that numerous studies exist that without doubt demonstrate that the presence of a growing neoplasm within a tissue determines a functional alteration of all the GMM elements, with a reduction of their chemotactic activity, their oxidative metabolism, the production of oxygen, and cytokine liberation.[46,47]

From what we have seen, it is obviously difficult to define exactly to what extent the GMM system constitutes a barrier to neoplastic growth and how the complex activity of the elements that make up this system, which are responsible for protecting the organism from endogenous and exogenous pathological agents, may be transferred and thus favor the expansion of the pathological process present. It is easy to see how a tumor may be responsible for important damage to the GMM system by reducing the specific functional activities.

Recently, we thought it useful to re-check, in particular, this aspect of the relationship between phagocytes and tumors, to see up to what point the variations of the principal functional activities of phagocytes could be associated with contemporary variations of a few of the most significative cell markers and of some of the correlated cytokines, including soluble adhesion molecules, that have an important place in the tumor growth and in GMM activity.[48–53]

METHODS

The research was conducted on circulating granulocytes and monocytes of normal subjects,[20] of subjects with carcinoma of the colon-rectum,[20] and carcinoma of the kidney.[5] In the subjects affected by malignant tumors the determination was carried out on peripheral venous blood and on venous blood deriving from the tumor taken during an operation.

Granulocytes, separated on Ficoll-Hypaque from other hematic elements, were studied to determine their functionality, in particular, chemotaxis, random migration (RM), and, after autologous (SA) serum, heterologous serum (SE), and casein (CAS) stimulation, the percentage of cells capable of phagocytosis and basal oxidative metabolism (evaluated as mean fluorescence of dichlorofluorescein-acetate-MFI of DCFH).

With immunofluorescent methods and cytofluorimetric analysis the manifestation of the following membrane cell markers were studied on the leukocyte population: CD2, CD19, CD3, DR, CD16, CD11b, CD14, CD54, IL-2r, IL-1ar, G-CSFr, GM-CSFr, TNFr, EGFr, IL-1r.

With the immunoenzymatic method (ELISA) the following plasmatic soluble factors were evaluated: sICAM-1, sELAM-1, sCD44vb, sIL-6r, sTNFr 60 kD, sTNFr 80 kD. Results have been reported in FIGURES 1–7.

RESULTS AND CONCLUSIONS

The results obtained from the study of peripheral granulocyte and monocyte function (FIG. 1) are, for the most part, in agreement with what has already been stated in current literature. The results confirm a reduction of the functional activity and in particular of phagocytosis and chemotaxis, in the presence of both autologous and heterologous serum, but not in the presence of casein.

The variations of chemotaxis seem to indicate a direct influence of the tumor on circulating granulocytes and monocytes, in that the reduction seen is more evident in the cells isolated from blood that derives directly from the tumor, than not in those present in the peripheral blood of the same patient. Basal production of hydrogen peroxide and RM values were within normal limits.

The degree of manifestation of the different cell markers examined varies for the different cell types.

The lymphocyte population examined presents a significant increase of NK cells (CD16) and of adhesion molecules CD11b, while mature T-lymphocytes (CD3) seem to be reduced (FIG. 2). These variations are clearly more evident in lymphocytes present in blood that derives directly from the tumor. IL-6r and IL-2r both showed a

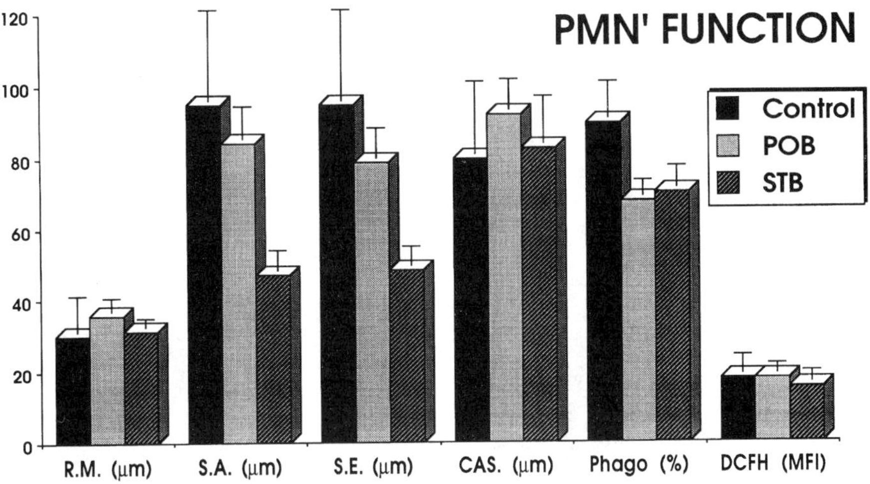

FIGURE 1. Peripheral granulocyte and monocyte function.

modest, but constant, increase compared with controls, with a higher intensity in those elements present in peripheral blood compared to those in the blood that derives from the neoplasm.

The most important result regarding monocytes (FIG. 3) was the increase of IL-6r, followed by an analogous, but less intense, increase of IL-1ar; the adhesion molecules CD11b were modestly reduced; and the variations of the other components examined (CD14, CD54, TNFr, G-CSFr, GM-CSFr) were not significant.

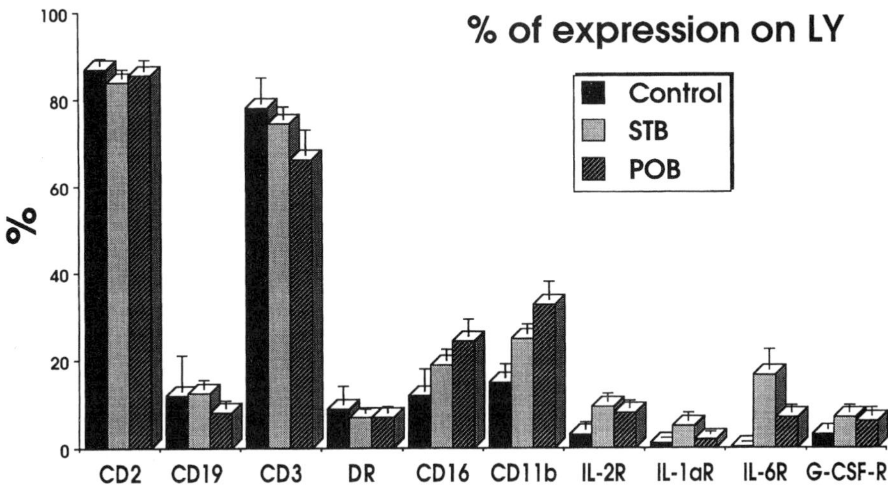

FIGURE 2. Results in lymphocyte population.

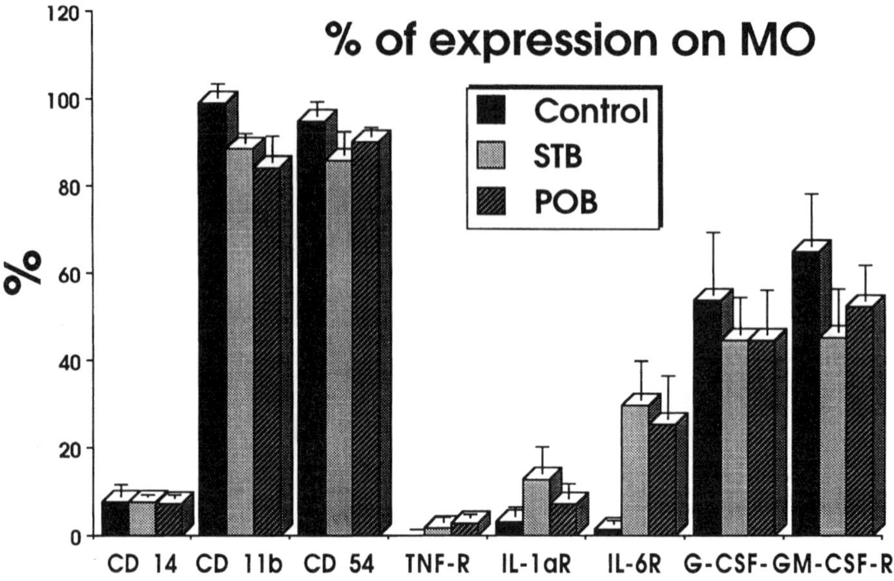

FIGURE 3. Percentage of expression on monocytes (MO).

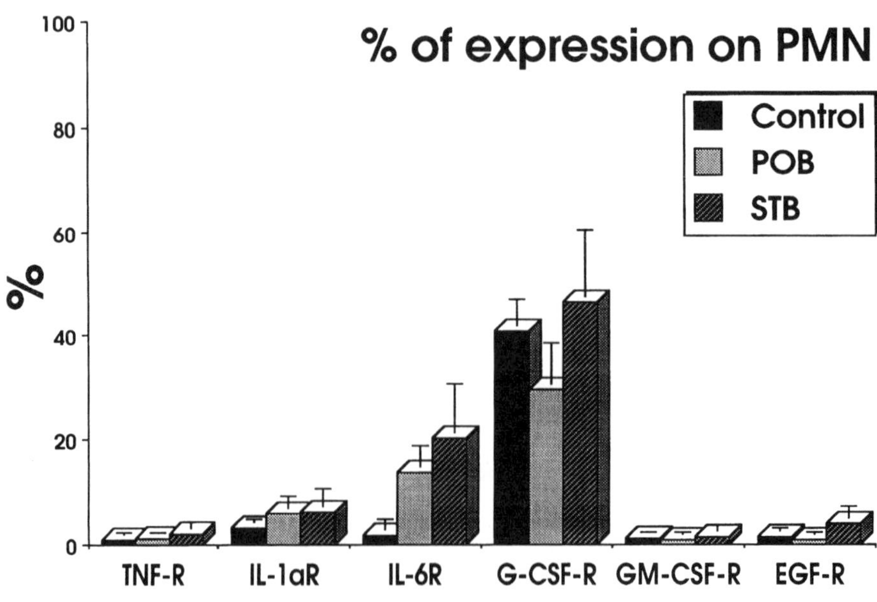

FIGURE 4. Percentage of expression on neutrophils (PMN).

There was also an analogous significant increase of IL-6r in neutrophils (FIGS. 4 and 5), but the increase in CD11b was less evident. The reduction of the granulocyte Fc receptor III (CD16) was also significant.

With respect to the soluble components of the serum, there was a more evident increase in the adhesion molecules of SICAM-1, of sTNFr-60kD, and sTNFr-80kD, while the variations of the other soluble components were less significant.

The results seem to confirm that the passage of blood through the tumoral mass determines functional alterations of leukocytes; alterations that, as far as neutrophils and monocytes are concerned, correspond to a reduction of phagocytosis function and chemotaxis, resulting from cell alterations, that do not depend on the presence, in the circulating blood, of tumor-produced inhibiting substances given that the variations are quantitatively superior in blood derived from the tumor and are similar in presence of SE and SA.

These functional alterations are associated with complex modifications of receptor distribution of these elements, which may also implicate modifications in the capability of answering to stimuli, with an exaltation of some adhesion molecules and a reduction of other important receptors, such as IL-6, that marks the Fc receptor III. With respect to this last fact, we should note that the concomitant decrease of the percentage of phagocytosing cells leads us to think of a possible direct effect of the neoplastic cells, which leads to a blinding of the phagocytes, which therefore become less active in the process of recognizing and attacking the neoplastic cells.

The increase of sICAM-1, associated with the increase of CD11b, indicates that the process of transmigration and accumulation of phagocytes in the inflammatory site has already taken place, while the increase of the two fractions of sTNF may indicate that the immune system has not been completely "put aside" by the tumoral cells, but that the production of antitumoral cytokines is present, even though it is difficult to determine if the increase is due to granulocyte stimulation or directly dependent on the tumoral cells.

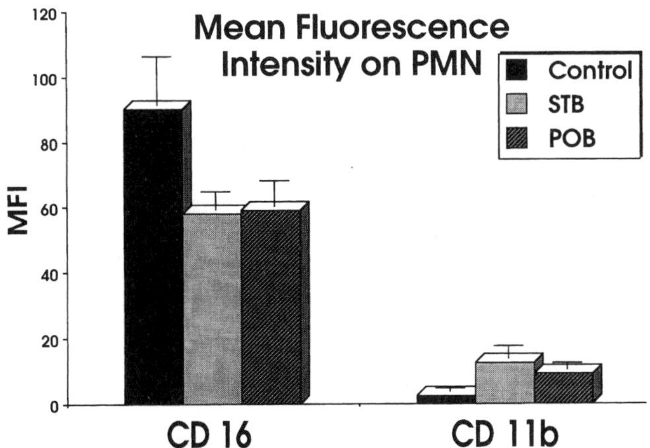

FIGURE 5. Mean fluorescence intensity on neutrophils (PMN).

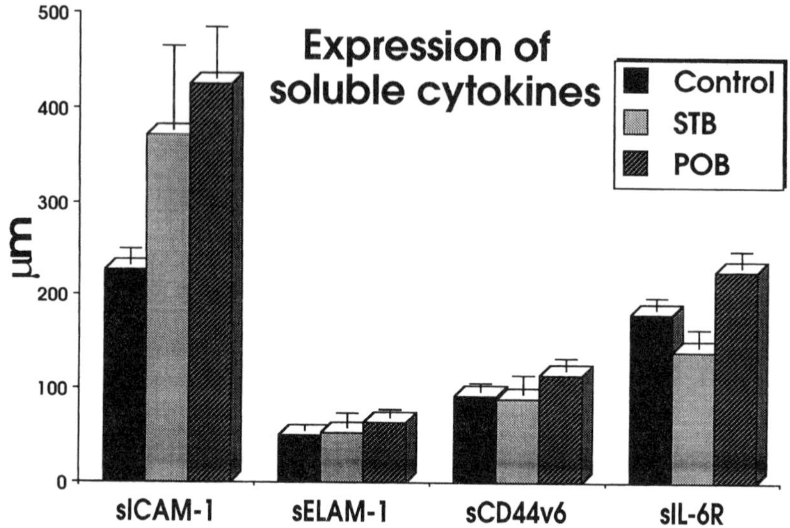

FIGURE 6. Expression of soluble cytokines.

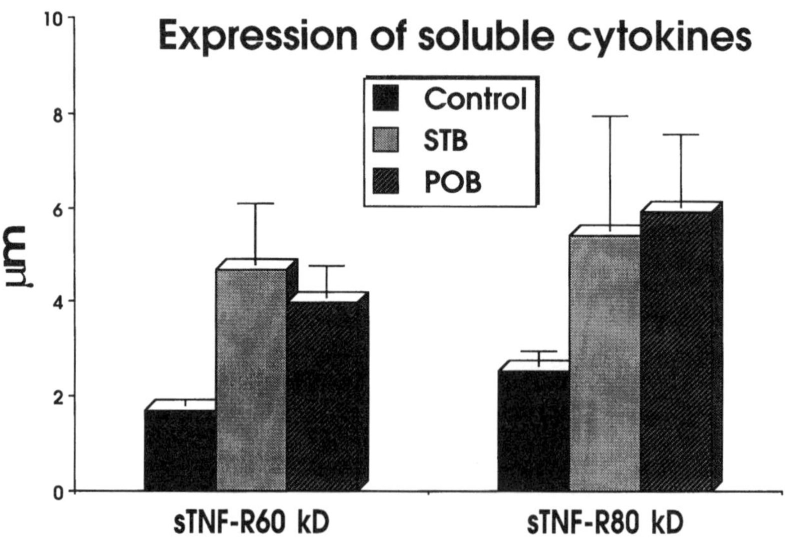

FIGURE 7. Expression of soluble cytokines.

The study conducted therefore demonstrates how the immune system becomes active, producing cytokines and NK cells, as an efficient response to the neoplastic cells, and yet the neoplastic cells seem to possess mechanisms capable of reducing the aggressiveness of phagocytes.

ACKNOWLEDGMENTS

A special thanks for the collaboration to the doctors: Donatella Gritti, Claudia Canale, Ocar Epis, Marilena Celano, Giovanni Evangelisti, MauroMorone, Camillo Porta, Adriana Lattanzi.

REFERENCES

1. FIDLER, I. J. & E. S. KLEINERMAN. 1993. Therapy of cancer metastasis by systemic activation of macrophages: from the bench to the clinic. Res. Immunol. **144:** 284–287.
2. KATANO, M. & M. TORISU. 1982. Neutrophil-mediated tumor cell destruction in cancer ascites. Cancer **50:** 62–68.
3. FURUKAWA, T., S. WATANABE, T. KODAMA, Y. SATO, Y. SHIMOSATO & K. SUEMASU. 1985. T-Zone histiocytes in adenocarcinoma of the lung in relation to postoperative prognosis. Cancer **56:** 2651–2656.
4. ADAMS, D. O., W. J. JOHNSON & P. A. MARINO. 1982. Mechanisms of target recognition and destruction in macrophage-mediated tumor cytotoxicity. Fed. Proc. **41:** 2212–2221.
5. COLOTTA, F., L. BERSANI, C. BALOTTA, J. M. WANG & A. MANTOVANI. 1987. The interaction of mononuclear phagocytes with neoplastic cells: regulation of tumor cells susceptibility to killing and monocyte chemotaxis. Adv. Biosci. **66:** 467–473.
6. CAMERON, D. J. 1982. In vivo macrophage-mediated tumor cytotoxicity in the mouse. Immunol. Lett. **4:** 321–325.
7. BARBERA-GUILLEM, E., I. SMITH & L. WEISS. 1993. Cancer-cell traffic in the liver. II. Arrest, transit and death of B16, F1O and M5076 cells in the sinusoids. Int. J. Cancer. **53:** 298–301.
8. WU, S., C. M. BOYER, R. S. WHITAKER, A. BERCHUCK, J. R. WIENER, J. B. WEINBERG & R. C. BAST, JR. 1993. Tumor necrosis factor alfa as an autocrine and paracrine growth factor for ovarian cancer: monokine induction of tumor cell proliferation and tumor necrosis factor alfa expression. Cancer Res. **53:** 1939–1944.
9. NATHAN, C. F., C. R. HOROWITZ, J. HARPE, S. VADHAN-RAJ, S. A. SHERWIN, H. F. OETTGEN & S. E. KROWN. 1985. Administration of recombinant interferon gamma to cancer patients enhances monocyte secretion of hydrogen peroxide. Proc. Natl. Acad. Sci. USA **82:** 8686–8690.
10. NAYLOR, M. S., G. W. H. STAMP, W. D. FOULKES, D. ECCLES & F. R. BALKWILL. 1993. Tumor necrosis factor and its receptors in human ovarian cancer. J. Clin. Invest. **91:** 2194–2206.
11. CARUSO, M., Y. PANIS, S. GAGANDEEP, D. HOUSSIN, J. P. SALZMANN & D. KLATZMANN. 1993. Regression of established macroscopic liver metastases after in situ transduction of a suicide gene. Proc. Natl. Acad. Sci. USA **90:** 7024–7028.
12. TEPPER, R. I., R. L. COFFMAN & P. LEDER. 1992. An eosinophil-dependent mechanism for the antitumor effect of interleukin-4. Science **257:** 548–551.
13. JAYARAM, Y., A. M. BUCKLE & N. HOGG. 1989. The Fc receptor, FCRI, and other activation molecules on human mononuclear phagocytes after treatment with interferon-gamma. Clin. Exp. Immunol. **75:** 414–420.

14. KUNDIG, T. M., M. F. BACHMANN, L. LEFRANCOIS, L. PUDDINGTON, H. HENGARTNER & R. M. ZINKERNAGEL. 1993. Nonimmunogenic tumor cells may efficiently restimulate tumor antigen-specific cytotoxic T cells. J. Immunol. **150:** 4450–4456.

15. LITTON, M. J., M. DOHLSTEN, P. A. LANDO, T. KALLAND, L. OHLSSON, J. ANDERSSON & U. ANDERSSON. 1996. Antibody-targeted superantigen therapy induces tumor-infiltrating lymphocytes, excessive cytokine production, and apoptosis in human colon carcinoma. Eur. J. Immunol. **26:** 1–9.

16. WING, E. J. M. MAGEE, T. L. WHITESIDE, S. S. KAPLAN & R. K. SHADDUCK. 1989. Recombinant human granulocyte/macrophage colony-stimulating factors enhances monocyte cytotoxicity and secretion of tumor necrosis factors alfa and interferon in cancer patients. Blood **73:** 643–646.

17. STOPPACCIARO, A., C. MELANI, M. PARENZA, A. MASTRACCHIO, C. BASSI, C. BARONI, G. PARMIANI & M. P. COLOMBO. 1993. Regression of an established tumor genetically modified to release granulocyte colony-stimulating factor requires granulocyte-T cell cooperation and T cell-produced interferon gamma. J. Exp. Med. **178:** 151–161.

18. LICHTENSTEIN, A. 1985. Rejection of murine ovarian cancer following treatment with regional immunotherapy: correlations with a neutrophil mediated activation of cytostatic macrophages. Cellular Immunol. **94:** 521–535.

19. MIZOI, T., H. OHTANI, K. MIYAZONO, M. MIYAZAWA, S. MATSUNO & H. NAGURA. 1993. Immunoelectron microscopic localization of transforming beta 1 binding protein in human gastrointestinal carcinomas. Qualitative difference between cancer cells and stromal cells. Cancer Res. **53:** 183–190.

20. CONKLING, P. R., C. C. CHUA, P. NADLER, C. S. GREENBERG, E. DOTY, M. A. MISUKONIS, A. F. HANEY, R. C. BAST, JR. & J. B. WEINBERG. 1988. Clinical trials with human tumor necrosis factor: In vivo and in vitro effects on human mononuclear phagocyte function. Cancer Res. **48:** 5604–5609.

21. BRAUN, D. P., M. C. AHN, J. E. HARRIS, E. CHU, L. CASEY, G. WILBANKS & K. P. SIZIO PIKOU. 1993. Sensitivity of tumoricidal function in macrophages from different anatomical sites of cancer patients to modulation of arachidonic acid metabolism. Cancer Res. **53:** 3362–3368.

22. SAGONE, A. L., JR., R. M. HUSNEY, P. L. TRIOZZI & J. RINEHART. 1991. Interleukin2 therapy enhances salicylate oxidation by blood granulocytes. Blood **78:** 2931–2936.

23. BOSCO, M. C., G. L. GUSELLA, I. ESPINOZA-DELGADO, D. L. LONGO & L. VARESIO. 1994. Interferon-gamma upregulates interleukin-8 gene expression in human monocytic cells by a posttranscriptional mechanism. Blood **83:** 537–542.

24. JOHNSON, G. S., R. M. FRIEDMAN & I. PASTAN. 1971. Restoration of several morphological characteristics of normal fibroblasts in sarcoma cells treated with adenosine-3′:5′-cyclic monophosphate and its derivatives. Proc. Natl. Acad. Sci. USA **68:** 425–429.

25. DONG, Z. X. QI, K. XIE & I. J. FIDLER. 1993. Protein tyrosine kinase inhibitors decrease induction of nitric oxide synthase activity in lipopolysaccharide-responsive and lipopolysaccharide-nonresponsive murine macrophages. J. Immunol. **151:** 2717–2724.

26. MELILLO, G., G. W. COX, D. RADZIOCH & L. VARESIO. 1993. Picolinic acid, a catabolite of L-tryptophan, is a costimulus for the induction of reactive nitrogen intermediate production in murine macrophages. J. Immunol. **150:** 4031–4040.

27. MELTZER, M. S., M. OCCHIONERO & L. P. RUCO. 1982. Macrophage activation for tumor cytotoxicity: regulatory mechanisms for induction and control of cytotoxic activity. Fed. Proc. **41:** 2198–2205.

28. AKAZA, H., A. IWASAKI, M. OHTANI, N. IKEDA, K. NIIJIMA, I. TOIDA & K. KOISO. 1993. Expression of antitumor response. Cancer **72:** 558–563.

29. SINGH, R. K., K. BERRY, K. MATSUSHIMA, K. YASUMOTO & I. J. FIDLER. 1993. Synergism between human monocyte chemotactic and activating factor and bacterial products for

activation of tumoricidal properties in murine macrophages. J. Immunol. **151:** 2786–2793.

30. WEITZMAN, S., C. SCHMEICHEL, P. TURK, C. STEVENS, S. TOLSMA & N. BOUCK. 1988. Phagocyte-mediated carcinogenesis: DNA from phagocyte-transformed C3H 1OT1/2 cells can transform NIH/3T3 Cells. Ann. N. Y. Acad. Sci. **551:** 103–110.

31. TRUSH, M. A., J. L. SEED & T. W. KENSLER. 1985. Oxidant-dependent metabolic activation of polycyclic aromatic hydrocarbons by phorbolester-stimulated human polymorphonuclear leukocytes: Possible link between inflammation and cancer. Proc. Natl. Acad. Sci. USA **82:** 5194–5198.

32. STRIETER, R. M., P. J. POLVERINI, D. A. ARENBERG, A. WALZ, G. OPDENAKKER, J. VAN DAMME & S. L. KUNKEL. 1995. Role of C-X-C chemokines as regulators of angiogenesis in lung cancer. J. Leukocyte Biol. **57:** 752–762.

33. LEWIS, C. E., R. LEEK, A. HARRIS & J. O. D. MCGEE. 1995. Cytokine regulation of angiogenesis in breast cancer: the role of tumor-associated macrophages. J. Leukocyte Biol. **57:** 747–751.

34. MUSSONI, L., M. RIGANTI, R. ACERO, A. ERROI, G. CONFORTI & A. MANTOVANI. 1988. Macrophages associated with murine tumours express plasminogen activator activity. Int. J. Cancer **41:** 227–230.

35. SEMERARO, N., O. DE LUCIA, A. LATTANZIO, P. MONTEMURRO, D. GIORDANO, M. LOIZZI & F. CARPAGNANO. 1986. Procoagulant activity of human alveolar macrophages: different expression in patients with lung cancer. Int. J. Cancer **37:** 525–529.

36. LORENZET, R., G. PERI, D. LOCATI, P. ALLAVENA, M. COLUCCI, N. SEMERARO, A. MANTOVANI & M. B. DONATI. 1983. Generation of procoagulant activity by mononuclear phagocytes: a possible mechanism contributing to blood clotting activation within malignant tissues. Blood **62:** 271–273.

37. PYKE, C., N. GRAEM, E. RALFKIAER, E. RONNE, G. HOYER-HANSEN, N. BRUNNER & K. DANO. 1993. Receptor for urokinase is present in tumor associated macrophages in ductal breast carcinoma. Cancer Res. **53:** 1911–1915.

38. ZIGHELBOIM, J., F. DOREY, N. H. PARKER, T. CALCATERRA, P. WARD & J. L. FAHEY. 1979. Immunologic evaluation of patients with advanced head and neck cancer receiving weekly chemoimmunotherapy. Cancer **44:** 117–123.

39. HARA, N., Y. ICHINOSE, H. ASOH, T. YANO, M. KAWASAKI & M. OHTA. 1992. Superoxide anion-generating activity of polymorhonuclear leukocytes and monocytes in patients with lung cancer. Cancer **69:** 1682–1687.

40. MANSON, L. A. 1991. Does antibody-dependent epitope masking permit progressive tumour growth in the face of cell-mediated cytotoxicity? Immunol. Today **12:** 352–355.

41. PEKAREK, L. A., B. A. STARR, A. Y. TOLEDANO & H. SCHREIBER. 1995. Inhibition of tumor growth by elimination of granulocytes. J. Exp. Med. **181:** 435–440.

42. TABUCHI, T., H. UBUKATA, S. SATO, I. NAKATA, Y. GOTO, Y. WATANABE, T. HASHIMOTO, T. MIZUTA, M. ADACHI & T. SOMA. 1995. Granulocytapheresis as a possible cancer treatment. Anticancer Res. **15:** 985–990.

43. STRASSMANN, G., C. O. JACOB, R. EVANS, D. BEALL & M. FONG. 1992. Mechanisms of experimental cancer cachexia. Interaction between mononuclear phagocytes and colon-26 carcinoma and its relevance to IL-6 mediated cancer cachexia. J. Immunol. **148:** 3674–3678.

45. STRASSMANN, G., Y. MASUI, R. CHIZZONITE & M. FONG. 1993. Mechanisms of experimental cancer cachexia. Local involvement of IL-1 in colon26 tumor. J. Immunol. **150:** 2341–2345.

46. GAVISON, R. & Z. BAR-SHAVIT. 1989. Impaired macrophage activation in vitamin D3 deficiency: differential in vitro effects of 1,25 dihydroxyvitamin D3 on mouse peritoneal macrophage functions. J. Immunol. **143:** 3686–3690.

47. SHIEH, J. H., R. H. F. PETERSON, D. J. WARREN & M. A. S. MOORE. 1989. Modulation of colony-stimulating factors-1 receptors on macrophages by tumor necrosis factor. J. Immunol. **143:** 2534–2539.

48. DE NICHILO, M. O. & G. F. BURNS. 1993. Granulocyte-macrophage and macrophage colony-stimulating factors differentially regulate alfa v integrin expression on cultured human macrophages. Proc. Natl. Acad. Sci. USA **90:** 2517–2521.

49. STEINBACH, F., K. TANABE, J. ALEXANDER, M. EDINGER, R. TUBBS, W. BRENNER, M. STOCKLE, A. C. NOVICK & E. A. KLEIN. 1996. The influence of cytokines on the adhesion of renal cancer cells to endothelium. J. Urol. **155:** 743–748.

50. MAYET, W. J., A. SCHWARTING, T. ORTH, R. DUCHMANN & K. H. DE MEYER ZUM BUSCHENFEL. 1996. Antibodies to proteinase 3 mediate expression of vascular cell adhesion molecule-1 (VCAM-1). Clin. Exp. Immunol. **103:** 259–267.

51. RAINGER, G. E., M. P. WAUTIER, G. B. NASH & J. L. WAUTIER. 1996. Prolonged E-selectin induction by monocytes potentiates the adhesion of flowing neutrophils to cultured endothelial cells. Br. J. Haematol. **92:** 192–199.

52. GORSKI, A. 1994. The role of cell adhesion molecules in immunopathology. Immunol. Today **15:** 251–255.

53. LESTER, B. R. & J. B. MCCARTHY. 1992. Tumor cell adhesion to the extracellular matrix and signal transduction mechanisms implicated in tumor cell motility, invasion and metastasis. Cancer Metastasis Rev. **11:** 31–44.

Cationic Protein-Rich Supernatants of Cultured Eosinophils from IL-2-Treated Patients Have No Cytotoxic Activity on Human Renal Cell Carcinoma and Melanoma Cells: A Preliminary Report

M. MORONI, C. PORTA, D. GRITTI, M. DE AMICI,[a] O. GIACOBBE,[a]
E. BOBBIO-PALLAVICINI,[b] AND A. NOTARIO

Istituto di Terapia Medica
I.R.C.C.S. Policlinico San Matteo
Università degli Studi di Pavia
I-27100 Pavia, Italy

[a]Clinica Pediatrica
I.R.C.C.S. Policlinico San Matteo
Università degli Studi di Pavia
I-27100 Pavia, Italy

[b]Divisione di Medicina Generale
Ospedale Maggiore di Crema
I-26013 Crema, Italy

INTRODUCTION

Nearly all cancer patients receiving recombinant interleukin-2 (IL-2), both intravenously and subcutaneously, develop marked peripheral blood eosinophilia.[1–4] The hypereosinophilia induced by IL-2 therapy is likely to result from secondary cytokine production by IL-2–stimulated lymphocytes. Although a number of soluble factors derived from T-cells, including interleukin-5 (IL-5), granulocyte-macrophage colony-stimulating factor (GM-CSF), interleukin-3 (IL-3), interferon-γ (IFN-γ), and transforming growth factor α (TNF-α), can modulate *in vitro* the maturation and the functional activity of eosinophils,[5–7] there is now good evidence that IL-5 is the major and possibly the only cytokine involved in the production of specific eosinophilia, even in patients treated with IL-2.[8,9]

Previous studies suggested a role of eosinophils in the anticancer mechanisms induced *in vivo* by the IL-2–activated immune system.[9,10] In particular, eosinophils may be involved in the anticancer activity as effectors of direct or antibody-dependent tumor lysis, or could interact with, and potentially present the antigen to, CD4[+] lymphocytes, since the expression of HLA-DR is inducible on eosinophils.[11] *In vitro,* eosinophils from subcutaneously IL-2–treated patients showed far greater cytotoxic activity against allogeneic tumor cells than eosinophils from healthy donors or from patients before IL-2 treatment. This non-specific direct cytolysis of target cells was significantly increased by the addition of an antibody specific for the relevant antigen of target neoplastic cells.[12]

As far as the potential mechanisms of direct tumor lysis by eosinophils is concerned, it is likely that the products of oxidative metabolism may be involved.[13] Even though the oxidative products of eosinophils, including superoxide anions, hydroxyl radicals, and singlet oxygen, can damage cells, evidence suggests that the eosinophil products damaging the host most are cationic proteins.[13] Indeed, in several human inflammatory and allergic diseases, the release of eosinophils' highly cationic intracellular granule proteins by degranulation or cytolysis can damage adjoining tissues.[13–15] We therefore decided to verify the hypothesis that cationic protein–rich supernatants of cultured eosinophils from IL-2–treated cancer patients could exert a direct cytotoxic effect on allogeneic human tumor cells *in vitro*.

MATERIALS AND METHODS

Patients and IL-2 Treatment Schedule

We obtained eosinophils from three patients affected with renal cell cancer and treated subcutaneously with very low doses of recombinant IL-2, according to the treatment protocol recently proposed by Buzio *et al.*[16]

Briefly, recombinant IL-2 was given subcutaneously for five days per week, together with recombinant IFN-α by intramuscular route twice weekly, for four consecutive weeks corresponding to one therapeutic cycle. The cycle was regularly repeated at four-month intervals. Recombinant IL-2 was administered at the dose of 1 MU/m^2 every 12 hours, on days 1 and 2, followed by 0.5 MU/m^2 twice daily on days 3–5 of each week; concomitantly, IFN-α was given as 1.8 MU/m^2 on days 3 and 5 of each week.

Controls

We selected three healthy controls, matching them for sex and age with our three cancer patients, within a population of 30 adult subjects, presenting with a normal hemochrome (without hypereosinophilia), no signs of allergic, parasitic, or neoplastic diseases, and serum titers of both eosinophil cationic protein (ECP) and eosinophil protein X (EPX) within the normal range for adult Caucasian subjects (20.3 ± 10.4 µg/l for EPX and 8.9 ± 5.1 µg/l for ECP).[17]

Purification and Culture of Eosinophils

Peripheral venous blood was drawn into preservative-free heparin, and leukocytes were collected after dextran sedimentation for 45 min at room temperature. The leukocyte-rich plasma (buffy coat) was removed and washed in a Tyrode's buffer. After lysis of contaminating blood cells, leukocytes were separated by centrifugation on discontinuous metrizamide gradients, according to the technique of Vadas and coworkers,[18] adapted as previously described by Prin and coworkers.[19]

After this step, cell fractions were collected from each density layer and washed in HBBS. The degree of purity and the morphology of the cells were evaluated on cytocentrifuge preparations stained with Giemsa. Cell viability, as assessed with the Trypan blue exclusion test, was superior to 90%. Only cell fractions containing more than 85% of eosinophils, recovered at the interface between 22% and 23% metrizamide solutions, were used.[20] Separated eosinophils were then incubated at 37°C, in 5% CO_2, 7% O_2, and 88% NO_2 atmosphere, in RPMI 1640 culture medium with gentamycin (50 μg/l), glutamine (2 mM) and human serum pools at 5% in 96-well flat dishes (10^5 eosinophils/well, 6 wells/time). Supernatants were collected after an 8-day incubation and both eosinophil cationic protein (ECP) and eosinophil protein X (EPX) were assayed on them.

ECP and EPX Assay in the Supernatants of Eosinophil Cultures[21]

A sensible radioimmune method (*Ria, Pharmacia*) was used to assay serum ECP and EPX in the supernatants of eosinophil cultures in both patients and controls. The technique is based on the double antibody. Sample ECP competes with an unvarying amount of ^{125}iodine-labeled ECP (or EPX). When an immunoadsorbent antibody is added, free myeloperoxidase can be separated from bound myeloperoxidase with centrifugation and then decantation. Pellet radioactivity is measured in a γ-counter and is inversely proportional to sample ECP (or EPX) amount. Concentration (mean of 6 wells) for each time is expressed as μg/l.

Target Tumor Cells

We used two human neoplastic cell lines derived from a malignant melanoma (A375) and a renal cell carcinoma (ACHN), extensively characterized and described elsewhere.[22,23] Both cell lines were purchased from American Type Culture Collection (Rockville, MD). A375 cells were cultured in D-MEM medium supplemented with 10% fetal bovine serum, 1% L-glutamine, and 1% streptomycin-penicillin. ACHN cells were cultured in MEM-Eagle medium supplemented as above. The cultures were maintained at 37°C in a humidified atmosphere containing 5% CO_2 and passaged once weekly using a solution of trypsin (1%) in HBSS for 2 minutes at 37°C, centrifuged and seeded in 25-cm^2 flasks. Periodically, cell lines were tested for the absence of Mycoplasma with the bis-benzimide staining test.[24]

Cytotoxicity Assays

The cells from 4- to 5-day-old cultures were seeded in 24-well culture dishes at the density of 2 × 10^5 cells per well. The volume of the medium in each well was 1 ml. In order to ensure uniform attachment of cells, experiments were performed 24 hours after seeding. Then, culture media were removed from each well, and three different concentrations (1/2, 1/4, and 1/8) of supernatants from each patient's and his/her age and sex-matched control's cultured eosinophils, diluted with adequate media, were added separately. Medium alone without supernatant was added to additional wells.

The cells were grown for four additional days, replacing both culture media and supernatant solutions every day. Cell growth was assessed by counting viable cells in a hemocytometer, using Trypan blue exclusion after trypsinization. Furthermore, the colorimetric tetrazolium (MTT) cytotoxic assay was also performed, as extensively described elsewhere.[25] All experiments were done in quadruplicate.

RESULTS

Eosinophil Count in Patients and Controls

As expected, significant eosinophilia developed during the first immunotherapy cycle in all the three cancer patients examined. Moreover, high eosinophil titers were still present at the end of the same treatment cycle, when venous blood was drawn (TABLE 1). In contrast, none of the three age- and sex-matched controls presented abnormal eosinophil counts; indeed, their leukocyte count was 6.07, 6.75, and 7.25 ($\times 10^3/\mu l$), respectively, while eosinophils were 0.06, 0.135, and 0.072 ($\times 10^3/\mu l$), respectively.

ECP and EPX Assay in the Serum

An increased serum level of both ECP and EPX, reflecting IL-2–driven eosinophilic stimulation and activation, was evidenced in the three cancer patients treated with IL-2. In contrast, controls presented with ECP and EPX titers within the normal range for an adult Caucasian population (TABLE 2).[17]

TABLE 1. Absolute Values of Both Total White Blood Cells (WBC) and Eosinophils Before and After the First Cycle of IL-2–Based Immunotherapy in the Three Renal Cell Cancer Patients Examined

Patients	WBC Count before IL-2 Treatment ($\times 10^3/\mu l$)	WBC Count after IL-2 Treatment ($\times 10^3/\mu l$)	Eosinophil Count before IL-2 Treatment ($\times 10^3/\mu l$)	Eosinophil Count after IL-2 Treatment ($\times 10^3/\mu l$)
T.M., ♂ 57 years	5.99	7.48	0.059	1.122
M.M., ♀ 49 years	7.07	13.26	0.141	3.182
C.A., ♂ 65 years	5.08	9.01	0.406	2.252

TABLE 2. ECP and EPX Titers Measured in the Serum of Both IL-2–Treated Renal Cell Cancer Patients and Their Age- and Sex-Matched Controls

Patient	ECP (μg/l)	EPX (μg/l)	Control	ECP (μg/l)	EPX (μg/l)
T.M., ♂ 57 years	100.29	460.39	A.G., ♂ 57 years	4.48	9.55
M.M., ♀ 49 years	88.26	425.55	N.M., ♀ 49 years	5.02	10.21
C.A., ♂ 65 years	99.79	320.76	A.B., ♂ 65 years	7.98	13.39

ECP and EPX Assay in the Supernatants of Eosinophil Cultures

In parallel with the above serum data, cultured eosinophils from IL-2–treated patients produced amounts of ECP and EPX that were higher than those produced from healthy controls' eosinophils (TABLE 3)

Cytotoxicity Assays

No signs of growth inhibition or of cytotoxicity were found when A375 or ACHN cancer cell lines were incubated with cationic protein–rich supernatants from IL-2–treated cancer patients' or healthy controls' cultured eosinophils. As a matter of fact, using the Trypan blue dye test, the number of cells grown with cationic proteins from IL-2 *in vivo* stimulated eosinophils did not differ significantly from the number of cells grown with cationic proteins from healthy donors' eosinophils in both cell lines. Moreover, the results did not differ depending on the different concentrations outlined above (FIGS. 1 and 2). Superimposable results were obtained when the most sensible MTT assay was used (data not shown). On the contrary, a minimal—but statistically not significant—stimulation of cell growth was documented, probably due to the presence of a number of growth factors in the supernatants of cultured eosinophils.

DISCUSSION

Eosinophils are known to play a pivotal role in allergy and helminthic infections with a number of functions, such as phagocytosis of immune-complexes or micro-or-

TABLE 3. ECP and EPX Titers Measured in the Supernatants of Eosinophil Cultures from Both IL-2–Treated Renal Cell Cancer Patients and their Age- and Sex-Matched Controls

Patient	ECP (μg/l)	EPX (μg/l)	Control	ECP (μg/l)	EPX (μg/l)
T.M., ♂ 57 years	108.25	558.66	A.G., ♂ 57 years	6.78	9.02
M.M., ♀ 49 years	215.19	337.50	N.M., ♀ 49 years	7.32	16.05
C.A., ♂ 65 years	113.75	456.16	A.B., ♂ 65 years	10.28	10.56

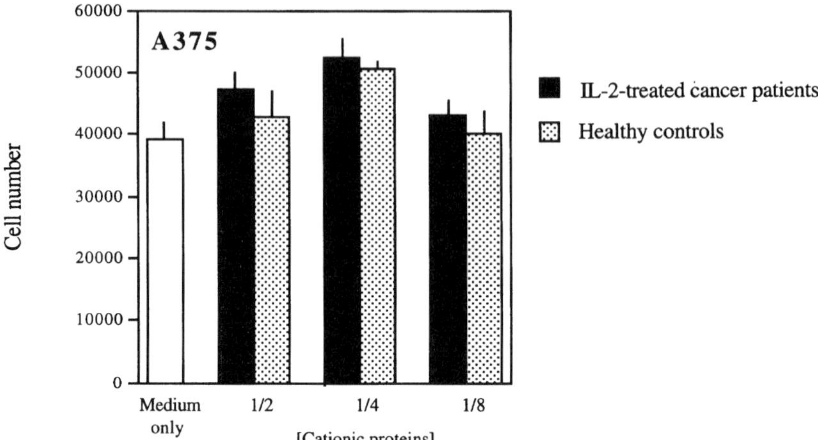

FIGURE 1. A375 melanoma cell growth was not significantly affected by the incubation with different concentrations of cationic-rich supernatants from eosinophils of IL-2–treated cancer patients or with supernatants from eosinophils of healthy controls. Results obtained with Trypan blue exclusion test and with the most specific and sensible MTT assay were superimposable.

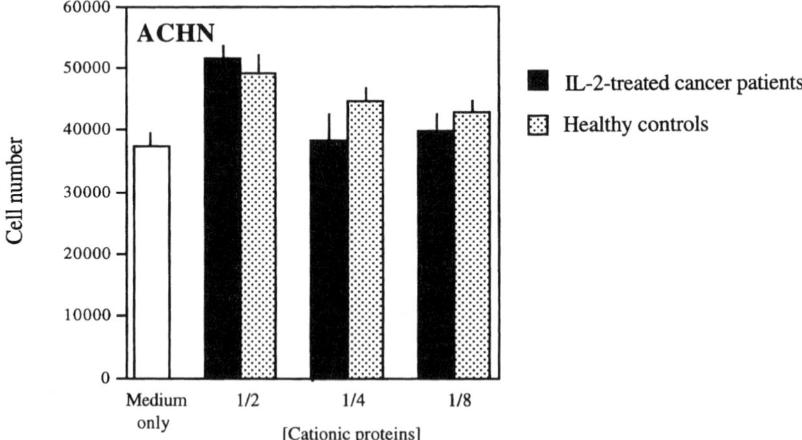

FIGURE 2. ACHN renal cell cancer growth was not significantly affected by the incubation with different concentrations of cationic-rich supernatants from eosinophils of IL-2–treated cancer patients or with supernatants from eosinophils of healthy controls. Again, results obtained with Trypan blue exclusion test and with the most specific and sensible MTT assay were superimposable.

ganisms, production of immunological regulatory factors, and secretion of toxic substances that can kill parasitic helminths or damage host tissues.[13]

Since hypereosinophilia was first described in cancer patients receiving IL-2, a possible role for eosinophils in IL-2–related anticancer activity has been postulated. In 1993, Rivoltini and colleagues demonstrated that eosinophils from cancer patients can mediate direct cytotoxicity and antibody-dependent cellular cytotoxicity *in vitro* against tumor cells after *in vivo* activation with IL-2.[12] Furthermore, one year later, Fabian and coworkers showed that the stimulating effect of IL-2/IFN-α therapy on *in vitro* eosinophils and neutrophils can mediate antileukemic activity[10] in addition to the well-known immunological effects of IL-2 on cytotoxic T-cells and natural killer cells.[26,27]

Even though the oxidative products of eosinophils, including superoxide anions, hydroxyl radicals, and singlet oxygen, can damage cells, both *in vitro* and *in vivo,* eosinophilic cationic proteins are the ideal mediators of a possible anticancer activity of eosinophils. However, such a role for these proteins has not been thoroughly investigated; as far as we know, only one report from Germany seems to support this hypothesis, revealing active degranulation of eosinophils on bladder tumor cells *in vitro.*[28] We therefore decided to challenge neoplastic cells *in vitro* with cationic protein–rich supernatants of cultured eosinophils from both IL-2–treated cancer patients and healthy controls. IL-2 treatment determined very high levels of cationic proteins in the supernatant of cultured eosinophils from our cancer patients, as demonstrated by the titration of both ECP and EPX by a sensitive radioimmunological method.[21] These data allowed us to concentrate on these attracting proteins within the likely great number of cell products present in the supernatants of cultured eosinophils.

On the basis of our preliminary results on a small sample, eosinophils seem unlikely to play a direct cytotoxic role on tumor cells *in vitro* through the release of their cationic proteins. Indeed, neither the supernatants of cultured eosinophils from IL-2–treated cancer patients nor those from healthy volunteers showed any sign of cytotoxicity on tumor cells, with no significant intergroup differences. Moreover, the number of cells grown with cationic protein–rich supernatants from both patients and healthy controls was higher than that of control cells grown with medium alone, but the difference did not reach statistical significance. This effect may be due to the presence, within the supernatants, of growth factors capable of stimulating cancer cell growth. However, the precise role of eosinophils in IL-2–treated cancer patients deserves further investigation and should and will be thoroughly addressed.

REFERENCES

1. LOTZE, M. T., Y. L. MATORY, S. E. ETTINGHAUSEN, A. A. RAYNER, S. O. SHARROW, C. A. SEIPP, M. C. CUSTER & S. A. ROSENBERG. 1985. *In vivo* administration of purified human Interleukin-2. II. Half-life, immunologic effects, and expansion of peripheral lymphoid cells *in vivo* with recombinant IL-2. J. Immunol. **135:** 2865–2875.

2. LOTZE, M. T., Y. L. MATORY, A. A. RAYNER, S. E. ETTINGHAUSEN, J. T. VETTO, C. A. SEIPP & S. A. ROSENBERG. 1986. Clinical effects and toxicity of Interleukin-2 in patients with cancer. Cancer **58:** 2764–2772.

3. ETTINGHAUSEN, S. E., J. G. MOORE, D. E. WHITE, L. PLATANIAS, N. S. YOUNG & S. A.

ROSENBERG. 1987. Hematologic effects of immunotherapy with lymphokine-activated killer cells and recombinant Interleukin-2 in cancer patients. Blood **69:** 1654–1660.

4. SCHNEEKLOTH, C., A. KÖRFER, M. HADAM, E. LOPEZ-HÄNNINEN, T. MENZEL, A. SCHOMBURG, I. DALLMANN, H. KIRCHNER, H. POLIWODA & J. ATZPODIEN. 1993. Low-dose interleukin-2 in combination with interferon-α effectively modulates biological response *in vivo.* Acta Haematol. **89:** 13–21.

5. YAMAGUCHI, Y., T. SUDA, J. SUDA, M. EGUCHI, Y. MIURA, N. HARADA, A. TOMINAGA & K. TAKATSU. 1988. Purified interleukin-5 supports the terminal differentiation and proliferation of murine eosinophilic precursors. J. Exp. Med. **167:** 43–56.

6. WELLER, P. F. 1992. Cytokine regulation of eosinophil function. Clin. Immunol. Immunopathol. **62:** S55–S59.

7. WALZ, T. M., B. K. NISHIKAWA, C. MALM, K. BRIHEIM & A. WASTESON. 1994. Transforming growth factor alpha expression in normal human blood eosinophils: differential regulation by granulocyte-macrophage colony-stimulating factor and interleukin-3. Leukemia **8:** 612–619.

8. MACDONALD, D., A. A. GORDON, H. KAJITANI, H. ENOKIHARA & J. BARRETT. 1990. Interleukin-2 treatment associated eosinophilia is mediated by interleukin-5 production. Br. J. Haematol. **76:** 168–173.

9. SANDERSON, C. J. 1992. Interleukin-5, eosinophils and disease. Blood **79:** 3101–3109.

10. FABIAN, I., V. KRAVTSOV, A. ELIS, O. GUREVITCH, A. ACKERSTEIN, S. SLAVIN & A. NAGLER. 1994. Eosinophils activation in post-autologous bone marrow transplanted patients treated with subcutaneous interleukin-2 and interferon-α2A immunotherapy. Leukemia **8:** 1379–1384.

11. LUCEY, D. R., A. NICHOLSON-WELLER & P. F. WELLER. 1989. Mature human eosinophils have the capacity to express HLA-DR. Proc. Natl. Acad. Sci. USA **86:** 1348–1351.

12. RIVOLTINI, L., V. VIGGIANO, S. SPINAZZÉ, A. SANTORO, M. P. COLOMBO, K. TAKATSU & G. PARMIANI. 1993. *In vitro* anti-tumor activity of eosinophils from cancer patients treated with subcutaneous administration of interleukin-2. Role of interleukin-5. Int. J. Cancer **54:** 8–15.

13. WELLER, P. F. 1991. The immunobiology of eosinophils. N. Engl. J. Med. **324:** 1110–1118.

14. GLEICH, G. J., A. L. SCHROETER, J. P. MARCOUX, M. I. SACHS, E. J. O'CONNELL & P. F. KOHLER. 1934. Episodic angioedema associated with eosinophilia. N. Engl. J. Med. **310:** 1621–1626.

15. VENGE, P., R. DAHL, K. FREDENS & G. B. PETERSON. 1988. Epithelial injury by human eosinophils. Am. Rev. Respir. Dis. **138:** S54–S57.

16. BUZIO, C., G. DE PALMA, R. PASSALACQUA, D. POTENZONI, F. FERROZZI, M. A. CATTABIANI, L. MANENTI & A. BORGHETTI. 1996. Effectiveness of very-low doses of immunotherapy in advanced renal cell cancer. Br. J. Cancer In press.

17. DE AMICI, M., L. VITALI, A. ALIPRANDI, G. D'ANNUNZIO, A. SCARAMUZZA & R. LORINI. 1994. Aumentati livelli di ECP e EPX in pazienti affetti da diabete mellito insulino-dipendente. *In* Immunitá ed allergia: nuovi percorsi per il Pediatra (Atti del VI Congresso Nazionale di Immunologia ed Allergologia Pediatrica, Brescia, Ottobre 1994): 65. Società Italiana di Immunologia ed Allergologia Pediatrica. (This paper contains normal range for ECP and EPX according to our laboratory data.)

18. VADAS, M. A., J. R. DAVID, A. E. BUTTERWORTH, N. J. PISANI & T. A. SIONGOK. 1979. A new method for the purification of human eosinophils and neutrophils and a comparison of the ability of these cells to damage schistosomula of *S. Mansoni.* J. Immunol. **122:** 1228–1236.

19. PRIN, L., M. CAPRON, A. B. TONNEL, O. BLETRY & A. CAPRON. 1983. Heterogeneity of human peripheral blood eosinophils: variability in cell density and cytotoxic ability in relation to the level and the origin of hypereosinophilia. Int. Arch. Allergy Appl. Immunol. **72:** 336–346.

20. TOMASSINI, M., A. TSICOPOULOS, P. CHUN-TAI, V. GRUART, A. B. TONNEL, L. PRIN, A. CAPRON & M. CAPRON. 1991. Release of granule proteins by eosinophils from allergic and non-allergic patients with eosinophilia on immunoglobulin-dependant activation. J. Allergy Clin. Immunol. **88:** 365–375.

21. CONFALONIERI, M., F. TACCONI, M. DE AMICI, R. MACCARIO, C. PORTA, L. GIOGLIO & E. BOBBIO-PALLAVICINI. 1995. Benign idiopathic hypereosinophilia: a feeble masquerader or a smoldering form of the hypereosinophilic syndrome? Haematologica **80:** 50–53.

22. GIARD, D. J., S. A. AARONSON & G. J. TODARO. 1973. *In vitro* cultivation of human tumors: establishment of cell lines derived from a series of solid tumors. J. Natl. Cancer Inst. **51:** 1417–1423.

23. CHANG, A. Y. & P. C. KENG. 1983. Inhibition of cell growth in synchronous human hypernephroma cells by recombinant interferon alpha-D and irradiation. J. Interferon Res. **3:** 379–385.

24. CHEN, T. R. 1977. In situ detection of mycoplasma contamination in cell culture by fluorescent Hoechst 33259 stain. Exp. Cell Res. **104:** 255–262.

25. ALLEY, M. C., C. M. PACULA-COX, M. L. HURSEY, L. R. RUBINSTEIN & M. R. BOYD. 1991. Morphometric and colorimetric analysis of human tumor cell line growth and drug sensitivity in soft agar culture. Cancer Res. **51:** 1257–1256.

26. GOTTLIEB, D., H. PRENTICE, H. HESLOP, C. BELLO-FERNANDEZ, A. BIANCHI, A. GALAZKA & M. BRENNER. 1989. Effects of recombinant interleukin-2 administration on cytotoxic function following high-dose chemo-radiotherapy for hematological malignancy. Blood **74:** 2335–2342.

27. BLAISE, D., D. OLIVE, A. M. STOPPA, P. VIENS, C. POURREAU, M. LOPEZ, M. ATTAL, C. JASMINE, G. MONGES, C. MAWAS, P. MANNONI, P. PALMER, C. FRANKS, T. PHILIP & D. MARANINCHI. 1990. Hematologic and immunologic effects of the systemic administration of recombinant interleukin-2 after autologous bone marrow transplantation. Blood **76:** 1092–1097.

28. HULAND, E. & H. HULAND. 1992. Tumor-associated eosinophilia in interleukin-2-treated patients: evidence of toxic eosinophil degranulation on bladder cancer cells. J. Cancer Res. Clin. Oncol. **118:** 463–467.

Phagocytes and the Lung

PETER A. WARD[a]

Department of Pathology
The University of Michigan Medical School
M5240 Medical Science I, Box 0602
1301 Catherine Road
Ann Arbor, Michigan 48109-0602

INTRODUCTION

Activation of lung phagocytes, whether involving residential or recruited phagocytic cells (macrophages, monocytes, neutrophils), results in a series of products important for development of inflammatory injury of the lung. An understanding of the mechanisms of cell activation as well as how products of these activated cells interact with cellular and non-cellular targets to bring about tissue damage is important for the ultimate use of blocking interventions in the treatment of human inflammatory diseases. In these considerations, we will discuss cytokine products of activated macrophages, including pro-inflammatory cytokines, anti-inflammatory cytokines, oxidants, and proteinases (TABLE 1). All of the information to be presented in this paper derives from the study of an animal model of acute lung injury induced by intrapulmonary deposition of IgG immune complexes. This deposition results in a complement-dependent activation of lung macrophages, recruitment of large numbers of neutrophils, and ultimate damage of lung cells and matrix as a result of numerous products from activated macrophages and recruited (and activated) neutrophils.[1] Damage in this lung model can be precisely quantitated by extravascular leakage of ^{125}I-labeled albumin from the blood, extravasation of ^{51}Cr-labeled rat RBC, and build-up of neutrophils (as measured by lung content of myeloperoxidase (MPO) or retrieval of neutrophils from bronchoalveolar lavage (BAL) fluids). Cytokine content is usually measured in BAL fluids, although whole lung homogenates can also be employed. The IgG immune complex model may provide information relevant to an understanding of human inflammatory diseases triggered by deposition of IgG immune complexes, such as rheumatoid arthritis, systemic lupus erythematosus, vasculitis, membranous glomerulonephritis, idiopathic pulmonary fibrosis, etc.

PRO-INFLAMMATORY CYTOKINES/CHEMOKINES

There are at least three different functional categories of cytokines/chemokines as defined by their pro-inflammatory effects: Cytokines include the traditional products such as TNFα, IL-1, interferon-gamma (IFNγ), etc., while chemokines include the

[a]Address correspondence to: Peter A. Ward, M.D., Professor and Chairman, Department of Pathology, The University of Michigan Medical School, M5240 Medical Science I, Box 0602, 1301 Catherine Road, Ann Arbor, Michigan 48109-0602.

TABLE 1. Inflammatory Products of Lung Macrophages in Lung Injury

A. Pro-inflammatory cytokines/chemokines
  i. Induction of endothelial adhesion molecules (TNFα, IL-1)
  ii. Chemotactic activity, especially the α chemokines of the IL-8 family (MIP-2, CINC, etc.)
  iii. Other activities of chemokines (e.g., the β chemokine, MIP-1α)
B. Anti-inflammatory cytokines (IL-4, IL-10)
C. Oxidants
  i. Products of inducible nitric oxide synthase (iNOS)
    a. Lung sources of iNOS
    b. Inducers of iNOS
    c. Evidence for *in vivo* role of ·NO
  ii. NADPH oxidase
D. Proteinases
  i. Metalloproteinases
    a. Collagenases
    b. Gelatinases
  ii. Serine proteinases
    a. Elastase
    b. Cathepsins

IL-8 family of α chemokines (chemically characterized by C-X-C linkages and including products such as IL-8; MIP-2; PF-4; GROα,β,γ; KC, etc.) and the β chemokines (chemically characterized by C-C linkages and including products such as MCP-1,2,3; MIP-1α,β; RANTES; Eotaxin; etc.). In the IgG immune complex model of acute lung injury, bronchoalveolar (BAL) fluids as a function of time contain large amounts of biologically active TNFα and IL-1. Although these cytokines are known to have the ability to activate macrophages and neutrophils, alone each cytokine has fairly limited *in vitro* activity, best described as "priming" of these cells for enhanced responses to other stimuli (e.g., cytokines, immune complexes, lipopolysaccharide, etc.). A major function of TNFα and IL-1 in lung appears to be induction of endothelial adhesion molecules, ICAM-1 and E-selectin, both of which are critical for the early steps required in neutrophil adhesion to the activated endothelium and eventual transmigration of neutrophils into the alveolar compartment in the inflammatory model described above.[2] Blocking of TNFα by antibody or by soluble TNFα receptor-I, or blocking of IL-1 by antibody or by IL-1 receptor antagonist resulted in dramatically diminished recruitment of neutrophils and reduced development of lung injury. In the case of blockade of TNFα, these results could be attributed to greatly reduced upregulation of lung vascular ICAM-1 as determined by the use of quantitative fixation of ^{125}I-anti-ICAM-1 to the lung vasculature. Although studies with blockade of IL-1 are incomplete, the trends also suggest that IL-1 functions in this model in a similar manner to that of TNFα. These data strongly suggest that the "early response cytokines," TNFα and IL-1, function in a pro-inflammatory manner by playing a key role in upregulation of lung vascular ICAM-1 and E-selectin, which are critically necessary for neutrophil recruitment.

Another functional classification of cytokines/chemokines derives from their chemotactic activity.[3,4] Some of the α chemokines (IL-8 or its family relatives, such as MIP-2 and CINC, KC and others) and some of the β chemokines (MIP-1α,β; MCP-1,2 and 3; RANTES; and others) are well known for the chemotactic activities, the α chemokine family being described as having activity chiefly for neutrophils (and to a lesser extent for T cell subsets), while the β chemokines are thought to be predominantly chemotactic for monocytes and lymphocytes. It is clear that this functional classification cannot be strictly relied upon for predictions of the *in vivo* role of these chemokines. In the IgG immune complex model of injury in rats, message for MIP-2 appears within 2 h and is maintained for the next 4 h, followed by decline. MIP-2 protein followed a similar, albeit slightly delayed, pattern of expression. Most importantly, blocking of rat MIP-2 by antibody was significantly protective, resulting in reduced influx of neutrophils and diminishing degree of lung damage, without affecting BAL levels of TNFα.[5] These data indicate that MIP-2 is important in this inflammatory model and may be functioning chiefly as a chemotactic attractant for neutrophils. A second α chemokine that seems to play an important role in this inflammatory model is the chemokine-induced neutrophil chemotactic factor (CINC), which is expressed in a manner similar to that described for MIP-2 (as above). Blocking of CINC similarly suppresses neutrophil recruitment and development of lung injury.[6] Thus, at least two α chemokines play important roles in these reactions and seem to function as neutrophil chemoattractants. A third proinflammatory function of the chemokines derives from our studies in the rat lung model of IgG immune complex injury, in which MIP-1α expression has been demonstrated (both by mRNA and by protein) in the first 2–6 h of the developing reaction. Antibody-induced blocking of MIP-1α results in suppressed recruitment of neutrophils and reduced leakage of ^{125}I-albumin. In striking contrast to the protective effects of blockade of MIP-2 and CINC, blockade of MIP-1α is also associated with substantial reductions in levels of TNFα in BAL fluids.[7] This has led to the conclusion that in this model the β chemokine MIP-1α functions as an autocrine regulator of TNFα production, the end result being enhanced upregulation of lung vascular ICAM-1 by tissue macrophages. Accordingly, as compared to MIP-2 and CINC, this chemokine appears to play a very different functional role in the inflammatory response.

ANTI-INFLAMMATORY CYTOKINES

Another functional classification of cytokines comes from the recognition that certain cytokines have very clearly been shown to have anti-inflammatory functions, especially IL-4 and IL-10. A major function of these cytokines has been suggested by their *in vitro* ability to suppress cytokine production by stimulated macrophages.[8,9] Our employment of these cytokines in the IgG immune complex lung injury model has verified that both IL-4 and IL-10 have very powerful anti-inflammatory effects.[10] When added to the airway with anti-bovine serum albumin in minute (nanogram) quantities, these cytokines are profoundly suppressive, causing dramatic reductions in albumin leak, in intraalveolar hemorrhage, and in neutrophil accumulation. Furthermore, there are profound reductions in BAL levels of TNFα, which, in turn, has been shown to result in greatly reduced lung vascular ICAM-1 expression. In the case of IL-10, *in vivo* blocking of this cytokine increases the level of TNFα in BAL fluids, accompanied by increased accumulation of neutrophils and intensified injury, whereas antibody to IL-4 has no effect.[11] These data suggest that, in this model of lung injury, intrinsic IL-10 regulates the intensity of inflammatory damage by controlling the level of TNFα produced, and, correspondingly, the upregulation of ICAM-1, an essential adhesion molecule in this inflammatory model. It seems likely that there may be additional intrinsic cytokines with anti-inflammatory activity, such as IL-6 and IL-13.

OXIDANT PRODUCTS OF PHAGOCYTIC CELLS

Using the IgG immune complex model of inflammatory lung injury, evidence suggests that two oxidant-generating pathways in lung macrophages and neutrophils contribute to development of lung injury. These pathways are described in FIGURE 1. The first oxidant-generating pathway features inducible nitric oxide synthase (iNOS). This enzyme is inducible in lung macrophages by the action of three cytokines: TNFα, IL-1, and interferon gamma (INFγ). In the *in vivo* model described above, blockade of any one of these three cytokines produces partial protection from

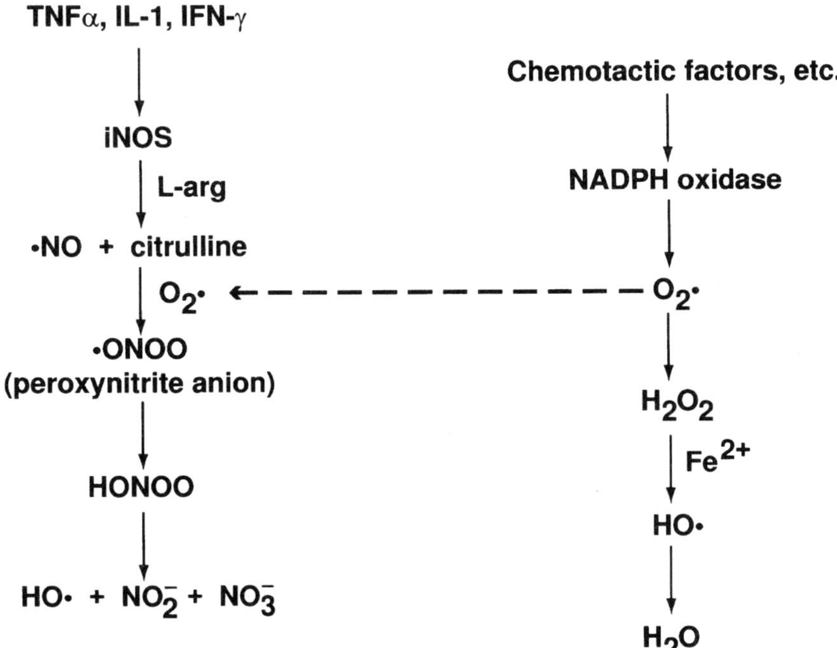

FIGURE 1. Sources of oxidants generated by activated phagocytic cells, featuring inducible nitric oxide synthase (iNOS) and NADPH oxidase. The intersection between the two pathways occurs between superoxide anion ($O_2\cdot$) and nitric oxide ($\cdot NO$).

lung injury and partial reduction in nitric oxide ($\cdot$NO) generation (as quantitated by formation of NO_2^- (NO_3^-), whereas *in vivo* blockade of all three cytokines (by antibodies) almost totally suppresses $\cdot$NO production and greatly attenuates development of lung injury.[12] In the $\cdot$NO generating pathway, iNOS converts L-arginine into $\cdot$NO and citrulline. $\cdot$NO can then react with available superoxide anion ($O_2\cdot$) to produce the highly reactive peroxynitrite anion ($\cdot$ONOO) which, when protonated (to form HONOO) in an acidic environment can undergo hemolytic cleavage to generate the hydroxyl radical (HO$\cdot$), which is also highly reactive. The ultimate breakdown products of this pathway are nitrite (NO_2^-) and nitrate (NO_3^-), which are the usual chemical surrogates for detection of $\cdot$NO. Evidence for the role of the $\cdot$NO pathway in this inflammatory model was obtained by the airway instillation of analogues of L-arginine, namely, L-N^G monomethyl arginine and related compounds.[13] Acting as competitive inhibitors of L-arginine, these analogues in a dose-dependent manner effectively inhibit $\cdot$NO production in lung and substantially reduce development of injury. These protective effects are *not* associated with any reduction in neutrophil accumulation in these inflammatory reactions, suggesting that the $\cdot$NO-generating pathway is a terminal effector mechanism for tissue injury. To date, there are two identified lung sources of iNOS in this model of lung injury: lung macrophages and type II alveolar epithelial cells.[12] This conclusion is based not only on immunostaining for iNOS, demonstrating its presence in these two cell types, but is also based on the finding that isolation from normal lung of either alveolar macrophages or type II alveolar epithelial cells and their subsequent *in vitro* stimulation with IFNγ or lipopolysaccharide (LPS) results in $\cdot$NO production that is suppressible in the presence of analogues of L-arginine.

A second oxidase-generating system, NADPH oxidase, is present in both lung macrophages and neutrophils.[14,15] Upon cell activation (with phorbol ester, immune complexes, etc.) cytoplasmic cofactors are transposed to the cell membrane to produce a protein complex that defines NADPH oxidase. This enzyme transfers single electrons, resulting in progressive reduction of O_2 to $O_2\cdot$ to H_2O_2, to HO$\cdot$, and finally, to H_2O. NADPH oxidase may be the key source for $O_2\cdot$ that intercalates with the iNOS pathway to react with $\cdot$NO, as described above. $O_2\cdot$ may play another important role in reducing Fe^{3+} in ferritin stores within cells to generate Fe^{2+}, a reactive transitional form that can interact with H_2O_2 to facilitate electron transport, reducing H_2O_2 to HO$\cdot$, thus regenerating $Fe^{3+}\cdot$ H_2O_2 can also be metabolized in the presence of chloride and MPO to generate hypochlorous acid (HOCl), which can convert procollagenase and progelatinase into their active enzyme forms (see below). The presumed role of NADPH oxidase in this lung injury model is not only to provide $O_2\cdot$, perhaps for the iNOS pathway (see above), but also to generate HO$\cdot$ from H_2O_2, as suggested by the protective effects of catalase and the iron chelator, deferoxamine.[16]

PHAGOCYTIC CELL PROTEINASES INVOLVED IN LUNG INJURY

Two categories of proteinases appear to be involved in lung injury in the IgG immune complex model: metalloproteinases and serine proteinases. The most direct experimental evidence incriminating these proteinases comes from the use of inhibitors. Metalloproteinases include collagenases and gelatinases, the latter having been identified in BAL fluids of animals developing IgG-immune complex–induced alveolitis. These enzymes derive chiefly from macrophages and, as the names imply, hydrolyze native or denatured collagens. Serine proteinases include elastase and cathepsins, derived both from macrophages and neutrophils. Elastolytic activity has been found in BAL fluids from inflamed rat lungs in the case of the IgG immune complex model (TABLE 2). The most compelling evidence for the role of these enzymes has been the demonstration that airway instillation of recombinant human tissue metalloproteinase inhibitor-2 (TIMP-2) or recombinant human secreted leukocyte proteinase inhibitor (SLPI) sharply reduces the intensity of injury.[17] Interestingly, these protective effects are associated with reduced neutrophil accumulation, suggesting that breakdown of lung connective matrix may reduce chemotactic peptides that facilitate neutrophil recruitment under the experimental conditions of inflammation. The extent to which either macrophage-derived matrix-destroying enzymes, such as cysteine proteinases (cathepsins B, H and L), may also be involved in these lung-damaging reactions remains unknown.

CONCLUSIONS

Products of activated phagocytic cells (lung macrophages and recruited neutrophils) represent a series of toxic factors that directly or indirectly injure both lung cells and matrix. Furthermore, there is evidence for synergy between the effects of oxidants and proteinases. The interplay of cytokines/chemokines in lung inflammatory reactions triggered by intrapulmonary deposition of IgG immune complexes is complicated. On the one hand, these inflammatory reactions cause production of a series of pro-inflammatory products that facilitate upregulation of endothelial adhesion molecules, chemotactic recruitment of neutrophils, and positive autocrine stimulation of macrophages productive of more cytokine generation. Yet these inflammatory reactions are also associated with macrophage products (cytokines) that downregulate the inflammatory response. Understanding the complex biological responses could set the stage for more specific approaches for blocking of the inflammatory response in a variety of human inflammatory diseases.

TABLE 2. Evidence for Role of Proteinases in IgG Immune Complex Alveolitis

Intervention	Reduction (%) in Lung Leak of Albumin
rhu TIMP-2 (0.5 mg)	33
rhu TIMP-2 (1.0 mg)	41
rhu SLPI (1.0 mg)	48
TIMP-2 (1.0 mg) + SLPI (1.0 mg)	65

REFERENCES

1. JOHNSON, K. J. & P. A. WARD. 1974. Acute immunologic pulmonary alveolitis. J. Clin. Invest. **54:** 349–357.
2. MULLIGAN, M. S., A. A. VAPORCIYAN, M. MIYASAKA, T. TAMATANI & P. A. WARD. 1993. Tumor necrosis factor α regulates *in vivo* intrapulmonary expression of ICAM-1. Amer. J. Pathol. **142:** 1739–1749.
3. SCHALL, T. J. 1991. Biology of the RANTES/SIS cytoking family. Cytokine **3:** 165–183.
4. OPPENHEIM, J. J., C. O. C. ZACHARIAE, N. MUKAIDA & K. MATSUSHIMA. 1991. Properties of the novel proinflammatory "intercrine" cytokine family. Ann. Rev. Immunol. **9:** 617.
5. SCHMAL, H., T. P. SHANLEY, M. L. JONES, H. P. FRIEDL & P. A. WARD. 1996. Role for macrophage inflammatory protein-2 in lipopolysaccharide-induced lung injury in rats. J. Immunol. **156:** 1963–1972.
6. SHANEY, T. P., H. SCHMAL, R. L. WARNER, E. SCHMID, H. P. FRIEDL & P. A. WARD. 1997. Requirement for C-X-C chemokines (macrophage inflammatory protein-2 and cytokine-induced neutrophil chemoattractant) in IgG immune complex–induced lung injury. J. Immunol. **158:** 3439–3448.
7. SHANLEY, T. P., H. SCHMAL, H. P. FRIEDL, M. L. JONES & P. A. WARD. 1995. Role of macrophage inflammatory protein-1α (MIP-1α) in acute lung injury in rats. J. Immunol. **154:** 4793–4802.
8. HART, P. H., G. F. VITTI, D. R. BURGESS, G. A. WHITTY, D. S. PICCOLI & J. A. HAMILTON. 1989. Potential anti-inflammatory effects of interleukin 4: suppression of human monocyte tumor necrosis factor alpha, interleukin 1, and prostaglandin E2. Proc. Natl. Acad. Sci. USA **86:** 3803.
9. DE WAAL MALEFYT, R., J. ABRAMS, B. BENNETT, C. G. FIGDOR & J. E. DE VRIES. 1991. Interleukin 10 (IL-10) inhibits cytokine synthesis by human monocytes: an autoregulatory role of IL-10 produced by monocytes. J. Exp. Med. **174:** 1209.
10. MULLIGAN, M. S., M. L. JONES, A. A. VAPORCIYAN, M. C. HOWARD & P. A. WARD. 1993. Protective effects of IL-4 and IL-10 against immune complex-induced lung injury. J. Immunol. **151:** 5666–5674.
11. SHANLEY, T. P., H. SCHMAL, H. P. FRIEDL, M. L. JONES & P. A. WARD. 1995. Regulatory effects of intrinsic IL-10 in IgG immune complex-induced lung injury. J. Immunol. **154:** 3454–3460.
12. WARNER, R. L., R. PAINE, III, P. J. CHRISTENSEN, M. A. MARLETTA, M. K. RICHARDS, S. E. WILCOXEN & P. A. WARD. 1995. Lung sources and cytokine requirements for *in vivo* expression of inducible nitric oxide synthase. Am. J. Resp. Cell Molec. Biol. **12:** 649–661.
13. MULLIGAN, M. S., J. M. HEVEL, M. A. MARLETTA & P. A. WARD. 1991. Tissue injury caused by deposition of immune complexes is L-arginine dependent. Proc. Natl. Acad. Sci. USA **88:** 6338–6342.
14. MOREL, F., J. DOUSSIERE & P. V. VIGNAIS. 1991. The superoxide-generating oxidase of phagocytic cells. Physiological, molecular and pathological aspects. Eur. J. Biochem. **201**(3): 523–546.
15. UMEKI, S. 1994. Mechanisms for the activation/electron transfer of neutrophil NADPH-oxidase complex and molecular pathology of chronic granulomatous disease. Ann. Hematol. **68**(6): 267–277.
16. JOHNSON, K. J. & P. A. WARD. 1981. Role of oxygen metabolites in immune complex injury of lung. J. Immunol. **126:** 2365–2369.
17. MULLIGAN, M. S., P. E. DESROCHERS, A. M. CHENNAIYAN, D. F. GIBBS, K. J. JOHNSON & S. J. WEISS. 1993. *In vivo* suppression of immune complex-induced alveolitis by secretory leukoproteinase inhibitor and tissue inhibitor of metalloproteinase-2. Proc. Natl. Acad. Sci. USA **90:** 11523–11527.

Leukocyte–Endothelial Cell Interactions in Ischemia-Reperfusion Injury

ROBERT K. WINN, CHANDRA RAMAMOORTHY,
NICHOLAS B. VEDDER, SAM R. SHARAR, AND JOHN M. HARLAN

*Department of Surgery
University of Washington
Seattle, Washington 98195*

INTRODUCTION

Neutrophils (PMNs) have been implicated as the cause of tissue injury leading to organ dysfunction and organ failure following a variety of insults. One of the first suggestions of a potential for injuries of this type was made by Metchnikoff in 1887 when he suggested that tissue injury could result during normal phagocytosis.[1] Subsequently, several studies have demonstrated the ability of stimulated PMNs to cause injury to endothelial cells *in vitro*.[2-7] In some of these studies it was shown that adherence of PMNs to the endothelial cells with the formation of a protected microenvironment was necessary before the endothelial cells were injured.[5,7] The leukocyte–endothelial cell adhesion results from specific molecular interactions between molecules on the surface of leukocytes and their counter-receptors on the endothelial cells.

The role of leukocytes in organ injury *in vivo* has been demonstrated by reducing the number of circulating PMNs with chemotherapeutic agents. PMN depletion reduced focal ischemia-reperfusion injury to the heart,[8,9] gut,[10] liver,[11,12] as well as the generalized ischemia-reperfusion injury resulting from resuscitation from hemorrhagic shock.[10,13]

Leukocyte Adhesion Molecules

Adhesion molecules responsible for leukocyte–endothelial cell adhesion are members of three families of adhesion molecules designated the selectin family, the integrin family, and the immunoglobulin (Ig) super family. Several reviews of adhesion molecules can be found in the literature, thus only a brief discussion will be given here.[14-19]

The selectin family consists of three molecules designated L-selectin (CD62L), P-selectin (CD62P), and E-selectin (CD62E). L-selectin is found only on leukocytes, E-selectin is restricted to endothelial cells, and P-selectin is found on both activated platelets and endothelial cells. L-selectin is constitutively expression on all leukocytes and is shed from their surface following activation of these cells with a variety

[a]Address correspondence to: Robert K. Winn, Ph.D., Department of Surgery ZA-16, Harborview Medical Center, 325 9th Avenue, Seattle, WA 98104.

of inflammatory stimuli. P-selectin is found in the Weibel-Palade bodies of endothelial cells and in the alpha granules of platelets and is rapidly expressed on the surface of these cells upon activation. P-selectin expression can also be increased by *de novo* protein synthesis in endothelial cells. E-selectin is produced only by *de novo* protein synthesis following stimulation by cytokines and lipopolysaccharide (LPS). All three of the selectins have been shown to recognize sialylated and fucosylated glycoconjugates, particularly sialyl Lewis^x (Sle^x, CD15s).[20,21] P- and E-selectin also recognize glycoconjugates expressed on the P-selectin glycoprotein ligand-1 (PSGL-1) on the surface of leukocytes.[22] E-selectin also recognizes glycoconjugates on the E-selectin ligand ESL-1 that is also found on leukocytes.[23] L-selectin recognizes glycoconjugates CD34, MadCAM-1, and GlyCAM-1.[24–26]

The members of the integrin family of molecules involved in leukocyte–endothelial cell adhesion are in the β_1- and β_2-families. They consist of distinct alpha chain non-covalently linked to a common beta chain. The β_2-family consists of three molecules designated CD11a/CD18, CD11b/CD18, and CD11c/CD18 and is found on some or all leukocytes.[27] CD11a/CD18 binds to the intercellular adhesion molecule-1 (ICAM-1, CD54) and ICAM-2 (CD102); CD11b/CD18 recognizes ICAM-1 as well as other proteins (C3bi, fibrinogen, Factor X).[16] The molecules in the β_1-family that are important in leukocyte–endothelial cell adhesion are VLA-4 and $\alpha_4\beta_7$.[16] VLA-4 is found on all leukocytes except PMNs and binds to vascular cell adhesion molecule-1 (VCAM-1, CD106) as well as the CS-1 fragment of fibronectin.[16] The $\alpha_4\beta_7$ molecule is expressed on some lymphocytes and binds to mucosal vascular addressin-1 (MadCAM-1) and, to a lesser extent, VCAM-1.

Members of the Ig-family that are important in leukocyte–endothelial cell adhesion include ICAM-1, ICAM-2, VCAM-1, MadCAM-1, and platelet–endothelial cell adhesion molecule-1 (PECAM-1). The leukocyte–endothelial cell interactions with these molecules were briefly described above with the exception of PECAM-1. This molecule is found on endothelial cells, platelets, and some leukocytes. It is constitutively expressed on endothelial cells and is localized to intracellular junctions and has been shown to play a role in diapedesis of PMNs and monocytes between endothelial cells.[28,29] VCAM-1, ICAM-1, and ICAM-2 are constitutively expressed on endothelial cells. VCAM-1 and ICAM-1 expression can be increased by *de novo* protein synthesis in response to cytokines or LPS stimulation.

Leukocyte Adhesion Cascade

Leukocyte–endothelial cell adherence is a prerequisite for tissue injury and occurs following a sequential cascade of distinct steps.[16,17] The initial event leading to adherence is the activation of adherence molecules on both the leukocyte and the endothelial cell as a result of a specific inflammatory event. Following activation, the next step is the random contact of circulating leukocytes with the endothelial surface that allows interactions of leukocyte and endothelial selectins with their counter receptors to produce leukocyte rolling along the endothelial surface. Next, firm adherence of the two cell types occurs, mediated by interactions between integrins on leukocytes with their counter structures in the Ig-family on endothelial cells. Adherent leukocytes then migrate along the endothelial surface to cell junctions where they migrate between endothelial cells using PECAM-1 and an undefined counter structure on leukocytes. Finally, extravascular localization to the inflammatory site occurs as the leukocyte migrates along chemotactic gradients.

Just as leukocyte–endothelial cell adherence is required for endothelial cell injury *in vitro* (described above) such adherence may also be necessary for injury to occur *in vivo*. If true, the cascade of adhesive events that occurs during inflammation must take place before tissues are injured. Therefore, interrupting the adhesion cascade may prevent leukocyte-mediated injury. Specifically, interruption of leukocyte rolling by blocking the appropriate selectin should prevent the initial molecular interaction between leukocytes and endothelial cells and the subsequent firm adhesion and tissue injury. Alternately, we and others have previously shown that interrupting CD18-Ig-superfamily interactions to prevent firm adhesion results in a reduction in subsequent tissue injury following ischemia and reperfusion.

Interrupting the adhesion cascade can be accomplished by targeting the receptor–counter receptor interaction with specifically designed molecules. Several monoclonal antibodies (mAb) have been developed that recognize functional epitopes on all three classes of adhesion molecules (selectins, integrins, Ig-superfamily) and have been used experimentally (reviewed in Harlan and colleagues[30]). Chimeric molecules consisting of the extracellular domain of P, E, and L-selectins have also been used as competitive inhibitors *in vivo*.[31–33] Also, there are a number of small molecular weight molecules that interrupt the action of adhesion molecule that have been shown effective in the experimental setting (reviewed in Cornejo and colleagues[34]).

ANTI-ADHESION THERAPY

Ischemia-Reperfusion Injury

The initial reports of anti-adhesion therapy following ischemia and reperfusion examined the effect of β_2-integrin blockade. Monoclonal antibodies provided protection from injury following ischemia-reperfusion of the gut[35] and the heart.[36] These studies were followed by a number of additional experiments in other organs.[34] Development and testing of mAbs that recognize selectins provided additional confirmation of the efficacy of this approach in ischemia-reperfusion injury. L-selectin mAb administration reduced injury to the heart,[37] rabbit ear,[38] and rat hind limb.[39] Two of the earliest studies using P-selectin mAbs showed protection in the heart[40] and rabbit ear.[41] Several other studies have shown protection in other organs.[34] Relatively little work has been reported using E-selectin mAbs in ischemia-reperfusion due to a lack of cross-reactivity in small laboratory animals. However, the results that are available are contradictory. E-selectin blockade failed to protect in the rat hind limb[39]; but protection was found in the heart[42] following administration of serum containing antibodies to E-selectin.

Hemorrhagic Shock

We have investigated the role of leukocyte adhesion molecules in generalized ischemia-reperfusion injuries associated with resuscitation from hemorrhagic shock.

New Zealand White rabbits were used in most experiments with Rhesus monkeys being used for one set of these experiments. New Zealand White rabbits had catheters placed in the vena cava via one femoral vein and in the aorta via one femoral artery. The arterial catheter had a thermistor at its tip and was used for measurement of pressure and the determination of cardiac output by thermal dilution. The venous catheter was used for injection of cold saline for cardiac output determinations, injection of mAb, and withdrawal of blood. Baseline cardiac output, arterial pressure, and arterial blood gas data were collected for at least one hour. Cardiac output was then reduced to 33% of baseline by withdrawal of blood. Cardiac output was maintained at that level by further withdrawal or reinfusion of shed blood for periods ranging from 60 to 120 minutes. Initial resuscitation was accomplished by returning the shed blood, followed by continued resuscitation with lactated Ringer's solution to maintain cardiac output within 90% of baseline.

CD18 mAb Treatment

Rabbits were subjected to the hemorrhagic shock for 2 h then treated with either the CD18 mAb 60.3 or saline prior to resuscitation with blood and lactated Ringer's solution.[43] Catheters were removed after 4 h of resuscitation and the animals returned to their cages with free access to food and water for the next 5 days. There were no differences in blood removed, systemic arterial pressure, or cardiac output during shock, or serum bicarbonate at the end of shock between the two groups of animals, suggesting that the degree of shock was equivalent in both groups. Mortality in these experiments was significantly different between the two groups and is shown in FIGURE 1. The volume of fluid required to maintain cardiac output was greater in the saline-treated group although it did not reach statistical significance at 4 hours.

Anesthetized Rhesus monkeys were subjected to hemorrhagic shock for 90 min then treated with either the CD18 mAb 60.3 or saline prior to resuscitation with their shed blood and additional lactated Ringer's solution as required for the next 24 hours.[44] The animals were allowed to wake up and were placed in the care of the Primate Center veterinarian staff who were unaware of their treatment. There was no difference in blood removed, systemic arterial pressure, or cardiac output during shock, or serum bicarbonate at the end of shock between the two groups of animals. The fluid requirements (FIG. 2) for the saline-treated animals were significantly greater than those for the mAb 60.3–treated group. In addition, five or seven of the animals (two animals were not examined) in the saline-treated group showed signs of hemorrhagic gastritis by endoscopsy (in four animals) or at autopsy (one additional animal). None of the animals that were examined (0/5) in the CD18-treated group showed these signs. Four of seven animals in the saline group and none of the CD18 mAb–treated group were killed as directed by the veterinarian.

Selectin mAb Treatment

Rabbits were subjected to hemorrhagic shock for 90 min then treated with either saline, anti-P-selectin mAb PB1.3, isotype-matched mAb PNB1.6, or CD18 mAb

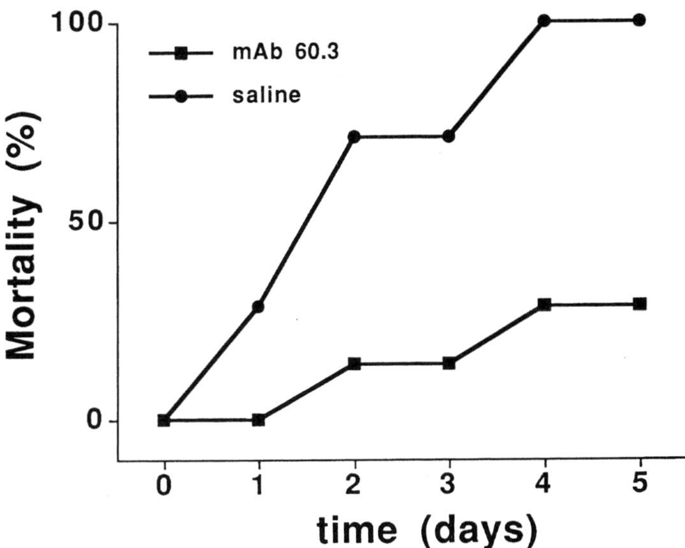

FIGURE 1. Rabbit mortality over a five-day observation period following hemorrhage to 33% of baseline for two hours. Rabbits were treated with either saline or the anti-CD18 mAb 60.3. The two groups were significantly different. (Adapted from Vedder *et al.*[43] with permission.)

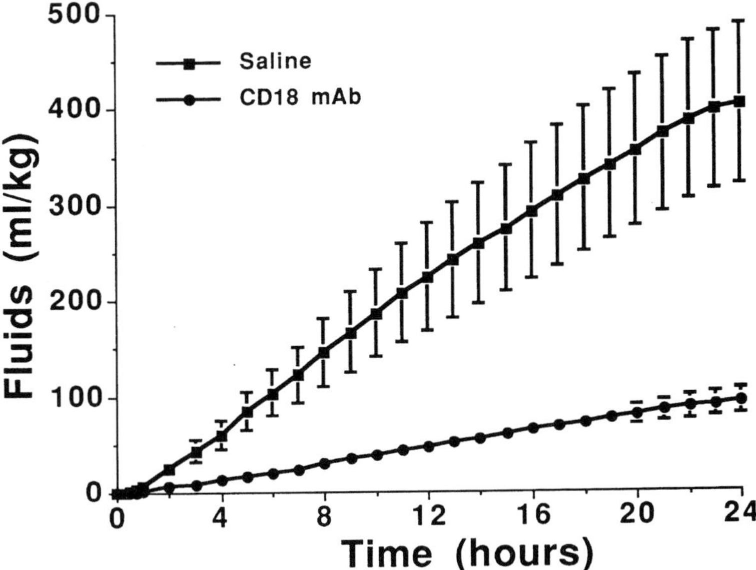

FIGURE 2. Fluid requirement in non-human primates during the 24-hour period following hemorrhage to 33% of baseline. Animals were treated with the anti-CD18 mAbs or saline just prior to resuscitation. Fluid requirements were significantly different between groups.

60.3. The animals were resuscitated with their shed blood and additional lactated Ringer's solution for the next 6 hours.[45] Again, there was no difference in blood removed, systemic arterial pressure, or cardiac output during shock, or serum bicarbonate at the end of shock between these groups of animals. The animals in the saline-treated group and the isotype-matched group were combined for analysis and this group was different from the mAb PB1.3 group (FIG. 3). The mAb 60.3-treated group was also different from the combined control group but was not different from the mAb PB1.3–treated group.

Rabbits were subjected to hemorrhagic shock for 2 h then treated with the anti-L-selectin mAb LAM1-3 (blocking), mAb LAM1-14 (non-blocking), saline, or the CD18 mAb 60.3. They were then resuscitated with their shed blood and additional lactated Ringer's solution for 6 hours.[46] As with the previous studies, there was no difference in blood removed, systemic arterial pressure, or cardiac output during shock, and serum bicarbonate at the end of shock between these groups of animals. There were deaths in the saline-treated group and in the non-blocking mAb LAM1-14 treated group and the fluid requirements for these animals were projected from the time of death to the end of the 6-h resuscitation period by linear regression. There was a significant difference in fluid requirements between the mAb LAM1-3-treated group and both the mAb LAM1-14–treated and saline-treated groups (FIG. 4). The mAb 60.3–treated group was also different from these two control groups but was not different from the mAb LAM1-3 group.

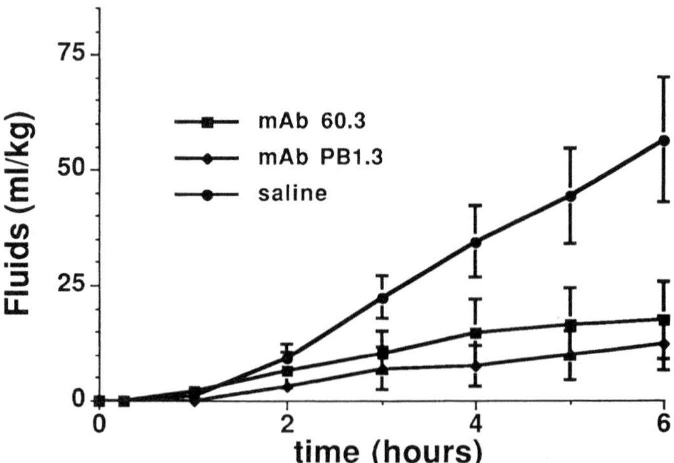

FIGURE 3. Fluid requirements in rabbits during the six-hour period following hemorrhage to 33% of baseline. Rabbits were treated with the anti-CD18 mAb 60.3, anti-P-selectin mAb PB1.3, the isotype-matched mAb PNB1.6, or saline. The isotype-matched and saline groups were not significantly different and were combined. The mAb 60.3- and PB1.3-treated groups were significantly different from the combined control group. (Adapted from Winn *et al.*[45] with permission.)

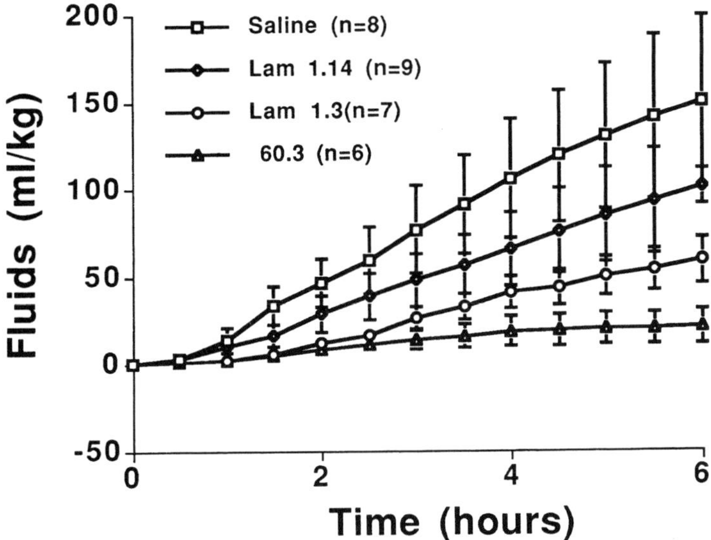

FIGURE 4. The six-hour fluid requirements for rabbits subjected to two hours of hemorrhagic shock. Animals were treated with saline, the non-blocking anti-L-section mAb LAM1-14, the anti-L-sectin mAb LAM1-3, or the anti-CD18 mAb 60.3. The mAb LAM1-3– and mAb 60.3–treated groups were both significantly different from the saline- and mAb LAM1-14–treated groups, but were not different from each other. (Adapted from Ramamoorthy *et al.*[46] with permission.)

CONCLUSIONS

The mAb PB1.3 was shown to attenuate leukocyte rolling when the shear rate was less than 250/sec in postcapillary venules of the cat mesentery.[47] Leukocytes roll spontaneously following exposure and preparation for intravital microscopic viewing. Also, this mAb reduced leukocyte rolling in the rat mesentery following stimulation with histamine, a drug known to cause surface expression of P-selectin.[48] Therefore, protection might result as a result of mAbP B1.3 blocking rolling.

The anti-L-selectin mAb LAM1-3 reduces non-static leukocyte interactions under a variety of *in vitro* conditions.[49–51] Brady and colleagues[49] showed that PMN adherence to activated glomerular endothelial cells subjected to shear stress *in vitro* by a rotational motion was reduced by LAM1-3. Rolling of PMNs on activated immobilized platelets was reduced by mAb LAM1-3,[50] as well as by the mAb G1 that recognizes the lectin domain of P-selectin, thus the interaction was presumable due to a P-selectin–L-selectin interaction. Thus, it is reasonable to conclude that L-selectin blockade reduces leukocyte rolling on endothelial cells *in vivo* and that is the mechanism of protection.

The CD18 mAb 60.3 has been shown to block leukocyte adherence in a variety of experimental settings clearly suggesting that the mechanism of protection following administration of this mAb is the result of this blockade.[16]

CLINICAL SIGNIFICANCE OF HEMORRHAGIC SHOCK

The results of a recent year-long epidemiologic study at Harborview Medical Center (Seattle, WA), which examined patients that suffered severe traumatic injuries and hemorrhagic shock, suggest that these patients may suffer from ischemia-reperfusion injuries (manuscript in preparation). In this study, patients were enrolled if they had suffered severe traumatic injury and if they had a systolic blood pressure of less than 90 torr during their initial hospitalization. Approximately 50% of these patients died and this entrance criteria alone allowed the enrollment of greater than 90% of all trauma patients that died. Therefore, since anti-adhesion therapy has been shown highly effective in preventing generalized ischemia-reperfusion injury it is reasonable to suggest that this therapy might improve outcome in severely injured patients.

REFERENCES

1. METCHNIKOFF, E. 1887. Sur lallutte des cellules de l'organisme contre l'invasion des microbes. Ann. Inst. Pasteur 1: 321.
2. SACKS, T., C. F. MOLDOW, P. R. CRADDOCK, T. K. BOWERS & H. S. JACOB. 1978. Oxygen radicals mediate endothelial cell damage by complement-stimulated granulocytes. J. Clin. Invest. 61: 1161–1167.
3. HARLAN, J. M., P. D. KILLEN, L. A. HARKER & G. E. STRIKER. 1981. Neutrophil-mediated endothelial injury in vitro. J. Clin. Invest. 68: 1394–1403.
4. CAMPBELL, E. J., R. M. SENIOR, J. A. McDONALD & D. L. COX. 1982. Proteolysis by neutrophils. Relative importance of cell-substrate contact and oxidative inactivation of proteinase inhibitors in vitro. J. Clin. Invest. 70: 845–852.
5. SHASBY, D. M., S. S. SHASBY & M. J. PEACH. 1983. Granulocytes and phorbol myristate acetate increase permeability to albumin of cultured endothelial monolayers and isolated perfused lungs. Role of oxygen radicals and granulocytes. Am. Rev. Respir. Dis. 127: 72–76.
6. MARTIN, W. J. 1984. Neutrophils kill pulmonary endothelial cells by a hydrogen-peroxide-dependent pathway. An in vitro model of neutrophil-mediated lung injury. Am. Rev. Respir. Dis. 130: 209–213.
7. DIENER, A. M., P. G. BEATTY, H. D. OCHS & J. M. HARLAN. 1985. The role of neutrophil membrane glycoprotein 150 (GP-150) in neutrophil-mediated endothelial cell injury in vitro. J. Immunol. 135: 537–543.
8. ENGLER, R. L., G. W. SCHMID-SCHONBEIN & R. S. PAVELEC. 1983. Leukocyte capillary plugging in myocardial ischemia and reperfusion in the dog. Am. J. Pathol. 111: 98–111.
9. ROMSON, J. L., B. G. HOOK, S. L. KUNKEL, G. D. ABRAMS, A. SCHORK & B. R. LUCCHESI. 1983. Reduction of the extent of ischemic myocardial injury by neutrophil depletion in the dog. Circulation 67: 1016–1023.
10. SMITH, S. M., R. L. HOLM, M. A. PERRY, M. B. GRISHAM, K. E. ARFORS, D. N. GRANGER & P. R. KVIETYS. 1987. Role of neutrophils in hemorrhagic shock-induced gastric mucosal injury in the rat. Gastroenterology 93(3): 466–471.

11. JAESCHKE, H., A. FARHOOD & C. W. SMITH. 1990. Neutrophils contribute to ischemia/reperfusion injury in rat liver in vivo. FASEB J. **4:** 3355–3359.

12. LANGDALE, L. A., L. C. FLAHERTY, H. D. LIGGITT, J. M. HARLAN, C. L. RICE & R. K. WINN. 1993. Neutrophils contribute to hepatic ischemia-reperfusion injury by a CD18-independent mechanism. J. Leukocyte Biol. **53**(5): 511–517.

13. BARROSO-ARANDA, J., G. W. SCHMID-SCHONBEIN, B. W. ZWEIFACH & R. L. ENGLER. 1988. Granulocytes and no-reflow phenomenon in irreversible hemorrhagic shock. Circ. Res. **63:** 437–447.

14. BEVILACQUA, M. P. 1993. Endothelial-leukocyte adhesion molecules. Annu. Rev. Immunol. **11:** 767–804.

15. BEVILACQUA, M. P. & R. M. NELSON. 1993. Selectins. J. Clin. Invest. **91**(2): 379–387.

16. CARLOS, T. M. & J. M. HARLAN. 1994. Leukocyte-endothelial adhesion molecules. Blood **84**(7): 2068–2101.

17. SPRINGER, T. A. 1994. Traffic signals for lymphocyte recirculation and leukocyte emigration: the multistep paradigm. Cell **76**(2): 301–14.

18. IMHOF, B. A. & D. DUNON. 1995. Leukocyte migration and adhesion. Adv. Immunol. **58:** 345–416.

19. TEDDER, T. F., D. A. STEEBER, A. CHEN & P. ENGEL. 1995. The selectins: vascular adhesion molecules. FASEB J. **9**(10): 866–873.

20. PHILLIPS, M. L., E. NUDELMAN, F. C. GAETA, M. PEREZ, A. K. SINGHAL, S. HAKOMORI & J. C. PAULSON. 1990. ELAM-1 mediates cell adhesion by recognition of a carbohydrate ligand, sialyl-Lex. Science **250**(4984): 1130–1132.

21. WALZ, G., A. ARUFFO, W. KOLANUS, M. BEVILACQUA & B. SEED. 1990. Recognition by ELAM-1 of the sialyl-Lex determinant on myeloid and tumor cells. Science **250**(4984): 1132–1135.

22. SAKO, D., X. J. CHANG, K. M. BARONE, G. VACHINO, H. M. WHITE, G. SHAW, G. M. VELDMAN, K. M. BEAN, T. J. AHERN, B. FURIE *et al.* 1993. Expression cloning of a functional glycoprotein ligand for P-selectin. Cell **75**(6): 1179–1186.

23. STEEGMAIER, M., A. LEVINOVITZ, S. ISENMANN, E. BORGES, M. LENTER, H. P. KOCHER, B. KLEUSER & D. VESTWEBER. 1995. The E-selectin-ligand ESL-1 is a variant of a receptor for fibroblast growth factor. Nature **373**(6515): 615–620.

24. BAUMHETER, S., M. S. SINGER, W. HENZEL, S. HEMMERICH, M. RENZ, S. D. ROSEN & L. A. LASKY. 1993. Binding of L-selectin to the vascular sialomucin CD34. Science **262**(5132): 436–438.

25. BERG, E. L., L. M. MCEVOY, C. BERLIN, R. F. BARGATZE & E. C. BUTCHER. 1993. L-selectin-mediated lymphocyte rolling on MAdCAM-1. Nature **366:** 695–698.

26. IMAI, Y., L. A. LASKY & S. D. ROSEN. 1993. Sulphation requirement for GlyCAM-1, an endothelial ligand for L-selectin. Nature **361:** 555–557.

27. ARNAOUT, M. 1990. Leukocyte adhesion molecule deficiency: its structural basis, pathophysiology and implication for modulating the inflammatory response. Immunol. Rev. **114:** 145–180.

28. MULLER, W. A., S. A. WEIGL, X. DENG & D. M. PHILLIPS. 1993. PECAM-1 is required for transendothelial migration of leukocytes. J. Exp. Med. **178**(2): 449–460.

29. VAPORCIYAN, A. A., H. M. DELISSER, H. C. YAN, I. I. MENDIGUREN, S. R. THOM, M. L. JONES, P. A. WARD & S. M. ALBELDA. 1993. Involvement of platelet-endothelial cell adhesion molecule-1 in neutrophil recruitment in vivo. Science **262**(5139): 1580–1582.

30. HARLAN, J. M., R. K. WINN, C. M. DOERSCHUK, N. B. VEDDER & C. L. RICE. 1992. In vivo models of leukocyte adherence to endothelium. *In* Adhesion: Its Role in Inflammatory Disease. J. M. Harlan & D. Liu, Eds.: 117–150. W.H. Freeman & Co. New York.

31. WATSON, S. R., Y. IMAI, C. FENNIE, J. GEOFFREY, M. SINGER, S. D. ROSEN & L. A. LASKY. 1991. The complement binding-like domains of the murine homing receptor facilitate lectin activity. J. Cell. Biol. **115**(1): 235–243.

32. MULLIGAN, M. S., S. R. WATSON, C. FENNIE & P. A. WARD. 1993. Protective effects of selectin chimeras in neutrophil-mediated lung injury. J. Immunol. **151**(11): 6410–6417.

33. LEE, W. P., P. GRIBLING, L. DE-GUZMAN, N. EHSANI & S. R. WATSON. 1995. A P-selectin-immunoglobulin G chimera is protective in a rabbit ear model of ischemia-reperfusion. Surgery **117**(4): 458–465.

34. CORNEJO, C. J., R. K. WINN & J. M. HARLAN. 1997. Anti-adhesion therapy. Adv. Pharmacol. **39**: 99–142.

35. HERNANDEZ, L. A., M. B. GRISHAM, B. TWOHIG, K.-E. ARFORS, J. M. HARLAN & D. N. GRANGER. 1987. Role of neutrophils in ischemia-reperfusion induced microvascular injury. Am. J. Physiol. **253**: H699–H703.

36. SIMPSON, P. J., R. F. TODD III, J. C. FANTONE, J. K. MICKELSON, J. D. GRIFFIN & B. R. LUCCHESI. 1988. Reduction of experimental canine myocardial reperfusion injury by a monoclonal antibody (Anti-Mo-1, Anti-CD11b) that inhibits leukocyte adhesion. J. Clin. Invest. **81**: 624–629.

37. MA, X. L., A. S. WEYRICH, D. J. LEFER, M. BUERKE, K. H. ALBERTINE, T. K. KISHIMOTO & A. M. LEFER. 1993. Monoclonal antibody to L-selectin attenuates neutrophil accumulation and protects ischemic reperfused cat myocardium. Circulation **88**(2): 649–658.

38. MIHELCIC, D., B. SCHLEIFFENBAUM, T. F. TEDDER, S. R. SHARAR, J. M. HARLAN & R. K. WINN. 1994. Inhibition of leukocyte L-selectin function with a monoclonal antibody attenuates reperfusion injury to the rabbit ear. Blood **84**(7): 2322–2328.

39. SEEKAMP, A., G. O. TILL, M. S. MULLIGAN, J. C. PAULSON, D. C. ANDERSON, M. MIYASAKA & P. A. WARD. 1994. Role of selectins in local and remote tissue injury following ischemia and reperfusion. Am. J. Pathol. **144**(3): 592–598.

40. WEYRICH, A. S., X.-L. MA, K. H. ALBERTINE & A. M. LEFER. 1993. In vivo neutralization of P-selectin protects feline heart and endothelium in myocardial ischemia and reperfusion injury. J. Clin. Invest. **91**: 2620–2629.

41. WINN, R. K., D. LIGGITT, N. B. VEDDER, J. C. PAULSON & J. M. HARLAN. 1993. Anti-P-selectin monoclonal antibody attenuates reperfusion injury to the rabbit ear. J. Clin. Invest. **92**: 2042–2047.

42. ALTAVILLA, D., F. SQUADRITO, M. IOCULANO, P. CANALE, G. M. CAMPO, B. ZINGARELLI & A. P. CAPUTI. 1994. E-selectin in the pathogenesis of experimental myocardial ischemia-reperfusion injury. Eur. J. Pharmacol. **270**(1): 45–51.

43. VEDDER, N. B., B. W. FOUTY, R. K. WINN, J. M. HARLAN & C. L. RICE. 1989. Role of neutrophils in generalized reperfusion injury associated with resuscitation from shock. Surgery **106**: 509–516.

44. MILESKI, W. J., R. K. WINN, N. V. VEDDER, T. H. POHLMAN, J. M. HARLAN & C. L. RICE. 1990. Inhibition of CD18-dependent neutrophil adherence reduces organ injury after hemorrhagic shock in primates. Surgery **108**: 205–212.

45. WINN, R. K., J. C. PAULSON & J. M. HARLAN. 1994. A monoclonal antibody to P-selectin ameliorates injury associated with hemorrhagic shock in rabbits. Am. J. Physiol. **267**: H2391–H2397.

46. RAMAMOORTHY, C., S. R. SHARAR, J. M. HARLAN, T. F. TEDDER & R. K. WINN. 1996. Blocking L-selectin function attenuates reperfusion injury following hemorrhagic shock in rabbits. Am. J. Physiol. **271**: H1871–H1877.

47. BIENVENU, K. & D. N. GRANGER. 1993. Molecular determinants of shear rate-dependent leukocyte adhesion in postcapillary venules. Am. J. Physiol. **264**(5 Pt 2): H1504–H1508.

48. ASAKO, H., I. KUROSE, R. WOLF, S. DEFREES, Z. L. ZHENG, M. L. PHILLIPS, J. C. PAULSON & D. N. GRANGER. 1994. Role of H1 receptors and P-selectin in histamine-induced leukocyte rolling and adhesion in postcapillary venules. J. Clin. Invest. **93**(4): 1508–1515.

49. BRADY, H. R., O. SPERTINI, W. JIMENEZ, B. M. BRENNER, P. A. MARSDEN & T. F. TEDDER. 1992. Neutrophils, monocytes, and lymphocytes bind to cytokine-activated kidney

glomerular endothelial cells through L-selectin (LAM-1) in vitro. J. Immunol. **149**(7): 2437–2444.

50. BUTTRUM, S. M., R. HATTON & G. B. NASH. 1993. Selectin-mediated rolling of neutrophils on immobilized platelets. Blood **82:** 1165–1174.

51. LAWRENCE, M. B., D. F. BAINTON & T. A. SPRINGER. 1994. Neutrophil tethering to and rolling on E-selectin are separable by requirement for L-selectin. Immunity **1:** 137–145.

Pharmacological Control of Phagocyte Function: Inhibition of Cholesterol Accumulation

R. PAOLETTI, S. BELLOSTA, AND F. BERNINI[a]

Institute of Pharmacological Sciences
University of Milan
Via Balzaretti, 9
20133 Milan, Italy

[a]*Institute of Pharmacology and Pharmacognosy*
University of Parma
Parma, Italy

INTRODUCTION

Atherosclerosis results from the interaction between blood elements and vessel wall abnormality involving several pathological processes, namely, increased endothelial permeability, monocyte recruitment, smooth muscle cell (SMC) proliferation and migration, matrix synthesis, lipid accumulation, tissue degeneration, and cell necrosis.[1–3] In addition, thrombosis may play a role during atherogenesis, but a flow-limiting thrombus develops only if mature plaques are present and represents a complication rather than a genuine component of atherosclerosis: in fact, atherosclerosis without thrombosis is in general a benign disease.

Advanced human atherosclerotic plaques are characterized by a lipid core covered by a fibrous cap composed of SMCs and extracellular matrix.[1] These lesions have chronic inflammatory infiltrates of macrophages and T lymphocytes.

The composition and vulnerability of plaque rather than its volume (i.e., severity of stenosis) is the most important determinant of atherosclerosis complications. Plaque disruption with superimposed thrombosis is the main cause for the acute coronary syndrome of unstable angina, myocardial infarction, and sudden death.[4]

Plaque instability, manifesting as ulceration of the fibrous cap, plaque rupture, and intraplaque hemorrhage, is characteristic of plaques with a high content of lipid and an excess of macrophages in the cap.[5,6]

The size and consistency of the atheromatous core, which is rich in extracellular lipid (i.e., cholesterol and its esters) are critical for the stability of individual lesions. A significant atheromatous component is often observed in culprit lesions responsible for acute coronary syndromes.[7] On the contrary the thickness and collagen content of the fibrous cap are important for the stability of a plaque.[8] Fibrous caps are often thin and macrophage-infiltrated at their shoulder regions, where disruption most frequently occurs.[9] Disrupted aortic caps contain fewer SMC (the collagen-synthesizing cells) and less collagen than intact caps.[5,10] Collagen is the main component of fibrous caps responsible for their tensile strength.[10] Macrophages are capable of degrading extracellular matrix by phagocytosis or by secreting proteolytic enzymes, in particular, a family of MMPs that may weaken the fibrous cap, predisposing it to rupture.[11]

PHARMACOLOGICAL CONTROL OF MACROPHAGE CHOLESTEROL ACCUMULATION

Effect of Calcium Antagonists

Several *in vivo* and *in vitro* studies suggest that calcium antagonists affect major processes involved in atheroma formation.[12] Although the relevance of these effects in humans remains to be established, they provide the opportunity to develop a class of compounds effective in reducing the progression or stimulating the regression of atherosclerotic lesions by a direct effect on the cellular components of atheroma. Among the possible mechanisms involved, recent reports indicate that calcium antagonists modulate cholesteryl ester homeostasis in macrophages in culture.[13] This effect may relate to the *in vivo* ability of calcium antagonists to reduce cholesterol accumulation in the arterial wall, a major event in atherogenesis.[1]

The calcium antagonist prototypes, nifedipine and verapamil, but not diltiazem, have been reported to inhibit cholesterol esterification induced by β-very-low-density lipoprotein (β-VLDL) in rabbit alveolar macrophages.[14] Stein and Stein[15] provided evidence that the inhibition of cholesterol esterification elicited by verapamil is not mediated by a direct effect of the drug on acyl-CoA: cholesterol acyltransferase (ACAT), the enzyme catalyzing the reaction, but involves an inhibition of cholesteryl ester hydrolysis in lysosomes and of cholesterol transport to the active site of esterification. The effect of nifedipine on cholesterol esterification in macrophages awaits clarification. Schmitz and coworkers[16] reported that nifedipine partially inhibits cholesterol esterification in macrophages previously loaded with cholesterol, but not when the drug is simultaneously incubated with acetyl-low-density lipoprotein (AcLDL), a potent activator of ACAT. On the contrary, Daugherty and coworkers[14] reported that in rabbit macrophages pre-treated for 2 h with nifedipine, the esterification activity induced by β-VLDL was almost halved. No effect of nifedipine on ACAT activity was also reported by Etinjin and Hajjar in rabbit arterial smooth muscle cells.[17]

In our laboratory, we compared the effect of verapamil and nifedipine on cholesterol esterification activity in mouse peritoneal macrophages in different conditions of ACAT activation.

Stimulation of cholesterol esterification by AcLDL in macrophages involves their receptor-mediated internalization, hydrolysis, and delivery of their cholesterol content formed to the esterification site of ACAT present on the endoplasmic reticulum.[18] In the cytoplasm, cholesterol undergoes a continuous cycle of esterification and de-esterification that causes a constant activation of ACAT.[19] In the absence of a cholesterol acceptor in the extracellular space, this cycle remains activated even after removal of AcLDL.[18] ACAT stimulation may also be achieved by incubation of cells with hydroxysterols, such as 25-hydroxycholesterol,[20] which does not involve the hydrolysis of cholesteryl ester in lysosomes. Our results confirm previous observations on the capacity of verapamil to inhibit the esterification of cellular cholesterol.[14,15] Verapamil (10 μM) was effective when simultaneously incubated with AcLDL, but not when cholesterol esterification was induced by 25-hydroxycholesterol; the drug was less active in macrophages preloaded with cholesterol. At the highest concentration tested (50 μM), an inhibitory effect also was observed under the latter two conditions (TABLE 1).

Stein and Stein observed a greater effect of verapamil in inhibiting ACAT activation induced by AcLDL compared to the enzyme stimulation obtained with cholesterol-rich liposomes.[15] Moreover, these authors demonstrated that verapamil did not affect cholesterol esterification in cell-free homogenate obtained from macrophages. In our studies, verapamil was completely inactive when added directly in the cell-free homogenate (data not shown). Our data are consistent with the hypothesis suggested by Stein and Stein[15] that inhibition of cholesterol esterification determined by verapamil involves an interference of the drug with cholesterol transport to the ACAT esterification site. As a simple inhibition of cholesteryl ester hydrolysis in lysosomes does not account for the complete abolition of ACAT stimulation by AcLDL, the different sensitivity of cells, under the different experimental conditions of ACAT activation, remains to be interpreted.

The results obtained with nifedipine indicate that this dihydropyridine has no major influence on cholesterol esterification activity in MPMs either stimulated by AcLDL or by 25-hydroxycholesterol. The slight inhibitory effect of the drug on this enzymatic system in preloaded cells may follow the stimulation of neutral cholesteryl ester hydrolase elicited by nifedipine, at least in arterial myocytes.[17] Under experimental conditions similar to ours, Daugherty and colleagues[14] demonstrated that nifedipine was very active in inhibiting cholesterol esterification induced by β-VLDL in rabbit alveolar macrophages. We could not confirm such results in MPMs and J774, a macrophage-like permanent cell line (data not shown). No effect of nifedipine on ACAT activity in MPMs during the simultaneous incubation of the drug with AcLDL was also reported by Schmitz and colleagues.[16] It is therefore probable that rabbit macrophages are particularly sensitive to nifedipine-induced inhibition of cholesterol esterification elicited by lipoproteins. Our results suggest that

TABLE 1. Effect of Verapamil, Nifedipine, and Progesterone on Cholesterol Esterification in Mouse Peritoneal Macrophages

	Conditions of ACAT Stimulation (% of control, mean ± SD)		
Drugs	Preloading	AcLDL	25-Hydroxycholesterol
Control	100.0 ± 2.2	100.0 ± 1.4	100.0 ± 11.0
Verapamil			
10 μM	28.2 ± 2.5[b]	21.1 ± 0.7b	100.1 ± 3.7
50 μM	84.9 ± 4.3[a]	1.1 ± 0.3b	37.9 ± 0.5[b]
Nifedipine 50 μM	79.1 ± 1.2[a]	88.1 ± 5.4	118.5 ± 4.7
Progesterone 30 μM	2.7 ± 0.6[b]	0.1 ± 0.01b	9.4 ± 0.6[b]

Values of control were as follows (pmol of cholesteryl oleate formed/mg of cell protein): cholesterol loaded, 2,468 ± 53; AcLDL, 2,988 ± 148; 25-hydroxycholesterol, 1,548 ± 58. Samples were run in triplicate [a]p < 0.01; [b]p < 0.001 versus control.

calcium antagonists of different classes may have different effects on cholesterol esterification.

Effect of HMG-CoA Reductase Inhibitors

Recently it was reported that vastatins are able to inhibit cholesterol esterification and deposition induced by AcLDL in human macrophages[21] and mouse peritoneal macrophages (MPM)[22] (TABLE 2). Since this inhibition did not occur in cell-free homogenates or in cholesterol preloaded cells, but was observed only when vastatins were simultaneously incubated with AcLDL, it was concluded that these drugs are not direct inhibitors of ACAT. Results obtained in our laboratory showed that inhibition of cholesterol esterification in MPM by vastatins could be fully reversed by exogenous mevalonate or by geranylgeraniol (a mevalonate metabolite), and took place in the presence of an excess of exogenous cholesterol.[22] These results provided the first evidence that the mevalonate pathway plays an essential role in the process of esterification of excess cholesterol delivered to macrophages by modified LDL.

Recently, we have repeated these data also in human macrophages incubated with oxidized LDL (manuscript in preparation), confirming that vastatins do not affect esterification by preventing the intracellular formation of substrate for ACAT (i.e., cholesterol), but rather by inhibiting the formation of non-sterol mevalonate product(s).

Inhibition of cholesterol esterification by another vastatin, lovastatin, has been reported in the CaCo-2 intestinal cell line.[23] Inhibition of intestinal ACAT activity has also been reported in rabbits given simvastatin.[24] In these cells the action of the drug is apparently linked to a mechanism different from that exerted in macrophages, since the inhibitory effect was not prevented by the addition of mevalonate,[23] and involved a direct inhibition of ACAT activity as tested in cell-free systems.[23,25] Fellermann and colleagues[26] showed that mevinolin failed to inhibit cholesterol esterification in enterocytes in the presence of high concentrations of exogenous mevalonate.

TABLE 2. Effect of Vastatins on Free, Esterified, and Total Cholesterol Content in MPM Incubated with AcLDL

Vastatins	Cellular Cholesterol (μg/mg cell protein)		
	Free	Esterified	Total
Basal	24.6	2.1	26.7
AcLDL (50 μg/ml)	37.0	30.9	67.9
AcLDL + Fluvastatin 0.5 μM	36.4	19.8	56.2
AcLDL + Fluvastatin 1 μM	41.9	15.3	57.2
AcLDL + Fluvastatin 5 μM	40.6	8.8	49.4
AcLDL + Simvastatin 0.5 μM	38.8	24.1	62.9
AcLDL + Simvastatin 1 μM	39.8	23.3	63.1
AcLDL + Simvastatin 5 μM	37.7	9.0	46.7

Cells were incubated with the indicated concentrations of drugs for 24 h, followed by a 24 h incubation in the same medium with AcLDL (50 μg protein/ml). Data are the mean of duplicate determinations not differing by more than 8%.

In these experiments the large amount of mevalonate supplied to cells produced sufficient cholesterol substrate to stimulate ACAT activity directly. These experiments demonstrate that mevinolin did not inhibit esterification of endogenously derived cholesterol, but did not provide any information on the involvement of mevalonate product(s) on esterification of lipoprotein-derived cholesterol.

More recently in our laboratory, we showed that HMG-CoA reductase inhibitors reduce *in vitro* cholesterol accumulation elicited by AcLDL in mouse peritoneal macrophages by inhibiting the endocytosis of these lipoproteins by cells.[27]

Inhibition of ^{125}I-labeled AcLDL degradation (TABLE 3) and fluorescent Dil-AcLDL internalization offered direct evidence for this conclusion. As mentioned above, the inhibition by vastatins of AcLDL-induced cholesterol esterification in human macrophages was previously reported by Kempen and coworkers.[21] These authors reported a slight, not statistically significant, effect of these drugs on AcLDL degradation, and concluded that the inhibitory effect of vastatins on cholesterol esterification could not be attributed to a decrease in receptor-mediated uptake or degradation of AcLDL. The reasons for this discrepancy are not clear. A species difference is possible; however, the results reported by Kempen and coworkers indicating a net reduction of total cellular cholesterol content in human macrophages are consistent with our observations. In any case, our results do not exclude additional mechanisms (such as an interference with the intracellular cholesterol trafficking)[21] that may contribute to the ability of vastatins to reduce cholesterol esterification.

The mechanism involved in fluvastatin action on AcLDL endocytosis needs clarification. The effect is not related to a decreased expression of the scavenger receptors since no decrease of cellular binding at 4°C could be detected. Although we cannot exclude an inhibitory effect of vastatins on the endocytosis of other ligands, the effect on AcLDL seems not due to a non-specific depression of cellular endocytotic functions, since in the condition in which AcLDL degradation was reduced, a slight but significant increase of native LDL degradation was observed (TABLE 4). Our results show that the inhibition by fluvastatin of AcLDL catabolism is reversed by mevalonate and its isoprenoid derivative geranylgeraniol (TABLE 3). This result suggests the involvement of non-sterol products of the mevalonate pathway in AcLDL endocytosis.

Interestingly, data from our laboratory indicate that the effects of fluvastatin are

TABLE 3. Effect of Fluvastatin and Fluvastatin Plus Mevalonate Derivatives on ^{125}I-Labeled AcLDL Degradation in Mouse Peritoneal Macrophages

	^{125}I-labeled AcLDL Degraded (ng/mg cell protein)
Control	$32,000 \pm 871$
Fluvastatin 5 µM	$18,000 \pm 1,590^{a}$
Fluvastatin 5 µM + Mevalonate 100 µM	$32,700 \pm 1,435^{b}$
Fluvastatin 5 µM + Geranylgeraniol 10 µM	$33,000 \pm 1,875^{b}$

Cells were incubated with the indicated compounds for 24 h, followed by a 24 h incubation in the same fresh medium with ^{125}I-labeled AcLDL (50 µg protein/ml). Data are the mean ± SD of triplicate samples.
$^{a}p < 0.05$ versus control; $^{b}p < 0.01$ versus fluvastatin alone

TABLE 4. Comparison of Fluvastatin Effect on ^{125}I-labeled AcLDL and ^{125}I-labeled LDL Degradation in MPM

	^{125}I-labeled Lipoproteins Degraded (ng/mg cell protein)	
	Control	Drug (5 μM)
[125]I-labeled AcLDL (40 μg/ml)	30,172 ± 186	21,093 ± 131[a]
[125]I-labeled-LDL (40 μg/ml)	1,992 ± 112	2,498 ± 178[a]

Cells were incubated with the indicated drugs for 24 h, followed by a 24 h incubation in the same fresh medium with radioactive lipoproteins added. Data are mean ± S.D. of triplicate samples.

[a] $p < 0.01$ versus control.

more pronounced in cholesterol-loaded cells. This result may be explained by the lower HMG-CoA reductase activity in cholesterol-rich cells as compared to unloaded cells.[28] This observation suggests the possibility that the mevalonate pathway in the arterial lesions may represent a selective target for pharmacological intervention. In conclusion, vastatin inhibition of AcLDL endocytosis might affect foam cells formation and have beneficial effects on atheroma generation not only by reducing plasma cholesterol levels, but also by directly acting on the arterial wall.

SUMMARY

Phagocytes play a major role in several diseases. In particular mononuclear phagocyte-derived foam cells have a prominent role in the development of the atherosclerotic lesions. Macrophages are present in all stages of atherogenesis: they internalize lipoproteins and accumulate cholesterol. Moreover, lipid-filled macrophages, by secreting extracellular matrix–degrading enzymes, may weaken rupture-prone atherosclerotic plaques, thus increasing the probability of precipitating atherosclerotic acute symptoms (i.e., myocardial infarction, angina, etc.). Therefore, control of cellular functions and cholesterol accumulation in macrophages represent pharmacological targets against atherosclerosis. In our laboratory we studied the effect of calcium antagonists on cellular cholesterol esterification in cultured macrophages. We also demonstrated that the HMG-CoA reductase inhibitors (vastatins) fluvastatin and simvastatin prevented cholesterol deposition in cultured human and murine macrophage by inhibiting modified LDL endocytosis. Interestingly, vastatin activity was more pronounced in cholesterol-loaded macrophages (i.e., foam cells) than in normal cells. In conclusion, *in vitro* pharmacological control of cholesterol accumulation in macrophages may be achieved with some calcium antagonists and vastatins independently of their effects on blood pressure or cholesterolemia.

REFERENCES

1. Ross, R. 1993. The pathogenesis of atherosclerosis: a perspective for the 1990s. Nature **362:** 801–809.

2. HANSSON, G. K. 1993. Immune and inflammatory mechanisms in the development of atherosclerosis. Br. Heart J. **69:** S38–S41.
3. BERLINER, J. A., M. NAVAB, A. M. FOGELMAN, J. S. FRANK, L. L. DEMER, P. A. EDWARDS, A. D. WATSON & A. J. LUSIS. 1995. Atherosclerosis: basic mechanisms: oxidation, inflammation, and genetics. Circulation **91:** 2488–2496.
4. FALK, E., P. K. SHAH & V. FUSTER. 1995. Coronary plaque disruption. Circulation **92:** 657–671.
5. DAVIES, M. J., P. D. RICHARDSON, N. WOOLF, D. R. KATZ & J. MANN. 1993. Risk of thrombosis in human atherosclerotic plaques: role of extracellular lipid, macrophage, and smooth muscle cell content. Br. Heart J. **69:** 377–381.
6. FERNANDEZ-ORTIZ, A., J. BADIMON, E. FALK, V. FUSTER, B. MEYER, A. MAILHAC, D. WENG, P. K. SHAH & L. BADIMON. 1994. Characterization of the relative thrombogenicity of atherosclerotic plaque components: implications for consequences of plaque rupture. Am. J. Coll. Cardiol. **23:** 1562–1569.
7. FALK, E. 1989. Morphologic features of unstable atherothrombotic plaques underlying acute coronary syndromes. Am. J. Cardiol. **63:** 114E–120E.
8. LOREE, H. M., R. D. KAMM, R. G. STRINGFELLOW & R. T. LEE. 1992. Effects of fibrous cap thickness on peak circumferential stress in model atherosclerotic vessels. Circ. Res. **71:** 850–858.
9. RICHARDSON, P. D., M. J. DAVIES & G. V. R. BORN. 1989. Influence of plaque configuration and stress distribution on fissuring of coronary atherosclerotic plaques. Lancet **2:** 941–944.
10. BURLEIGH, M. C., A. D. BRIGGS, C. L. LENDON, M. J. DAVIES, G. V. BORN & P. D. RICHARDSON. 1992. Collagen types I and II, collagen content, GAGs and mechanical strength of human atherosclerotic plaque caps: snap-wise variations. Atherosclerosis **96:** 71–81.
11. DOLLERY, C. M., J. R. McEWAN & A. M. HENNEY. 1995. Matrix metalloproteinases and cardiovascular disease. Circ. Res. **77:** 863–868.
12. WEINSTEIN, D. B. 1988. The antiatherogenic potential of calcium antagonists. Cardiovasc. Pharmacol. **12:** S29–S35 (Abstract).
13. BERNINI, F., A. L. CATAPANO, A. CORSINI, R. RUMAGALLI & R. PAOLETTI. 1989. Effects of calcium antagonists on lipids and atherosclerosis. Am. J. Cardiol. **64:** 1291–1341.
14. DAUGHERTY, A., D. L. RATERI & S. B. SCHONFELD. 1987. Inhibition of cholesteryl ester deposition in macrophages by calcium entry blockers: an effect dissociable from calcium entry blockade. Br. J. Pharmacol. **91:** 113–118.
15. STEIN, O. & Y. STEIN. 1987. Effect of verapamil on cholesteryl ester hydrolysis and reesterification in macrophages. Arteriosclerosis **7:** 578–584.
16. SCHMITZ, G., H. ROBENEK, M. BEUCK, R. KRAUSE, A. SCHUREK & R. NIEMANN. 1988. Ca^{2+} antagonists and ACAT inhibitors promote cholesterol efflux from macrophages by different mechanisms. Arteriosclerosis **8:** 46–56.
17. ETINJIN, O. R. & D. P. HAJJAR. 1985. Nifedipine increases cholesteryl ester hydrolytic activity in lipid-laden rabbit arterial smooth muscle cells. A possible mechanism for its antiatherogenic effect. J. Clin. Invest. **75:** 1554–1558.
18. SUCKLING, K. & E. STANGE. 1985. Role of acyl-CoA: cholesterol acyl-transferase in cellular cholesterol metabolism. J. Lipid Res. **26:** 647–671.
19. BROWN, M. S., Y. K. HO & J. L. GOLDSTEIN. 1980. The cholesteryl ester cycle in macrophage from cells: continual hydrolysis and re-esterification of cytoplasmic cholesteryl esters. J. Biol. Chem. **255:** 9344–9352.
20. BROWN, M. S., S. E. DANA & J. L. GOLDSTEIN. 1975. Cholesterol ester formation in cultured human fibroblasts. J. Biol. Chem. **250:** 4025–4027.
21. KEMPEN, H. J. M., M. VERMEER, E. DE WIT & L. M. HAVEKES. 1991. Vastatins inhibit cholesterol ester accumulation in human monocyte-derived macrophages. Arterioscl. Thromb. **11:** 146–153.

22. BERNINI, F., G. DIDONI, G. BONFADINI, S. BELLOSTA & R. FUMAGALLI. 1993. Requirement for mevalonate in acetylated LDL induction of cholesterol esterification in macrophages. Atherosclerosis **104:** 19–26.

23. KAM, N., E. ALBRIGHT, S. MATHUR & F. FIELD. 1990. Effect of lovastatin on acyl-CoA: cholesterol O-acyltransferase (ACAT) activity and the basolateral-membrane secretion of newly synthesized by CaCo-2 cells. Biochem. J. **272:** 427–433.

24. ISHIDA, F., A. SATO, Y. IIZUKA, K. KITANI, Y. SAWASAKI & T. KAMEI. 1989. Effects of MK-733 (simvastatin), an inhibitor of 3-hydroxy-3-methylglutaryl coenzyme A reductase, on intestinal acylcoenzyme A: cholesterol acyltransferase activity in rabbit. Biochim. Biophys. Acta **1004:** 117–123.

25. ISHIDA, F., A. SATO, Y. IZUKA & T. KAMEI. 1989. Inhibition of acyl coenzyme A: cholesterol acyltransferase by 3-hydroxy-3-methylglutaryl coenzyme A reductase inhibitors. Chem. Pharm. Bull. **37:** 1635–1636.

26. FELLERMANN, K., F. M. REIMANN, J. HEROLD & E. F. STANGE. 1992. Mevinolin, a competitive inhibitor of hydroxymethylglutaryl coenzyme A reductase, suppresses enterocyte esterification of exogenous but not endogenous cholesterol. Bichim. Biophys. Acta **1165:** 78–83.

27. BERNINI, F., N. SCURATI, G. BONFADINI & R. FUMAGALLI. 1995. HMG-CoA reductase inhibitors reduce acetyl LDL endocytosis in mouse peritoneal macrophages. Arterioscl. Thromb. Vasc. **15:** 1352–1358.

28. GOLDSTEIN, J. L. & M. S. BROWN. 1990. Regulation of the mevalonate pathway, Nature **343:** 425–430.

Pentoxifylline Differentially Regulates Migration and Respiratory Burst Activity of the Neutrophil[a]

STEFAN DUNZENDORFER, PETER SCHRATZBERGER,
NORBERT REINISCH, CHRISTIAN M. KÄHLER,
AND CHRISTIAN J. WIEDERMANN[b]

Department of Internal Medicine
Medical Faculty
University of Innsbruck
Anichstraße 35
A-6020 Innsbruck, Austria

INTRODUCTION

Tumor necrosis factor (alpha) (TNF), a well-known pro-inflammatory cytokine, is mainly produced by mononuclear leukocytes in response to numerous agents, including microorganisms, microbial products (e.g., lipopolysaccharide), C5a, and cytokines.[1] In patients suffering from systemic inflammatory response syndrome (SIRS)/sepsis, elevated serum levels of TNF have been reported[2] and there is abundant evidence that TNF leads to tissue damage via enhanced neutrophil (PMNL) degranulation, superoxide production, and altered PMNL chemotaxis. Inhibition of the effects of this cytokine on PMNL may be beneficial in a variety of inflammatory diseases, including SIRS and septic shock due to bacterial infection. Therapies against TNF have been developed but none of the agents tested demonstrated any clearcut beneficial effects or reduced mortality in clinical trials.[3]

Colony-stimulating factors were originally identified as hematopoetic growth factors. The fact that endogenous granulocyte colony-stimulating factor (G-CSF) serum levels are increased 30-fold in patients with severe infections supports the interpretation that G-CSF is part of a physiologic defense mechanism and that it should be possible to reinforce or shift this mechanism by pharmacologic intervention.[4] The therapeutic effects of G-CSF include the recruitment of PMNL from the bone marrow, shortening of a neutropenic period, and priming of PMNL for enhanced bactericidal activity.[5–7] Recent animal studies showed that G-CSF pretreatment attenuated lipopolysaccharide-inducible serum TNF concentrations *in vivo*, while no such effect could be observed on macrophage cultures *in vitro*.[8] Elevated levels of G-CSF during bacterial infection suggest that G-CSF may be involved in the primary host response

[a]This work supported by the Austrian Science Funds grant number 09977 (C. J. W.) and by Hoechst-Marion-Roussel Pharmaceuticals (Vienna, Austria).
[b]Address all correspondence to Christian J. Wiedermann, M.D., Department of Internal Medicine, University of Innsbruck, Anichstraße 35, A-6020 Innsbruck, Austria. Telephone, 43-512-504-3255. Fax, 43-512-504-4201.

and in addition some evidence renders G-CSF a candidate drug for the prevention and treatment of its systemic responses.[9,10]

Pentoxifylline (PTX) [1-(5-oxyohexyl)-3,7-dimethylxanthine], a methylxanthine derivative, is a well-known rheologically active drug and is used in therapy of peripheral vascular disease and intermittent claudication. It has also been reported to suppress transcription of TNF mRNA and thereby to inhibit subsequent TNF production by human monocytes.[11] However, in another study no reduction of circulating levels of TNF was found after treatment with PTX.[12] The substance has been extensively used in animal models in which an amelioration of clinical parameters of sepsis was observed, but again results contradicting these observations have also been reported.[13–15] Many studies focused on the effects of the drug on PMNL function. Briefly, PTX is reported to block the effect of TNF in adherence assays,[16] to prevent degranulation of myeloperoxidase and lysozyme, to inhibit stimulated superoxide production without affecting phagocytosis,[17] and to improve PMNL motility and chemotaxis.[18] However, other *in vitro* studies have reported observations that contradict the above-mentioned effects of PTX.[19,20]

Despite these conflicting results of animal and *in vitro* experiments, PTX has been suggested as a treatment for several diseases connected with elevated TNF serum levels based on its ability to inhibit TNF mRNA transcription.[11]

With reference to the scheme of therapy in SIRS/sepsis using G-CSF, the aim of our *in vitro* investigation was to determine whether there are interactions between PTX and G-CSF at the level of PMNL functions. On the one hand, it could be beneficial to attenuate the pro-inflammatory action of TNF and, on the other, this should not lessen a positive outcome of G-CSF therapy.

MATERIALS AND METHODS

Materials

Materials used in this study include PTX (Hoechst-Marion-Roussel Pharmaceuticals, Vienna, Austria), recombinant human tumor necrosis factor-alpha (TNF) (specific activity 4×10^7 U/mg protein, Genentech Inc., South San Francisco, CA), human recombinant granulocyte-colony stimulating factor (hrG-CSF) (Neupogen®; Amgen, Vienna, Austria), N-formyl-Met-Leu-Phe (fMLP), interleukin-8 (IL-8), cytochrome *c* (type III from horse heart), gelatin, dextran 460.500, and Percoll (all from Sigma Corp., St. Louis, MO), RPMI-1640, trypan blue (both from Biological Industries, Kibbutz Beit Heamek, Israel), and bovine serum albumin (BSA) (Behringwerke AG, Marburg, Germany).

Preparation of PMNL

From the peripheral blood (anticoagulated with EDTA) of healthy volunteers, PMNL were obtained after discontinuous density gradient centrifugation of whole blood on Percoll followed by hypotonic lysis of contaminating erythrocytes. The cell preparations (> 95% PMNL by morphology in Giemsa stains; > 98% viability by trypan blue dye exclusion) were resuspended in RPMI-1640 containing 0.5% BSA for chemotaxis experiments or Hanks' balanced salt solution without phenol red (HBSS; containing 0.05% BSA) for respiratory burst assays.

Chemotaxis Experiments

Chemotaxis of PMNL through cellulose nitrate to gradients of soluble attractants was measured using a 48-well microchemotaxis chamber (Neuroprobe, Bethesda, MD) in which a 5-μm pore cellulose nitrate filter (Sartorius, Göttingen, Germany) separates the upper and lower chamber. Cells were preincubated for 15 min with PTX (1 mM), washed, and then stimulated with TNF (10 ng/ml) or hrG-CSF (3,000 U/ml). After 45 min, cells were washed twice and placed into the upper chamber (5×10^4 per well in RPMI 1640/BSA 0.5%). PMNL were allowed to migrate towards the soluble attractants in the lower chamber for 35 min at 37°C in humidified atmosphere (5% CO_2). After this incubation time the nitrocellulose filters were dehydrated, fixed, and stained with hematoxylin-eosin. Migration depth of PMNL into the filter was quantified by microscopy, measuring the distance (μm) from the surface of the filter to the leading front of three cells. Data are expressed as chemotaxis index, which is the ratio between the distances of directed and undirected migration of PMNL into the nitrocellulose filters.

Respiratory Burst of PMNL

Measurement of the production of extracellular superoxide anion was based on the reduction of cytochrome c and specificity was demonstrated via its inhibition by superoxide dismutase (data not shown). PMNL were primed for 45 min at 37°C (5% CO_2 atmosphere) with TNF (10 ng/ml) or hrG-CSF (3000 U/ml) with or without PTX at various concentrations. To determine the effect of PTX alone, the drug was added for an incubation period of 15 min. Then 100 μl/well (96-well plate; Falcon® 3072) of 2×10^6 PMNL/ml were immersed at 37°C in a 160 μmol/l solution of cytochrome c in phenol red–free HBSS containing 1 μmol/l of fMet-Leu-Phe (fMLP) or medium. The plates were covered with lids and placed in a humidified incubator (95% air-5% CO_2) and after 10 min transferred to the ELISA reader (Labsystems Multiscan, Helsinki, Finland) and absorbances were read at 550 nm. Data are given as the index that describes the quotient of basal and formyl-peptide–stimulated reduction of cytochrome c.

RESULTS

Chemotaxis Experiments

Random migration of PMNL into nitrocellulose remained unaffected after pretreatment of the cells with PTX (1 mM), whereas fMLP- and IL-8–stimulated chemotaxis was significantly reduced. Preincubation of PMNL with TNF (10 ng/ml) for 45 min significantly decreased PMNL non-directed and directed migration towards fMLP (10 nM) or IL-8 (1 nM). Only directed migration to fMLP or IL-8 was diminished by preincubation of the PNML with 3,000 U/ml G-CSF. Incubation of PMNL with PTX (1 mM) for 15 min prior to stimulation with TNF or G-CSF abolished the inhibition by TNF of both undirected and directed migration but failed to counteract the G-CSF inhibition of directed migration (FIG. 1).

Respiratory Burst Assays

After a 45-min incubation of PMNL with TNF (10 ng/ml) or a 15-min incubation with G-CSF (3000 U/ml), fMLP (10 nM) was added simultaneously with various concentrations of PTX (0.1 nM–10 mM). Priming of PMNL with TNF or G-CSF led to a significant increase in triggered oxygen-derived radical production compared to the control experiment without TNF or G-CSF priming. Addition of PTX resulted in a highly significant reduction of radical production in a dose-dependent manner (1 mM to 10 mM), whereas at concentrations of less than 1 mM, PTX failed to exert significant effects on respiratory burst. At the highest concentration of the drug, triggered free oxygen radical production was reduced to below baseline levels in both TNF- and G-CSF-primed PMNL (FIG. 2).

In the following experiments we preincubated PMNL with PTX (1 μM–10 mM) for 15 min before cells were primed with TNF (10 ng/ml) or G-CSF (3,000 U/ml) and subsequently triggered respiratory burst with fMLP (10 nM). Data shown in FIGURE 3 are expressed as an index describing the ratio of superoxide anion production of primed but unstimulated cells to that of primed and fMLP-stimulated ones. Data indicate that PTX enhanced superoxide anion production of TNF- or G-CSF-primed PMNL in response to fMLP. This effect was significant at a concentration range of 1–10 mL PTX. This effect was not significant at concentrations below 1 mM of PTX. Respiratory burst activity of unprimed PMNL stimulated with fMLP remained unaffected by PTX preincubation at various concentrations of PTX (FIG. 3).

DISCUSSION

In the management of severe sepsis, many agents blocking pro-inflammatory mediators were tested for their effectiveness in the amelioration of clinical signs occurring during this syndrome. None of these agents, however, reduced mortality.[21] In an attempt to restore homeostasis, anti-inflammatory components are released in response to a pro-inflammatory systemic response[22] and inflammatory components are released in reaction to an initially anti-inflammatory systemic response. Since persistent levels of anti-inflammatory mediators will cause anergy and/or immune dysfunction, agents that stimulate the immune system, such as G-CSF, may be helpful in the treatment of patients with a massive or persistent anti-inflammatory reaction. As PTX was reported to cause clinical improvement in animal models of SIRS/sepsis,[13] our interest focused on possible drug interactions between PTX and G-CSF when PMNL are exposed to both agents.

TNF is reported to initiate PMNL shape changes combined with decreased plas-

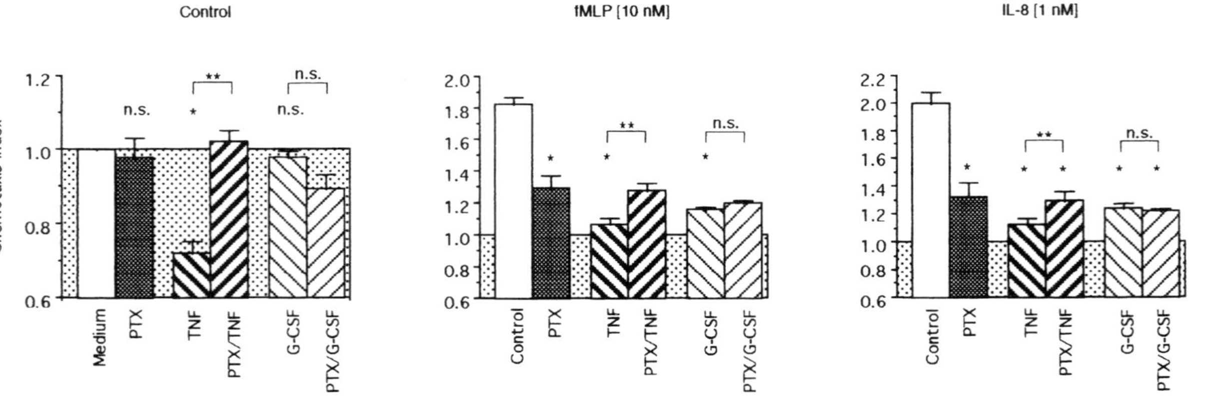

FIGURE 1. Migration of human PMNL into nitrocellulose filters (5 μm pore size). Cells were preincubated for 15 min with PTX (1 mM) prior to incubation with TNF (10 ng/ml) or G-CSF (3,000 U/ml) at 37°C in humidified atmosphere. After the incubation period, PMNL were washed twice and allowed to migrate for 35 min. Data are expressed as mean ± SEM of the chemotaxis index (distance of migration toward attractant divided by that toward medium). N = 5. Statistical analysis: Student's *t* test; *$p< 0.05$; **$p<0.01$; n.s., not significant.

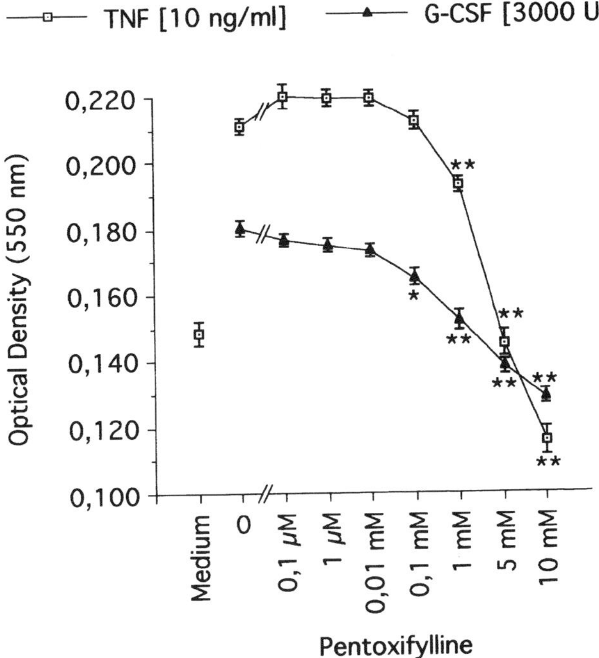

FIGURE 2. Measurement of fMLP-triggered superoxide anion production of PMNL by reduction of cytochrome *c*. Cells were primed with TNF (10 ng/ml; 45 min) or G-CSF (3,000 U/ml; 15 min) followed by concomitant addition of fMLP (10 nM) and PTX at various concentrations. Reduction of cytochrome *c* was measured after 10 min with an ELISA reader. Data are given as mean ± SEM of the optical density. N = 3. Statistical analysis: Student's *t* test; *$p<0.05$; **$p<0.01$.

ma membrane fluidity and cytoskeletal polymerization.[23] Such TNF effects on PMNL could result in decreased flux of plasma membrane adhesion elements important for PMNL migration. In addition, TNF-induced up-regulation of adhesion molecules may also be important for PMNL migration. It has been reported that CD 11b up-regulation together with loss of CD 62-L is induced by TNF.[24] Sullivan and colleagues[23] demonstrated that hyperadherence and increased oxidative activity of PMNL have little effect on TNF inhibition of directed and non-directed migration. So PTX is thought to restore the migratory properties of PMNL via its ability to increase the fluidity of the plasma membrane combined with depolymerization of F-actin.[23,25] PTX is also reported to decrease CD 11b on the surface of TNF-stimulated PMNL[17] and this may contribute to the restoring of TNF-induced inhibition of PMNL migration.

Since in contrast to TNF, G-CSF has been shown to be a chemotactic signal for PMNL,[26] G-CSF–induced deactivation of PMNL chemotaxis towards fMLP or IL-8 may be due to chemotaxis receptor cross-desensitization.[27] The biologic activities of

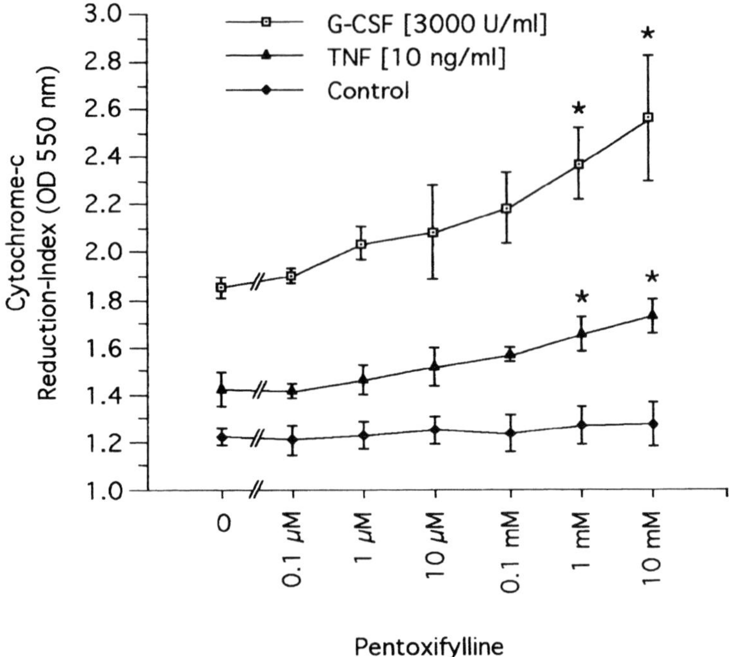

FIGURE 3. Measurement of fMLP-triggered superoxide anion production of PMNL by reduction of cytochrome *c*. Cells were preincubated with various concentrations of pentoxifylline for 15 min, washed, and stimulated either with TNF (10 ng/ml; 45 min) or G-CSF (3,000 U/ml; 15 min). After these periods, cells were either stimulated with fMLP (10 nM) or remained unstimulated. Reduction of cytochrome *c* was measured after 10 min with an ELISA reader. Data are given as mean ± SEM of an index that describes the quotient of fMLP-stimulated and unstimulated O_2 release. N = 3. Statistical analysis: Student's *t* test; * $p < 0.05$; ** $p < 0.01$.

G-CSF are mediated by specific receptors on the surface of responsive cells. Various agents that activate PMNL, including GM-CSF, TNF, lipopolysaccharide, C5a, and fMLP have been reported to downregulate G-CSF receptor expression on PMNL.[28] Our observation that PTX fails to affect G-CSF–induced modulation of PMNL chemotaxis indicates that the drug does not influence receptor regulation or G-CSF receptor–dependent signaling pathways, which are responsible for inhibition of migration. In contrast to migration experiments, pathways that mediate G-CSF–induced priming of the PMNL for enhanced respiratory burst appear to be influenced by PTX, as it significantly augmented G-CSF–induced priming. No conclusion on the precise mechanisms of interactions of PTX and G-CSF of PMNL can be drawn.

Simultaneous administration of PTX and fMLP after PMNL priming with TNF or G-CSF led to a significant decrease in free oxygen–derived radicals. This effect has also been observed by other investigators[29] and is consistent with the observation that PTX functions as an oxygen-radical scavenger.[30] The result that preincubation with PTX for 15 min, removal of PTX, and washing of PMNL before stimulation with fMLP does not have an influence on superoxide anion detection is also in accordance with another previous report.[31] However, we were surprised to see that PTX even enhanced the priming effects of TNF and G-CSF on PMNL respiratory burst activity in response to fMLP.

The mechanism by which TNF activates PMNL remains unclear, but ligation of TNF receptors leads to rapid increase in diacylglycerol (DAG) and ceramide in PMNL.[32] It is quite possible that PTX may also elevate intracellular DAG levels via its reported property to augment DAG precursors, such as phosphatidylinositol 4-phosphate or phosphatidylinositol 4,5-biphosphate,[33] which in turn possibly lead to the augmented response of PMNL respiratory burst priming by TNF. Mechanisms involved in a possibly additive interaction with G-CSF are unknown. Our data show that exposure of PMNL to PTX augment free oxygen radical production primed by pro-inflammatory cytokines. As PTX is an oxygen-radical scavenger, this effect is completely blunted by the continuous presence of PTX.

PTX may have beneficial effects in SIRS/sepsis due to its function as an oxygen-radical scavenger and as a blocker of TNF synthesis. Restoration of TNF-induced inhibition of PMNL migration by PTX may ameliorate impairment of endothelial cells. TNF-induced impairment of PMNL migration may, on the other hand, be beneficial for antagonizing the spread of focal inflammation by arresting PMNL at the site of highest TNF concentrations. Such a beneficial role of TNF would then also be affected by PTX.

Timing and duration of the presence may be critical determinants of the effects of PTX on TNF and G-CSF actions on PMNL. Our finding is in agreement with studies on animal models that demonstrated that application of PTX after the beginning of group B streptococcal infusion was able to ameliorate the decline in cardiac output, stroke volume, and the increase in pulmonary and systemic vascular resistance.[13] If PTX is given prior to administration of G-CSF or before the initial elevated TNF levels in sepsis, the beneficial effects of G-CSF might be negated and TNF-induced PMNL toxicity on endothelial cells might be enhanced. Perhaps it would be better to take advantage of the ability of PTX to scavenge oxygen-derived radicals. Only high-dose PTX is able to exert this effect but administration of high-dose PTX is also reported to be associated with systemic hypotension and deterioration of clinical parameters when given in established sepsis.[34] In conclusion, as the therapeutic range of PTX is narrow, caution is advised. The complexity of PTX actions and of the mechanisms involved does not as yet allow formulation of simple and straightforward concepts that help define effective indications of PTX in SIRS/sepsis.

SUMMARY

TNF is produced by monocytes/macrophages in response to endotoxin, which may lead to septic shock. TNF stimulates neutrophil adherence, degranulation, and superoxide production, but inhibits neutrophil migration. A mitigating anti-inflammatory effect can be experimentally induced in septic shock by TNF blockers, such as pentoxifylline, and is also suggested for treatment with hrG-CSF. With regard to the combination of pentoxifylline and hrG-CSF, the purpose of this investigation was to explore whether and in what way the effects of hrG-CSF and pentoxifylline interact with each other in neutrophils. To this end, we studied the effects of pentoxifylline on TNF- and G-CSF–induced modulation of neutrophil chemotaxis and O_2 release. TNF and G-CSF decreased directed migration of neutrophils to FMLP or IL-8. High-dose pentoxifylline (1 mM) was able to counteract the effect of TNF but not that of G-CSF on neutrophil migration. In the presence of pentoxifylline, TNF and G-CSF were unable to stimulate respiratory burst. In contrast, pre-exposure of cells to pentoxifylline followed by washing increased the priming effect of TNF or hrG-CSF on neutrophil respiratory burst activity. The methylxanthine derivative by itself showed no effect on spontaneous and fMLP-stimulated O_2 release by neutrophils. Stimulation of neutrophil respiratory burst by pentoxifylline may not be detectable in the presence of pentoxifylline due to its known oxygen-radical scavenging function. Results suggest that by blocking the inflammatory action of TNF on neutrophils, pentoxifylline may diminish endothelial cell damage caused by inhibited neutrophil chemotaxis. On the other hand, since transiently present pentoxifylline may enhance the respiratory burst activity of TNF- or hrG-CSF-primed neutrophils, concomitant administration of pentoxifylline and hrG-CSF to patients with SIRS/sepsis might diminish beneficial effects of the latter and additional deleterious effects might occur.

REFERENCES

1. BEUTLER, B. & A. CERAMI. 1986. Cachectin and tumor necrosis factor as two sides of the same biological coin. Nature **320:** 584–588.
2. THIJS, L. G. & C. E. HACK. 1995. Time course of cytokine levels in sepsis. Intens. Care Med. **21:** S258–S263.
3. ABRAHAM, E., R. WUNDERINK, H. SILVERMANN, T. M. PERL, S. NASRAWAY, H. LEVY, R. BONE, R. P. WENZEL, R. BALK & R. ALLRED. 1995. Efficacy and safety of monoclonal antibody to human tumor necrosis factor-alpha in patients with sepsis syndrome. J. Am. Med. Assoc. **273:** 931–934.
4. KAWAKAMI, M., H. TSUTSUMI, T. KUMAKAWA, H. ABE, M. HIRAI, S. KUROSAWA, M. MORI & M. FUKUSHIMA. 1990. Levels of serum granulocyte colony-stimulating factor in patients with infections. Blood **76:** 1962.
5. LANG, C. H., G. J. BAGBY, C. DOBRESCU, S. NELSON & J. J. SPITZER. 1992. Effect of granulocyte colony-stimulating factor on sepsis-induced changes in neutrophil accumulation and organ glucose uptake. J. Infect. Dis. **166:** 336.
6. ROILIDES, E., T. J. WALSH, P. A. PIZZO & M. RUBIN. 1991. Granulocyte colony-stimulating factor enhances the phagocytotic and bactericidal activity of normal and defective human neutrophils. J. Infect. Dis. **163:** 579.
7. YUO, A., S. KITAGAWA, A. OHSAKA, M. OHTA, K. MIYAZONO, T. OKABE, A. URABE, M. SAITO & F. TAKAKU. 1989. Recombinant human granulocyte colony-stimulating factor as an activator of human granulocytes: Potentiation of responses triggered by receptor-mediated agonists and stimulation of C3bi receptor expression and adherence. Blood **74:** 2144–2149.
8. HARTUNG, T., W. D. DÖCKE, F. GANTNER, G. KRIEGER, A. SAUER, P. STEVENS, H. D. VOLK & A. WENDEL. 1995. Effect of granulocyte colony-stimulating factor treatment on ex vivo blood cytokine response in human volunteers. Blood **85:** 2482–2489.
9. HEBERT, J. C., M. O'REILLY & R. L. GAMELLI. 1990. Protective effect of recombinant human granulocyte colony-stimulating factor against pneumococcal infections in splenectomized mice. Arch. Surg. **125:** 1075.

10. POLLMÄCHER, T., C. KORTH, J. MULLINGTON, W. SCHREIBER, J. SAUER, H. VEDDER, C. GALANOS & F. HOLSBOER. 1996. Effects of granulocyte colony-stimulating factor on plasma cytokine and cytokine receptor levels and on the in vivo host response to endotoxin in healthy men. Blood **87:** 900–905.

11. DOHERTY, G. M., J. C. JENSEN, H. R. ALEXANDER, C. M. BURESH & J. A. NORTON. 1991. Pentoxifylline suppression of tumor necrosis factor gene transcription. Surgery **21:** S423–435.

12. REMICK, D., Y. NEGUSSIE, D. FEKADE & G. GRIFFIN. 1996. Pentoxifylline fails to prevent the Jarisch-Herxheimer reaction or associated cytokine release. J. Infect. Dis. **174:** 627–630.

13. DEL MORAL, T., R. GOLDBERG, J. URBON, C. SUGUIHARA, O. MARTINEZ, J. STEIN-STREILEIN, W. J. FEUER & E. BANCALARI. 1996. Effects of treatment with pentoxifylline on the cardiovascular manifestations of *group B streptococcal* sepsis in the piglet. Pediatr. Res. **40:** 469–473.

14. LECHNER, A. J., L. R. ROUBEN, L. H. POTTHOFF, T. L. TREDWAY & G. M. MATUSCHAK. 1993. Effects of pentoxifylline on tumor necrosis factor production and survival during lethal *E. coli* sepsis vs. Disseminated candidiasis with fungal septic shock. Circ. Shock **39:** 306–315.

15. TIGHE D., R. MOSS, J. HYND, S. BOGHOSSIAN, N. AL-SAADY, M. F. HEATH & E. D. BENNETT. 1990. Pretreatment with pentoxifylline improves the hemodynamic and histologic changes and decreases neutrophil adhesiveness in a pig fecal peritonitis model. Crit. Care Med. **18:** 184–189.

16. SALYER, J. L., J. F. BOHNSACK, W. A. KNAPE, A. O. SHIGEOKA, E. R. ASHWOOD & H. R. HILL. 1990. Mechanisms of tumor necrosis factor-alpha alteration of PMN adhesion and migration. Am. J. Pathol. **136:** 831–841.

17. CURRIE, M. S., K. M. RAO, J. PADMANABHAN, A. JONES, J. CRAWFORD & H. J. COHEN. 1990. Stimulus-specific effects of pentoxifylline on neutrophil CR3 expression, degranulation, and superoxide production. J. Leuk. Biol. **47:** 244–250.

18. SULLIVAN, G. W., T. N. PATSELAS, J. A. REDICK & G. L. MANDELL. 1984. Enhancement of chemotaxis and protection of mice from infection. Trans. Assoc. Am. Physicans **97:** 337–345.

19. DEISHER, TA., I. GARCIA & J. M. HARLAN. 1993. Cytokine-induced adhesion molecule expression on human umbilical vein endothelial cells is not regulated by cyclic adenosine monophosphate accumulation. Life Sci. **53:** 365–370.

20. MORANDINI, R., G. GHANEM, A. PORTIER-LEMARIÉ, B. ROBAYE, A. RENAUD & J. M. BOEYNAEMS. 1996. Action of cAMP on expression and release of adhesion molecules in human endothelial cells. Am. J. Physiol. **270:** H807–H816.

21. BONE, R. C. 1996. Why sepsis trials fail. J. Am. Med. Assoc. **276:** 565–566.

22. GOLDIE, A. S., K. C. H. FEARON, J. A. ROSS, G. R. BARCLAY, R. E. JACKSON, I. S. GRANT, G. RAMSAY, A. S. BLYTH & J. C. HOWIE. 1995. Natural cytokine antagonists and endogenous antiendotoxin core antibodies in sepsis syndrome. J. Am. Med. Assoc. **274:** 172–177.

23. SULLIVAN, G. W., H. T. CARPER, J. B. HYLTON, W. J. NOVICK, JR. & G. MANDELL. 1990. Lack of correlation between TNF-inhibition and enhanced PMN oxidative activity and adherence: Implications for mechanisms of pentoxifylline action. *In* Pentoxifylline and Analogues: Effects on Leukocyte Function. pp. 1–8. Karger. Basel.

24. CONDLIFFE, A. M., E. R. CHILVERS, C. HASLETT & I. DRANSFIELD. 1996. Priming differentially regulates neutrophil adhesion molecule expression/function. Immunology **89:** 105–111.

25. RAO, K. M. K., J. PADMANABHAN, H. J. COHEN & M. S. CURRIE. 1990. Effect of pentoxifylline and analogs on actin state and cell surface receptor expression in human leukocytes. *In* Pentoxifylline and Analogues: Effects on Leukocyte Function. pp. 64–70. Karger. Basel.

26. WANG, J. M., Z. G. CHEN, S. COLELLA, M. A. BONILLA, K. WELTE, C. BORDIGNON & A. MANTOVANI. 1988. Chemotactic activity of recombinant granulocyte-stimulating factor. Blood **72:** 1456–1460.

27. TOMHAVE, E. D., R. M. RICHARDSON, J. R. DIDSBURY, L. MENARD, R. SNYDERMAN & H. ALI. 1994. Cross-desensitization of receptors for peptide chemoattractants. J. Immunol. **153:** 3267.

28. KHWAJA, A., J. CARVER, H. M. JONES, D. PATERSON & D. C. LINCH. 1993. Expression and dynamic modulation of the human granulocyte colony-stimulating factor receptor in immature and differentiated myeloid cells. Brit. J. Haematol. **85:** 254.

29. SULLIVAN, G. W., H. T. CARPER, W. J. NOVICK & G. L. MANDELL. 1988. Inhibition of the inflammatory action of interleukin-1 and tumor necrosis factor (alpha) on neutrophil function by pentoxifylline. Infect. Immun. **56:** 1722–1729.

30. FREITAS, J. P. & P. M. FILIPE. 1995. Pentoxifylline, a hydroxyl radical scavanger. Biol. Trac. Elem. Res. **47:** 307–311.

31. CROUCH, S. P. M. & J. FLETCHER. 1992. Effect of ingested pentoxifylline on neutrophil superoxide anion production. Infect. Immun. **60:** 4504–4509.

32. BALAZOVICH, K. J., S. J. SUCHARD, D. G. REMICK & L. A. BOXER. 1996. Tumor necrosis factor-α and FMLP receptors are functionally linked during FMLP-stimulated activation of adherent human neutrophils. Blood **88:** 690–696.

33. SATO, Y., T. MIURA & Y. SUZUKI. 1990. Interaction of pentoxifylline with human erythrocytes. II. Effects of pentoxifylline on the erythrocyte membrane. Chem. Pharm. Bull. Tokyo **38:** 555–558.

34. RIDINGS, P. C., C. J. WINDSOR, H. J. SUGERMAN, E. KENNEDY, M. M. SHOLLY, C. R. BLOCHER, B. J. FISHER & A. A. FOWLER. 1994. Beneficial cardiopulmonary effects of pentoxifylline in experimental sepsis are lost once septic shock is established. Arch. Surg. **129:** 1144–1152.

Activation of Human Neutrophils by Soluble Immune Complexes: Role of FcγRII and FcγRIIIb in Stimulation of the Respiratory Burst and Elevation of Intracellular Ca²⁺[a]

STEVEN W. EDWARDS,[b] FIONA WATSON, LAKHDAR GASMI,
DALE A. MOULDING, AND JULIE A. QUAYLE

School of Biological Sciences
Life Sciences Building
University of Liverpool
P.O. Box 147
Liverpool L69 7XB, United Kingdom

INTRODUCTION

Human neutrophils express three types of receptor for IgG, namely FcγRI, FcγRII, and FcγRIIIb.[1–4] Whilst these appear to have overlapping activities, it is clear that they may mediate different functions that are appropriate under different physiological or pathological conditions. The expression of these three receptors can vary considerably depending upon the past history of the neutrophils. For example, FcγRI is only expressed on neutrophils after exposure to certain cytokines, such as γ-interferon, whereas the expression of FcγRIIIb can be upregulated (via the translocation of pre-formed intracellular pools to the plasma membrane) or downregulated via shedding from the cell surface.[1] There is considerable evidence to suggest that, as with the complement receptors, the function of these receptors can be modulated (in the absence of a change in receptor number) so that the affinity of binding to the ligand is altered.[5]

FcγRI is a heavily glycosylated, 72 kD transmembrane protein. cDNA sequence analysis predicts a mature protein of 40 kD and six potential glycosylation sites. Circulating bloodstream neutrophils do not express FcγRI, but its expression is upregulated *in vitro* by exposure to γ-interferon (up to 100 U/ml for 24 h).[6,7] This treatment results in the expression of about 10^4 receptors/cell (a value comparable to that found on freshly isolated blood monocytes), but has no effect on the expression of FcγRII or FcγRIIIb. FcγRI expression has also been reported on neutrophils of patients undergoing G-CSF therapy,[8,9] but it is unknown if this upregulation is due to the G-CSF itself or to the generation of some other cytokine (e.g., γ-interferon) that has been

[a]This work supported by the Arthritis and Rheumatism Council and North West Cancer Research Fund.

[b]Address correspondence to Dr. Steven W. Edwards, School of Biological Sciences, Life Sciences Building, University of Liverpool, P.O. Box 147, Liverpool L69 7XB, U.K. Telephone, 44 151 794 4363; Fax, 44 151 794 4349; and Email, sbirl2@liverpool.ac.uk.

generated secondary to the G-CSF. This receptor is also present at low levels on neutrophils isolated from the synovial fluid of patients with rheumatoid arthritis.[10]

The increase in expression of FcγRI on neutrophils results from the enhanced transcription and translation of the gene for this receptor.[11,12] Whilst three transcripts for this gene have been cloned, Southern analyses reveal a single gene for this receptor, which is present on chromosome 1q. Two of the transcripts arise from polymorphisms, whilst the third represents diversity in the predicted cytoplasmic domain. The transcript size is 1.7 kb. This increase in FcγRI expression on neutrophils and monocytes is associated with an enhancement of antibody-dependent cellular cytotoxicity (ADCC) and phagocytosis. Co-treatment of neutrophils or monocytes with γ-interferon and dexamethasome (200 nM) largely prevents the upregulation in FcγRI expression (by 40–75% dependent upon the donor) and also decreases ADCC and phagocytosis.[13]

FcγRI (unlike FcγRII and FcγRIII) binds monomeric IgG with high affinity (K_d = 10^{-8} to 10^{-9} M). Thus, bloodstream neutrophils, which lack this receptor, do not bind monomeric IgG. The affinity of binding of murine monomeric IgG is IgG_{2a}= IgG_3≫IgG_1 = IgG_{2b}, whilst that for human monomeric IgG is IgG_1 = IgG_3> IgG_4≫IgG_2. The molecule comprises an extracellular domain consisting of three immunoglobulin-like domains, the structures of which are maintained by disulfide bridges. Two of these domains share homology to the two extracellular, immunoglobulin-like domains of FcγRII and FcγRIII. The third domain does not, however, share homology with these structures and it is likely that this extra domain confers upon FcγRI the ability to bind monomeric IgG with high affinity. The murine gene is 65–70% homologous with the human gene in the extracellular and transmembrane domains, but the human cytoplasmic domain is 25 amino acids shorter and is only 25% homologous with its murine counterpart.[1–4]

FcγRII is a 40 kD transmembrane glycoprotein present on a variety of immune cells, such as neutrophils, B lymphocytes, platelets, eosinophils, monocytes, and macrophages, but it is not expressed on NK cells. It binds monomeric IgG with very low affinity but binds well to dimers, trimers, or aggregated IgG (K_d>10^{-7} M). There are about 10^3 receptors per platelet, 10^5 per monocyte, and $1–2 \times 10^4$ per neutrophil.

In humans, three different forms of the receptor exist (FcγRIIA, FCγRIIB, and FcγRIIC) and these are encoded by three separate genes located on chromosome 1q23. These three separate genes give rise to six separate transcripts. FcγRIIA gives rise to two transcripts (HR, LR) of 1.8 and 2.5 kb due to alternative polyadenylation sites, FcγRIIC gives rise to a single (1.8 kb) transcript whilst FcγRIIB generates three transcripts. These three latter transcripts, b1, b2, and b3, arise from alternative splicing: b1 and b2 are generated from alternative splicing of exons encoding the signal sequence. The mature proteins of FcγRIIA and FcγRIIC are 95% homologous in the extracellular and transmembrane domains, and 100% identical in the intracytoplasmic domain. The FcγRIIB proteins, b1, b2, and b3, are 95% homologous to FcγRIIC in the extracellular and transmembrane domains, but the FcγRIIB intracytoplasmic domain is unrelated to FcγRIIA and FcγRIIC. Furthermore, there is a 19 amino acid insertion into the cytoplasmic domains of b1 and b3 (not b2) that is due to an alternative splicing event.

These forms of human FcγRII are differentially expressed in immune cells.[1–4] For example, FcγRIIB transcripts are detectable in monocytes, macrophages, and lymphocytes, but not on neutrophils, NK cells, or T cell lines. Alternatively, FcγRIIA and FcγRIIC are expressed on monocytes, macrophages, and neutrophils but not on NK cells nor lymphocytes. FcγRIIA possesses two potential glycosylation sites whilst FcγRIIB and FcγRIIC possess three and the murine receptors have four potential sites. The specificity of binding of IgG for the murine receptor is $IgG_{2b}>IgG_{2a}>IgG_1\gg IgG_3$, whilst that of the human receptor is $IgG_1=IgG_3\gg IgG_2=IgG_4$.

FcγRIII is a glycoprotein appearing as a broad band of 50–70 kD in SDS-PAGE and is expressed on neutrophils, eosinophils, macrophages, and NK cells. It is not expressed on blood monocytes, but macrophages derived from cultured monocytes and macrophages isolated from the peritoneum, lung, and liver are found to express FcγRIII. The protein backbone of the molecule (predicted from cDNA analysis or after removal of the sugars) is 29 or 33 kD. The murine receptor has four potential glycosylation sites, whereas the two human forms have five or six. It binds IgG complexes with low affinity ($K_d<10^{-7}$ M in humans, 10^{-6} M in murine cells), but is present on the cell surface in large numbers. In human neutrophils there are between 100,000 and 200,000 receptors per cell and so it is by far the most abundant Fcγ receptor on these cells. It is present on the plasma membrane, but additionally subcellular pools of this receptor exist and these may be mobilized to the plasma membrane in order to maintain or augment expression.[14] On human neutrophils it binds IgG molecules with the following specificity: $IgG_1=IgG_3\gg IgG_2=IgG_4$. On murine cells it binds IgG molecules with the specificity: $IgG_3>IgG_{2a}>IgG_{2b}\gg IgG_1$.

The murine and human genes for FcγRIII are homologous in terms of sequence, genomic organization, cellular distribution, and function.[1–4] In murine cells, the single gene gives rise to a single transcript of 1.6 kb, and the extracellular domain is 95% homologous with that of FcγRII. The transmembrane and cytoplasmic domains are, however, unrelated. Transfection of COS cells or L cells with the murine cDNA for FcγRIII results in the appearance of low affinity binding sites for IgG complexes, but these receptors are only expressed at low levels. It was found that the coexpression of another molecule, the γ-chain of FcεR1 are found in NK cells and macrophages, even though these cells do not express FcεR, but they do express FcγRIII. Thus, it appears that the expression of this γ-chain somehow affects the expression, structure, or stability of FcγRIII.

In human cells, two forms of FcγRIII exist, encoded for by two separate genes, FcγRIIIA and FcγRIIIB. A single size of mRNA is detected in Northern analyses of 2.2 kb. The gene is mapped to chromosome 1 and both FcγRII and FcγRIII are located within 200 kb of the genome. The existence of two forms of FcγRIII was predicted from studies of patients with paroxysmal nocturnal hemoglobinuria (PNH). These patients have a greatly decreased expression of FcγRIII on their neutrophils (only 10–15% of that on normal neutrophils), but the expression of this receptor on NK cells from these patients is normal. It has been shown that FcγRIIIA, which is present on the surface of NK cells, macrophages, and cultured monocytes comprises extracellular, transmembrane, and cytoplasmic domains, whereas that present on neutrophils comprises an extracellular domain anchored to the membrane via a glycosylphosphatidylinositol (GPI) linkage.[15–17] This linkage is cleaved by proteases such as elastase and pronase or by phosphatidylinositol-specific phospholipase C. Thus, the receptor may be shed from the neutrophil membrane upon activation. This switch from the receptor having a transmembrane domain or a GPI linkage results from a change in amino acid 203 of the sequence: in FcγRIIIB, residue 203 is Ser (which is followed by a termination codon) and results in a GPI linkage, whereas in FcγRIIIA residue 203 is phenylalanine and this results in a transmembrane linkage. The cytoplasmic domain of FcγRIIIA is a 25 amino acid sequence that arises from a T→C transition in the TGA stop sequence present in FcγRIIIB. Transfection experiments of cell lines with cDNA molecules for FcγRIII indicate that, as for the murine gene, co-infection with either the γ-chain of FcεR1 or the ζ-chain of the CD3/TcR (T cell receptor) is required for maximal expression of FcγRIIIA. Co-infection with these molecules is not required, however, for expression of FcγRIIIB. Thus, FcγRIIIA molecules are designated FcγRIIIAγ or FcγRIIIAζ depending upon the nature of the subunit associated with them: FcγRIIAα is not associated with either a γ-chain or a ζ-chain.

Allogenic forms of FcγRIIIB also exist. These are recognized by an antibody present in the serum of patients with a form of autoimmune neutropenia, and separate monoclonal antibodies recognize these allotypic forms (NA1 and NA2) of the receptor. The two allotypic forms can also be recognized by different mobilities on gels. Whilst cDNA for both NA1 and NA2 have been cloned and sequenced, both molecules predict primary translation products of equal size. However, when the immunoprecipitated NA1 and NA2 molecules are de-glycosylated, the apparent relative molecular masses are 29 and 33 kD. Similarly, *in vitro* translation of mRNA for these two allotypic forms yields proteins of 24 and 26 kD for NA1 and NA2, respectively. Such a translation system would not be expected to glycosylate the newly made proteins and so these differences in apparent size cannot be accounted for by differential glycosylation. These cDNA molecules differ in only five nucleotides, which predict four amino acid substitutions. These substitutions account for the fact that there are six potential glycosylations sites on NA2, but only four in NA1. The anomalous mobility of these two non-glycosylated or de-glycosylated proteins on SDS-PAGE yielding different apparent molecular masses (even though amino acid prediction of cDNA molecules suggests that this should not be the case) may thus result from conformational differences in these two proteins due to the small differences in their amino acid composition. It is also reported that NA2 type FcγRIII receptors have a lower capacity to mediate phagocytosis than the NA1 counterparts.

There is much debate in the literature as to the roles of FcγRII and FcγRIIIb in neutrophil activation.[18–20] There are reports indicating that occupancy of FcγRII leads to activation of the respiratory burst and degranulation,[21–24] whilst FcγRIIIb may enhance immune complex binding and augment FcγRII function. The intracellular signaling events following FcγRII and FcγRIIIb binding are also undefined, and it is unclear how FcγRIIIb, which lacks a cytoplasmic tail, can actually generate intracellular signals. Ligation of either FcγRII or FcγRIIIb using monoclonal antibodies can generate intracellular Ca^{2+} transients,[25–29] but care must be taken in such experiments if whole antibody molecules are used. For example, ligation of FcγRIIIb on one cell can activate FcγRII on an adjacent cell via the exposed Fc region of the antibody. Such experiments should therefore use Fab or $F(ab')_2$ fragments of antibodies prior to cross-linking. Both FcγII and FcγRIIIb are associated with tyrosine kinase activity[30–35]: FcγRII function is associated with translocation and activation of the *src*-like tyrosine kinase, Fgr, whilst FcγRIIIb function is associated with Hck activation.

In this study we have investigated the expression of FcγRs on neutrophils that have been primed *in vivo* (i.e., within rheumatoid joints) and *in vitro* (using GM-CSF and TNFα) and activated the cells with soluble immune complexes. Additionally, we have probed the function of FcγRII and FcγRIIIb by cross-linking anti-Fab/F(ab′)$_2$ fragments and measured changes in intracellular Ca^{2+} and activation of the respiratory burst. Finally, we have probed the function of FcγRIIIb by measuring responses of neutrophils isolated from an individual with a gene deficiency in FcγRIIIb.

EXPERIMENTAL

Materials

Neutrophil isolation medium (NIM) was from Cardinal Associates Inc., RPMI 1640 medium from Flow Laboratories; Fluo-3-AM was from Calbiochem. rGM-CSF was a non-glycosylated peptide from Glaxo and had an activity of $\geq$ 1.5 mU/mg protein in the AML-193 proliferation assay. Zetaprobe was from Bio-Rad and [^{32}P]CTP was from ICN. The monoclonal antibodies IV3, 197, and 322 were from Mederex whilst Leu 11b and FITC-labeled goat-(anti-mouse) immunoglobulin were from Becton and Dickinson. TNFα was from National Institute for Biological Standards and Controls (Potters Bar, U.K.). F(ab′)$_2$ fragments of monoclonal antibody 3G8 (recognizing FcγRIIIb) and Fab fragments of IV.3 (recognizing FcγRII) were from Medarex, Inc. PI-PLC was from Boehringer. All other specialist reagents were from Sigma Chemical Co.

Neutrophil Isolation

Neutrophils were isolated from the venous blood of healthy volunteers by centrifugation on NIM for 15 min at 400 g.[36] After removal of contaminating erythrocytes by hypotonic lysis, purified neutrophils were suspended in RPMI 1640 medium and counted. Neutrophil purity (assessed by Wright's staining) and viability (assessed by trypan blue exclusion) were >97% and >95%, respectively.

Neutrophil Priming

Neutrophils were primed using either GM-CSF or TNFα. Cells (10^7/ml) were incubated in the presence and absence of GM-CSF (50 U/ml) for 1 h at 37°C, whilst TNFα (50 ng/ml) was added 10 min prior to stimulation.

Immune Complex Preparation

Synthetic immune complexes were made from human serum albumin (HSA) and rabbit anti-(HSA) antibodies as previously described.[37,38] The antigen was titrated against constant antibody concentration and the $A_{450\,nm}$ measured to identify equivalence. The soluble complexes were formed at 6 × antigen equivalence and were briefly centrifuged (2 min at 13,000 g in a microfuge) to remove any contaminating insoluble immune complexes that may have been present. Soluble complexes were formed at 180 μg/ml antigen and 125 μg/ml of antibody. A 10% (vol/vol) solution of complexes was used routinely for neutrophil stimulation.

Reactive Oxidant Production

Chemiluminescence was measured at 37°C in neutrophil suspensions (5×10^5/ml) in RPMI 1640 medium that was supplemented with 10 μM luminol using an LKB 1251 luminometer.[36,39] For measurements of superoxide secretion, neutrophils were suspended in RPMI 1640 supplemented with 75 μM cytochrome c.[40] Absorption changes were recorded at 550 nm using a Bio-Rad 3550 kinetic plate reader. Reference wells contained 30 μg/ml superoxide dismutase.

Intracellular Free Ca²⁺

Changes in intracellular Ca^{2+} concentration $[Ca^{2+}]_i$ were monitored with the fluorescent probe fluo-3. Neutrophils in RPMI 1640 (2×10^7/ml) were loaded by incubation at 37°C for 30 min with 2 μM Fluo-3 AM. The cells were then washed twice and resuspended at 2×10^6/ml in Ca^{2+} free medium (NaCl, 145 mM; $Na_2HPO_4 \cdot 2H_2O$, 1 mM; $MgSO_4 \cdot 7H_2O$, 0.5 mM; glucose, 5 mM; HEPES 20 mM, pH 7.4) to which 1 mM $CaCl_2$ was added as required. In some experiments, 1 mM EGTA was added to media devoid of Ca^{2+}. Fluorescence was then measured at 505 nm excitation and 530 nm emission. Calibration of changes in intracellular Ca^{2+} levels was as described in using a K_d for Fluo-3 of 864 nM at 37°C.[41]

Receptor Cross-linking and Mab Blocking Studies

For measurements of intracellular Ca^{2+} following the cross-linking of receptors, Fluo-3 loaded neutrophils (2×10^6/ml) were incubated with 1 μg/ml of Fab/F(ab′)$_2$ fragments of appropriate monoclonal antibodies at 37°C prior to cross-linking with 40 μg/ml F(ab′)$_2$ fragments of goat anti-mouse IgG. For Mab blocking studies 3×10^6 neutrophils were incubated with 3 μg Fab/F(ab′)$_2$ fragments in a volume of 250 μl for 10 min at 37°C prior to dilution (to 5×10^5 cells/ml) and stimulation of cells with soluble immune complexes.

Receptor Expression by FACS Analysis

The monoclonal antibodies used were IV3 (anti-CD32, FcγRII) and Leu 11b (anti-CD16, FcγRIIIb). Expression of FcγRI (the high affinity receptor for monomeric IgG) was measured using the anti-CD64 monoclonal antibodies 32.2 and 197. For immunostaining, isolated neutrophils were suspended in PBS/1% BSA (globulin-free)/0.1% sodium azide, pH 7.2, and receptor expression was measured using a standard indirect immunofluorescence technique using FITC-labeled goat-(anti-mouse) immunoglobulin as a second layer.[10,42] Both first and second layer antibodies were added at saturating concentrations, and in all experiments non-immune mouse IgG of the appropriate isotype was included as a class-specific first-layer control. Stained cells were fixed in 1% paraformaldehyde in PBS and analyzed using a Becton-Dickinson Ortho Diagnostics Cytron analyzer. Fluorescence distributions represent a total of 5,000 gated events (cells), with the mean fluorescence proportional to the number of specific antigenic sites per cell. The number of binding sites for anti-FcγRI antibodies was determined using the Quantum Simply Cellular Microbeads kit from Sigma. In all experiments, the number of binding sites for anti-FcγRI antibodies (equivalent to the number of FcγRI molecules on the cell surface) on blood and synovial fluid neutrophils, or on synovial fluid–treated neutrophils, is expressed as a percentage of the number of binding sites induced by treatment of control blood neutrophils with 100 U/ml γ-interferon for 24 h at 37°C, which was taken as 100%.

RNA Extraction

RNA was isolated from control blood neutrophils that had been incubated at 37°C for periods of up to 24 h in the absence or presence of γ-interferon or cell-free synovial fluid.[43] RNA was also extracted from blood neutrophils (patient or control) and synovial fluid neutrophils immediately after isolation. Cell pellets were suspended in 4 M guanidinium isothiocyanate, 5% β-mercaptoethanol, 50 mM EDTA, 50 mM Tris, pH 7.0. Cells were lysed by drawing them through a 23-gauge needle to shear chromosomal DNA. The suspension was then layered onto a CsCl/EDTA gradient (5.7 M CsCl, 50 mM EDTA, density = 1.3995 ± 0.001) and centrifuged at 100,000 *g* for 16 h at 14°C. The RNA pellet was then suspended in diethylpyrocarbonate (DEPC)-treated water and precipitated overnight with 0.1 vol of 3 M sodium acetate (pH 5.5) and 2.5 vol ethanol at –80°C. The recovered RNA was then quantified by UV spectroscopy (typically 2 μg RNA recovered/10^7 neutrophils) and stored in aliquots at –80°C as ethanol precipitates.

Northern Blot Analyses

Aliquots of RNA (10 μg) were electrophoresed on 1.2% agarose gels (containing 1% (vol/vol) formaldehyde, 20 mM 3-*N*-morpholinopropane sulfonic acid, 1 mM EDTA, 5 mM sodium acetate, pH 8.0) for 16 h at 5 mA. The gels were then stained in ethidium bromide and RNA visualized by UV illumination. The RNA was then transferred by capillary blotting onto Zetaprobe GT nylon membrane in 20 × SSC (3 M NaCl, 0.3 M sodium citrate, pH 7.0). The filter was then baked at 80°C for 30 min and stored at room temperature wrapped in Saranwrap® until use. The filters were probed with cDNA clones FcγRI (a kind gift from Dr. B. Seed, Department of Molecular Biology, Massachusetts General Hospital, Boston, MA) and β-actin (ATCC 65128). The cDNA inserts were excised using appropriate restriction endonucleases and isolated from vector DNA by electrophoresis in low melting point agarose. Then 50–100 ng of each insert was radiolabeled using a random-primed labeling system using 25 μCi [^{32}P]CTP. Labeling proceeded for 20 h at 16°C and unincorporated [^{32}P]CTP was removed from the labeled cDNA using Nuctrap columns (Stratagene). The amount of radioactivity incorporated was typically $>10^8$ cpm/μg DNA. The filters were pre-hybridized for 30 min at 65°C in 0.25 M Na$_2$HPO$_4$·7H$_2$O/7% SDS, pH 7.2, and then hybridized with the probe for 16–20 h in the same buffer at 65°C. The filters were washed in 20 mM Na$_2$HPO$_4$·7H$_2$O/5% SDS, pH 7.2 for 2 × 30 min at 65°C, followed by 2 × 10 min washes in 20 mM Na$_2$HPO$_4$·7H$_2$O/0.1% SDS at the same temperature. The filters were blotted dry, wrapped in Saranwrap®, and exposed to X-ray film (Fuji RX) for 24–48 h. After radiography, the probes were removed by heating the filters to 95°C in 0.1% SSC containing 0.5% SDS for 2 × 20 min. After checking for removal of the probe by autoradiography, the filters were then re-probed. Hybridization signals were quantified by densitometry of autoradiographs: films were digitized and analyzed using Image software.

RESULTS

FcγRI Expression in Blood and Synovial Fluid Neutrophils

Neutrophils isolated from the blood of healthy volunteers do not express FcγRI on their cell surface, as determined by FACS analysis (FIG. 1, A). Similarly, in control bloodstream neutrophils, no mRNA for this receptor could be detected by Northern blotting (FIG. 1, C). However, when neutrophils were incubated with 100 U/ml γ-interferon, both mRNA and surface expression were detected: levels of mRNA were detected within 4 h of incubation with γ-interferon, whilst surface expression was detected 24 h after addition of cytokine. Similarly, blood neutrophils isolated from patients with rheumatoid arthritis did not express FcγRI (either mRNA or mature protein on the cell surface), whilst transcripts and surface expression were detected in the synovial fluid neutrophils from 12/15 and 16/24 patients, respectively (FIG. 1, B).

Activation of Neutrophils by Soluble Immune Complexes

The addition of soluble immune complexes to control bloodstream neutrophils failed to activate a respiratory burst (FIG. 2), as assessed by either luminol chemiluminescence (which measures both intra- and extracellular reactive oxidant generation) or cytochrome c reduction (which measures O$_2^-$ secretion). However, when neutrophils were primed (with either GM-CSF (45 min with 50 U/ml) or TNFα (10 min at 50 ng/ml)) prior to addition of soluble immune complexes, then a rapid activation of the oxidase was observed. The reactive oxidants were produced transiently (maximal production was observed 3 min after stimulation) and the cytochrome c reduction assay indicated that many of these oxidants were secreted.

Addition of soluble immune complexes to unprimed neutrophils resulted in a transient, monophasic increase in intracellular Ca^{2+} that was detected by Fluo-3 fluorescence (FIG. 3). Intracellular Ca^{2+} began to rise within 30 sec of addition, reached a

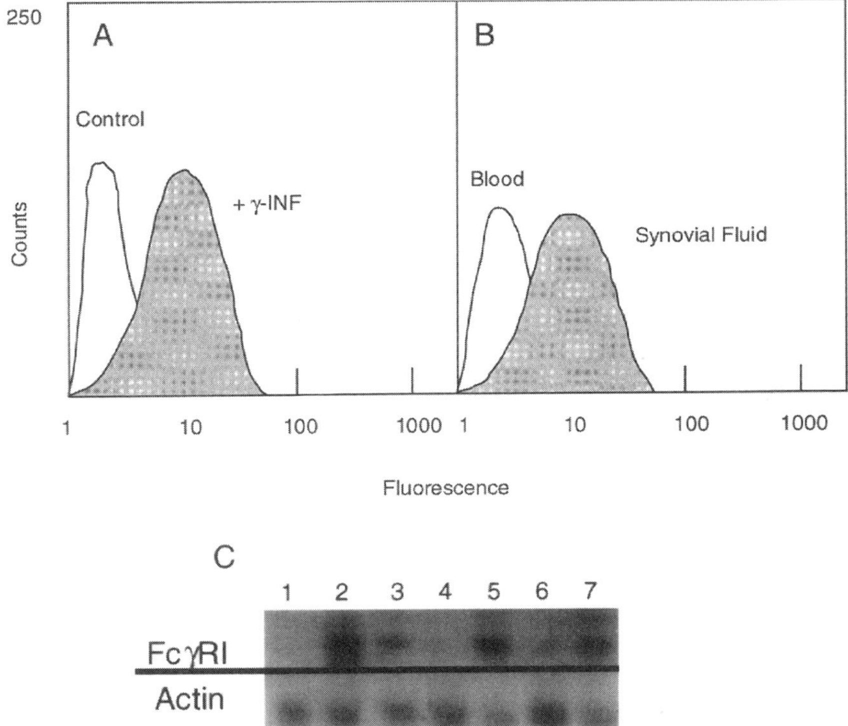

FIGURE 1. FcγRI expression by blood and synovial fluid neutrophils. In **A** and **B**, FcγRI expression was determined by FACS. **(A)** Expression of control blood neutrophils incubated for either 0 or 20 h in the absence (*unshaded*) or presence (*shaded*) of 100 U/ml γ-interferon. **(B)** FcγRI expression of blood (*unshaded*) or synovial fluid (*shaded*) neutrophils isolated from a patient with rheumatoid arthritis. **(C)** A northern blot of RNA isolated from neutrophils: 1, control blood neutrophils, no additions; 2, control blood neutrophils incubated for 4 h with 100 U/ml γ-interferon; 3, synovial fluid neutrophils from patient 1; 4, blood neutrophils from patient 2; 5, synovial fluid neutrophils from patient 2; 6, blood neutrophils from patient 3; synovial fluid neutrophils from patient 3. After probing for transcripts for FcγRI, filters were stripped and probed for actin mRNA.

maximum by 1 min, and then declined to basal levels. When the cells were primed (with either GM-CSF or TNFα) prior to stimulation, the soluble immune complexes elicited a different pattern of intracellular Ca^{2+}. The initial peak of intracellular Ca^{2+} was largely unaffected, whilst a second, more sustained Ca^{2+} transient was seen in the primed cells. This "extra" intracellular Ca^{2+} signal was not observed in primed cells that were stimulated in Ca^{2+} free medium (containing 1 mM EGTA) indicating that it arose from Ca^{2+} influx (data not shown). In contrast, the initial Ca^{2+} signal seen in primed or unprimed cells was not affected by incubation of cells in Ca^{2+} free medium and is therefore likely to arise from the mobilization of intracellular stores.

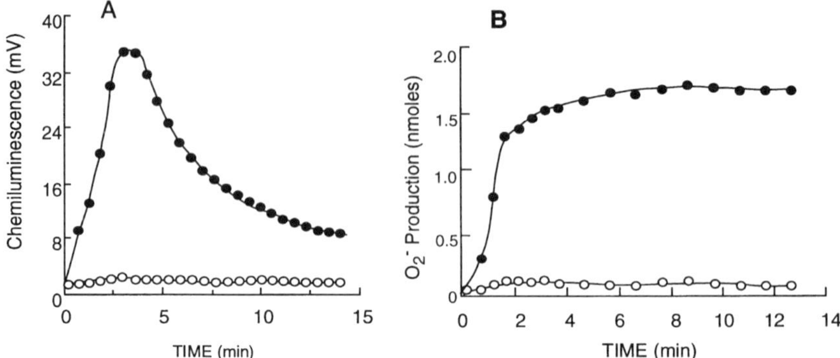

FIGURE 2. Activation of the respiratory burst by soluble immune complexes. Neutrophils were incubated for 10 min in the absence (○) or presence (●) of 50 ng/ml TNFα prior to addition of soluble immune complexes (10%, vol/vol). **(A)** Samples were supplemented with 10 μM luminol prior to measurement of chemiluminescence. **(B)** Samples were supplemented with 75 μM cytochrome c prior to measurement of superoxide secretion. Typical results of at least eight separate measurements.

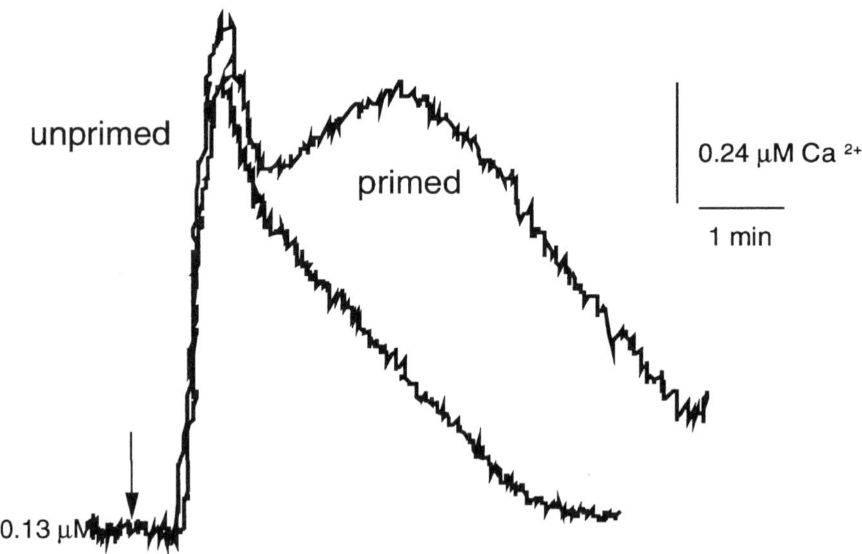

FIGURE 3. Changes in intracellular Ca^{2+}. Neutrophils were loaded with Fluo-3 and then incubated for 10 min in the absence (unprimed) or presence (primed) of 50 ng/ml TNFα. As indicated by the arrow, the cells were stimulated by the addition of 10% (vol/vol) soluble immune complexes. Typical result of at least 10 separate experiments.

Roles of FcγRII and FcγRIIIb in Neutrophil Activation by Soluble Immune Complexes

FcγRIIIb is anchored to the neutrophil plasma membrane via a GPI linkage that can be cleaved by mild protease treatment or incubation with PI-PLC. Incubation of neutrophils with 0.25 U/ml phosphoinositide-phospholipase C (PI-PLC) for 30 min resulted in a marked removal of FcγRIIIb from the cell surface, whilst having little, if any, effect on FcγRII surface expression (FIG. 4, A). However, when PI-PLC–treated

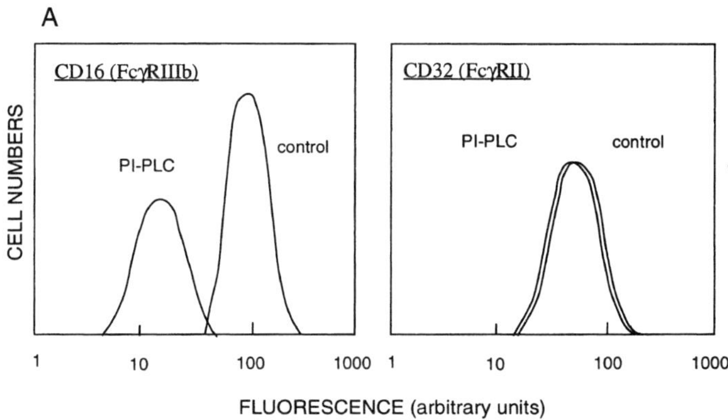

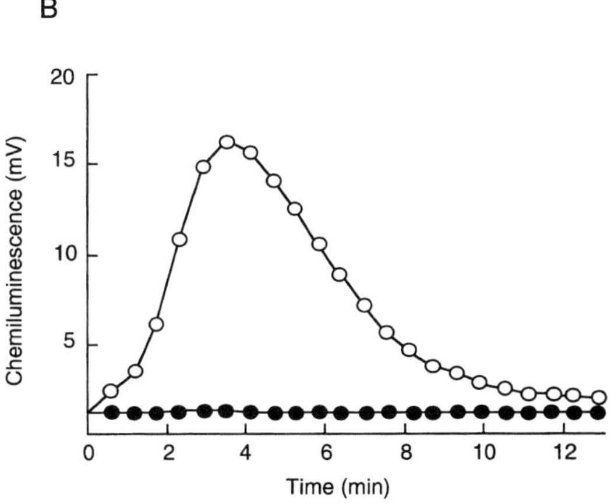

FIGURE 4. FcγRIIIb depletion of neutrophils. Neutrophils were incubated in the absence (control, ○) or presence (PI-PLC, ●) of PI-PLC (0.25 U/ml) for 30 min. After this incubation cells were washed and resuspended in RPMI 1640 medium. Expression of FcγRIIIb and FcγRII was measured by FACS **(A)** whilst in **(B)**, suspensions were primed with TNFα (50 ng/ml for 10 min), supplemented with 10 μM luminol and chemiluminescence in response to 10% (vol/vol) soluble immune complexes was measured.

neutrophils, devoid of FcγRIIIb were primed, they could not generate reactive oxygen metabolites in response to soluble immune complexes (FIG. 4, B). This indicates a crucial role for FcγRIIIb in the control of reactive oxidant generation in response to soluble immune complexes. In PI-PLC–treated neutrophils the "extra" intracellular Ca^{2+} signal normally seen in primed cells was not observed (data not shown). These results indicate that the priming-dependent increase in Ca^{2+} influx in primed cells required FcγRIIIb and not FcγRII. In contrast, in PI-PLC–treated neutrophils, the initial rise in intracellular Ca^{2+} due to store mobilization seen in unprimed cells was completely unaffected (data not shown). This mobilization of intracellular Ca^{2+} must therefore be due to the activity of FcγRII.

When neutrophils were incubated with Fab and $F(ab')_2$ fragments of IV3 (FcγRII) and 3G8 (FcγRIIIb), respectively, followed by crosslinking with goat anti-mouse $F(ab')_2$, the oxidase was not activated in unprimed cells (FIG. 5). In contrast, if the cells were primed (with TNFα or GM-CSF) prior to crosslinking, then both receptors could independently generate signals leading to activation of the NADPH oxidase.

A similar experimental approach was then taken to investigate the roles of FcγRII and FcγRIIIb in regulation of intracellular Ca^{2+} levels. Ligation of FcγRIIIb in unprimed cells failed to generate an intracellular Ca^{2+} transient (FIG. 6) whereas if the cells were primed prior to crosslinking, then a transient was observed that peaked 2 min after crosslinking. Ligation of FcγRII in either primed or unprimed cells resulted in an elevation in intracellular Ca^{2+} within 1 min of crosslinking, although maximal levels observed were higher in primed cells. When cells were incubated in Ca^{2+} free medium, no intracellular Ca^{2+} transients were observed following the crosslinking of FcγRIIIb (indicating the dependency upon Ca^{2+} influx), whilst incubation in Ca^{2+} free medium had little effect on the intracellular Ca^{2+} transients observed following

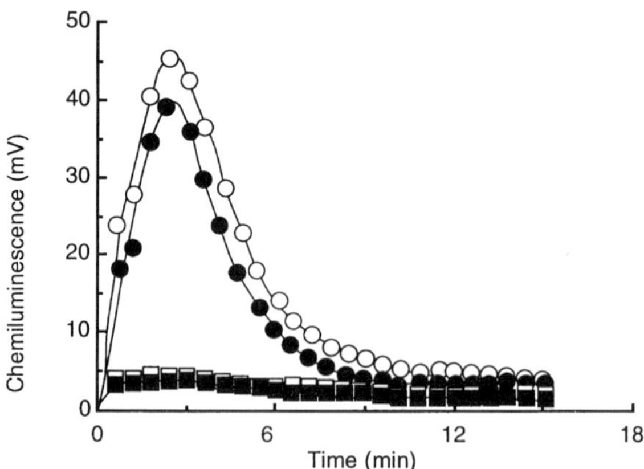

FIGURE 5. Role of FcγRII and FcγRIIIb in activation of the respiratory burst. Neutrophils were incubated in the absence (■, □) and presence (○, ●) of 50 ng/ml TNFα for 10 min and then incubated with either Fab fragments of IV.3 (anti-FcγRII, ■, ●) or $F(ab')_2$ fragments of 3G8 (anti-FcγRIIIb, □, ○). Suspensions were supplemented with 10 μM luminol and receptors were crosslinked, as described in *Experimental*.

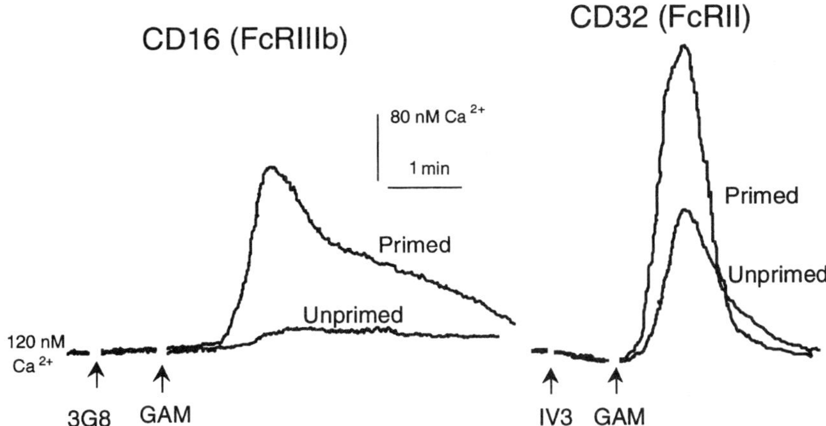

FIGURE 6. Role of FcγRII and FcγRIIIb in regulation of intracellular Ca^{2+} transients. Neutrophils were loaded with Fluo-3 and then incubated in the absence (unprimed) and presence (primed) of 50 ng/ml TNFα. After crosslinking receptors with $Fab/(Fab')_2$ fragments, intracellular Ca^{2+} levels were measured. Typical result of five separate experiments.

crosslinking of FcγRII (data not shown).

When unprimed neutrophils from an individual with FcγRIIIb deficiency were stimulated with soluble immune complexes, no generation of reactive oxidants was observed (FIG. 7). In contrast to the marked generation of reactive oxidants seen in control primed neutrophils, FcγRIIIb-deficient primed neutrophils also failed to generate reactive oxidants following stimulation with soluble immune complexes. These neutrophils could, however, generate normal amounts of reactive oxidants in response to the phorbol ester PMA.

These experiments thus indicate a key role for the role of FcγRIIIb in the generation of reactive oxidants in response to soluble immune complexes by primed neutrophils.

DISCUSSION

Fcγ receptors on neutrophils play important roles in the recognition and phagocytosis of IgG-opsonized bacteria, but also in responses of neutrophils to immune complexes that are either free in solution or deposited on surfaces. In this way, Fcγ receptors play a role in host defense against infections and are implicated in neutrophil-mediated tissue damage in inflammatory diseases that involve either immune complex production or IgG coating of tissues. In inflammatory joint disease, therefore, FcγR-dependent neutrophil activation can occur in response to soluble immune complexes that are present within diseased synovial fluid, or else in response to IgG/immune complex deposition on joint structures such as cartilage. In rheumatoid arthritis, neutrophils have an additional mechanism by which they can respond to these ag-

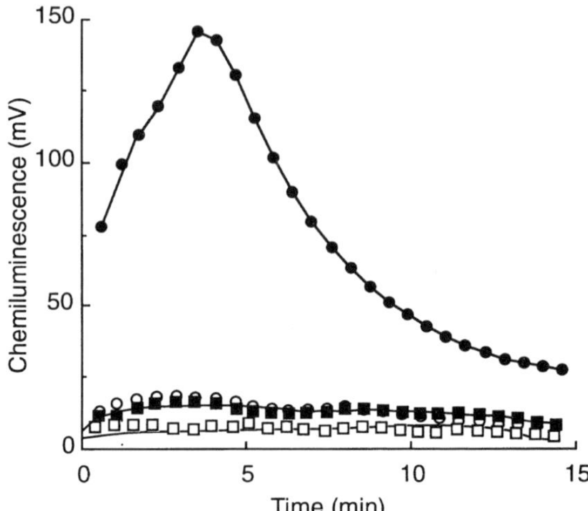

FIGURE 7. Stimulation of FcγRIIIb gene–deficient neutrophils with soluble immune complexes. Neutrophils were isolated from the blood of either healthy controls (●, ○) or an individual with FcγRIIIb gene deficiency (■, □). Suspensions were incubated for 10 min in the absence (○, □) and presence (●, ■) or TNFα (50 ng/ml) and luminol chemiluminescence in response to soluble immune complexes (10%, vol/vol) was measured.

onists because they express FcγRI,[10] in addition to FcγRII and FcγRIIIb. This former receptor is not normally expressed by control blood neutrophils and its function in neutrophils is unknown. It has been proposed to play a role in ADCC in *in vitro* experiments, but its expression on neutrophils within diseased joints will undoubtedly affect the ability of these cells to respond to immune complexes or IgG-coated surfaces.

We have previously shown that the receptor/signal transduction mechanisms that regulate neutrophil activation by soluble and insoluble immune complexes are distinct.[38,44,45] Insoluble immune complexes are largely phagocytosed and most of the reactive oxidants that are generated are intracellular, i.e., contained within phagolysosomes. Neutrophil activation via these large insoluble complexes is hardly affected when FcγRIIIb is removed from the cell surface by treatment of neutrophils with pronase.[46] In contrast, soluble immune complexes only activate neutrophils that have previously been primed and they activate *secretion* of granule enzymes and reactive oxidants; this response is almost completely abolished when FcγRIIIb is experimentally removed from the cell surface. Of great interest has been the recent discovery of individuals with a gene defect in FcγRIIIb, which results in a complete lack of expression of this receptor on their neutrophils.[47,48] Curiously, these individuals are generally asymptomatic and do not have an increased risk of infections. Hence, FcγRIIIb expression cannot play a major role in protection against infections, a conclusion supported by our experimental findings. However, we would predict that FcγRIIIb plays a key role in the events that lead to tissue damage following the binding of soluble immune complexes to primed neutrophils via their ability to induce secretion of tissue-damaging products. Whilst soluble immune complexes failed to activate a respiratory burst in unprimed neutrophils, they did stimulate an intracellular Ca^{2+} transient, which arose from mobilization of intracellular stores. This indicates that these complexes must bind to functional receptors. Our data indicate that these receptors must be FcγRII, because this event was completely unaffected when FcγRIIIb was experimentally removed by treatment of neutrophils with pronase or PI-PLC. In contrast, when the cells were primed, an "extra" intracellular Ca^{2+} signal was observed, which arose from Ca^{2+} influx and this was not observed when the cells were depleted of FcγRIIIb. Thus, we propose that during priming, FcγRIIIb is functionally activated and its ligation leads to elevation in intracellular Ca^{2+} via stimulated Ca^{2+} influx. Experiments independently ligating FcγRII or FcγRIIIb appear to confirm this hypothesis. Indeed, ligation of either FcγRII or FcγRIIIb failed to activate the NADPH oxidase in unprimed cells, whereas in primed cells, both receptors could generate signals that resulted in oxidase activation.

In conclusion, ligation of both FcγRII and FcγRIIIb can independently generate signals that lead to neutrophil activation. However, major differences in their functional properties exist. FcγRII function is largely unaffected by priming and it is coupled to a signal transduction pathway that results in mobilization of intracellular Ca^{2+} stores via an inositol 1,4,5-trisphosphate independent pathway.[49–51] In contrast, FcγRIIIb appears to be non-functional in unprimed cells, but following priming its ligation becomes coupled to a signaling pathway that results in Ca^{2+} influx and activation of the NADPH oxidase. Because FcγRIIIb is anchored to the outer leaflet of the plasma membrane via a GPI linkage, some membrane-spanning molecule must form a bridge between the receptor and the inner leaflet, which then physically links the receptor to inner membrane–bound signaling molecules.[5]

SUMMARY

Activation of control, unprimed neutrophils with soluble immune complexes fails to generate a respiratory burst. However, if the cells are primed with either tumor necrosis factor-α or granulocyte-macrophage colony-stimulating factor prior to addition of soluble immune complexes, then a rapid and transient burst of reactive oxidant secretion is observed. In unprimed neutrophils the soluble immune complexes stimulate an intracellular Ca^{2+} transient that arises from the mobilization of intracellular Ca^{2+}. However, in primed cells, an "extra" intracellular Ca^{2+} signal is observed that arises from Ca^{2+} influx. After removal of FcγRIIIb by treatment with pronase or PI-PLC, the soluble immune complexes fail to activate a respiratory burst in unprimed neutrophils and the "extra" Ca^{2+} signal is not observed. These results indicate that during priming FcγRIIIb becomes functionally activated and thence its ligation leads to stimulated Ca^{2+} influx and the generation of intracellular signals that lead to NADPH oxidase activation. Experiments using Fab/F(ab$'$)$_2$ fragments to specifically crosslink either FcγRII or FcγRIIIb and experiments with neutrophils from an individual with FcγRIIIb gene deficiency confirm this important function for FcγRIIIb in neutrophil activation.

REFERENCES

1. EDWARDS, S. W. 1994. Biochemistry and Physiology of the Neutrophil. Cambridge University Press. Cambridge, U.K.
2. FANGER, M. W., L. SHEN, R. F. GRAZIANO & P. M. GUYRE. 1989. Immunol. Today **10:** 92–99.
3. HUIZINGA, T. W. J., D. ROOS & A. E. G. K. VON DEM BORNE. 1990. Blood **75:** 1211–1214.
4. RAVETCH, J. V. & J.-P. KINET. 1991. Ann. Rev. Immunol. **9:** 457–492.
5. EDWARDS, S. W. 1995. Trends Biochem. Sci. **20:** 362–367.
6. PERUSSIA, B., E. T. DAYTON, R. LAZARUS, V. FANNING & G. TRINCHIERI. 1983. J. Exp. Med. **158:** 1092–1113.
7. PERUSSIA, B., M. KOBAYASHI, M. E. ROSSI, I. ANEGON & G. TRINCHIERI. 1987. J. Immunol. **138:** 765–774.
8. REPP, R., T. VALERIUS, A. SENDLER, M. GRAMATZKI, H. IRO, J. R. KALDEN & E. PLATZER. 1991. Blood **78:** 885–889.
9. VALERIUS, T., R. REPP, T. P. DE WIT, S. BERTHOLD, E. PLATZER, J. R. KALDEN, M. GRAMATZKI & J. G. VAN DE WINKEL. 1993. Blood **82:** 931–939.
10. WATSON, F., J. J. ROBINSON, M. PHELAN, R. C. BUCKNALL & S. W. EDWARDS. 1993. Ann. Rheum. Dis. **52:** 353–359.
11. CASSATELLA, M. A., F. BAZZONI, F. CALZETTI, I. GUASPARRI, F. ROSSI & G. TRINCHIERI. 1991. J. Biol. Chem. **266:** 22079–22082.
12. CASSATELLA, M. A., R. M. FLYNN, M. A. AMEZAGA, F. BAZZONI, F. VICENTINI & G. TRINCHIERI. 1990. Biochem. Biophys. Res. Commun. **170:** 582–588.
13. PETRONI, K. C., L. SHEN & P. M. GUYRE. 1988. J. Immunol. **140:** 3467–3472.
14. TOSI, M. F. & H. ZAKEM. 1992. J. Clin. Invest. **90:** 462–470.
15. HUIZINGA, T. W. J., C. E. VAN DER SCHOOT, C. JOST, R. KLAASSEN, M. KLEIJER, A. E. G. K. VON DEM BORNE, D. ROOS & P. A. T. TETTEROO. 1988. Nature **333:** 667–669.
16. SELVARAJ, P., W. F. ROSSE, R. SILBER & T. A. SPRINGER. 1988. Nature **333:** 565–567.
17. SIMMONS, D. & B. SEED. 1988. Nature **333:** 568–570.
18. HUIZINGA, T. W. J., M. KERST, J. H. NUYENS, A. VLUG, A. E. G. K. VON DEM BORNE, D. ROOS & P. A. T. TETTEROO. 1989. J. Immunol. **142:** 2359–2364.
19. HUIZINGA, T. W. J., F. VAN KEMENADE, L. KOENDERMAN, K. M. DOLMAN, A. E. G. K. VON DEM BORNE, P. A. T. TETEROO & D. ROOS. 1989. J. Immunol. **142:** 2365–2369.
20. HUNDT, M. & R. E. SCHMIDT. 1992. Eur. J. Immunol. **22:** 811–816.
21. KIMBERLEY, R. P., J. W. AHLSTROM, M. E. CLICK & J. C. EDBERG. 1990. J. Exp. Med. **171:** 1239–1255.
22. BRUNKHORST, B. A., G. STROHMEIER, K. LAZZARI, G. WEIL, D. MELNICK, H. B. FLEIT & E. R. SIMONS. 1992. J. Biol. Chem. **267:** 20659–20666.
23. ROSALES, C. & E. J. BROWN. 1991. J. Immunol. **146:** 3937–3944.
24. SALMON, J. E., N. L. BROGLE, J. C. EDBERG & R. P. KIMBERLEY. 1991. J. Immunol. **146:** 997–1004.
25. MACKENZIE, S. J. & M. A. KERR. 1995. Biochem. J. **306:** 519–523.
26. LUND-JOHANSEN, F., J. OLWEUS, A. AARLI & R. BJERKNES. 1991. Scand. J. Immunol. **33:** 261–266.
27. MORGAN, B. P., C. W. VANDENBERG, E. V. DAVIES, M. B. HALLETT & V. HOREJSI. 1993. Eur. J. Immunol. **23:** 2841–2850.
28. NAZIRUDDIN, B., B. F. DUFFY, J. TUCKER & T. MOHANAKUMAR. 1992. J. Immunol. **149:** 3702–3709.
29. VOSSEBELD, P. J. M., J. KESSLER, A. E. G. K. VON DEM BORNE, D. ROOS & A. J. VERHOEVEN. 1995. J. Biol. Chem. **270:** 10671–10679.
30. DUSI, S., M. DONINI, V. DELLA BIANCA, G. GANDINI & F. ROSSI. 1994. Biochem. Biophys. Res. Commun. **201:** 30–37.

31. Dusi, S., M. Donini, V. Dellabianca & F. Rossi. 1994. Biochem. Biophys. Res. Commun. **201:** 1100–1108.

32. Hamada, F., M. Aoki, T. Akiyama & K. Toyoshima. 1993. Proc. Natl. Acad. Sci. USA **90:** 6305–6309.

33. Huang, M. M., Z. Indik, L. F. Brass, J. A. Hoxie, A. D. Schreiber & J. S. Brugge. 1992. J. Biol. Chem. **267:** 5467–5473.

34. Zhou, M. J. & E. J. Brown. 1994. J. Cell Biol. **125:** 1407–1416.

35. Zhou, M., D. M. Lubin, D. C. Links & E. J. Brown. 1995. J. Biol. Chem. **270:** 13553–13560.

36. Edwards, S. W. 1996. Methods: A Companion to Methods in Enzymology **9:** 563–578.

37. Crockett-Torabi, E. & J. C. Fantone. 1990. J. Immunol. **145:** 3026–3032.

38. Robinson, J. J., F. Watson, R. C. Bucknall & S. W. Edwards. 1994. FEMS Immunol. Med. Microbiol. **8:** 247–258.

39. Edwards, S. W. 1987. J. Lab. Clin. Immunol. **22:** 35–39.

40. Babior, B. M., R. S. Kipnes & J. T. Curnutte. 1973. J. Clin. Invest. **52:** 741–747.

41. Merrit, J. E., S. A. McCarthy, M. P. A. Davies & K. E. Moores. 1990. Biochem. J. **269:** 513–519.

42. Edwards, S. W., F. Watson, R. Macleod & J. M. Davies. 1990. Biosci. Rep. **10:** 393–401.

43. Quayle, J. A., S. Adams, R. C. Bucknall & S. W. Edwards. 1994. FEMS Immunol. Med. Microbiol. **8:** 233–240.

44. Robinson, J. J., F. Watson, R. C. Bucknall & S. W. Edwards. 1992. Biochem. J. **286:** 345–351.

45. Robinson, J. J., F. Watson, R. C. Bucknall & S. W. Edwards. 1994. Ann. Rheum. Dis. **53:** 515–520.

46. Robinson, J. J., F. Watson, M. Phelan, R. C. Bucknall & S. W. Edwards. 1993. Ann. Rheum. Dis. **52:** 347–353.

47. De Haas, M., M. Kliejer, R. Van Zwieten, D. Roos & A. E. K. Van Dem Borne. 1995. Blood **86:** 2403–2413.

48. Veys, P. A., S. A. Wilkes & A. V. Hoffbrand. 1991. Blood **78:** 852–853.

49. Rosales, C. & E. J. Brown. 1992. J. Biol. Chem. **267:** 5267–5271.

50. Rosales, C., S. L. Jones, D. McCourt & E. J. Brown. 1994. Proc. Natl. Acad. Sci. USA **91:** 3534–3538.

51. Walker, B. A. M., B. E. Hagenlocker, E. B. Jr. Stubbs, R. R. Sandborg, B. W. Agranoff & P. A. Ward. 1991. J. Immunol. **146:** 735–741.

Phagocytic Activity of Bronchoalveolar Lavage Neutrophils in Intensive Care Unit Patients on Mechanical Ventilation

E. PIVA,[a] S. DE TONI, G. SERVIDIO, P. BORIN,[b] AND M. PLEBANI

Department of Laboratory Medicine
University of Padua
Padua, Italy

[b]*ICU (Intensive Care Unit)*
Azienda Ospedaliera
Padua, Italy

INTRODUCTION

In patients on mechanical ventilation (MV) it is difficult to identify pulmonary infiltrates, which have different causes but are mainly due to infection. Despite many advances in infection control practices and antimicrobial therapy, nosocomial pneumonia is still a frequent complication in patients in intensive care units (ICUs), and it has been estimated that 15% of all deaths of hospitalized patients are directly related to nosocomial pneumonia.

Traditional criteria commonly used to diagnose pneumonia do not enable a distinction between patients with and those without bacterial pneumonia. Moreover routine clinical and radiographic criteria for diagnosing bacterial lung infection are unreliable in critically ill patients on MV, making an accurate diagnosis of pneumonia difficult in this setting. There is also considerable controversy regarding the diagnostic techniques used to identify the causal pathogen. Conventional bacteriologic methods are also of limited value in distinguishing between tracheobronchial colonization and pulmonary infection.

Using bronchoscopic techniques, a bronchoalveolar lavage specimen (BAL) can be obtained from the affected pulmonary area. There is currently an increasing recognition of the value of quantitative cultures of lower respiratory tract secretions obtained by BAL in the diagnosis of ventilator-associated pneumonia, for which, moreover, early markers of pneumonia are needed. Since polymorphonuclear neutrophils (PMN) are important for lung defense and are found in increased numbers in BALs from MV patients, we evaluated the phagocytic activity of PMN against bacteria and fungi by microscopic examination to discriminate between with and those without pneumonia. The utility of the quantification of BAL cells containing intracellular bacteria (ICB) in making an early diagnosis of MV-associated pneumonia was studied with a view to deciding upon the appropriate treatment for this frequent complication.

[a]Address all correspondence to: Dr.ssa Elisa Piva, Servizio di Medicina di Laboratorio, Laboratorio Centrale, Azienda Ospedaliera di Padova, Via Giustiniani, 2, 35128 Padova, Italy. Phone, 00 39 49 8212792; Fax, 00 39 49 663240.

MATERIAL AND METHODS

Patients

From March 1996 to July 1996 at the Intensive Care Unit of Padua University Hospital, thirteen patients (10 males and 3 females) who had been on mechanical ventilation for at least 72 hours were studied using BAL. All patients had suspected pneumonia, with fever (>38°C), purulent tracheal secretions, and a radiographic finding of an infiltrate, still present after 24 hours at repeat x-ray and/or acute respiratory failure. Underlying conditions included chronic obstructive pulmonary disease ($n=1$), postoperative respiratory failure ($n=5$), systemic lupus erythematosus ($n=1$), multitrauma ($n=1$), head injury ($n=2$), leukemia ($n=1$), coma ($n=1$), and burn injury ($n=1$).

Bronchoalveolar Lavage

A fiberoptic bronchoscope (Olympus model BF-IT, New Hyde Park, NY) was introduced through a special sterile adaptor to minimize air leakage (Bodai Suction-Safe Y; Sontek Medical, Lexington, MA), and advanced into the bronchial orifice of a lung segment identified radiographically as that containing the new infiltrate. BAL was obtained by infusion and aspiration of three 50 ml aliquots of a sterile physiologic solution, and specimens were collected and filtered through a surgical gauze.

The first aliquot was discarded, and further aliquots, considered as alveolar fractions, were pooled and used for cytology, quantitative culture, and analysis for mycobacteria, fungi, and viruses.

Cytology

In one aliquot of BAL, the fluid cell count was performed using a Bürker hemocytometer; BAL fluid was then cytocentrifuged for 10 minutes at 1,800 rpm. The air-dried slides were stained using May-Grünwald-Giemsa stain (Merck Diagnostics, Darmstadt, Germany) and a differential cell count was made. The percentage of infected cells and the presence and type of extracellular and/or intracellular bacteria, whatever their number, were determined by means of microscopic examination. A polymorphonuclear leukocyte or an alveolar macrophage containing at least one microorganism was considered an infected cell. BAL samples were considered technically invalid and excluded when more than 5% of the cells counted consisted of ciliated bronchial cells.

Bacteriology

BAL fluid was processed for microbiologic analysis. After incubation, the colonies were counted and identified using traditional methods. Colonies were enumerated, and the results expressed as CFU/ml.

RESULTS

The mean age of patients was 57.8±19.3, the mean simplified acute physiologic score (SAPS) 32.7±8.6, the mean lung injury score (LIS) 1.8±0.6, and the mean multiple organ failure score (MOFs) 3.6±1.6. No differences were found between the group with and that without for age, SAPS, or extent of the infiltrate. One BAL sample were considered technically invalid and excluded.

BAL PMN count failed to distinguish between the presence or absence of pneumonia, so it was not possible to identify a clinically useful cut-off point. On the other hand, the mean percentage of infected cells was greater in the pneumonia group. The values of a cut-off ≥5% for the mean percentage of infected cells and microscopic examination of extracellular bacteria (ECB) were later confirmed by culture results, and four of the patients were found to have bacterial pneumonia. ICB values were in fact related to quantitative cultures (cut-off=CFU≥10^4/ml), as shown in TABLE 1. When using a cut-off point value of 5% infected cells, the test had a sensitivity of 71% and a specificity of 100%.

DISCUSSION

Nosocomial pneumonia during mechanical ventilation is associated with an extremely high mortality rate. The diagnosis often remains doubtful, and this uncertainty has an important impact on clinical research and practice. It may, moreover, lead to the unnecessary administration of antibiotics to patients with suspected ventilator-acquired pneumonia, thus encouraging the development of antibiotic resistance in the

TABLE 1. BAL Cytology and Bacteriology of Patients

Patients	Cells/µl	% PMN	% Infected Cells	BAL Smear (ECB)	BAL Culture
C. B.	360	97	0	Negative	Not identified
C. L.	2,080	99	7	Cocci	Not determined
P. L.	640	76	24	Cocci	*Pseudomonas aeruginosa* (≥10^4)
Z. G.	400	90	1	Negative	*S. aureus* (5×10^3)
M. R.	800	97	3	Negative	Negative
B. I.	720	96	6	Cocci yeasts	*Pseudomonas aeruginosa* (≥10^4) Aspergillus f.
B. I.	40	89	0	Negative	Negative
F. G.	40	95	0	Negative	Negative
S. G.	1,000	98	0	Negative	*Pseudomonas aeruginosa* (0.1×10^3)
T. O.	56	97	8	Cocci	*S. aureus* (≥10^4)
M. A.	4,000	98	5	Cocci	*S. epidemidi.* (≥10^4)
G. R.	300	98	0	Negative	Negative

hospital environment. While traditional clinical criteria (fever, purulent sputum, and leukocytosis, together with the appearance of new radiographic infiltrates) have an acceptable accuracy in the diagnosis of nosocomial pneumonia in non-intubated patients, these criteria have repeatedly been shown to have a low sensitivity and to be non-specific in mechanically ventilated patients. The optimal technique for diagnosing nosocomial bacterial pneumonia in patients on mechanical ventilation has yet to be clearly identified. It was recently suggested that bacterial phagocytosis by neutrophils or macrophages may be a useful marker of parenchymal lung infection.

Data reported in recent literature have shown that the microscopic identification of microorganisms within cells recovered by BAL may be a useful means for the early and rapid diagnosis of pneumonia in MV patients. Results obtained by different diagnostic techniques have been compared and the reliability of cytologic analysis has been assessed with respect to protected specimen brush and BAL quantitative cultures.[1,2]

In mechanically ventilated patients, culture techniques have been compared with other accepted methods, and the analysis of ROCs (receiver operator characteristics) has shown that these tests have a discriminating power comparable or superior to that of many widely accepted and routinely used tests.[3] Using the histopathology of bronchoscopically guided open-lung biopsies as the gold standard, the detection of intracellular organisms in protected and conventional BAL≥5% yielded 75% and 57% positive predictive values, respectively.[4] Our results confirm this observation, and a cut-off value ≥5% of ICB seems to be more suitable for the diagnosis of pneumonia. The microscopical identification of ICB in PMN recovered in BAL allows the early and accurate diagnosis of pneumonia in MV patients. While final culture results are being analyzed, the ICB cut-off of ≥5% appears useful in detection of pneumonia, enabling prompt management and in guiding antimicrobial therapy for this frequent complication from mechanical ventilation.

SUMMARY

In ventilator-dependent patients the management of clinically suspected nosocomial pneumonia is often difficult. A diagnosis of pneumonia is based upon findings including pulmonary infiltrate, fever, leukocytosis, or purulent secretions. By using bronchoscopic techniques, we can obtain bronchoalveolar lavage specimens (BAL) from the affected area of the lung. Neutrophils (PMN), which are important for lung defense, are found in increased numbers in BAL of these patients. We therefore ascertained the phagocytic activity of PMN against bacteria and fungi by microscopic examination. BAL specimens from ten mechanically ventilated patients were evaluated to assess the cellular counts using a Bürker hemocytometer, the differential cell counts by cytospin preparations (MGG stain), and the phagocytic activity of PMN and macrophages using the intracellular bacteria index (ICB) values. Microscopical examination of BAL cells and evaluation of ICB values (cut-off>5%) were higher in four out of twelve patients and the quantitative assessment of bacteria in PMN cytoplasm on cytospin preparations was found to be useful for the diagnosis of pneumonia. In these patients, pneumonia was suspected (in one patient fungal pneumonia) on the basis of microscopical examination of BAL cells and ICB values and the findings were confirmed later by microbiological cultures. In conclusion, in patients on mechanical ventilation a rapid diagnosis of bacterial or fungal pneumonia can be made using BAL cytology and by ICB values, and this in turn allows appropriate therapy to be initiated at an early stage. However, further studies of neutrophil functions are required to improve our understanding of the increased incidence of pulmonary infections in these patients.

REFERENCES

1. VIOLAN, J. S., F. RODRIGUEZ DE CASTRO, A. REY, J. C. MARTIN-GONZALES & P. CABRERA-NAVARRO. 1994. Usefulness of microscopic examination of intracellular organisms in lavage fluid in ventilator-associated pneumonia. Chest **106:** 889–894.
2. ALLEN, R. M., W. F. DUNN & A. H. LIMPER. 1994. Diagnosing ventilator-associated pneumonia: the role of bronchoscopy. Mayo Clin Proc. **69:** 962–968.
3. BAKER, A. M., D. L. BOWTON & E. F. HAPONIK. 1995. An analytic approach to the interpretation of quantitative bronchoscopic cultures. Chest **107:** 85–95.
4. TORRES, A., M. EL-EBIARY, N. FABREGAS, J. GONZALEZ, J. PUIG DE LA BELLACASA, C. HERNANDEZ, J. RAMIREZ & R. RODRIGUEZ-ROISIN. 1996. Value of intracellular bacteria detection in the diagnosis of ventilator associated pneumonia. Thorax **51:** 378–384.

Respiratory Burst of Neutrophils in Diabetic Patients with Periodontal Disease

S. DE TONI,[a] E. PIVA, A. LAPOLLA,[b] G. FONTANA,[b]
D. FEDELE,[b] AND M. PLEBANI

Department of Laboratory Medicine
[b]Clinical Medicine Institute
Chair in Metabolic Diseases
University of Padua
Padua, Italy

INTRODUCTION

Many studies suggest that diabetes mellitus leads to an increased prevalence and severity of periodontal disease. Diabetes mellitus is one of the most important metabolic disorders affecting cellular and biochemical processes within the body. Patients with diabetes often present depressed host defenses that result in increased susceptibility to infection. The mechanism underlying increased susceptibility may include the development of microangiopathy and sialadenosis, leading to xerostomia in diabetics. A more important contribution may be the effect of diabetes on the function of polymorphonuclear leukocytes (PMN). Defects in chemotaxis, phagocytosis, and bacterial killing have been observed in diabetic PMN.

The above observations, together with the evidence that PMN have an important protective function in the periodontium, suggest that increased host susceptibility may stem from bacterial-PMN interaction.

MATERIALS AND METHOD

Patients

The study was carried out on 40 diabetic patients (20 men and 20 women; mean age 59 ± 8 years) and 40 sex-matched non-diabetic subjects (56 ± 6 years). At preliminary screening, patients met the following entry criteria: a minimum of 16 teeth excluding third molars and the absence of systemic illness. The periodontal status was evaluated on the basis of alveolar bone level measurements (bone level as a percentage of total tooth length). Metabolic control was ascertained on the basis of findings for fasting plasma glucose, HbA_{1c}, cholesterol, and triglycerides.

[a]Address all correspondence to: Dr.ssa Stefania De Toni, Servizio di Medicina di Laboratorio, Laboratorio Centrale, Azienda Ospedaliera di Padova, Via Giustiniani, 2, 35128 Padova, Italy. Phone, 00 39 49 8212792; Fax, 00 39 49 663240.

Reagents

Ficoll-Hypaque (Histopaque-1077, Histopaque-1119, Sigma Diagnostics, St. Louis, MO); nitro blue tetrazolium MW 817.6 (NBT, Sigma Chemical Co., St. Louis, MO); phorbol myristate acetate MW 616.8 (PMA, Sigma Chemical Co.); phosphate-buffered saline 1 × pH 7.4 (PBS, from the hospital pharmacy); May-Grünwald-Giemsa stain (Merck Diagnostics, Darmstadt, Germany).

PMN Isolation

PMNs, obtained from whole blood samples collected by venipuncture and anticoagulated with EDTA (Vacutainer Systems, Becton-Dickinson, Meylan, France), were separated on a Ficoll-Hypaque density gradient (Histopaque-1077, Histopaque-1119, Sigma Diagnostics, St. Louis, MO) and the upper leukocyte-enriched population was collected and washed twice with phosphate-buffered saline solution (PBS, pH 7.4). PMNs were resuspended in PBS, counted by the hematological system Technicon H*2 (Technicon Bayer System, Tarrytown, NY), and diluted in an appropriate volume of PBS to obtain 5×10^9 PMNs/L. The test was performed within five hours after blood collection.

NADPH Oxidase Activity and Oxidative Burst Response by PMNs with a Quantitative Photometric Assay

A 50-µl aliquot of the PMN suspension at 5×10^9 neutrophils/L were incubated at room temperature in individual flat-bottom wells of a polystyrene microtiter plate (Kima, Piove di Sacco, Padua, Italy) with 50 µl of PBS and 50 µl of phorbol myristate acetate (PMA) (1.625 µmol/L) to initiate the respiratory burst. After 10 min of mixing, 50 µl of NBT (2.4 mmol/L) were added to each individual well. The rate of NBT reduction was monitored at 490 nm for 30 min, directly in the cells present in the wells, without prior solubilization. Starting immediately after the addition of NBT, optical density was recorded every 5 min by a photometer for microplates (Autoreader II, Ortho Diagnostic Systems, Milan, Italy). For each patient, the test was made in five replicates and also performed in resting PMNs, without stimulating the respiratory burst. NADPH oxidase activity, expressed as the mean of absorbance (A) values in the 30-min period, was measured as $A \times 10^{-3}$/min. To ascertain the precision of the method, the coefficient of variation (CV%) of five replicates for twenty samples was calculated. The mean CV was 5.09%, and the range for individual samples was 1.41 to 10.55%.

Neutrophil Chemotaxis

Cell migration was measured following the modified double-chamber filter method of Boyden, using blind well chambers (Costar, Nucleopore Italia, Concorezzo, Milan) with a volume of 200 µl zymosan-activated serum (ZAS) or control medium (PBS) in the bottom compartment and a 200-μl PMNs suspension containing 500 cells/μl in the top compartment, separated by 3-μm pore polycarbonate filters (Costar, Nucleopore Italia, Concorezzo, Milan). After a 60-min incubation at 37°C, the filters were fixed in methanol, stained with May-Grünwald-Giemsa solution, and dried and mounted on a Bürker hemocytometric chamber for counting. The results were expressed as neutrophil number/mm^3 (mean±SD) in the under side of the filter.

Statistical Analysis

Results were expressed as mean±SD and the statistical significance was determined using Student's *t* test.

RESULTS

Type 2 diabetic patients showed significantly higher levels of fasting plasma glucose (10.5±3.8 versus 5.5±1 mmol/L; $p<0.001$) and HbA$_{1c}$ (8.1±1.6 versus 5.4± 0.5%; $p<0.001$), but no differences in mean cholesterol (5.7±0.9 versus 5.7± 0.1 mmol/L) or triglyceride values (1.8±0.9 versus 1.7±1.4 mmol/L) were found with respect to normal controls.

Statistically significant differences were found between the periodontal status of diabetics and that of controls, especially on the mesial sites of the mandibular bone. When patients with more severe stages of the disease were considered, the prevalence of attachment loss and alveolar bone loss was statistically higher in diabetics (18.0% and 48.8%, respectively) than in normal controls (2.5% and 16.6%, respectively).

In all patients, results from tests for other diseases on admission were negative and, in particular, all had normal leukocyte counts, showing that they had neither infection nor inflammation. When the respiratory burst was activated by PMA, no difference was found between superoxide production, measured by the photometric method, of diabetics (4.31±1.67 A×10^{-3}/min) and that of normal subjects (4.25±1.25 A×10^{-3}/min), whereas significantly defective responses to opsonized zymosan were observed when using the microscopic method (58±17% in diabetics and 66±18% in controls; $p=0.05$). Our findings are reported in TABLE 1.

No quantitative difference was found in the neutrophil chemotactic response to zymosan-activated serum (ZAS) of diabetics and that of healthy controls. The data are shown in TABLE 2.

DISCUSSION

When the respiratory burst was activated by phorbol myristate acetate (PMA), a protein kinase C soluble activator, we found no difference between the PMN superoxide production of diabetics and that of healthy controls, whereas a significantly reduced response to opsonized zymosan was observed in diabetics. No quantitative difference was found in the neutrophil chemotactic response to zymosan-activated serum (ZAS) of diabetics and that of healthy controls. This finding shows that the

TABLE 1. NADPH Oxidase Activity in Neutrophils of Diabetics and Controls

	NADPH Oxidase Activity in Isolated PMNs by Photometric Method		NADPH Oxidase Activity in PMN Whole Blood by Microscopic Method		
	Resting PMNs	PMA-stimulated PMNs	Resting PMNs	PMA-stimulated PMNs	Zymosan-stimulated PMNs
Diabetics	0.70±0.58	4.31±1.67	4±2.8	74±35	58±17[a]
Controls	0.90±0.58	4.25±1.25	6.3±5	85±22	66±18[a]

Note: Superoxide anion production was measured as the NBT reduction at 490 nm in a microplate reader by the photometric method and as the percentage of positive PMNs with granules of formazan in the cytoplasm by a microscopic method. The absorbance values are expressed as $A \times 10^{-3}$/min (mean±SD).

[a]$p=0.05$, unpaired Student's t test.

impact on PMN function in diabetes is of multifactorial origin and is probably correlated to the glucose level and to the glycation of PMN protein, such as NADPH oxidase or myeloperoxidase.[1] Alternatively, glucose in PMN may be reduced by aldose reductase to polyols, and this pathway requires NADPH, the coenzyme for the respiratory burst. Moreover, we found that superoxide production in response to unopsonized zymosan was reduced in diabetic patients. The activation of protein tyrosine kinase (PTK) is probably an important mechanism underlying transmembrane signaling, and protein tyrosine phosphorylation stimulated by zymosan receptor–mediated activation may depend on the activation of specific PTK, whereas activation by PMA is thought to be mediated through protein kinase C (PKC).[2] There is a higher prevalence and severity of periodontal disease in type 2 diabetics. However, the results of the present study demonstrate that diabetes is not a direct cause of periodontal disease but a systemic promoting factor, creating suitable conditions for local pathological alterations that produce gingivitis and periodontitis. According to Oliver and colleagues it is likely that many diabetics have no defects in their neutrophil response.[3]

In conclusion, further studies on gingival tissues and pocket fluids are needed to explain how diabetes contributes to periodontal inflammation.

TABLE 2. Chemotaxis in 20 Diabetics and 20 Healthy Controls[a]

	Migration without Stimulation	Migration with ZAS Stimulation
Diabetics	47.55±63.11	107.75±146.05
Controls	52.26±79.44	88.21±128.43

[a]Chemotaxis measured as the number of PMNs/mm^3 that penetrated a polycarbonate filter separating the cells from a chemoattractant.

SUMMARY

Periodontal disease, a frequent complication of diabetes mellitus, is the major cause of tooth loss. However, studies on neutrophil function in patients with this condition have yielded contradictory findings. The NADPH oxidase activity of 40 diabetic patients with periodontosis who were on metabolic control was evaluated and compared with that in 40 healthy subjects. Superoxide anion production was measured by a photometric method, with NBT reduction at 490 nm in a microplate reader and by a microscopic method, with a percentage of positive PMNs with granules of formazan in the cytoplasm. When the PMN respiratory burst was activated by phorbol myristate acetate (PMA), a protein kinase C (PKC) soluble activator, superoxide production of diabetics (4.31 ± 1.67 $A\times10^{-3}$/min) and normal subjects (4.25 ± 1.25 $A\times10^{-3}$/min) was comparable by photometric method, whereas a significantly defective response to opsonized zymosan was observed when the microscopic method was used ($58\pm17\%$ in diabetics and $66\pm18\%$ in controls; $p=0.05$). Therefore in patients with diabetes the impact on PMN function is of multifactorial origin, and is probably correlated to the glucose level and to glycation of PMN protein, such as NADPH oxidase or myeloperoxidase. Alternatively, glucose in PMN may be reduced by aldose reductase to polyols, and this pathway requires NADPH, the coenzyme for the respiratory burst. Moreover, we found that superoxide production in response to opsonized zymosan was reduced in diabetic patients. The activation of protein tyrosine kinase (PTK) is an important mechanism underlying transmembrane signaling and, moreover, protein tyrosine phosphorylations, stimulated by zymosan receptor–mediated activation, might be caused by the activation of specific PTK, whereas activation by PMA is probably mediated through another PKC type.

REFERENCES

1. Lin Mbbs, X., J. K. Candlish & A. C. Thai. 1993. Effect of glucose on the respiratory burst of neutrophils from normal and diabetic subjects. Clin. Lab. Haemat. **15:** 203–210.
2. Sanguedolce, M., C. Capo, M. Bouhamdan, P. Bongrand, C. K. Huang & J. L. Mege. 1993. Zymosan-induced tyrosine phosphorylations in human monocytes. J. Immunol. **151:** 405–414.
3. Oliver, R. C. & T. Tervonen. 1994. Diabetes—A risk factor for periodontis in adults? J. Periodontal. **65:** 530–538.

G-Protein Coupled Receptor–Mediated Activation of PI 3-Kinase in Neutrophils[a]

MARCUS THELEN[b] AND SVETLANA A. DIDICHENKO

Theodor Kocher-Institute
University of Bern
CH-3000 Bern 9, Switzerland

INTRODUCTION

Neutrophil leukocytes are required for an efficient host defense against invading microorganisms and contribute to the inflammatory responses in mammals. Resting neutrophils circulate in the blood but when sensing a chemotactic signal the cells marginate to the endothelium and migrate to the inflammatory site.[1] Release of superoxide anions by a membrane-bound NADPH oxidase, exocytosis of proteolytic enzymes from storage organelles, and phagocytosis of the microorganisms are the hallmarks of the neutrophil inflammatory responses.[2,3] The secretory products are also toxic to the host tissue, thus the activation of neutrophils must be firmly controlled.[4,5]

Chemoattractants ligate to G-protein–coupled receptors of neutrophils and initiate a poorly characterized signal transduction cascade. Binding of the chemotactic agonists stimulates the dissociation of $\beta\gamma$ subunits from the $G_{i\alpha}$ subunit of the receptor-coupled heterotrimeric G_i protein.[3] The signal then branches into at least two transduction pathways leading to the activation of phospholipase $C\beta_2$ (PLC) and phosphatidylinositide 3-kinase (PI 3-kinase).[6–10] The activities of the calcium-dependent PLC and of a wortmannin-sensitive PI 3-kinase are both necessary to stimulate the NADPH oxidase.[11] Activation of the PLC by $\beta\gamma$ subunits of heterotrimeric G-proteins is well established,[6,7,12] by contrast, activation of PI 3-kinase by G-protein–coupled receptors is controversial.[13–16]

Three heterodimeric PI 3-kinase isoforms that accept $PI(4,5)P_2$, $PI(4)P$, and PI as substrate (type I PI 3-kinase) have been characterized from mammalian tissue. PI 3-kinase$_\alpha$ and PI 3-kinase$_\beta$ are composed of distinct catalytic subunits p110α[17] and p110β[18] and associate with the regulatory subunit, p85.[19–21] PI 3-kinase$_\gamma$ consists of the catalytic subunit p120 and the regulatory subunit p101.[22] Stephens and colleagues originally described a PI 3-kinase activity that is strongly activated by the $\beta\gamma$ subunits of heterotrimeric G-proteins.[15] The kinase was assumed to account for the rapid PIP_3 formation observed in myeloid-derived cells stimulated with agonists of G-protein–coupled receptors.[16] Cloning of PI 3-kinase$_\gamma$ revealed a high degree of ho-

[a]This work supported by the Swiss National Science Foundation. M. T. is a recipient of a career development award from the Swiss National Science Foundation.

[b]Address all correspondence to: Dr. Marcus Thelen, Theodor Kocher-Institute, University of Berne, PO Box, CH-3000 Bern 9, Switzerland. Phone, +41 31 631 4154; Fax, +41 31 631 3799; and Email. Thelen@tki.unibe.ch.

mology over the kinase domain located near the C-terminus of p120 and p110α. Otherwise p101/p120 and p85/p110 are very distinct.[22,23] The most abundantly expressed form in neutrophils is the p85/p110 PI 3-kinase$_\alpha$.[24]

The regulatory subunit p85 comprises a SH$_3$ domain (Src homology domain),[25] two SH$_2$ domains,[26–28] proline-rich regions,[29,30] and sequence with high homology to the C-terminus of the bcr gene product.[31] Phosphotyrosines that are located within a Y(P)XXM consensus bind tightly to p85 and activate the PI 3-kinase.[32] Similarly, SH$_3$ domains of several Src-related tyrosine kinases bind to the proline-rich domains of p85 stimulating the catalytic activity of p110.[33–35] The small GTPases CDC42Hs and Rac1 have been shown to stimulate PI 3-kinase through binding to the bcr-domain of p85[36] and Ras in its GTP-bound form stimulates PI 3-kinase by associating with p110.[37] The subunits of PI 3-kinase$_\alpha$ interact with each other through the inter-SH2 domain (iSH2) of p85 and the N-terminus of p110.[19,38] Overexpression of p85 with a deleted iSH2 domain (△p85) blocks stimulation of PI 3-kinase by trapping incoming signals without activating the catalytic subunit.[39,40]

The fungal metabolite wortmannin is the most powerful inhibitor of the agonist-dependent respiratory burst in neutrophils.[11] In intact neutrophils inhibition of the respiratory burst perfectly matches binding of wortmannin to the catalytic subunit of PI 3-kinase$_\alpha$.[24] Inhibition of PI 3-kinase$_\gamma$ activity appears to require slightly higher concentrations of wortmannin.[15] In the present study we used two independent approaches to test activation of PI 3-kinase$_\alpha$ by G-protein–coupled receptors. Genistein, a protein tyrosine kinase inhibitor,[41] was found to inhibit PIP$_3$ formation in neutrophils stimulated with fMet-Leu-Phe. Expression of the dominant negative △p85 in GM-1 cells impaired IL-8–induced PIP$_3$ production, suggesting that PI 3-kinase$_\alpha$ significantly contributes to the PIP$_3$ formation observed upon stimulation of myeloid cells with agonists of G-protein–coupled receptors.

MATERIALS AND METHODS

Materials

RPMI-1640 media, Hank's balance salt solution, antibiotics, additional cell culture reagents, and genistein were from GIBCO (Basel, Switzerland); cytochrome *c* from Sigma (St. Louis, MO), fMet-Leu-Phe from Bachem (Bubendorf, Switzerland); and [^{32}P]γ-ATP (5000 Ci/mmol) and [^{32}P]orthophosphate (10 mCi/ml) from Amersham, UK. 17-Hydroxywortmannin (wortmannin) was a gift from Dr. T. Payne (Sandoz Ltd., Basel, Switzerland).

GM-1 Cells

A lac-switch inducible expression system (Stratagene) was introduced into GM-1 cells.[42] GM-1 cells were transfected with the gene for the lac repressor in the pCMVLacI vector (Stratagene) carrying hygormycin B resistance. Constitutive expression of high levels of the repressor appeared not to alter the phenotype of stable clones (not shown). △p85 gene was obtained by removing 179 amino acids

(Tyr^{416}–Thr^{585}) located between the two SH_2 domains of human p85α.[8] The construct was inserted downstream of the strong CMV1E1-promoter and the lac repressor binding site in the pcDNA3 expression vector conferring G418 resistance.[39,43] The CXCR1 gene was inserted into pPUR (Clontech) under the control of the CMV1 promoter (pPUR/IL-8R1). GM-1 cells[42] were transfected as described.[44] Resistant clones were selected in RPMI-1640 media supplemented with 10% FCS and 110 U/ml hygromycin 0.8 mg/ml G418 or 0.2 µg/ml puromycin. Expression of $\triangle$p85 was induced by adding 5 mM IPTG to the cell cultures for 4 hours. If indicated, cells were pretreated with 100 µM $ZnCl_2$ and 2 nM phorbol myristate acetate to enhance the CMV1E1 promoter activity.

Neutrophils

Neutrophils were prepared from fresh donor blood as previously described by dextran sedimentation, hypotonic lysis of contaminating erythrocytes, and centrifugation in a Ficoll gradient.[5] Labeling of 4×10^7 cells/ml with 2 mCi/ml [^{32}P]orthophosphate was performed at 37°C for 60 min in calcium-free Hank's HEPES-buffered salt solution (HBSS) (140 mM NaCl, 5 mM KCl, 2.8 mM $NaHCO_3$, 1 mM $MgCl_2$, 0.06 mM $MgSO_4$, 5.6 mM glucose, 0.1% bovine serum albumin, and 15 mM HEPES, pH 7.2). The cells were washed three times in cold HBSS and finally resuspended in HBSS containing 1.5 mM $CaCl_2$. Treatment of prewarmed (5 min at 37°C) neutrophils with genistein or wortmannin was performed at 37°C for 10 min.

Assays

Phosphatidylinositol (3,4,5)-trisphosphate content of neutrophils and GM-1 transfectants was measured as previously described.[44] Superoxide formation was measured in calcium-containing HBSS without serum albumin as cytochrome *c* reduction.[6]

RESULTS

Stimulation of human neutrophils with the chemotactic agonist fMet-Leu-Phe induces a transient respiratory burst that results in the release of superoxide anions. FIGURE 1 shows the effect of the protein tyrosine kinase inhibitor genistein on fMet-Leu-Phe–stimulated superoxide production. Genistein inhibits superoxide formation in a concentration-dependent manner becoming apparent at concentrations as low as 100 nM. At 100 µM genistein maximum inhibition was obtained resulting in a 80–90% decrease of the superoxide production observed with control cells.

Similarly, preincubation of neutrophils with 0.1 to 100 µM genistein leads to a marked inhibition of G-protein–coupled receptor–mediated PIP$_3$ formation. FIGURE 2 illustrates the effect of genistein on PIP$_3$ formation in neutrophils stimulated for 15 sec with fMet-Leu-Phe. In the presence of 100 µM genistein agonist-dependent PIP$_3$ production was attenuated by more than 80%, comparable with the inhibitory effect

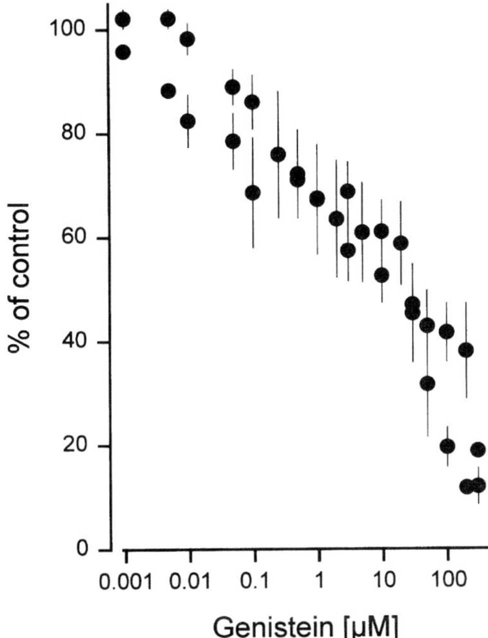

FIGURE 1. Effect of genistein on the neutrophil respiratory burst. Prewarmed cells $(2.5 \times 10^6/\text{ml})$ were incubated for 10 min at 37°C with the indicated concentrations of genistein and then stimulated with 1 μM fMet-Leu-Phe. Cytochrome c reduction was measured continuously.[46] Percent inhibition was calculated from the superoxide production obtained in the absence of genistein (7.8 ± 0.8 nmol/5 min $\times 10^6$ cells). Results are mean values $\pm$ SD of 2–4 determinations.

on the respiratory burst. FIGURE 3 shows PI(3)P formation by purified neutrophil p85/p110[24] in the presence of genistein or wortmannin. Phosphorylation of PI to PI(3)P was virtually unchanged if the PI 3-kinase was preincubated with genistein (up to 100 μM). By contrast, wortmannin (100 nM) fully inhibited the kinase activity. The results indicate that genistein interferes with a target that is upstream of PI 3-kinase in G-protein–coupled receptor signaling.

Activation of PI 3-kinase in neutrophils with fMet-Leu-Phe causes a rapid rise in PIP₃ levels with a maximum PIP₃ formation observed 10–15 sec after stimulation that is followed by a somewhat protracted decay (FIG. 4). In neutrophils that were pretreated with genistein and then stimulated with fMet-Leu-Phe, this transient rise in PIP₃ was strongly inhibited (FIG. 4). The results indicate that the bulk of agonist-stimulated PIP₃ formation is mediated through a genistein-sensitive signaling step.

An attempt was made to test the relative contribution of PI 3-kinase$_\alpha$ and PI 3-kinase$_\gamma$ to the PIP₃ production stimulated with agonists of G-protein–coupled receptors.[2] Promyelocytic GM-1 cells were first transformed with a lac-switch system, that allows inducible gene expression.[47] The cells were then transfected with a regulatory

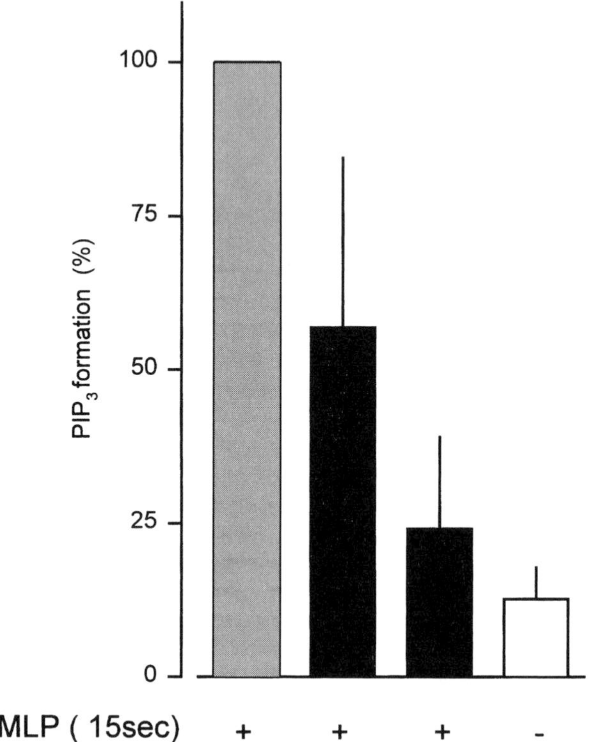

FIGURE 2. Effect of genistein on PIP$_3$ formation in neutrophils. [^{32}P]othophosphate loaded cells (5×10^6) were treated for 10 min at 37°C with the indicated concentrations of genistein and then stimulated with 1 μM fMet-Leu-Phe. Reactions were terminated after 15 sec, lipids extracted, and resolved on TLC plates. PIP$_3$ formation was quantified using a PhosphorImager. Duplicate determinations of two independent experiments.

subunit of PI 3-kinase$_\alpha$ $\triangle$p85, of which 179 amino acids were deleted that form the binding site for the catalytic subunit p110$_\alpha$.[48,49] Expression of $\triangle$p85 is expected to sequester stimulatory signals without activating the catalytic subunit, thus resulting in a dominant negative phenotype. Stable GM-1/$\triangle$p85 clones were selected and analyzed for the expression of $\triangle$p85 upon treatment with 5 nM IPTG in the presence of 100 μM ZnCl$_2$ and 2 nM phorbol myristate acetate. The latter were added to enhance promoter activity. The Western blot shown in FIGURE 5 indicates that in non-induced GM-1/$\triangle$p85 cells the mutated regulatory subunit is silent. However, following treatment of the cells with IPTG, ZnCl$_2$, and phorbol myristate acetate a massive expression of $\triangle$p85 is observed. A clone with high inducible expression of $\triangle$p85 was selected and transfected with the IL-8 receptor CXCR1.[50] Stable GM-1/$\triangle$p85/CXCR1 transfectants were cloned and tested for IL-8–stimulated chemotaxis and calcium elevations (not shown).

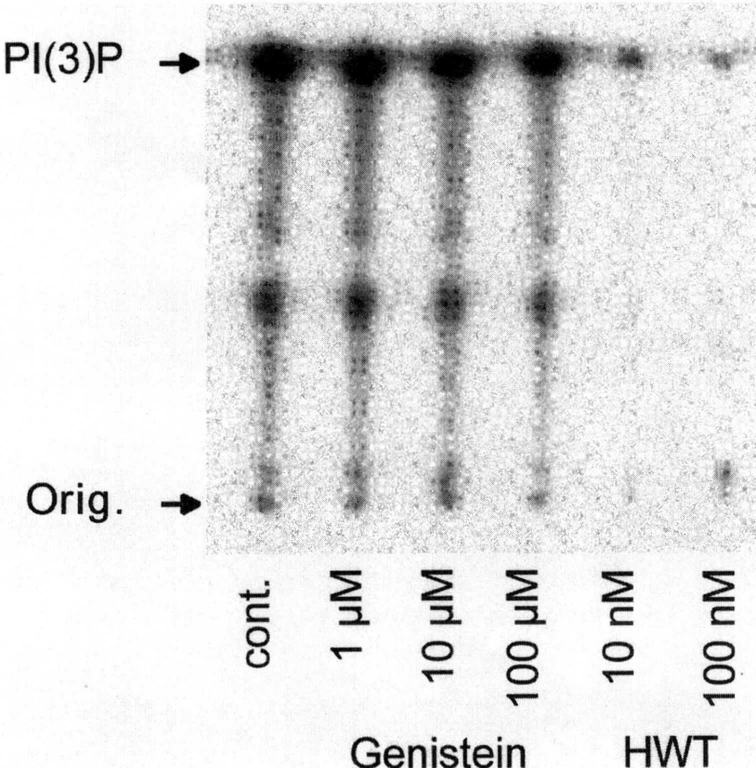

FIGURE 3. Effect of genistein and wortmannin on PI 3-kinase activity. Approximately 5 ng human neutrophil PI 3-kinase were incubated for 10 min in the presence of buffer (cont.), genistein (1–100 µM), or wortmannin (10 nM and 100 nM). Kinase reaction was initiated by the addition of [^{32}P]ATP and was terminated after 10 min. Lipids were extracted, resolved on silica-plates, and visualized as in FIGURE 2.

GM-1/$\triangle$p85/CXCR1 were loaded with [^{32}P], stimulated with 1 µM IL-8 and the PIP$_3$ formation measured. Similarly as described for neutrophils (FIG. 4), GM-1 cells show a bimodal PIP$_3$ formation, with a maximum observed 15–20 sec followed by a more protracted lower level of PIP$_3$ formation. After 4–5 min, the agonist-stimulated PIP$_3$ production returns to basal levels (data not shown). FIGURE 6 illustrates PIP$_3$ production in GM-1/$\triangle$p85/CXCR1 cells 15 sec after stimulation with IL-8. In control GM-1/CXCR1 cells (not transfected with $\triangle$p85) and non-induced GM-1/$\triangle$p85/CXCR1 cells IL-8 stimulated a two- to threefold increase of PIP$_3$. Treatment of the GM-1/$\triangle$p85/CXCR1 cells with ZnCl$_2$ or PMA in the absence of IPTG had only minor effects on IL-8–stimulated PIP$_3$ formation. However, when maximum expression of $\triangle$p85 was induced (FIG. 5) a marked inhibition of IL-8–stimulated PIP$_3$ formation was measured. The results demonstrate that expression of the dominant

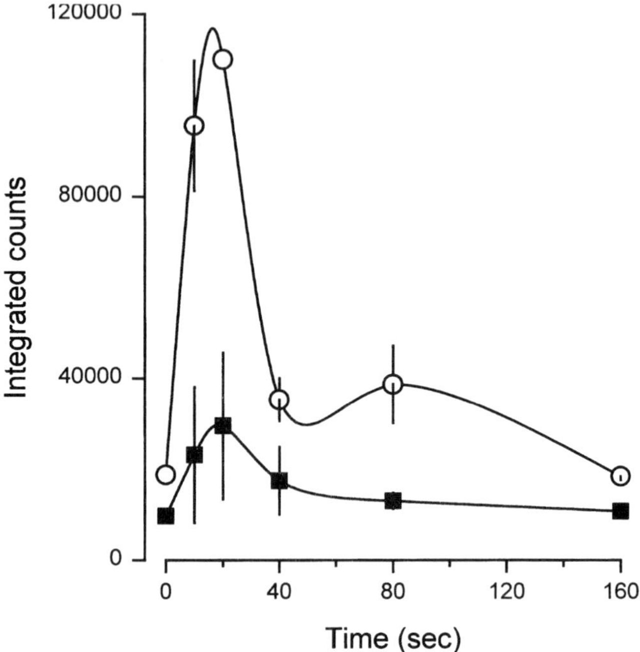

FIGURE 4. Time course of PIP_3 formation in neutrophils. Neutrophils (5×10^6/ml) were incubated for 10 min at 37°C with buffer alone (*open symbols*) or with 100 μM genistein (*closed symbols*) and were then stimulated with 1 μM fMet-Leu-Phe for the indicated times. PIP_3 formation was measured as in FIGURE 2.

negative $\triangle$p85 inhibits IL-8–stimulated PIP_3 formation. Thus it can be assumed that PI 3-kinase$_\alpha$ significantly contributes to the early PIP_3 production observed in phagocytic cells.

DISCUSSION

Stimulation of neutrophils with receptor agonists results in the rapid and transient formation of PIP_3 (FIG. 4).[16] Maximum PIP_3 elevation occurs after 10–15 sec, supporting the view that activation of PI 3-kinase is an early event in receptor-mediated signaling. *B. pertussis* toxin treatment of neutrophils completely inhibits the rapid chemoattractant-stimulated PIP_3 formation.[16,51] Thus activation of PI 3-kinase requires coupling of the fMet-Leu-Phe receptor to a heterotrimeric G_i protein.[3,52]

Inhibition of PI 3-kinase with wortmannin blocks neutrophil respiratory burst and exocytosis.[11] Binding studies and purification of the wortmannin target revealed that in neutrophils the predominant PI 3-kinase isoform is p85/p110.[24] The mechanism of activation, however, remains elusive. Stimulation of PI 3-kinase is well characterized

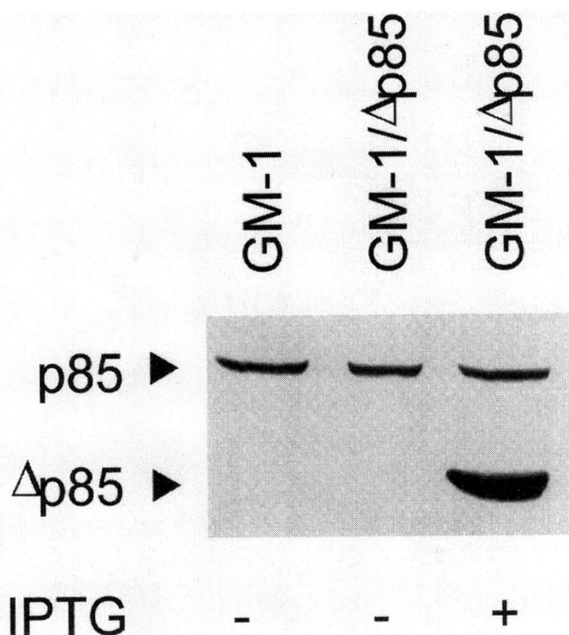

FIGURE 5. Expression of Δp85 in GM-1 transfectants. Western blot of lysates of GM-1 cells and GM-1/Δp85. The right lane shows lysates from GM-1/Δp85 which were induced with 5 mM IPTG, 100 μM ZnCl$_2$, and 2 nM PMA for 4 h in culture medium. The positions of wild type p85 and of Δp85 are indicated.

in growth factor receptor signaling.[53] Autophosphorylation of tyrosines 740 and 751 of the PDGF receptor provides docking sites for the SH$_2$ domains of p85 leading to the activation of the catalytic subunit p110.[9,54] By contrast, immunoprecipitates of p85 from stimulated neutrophils were devoid of associated tyrosine phosphorylated proteins,[55,56] suggesting that the rapid activation of PI 3-kinase does not occur via the SH$_2$ domains of p85.

The present studies suggest that activation of PI 3-kinase is mediated by a genistein-sensitive intermediate. The compound is a widely accepted inhibitor of protein tyrosine kinases that has minor effects on serine/thronine kinases.[41,57] Genistein treatment was reported to reduce the PI(4,5)P$_2$ content of neutrophils. In consequence the reduced substrate availability for PI 3-kinase was assumed to cause the apparent inhibition of fMet-Leu-Phe–stimulated PIP$_3$ formation.[58] Our results and observations by others,[14] however, indicate that genistein has a marked effect on the agonist-stimulated PIP$_3$ production. We could not detect a significant inhibition of purified p85/p110 at concentrations where genistein markedly attenuated PIP$_3$ formation or agonist-stimulated superoxide production, indicating that the compound does not interfere with PI 3-kinase$_\alpha$. Some effects of elevated genistein concentrations on PI 3-kinase$_\gamma$ activity were reported, but could not account for the dramatic

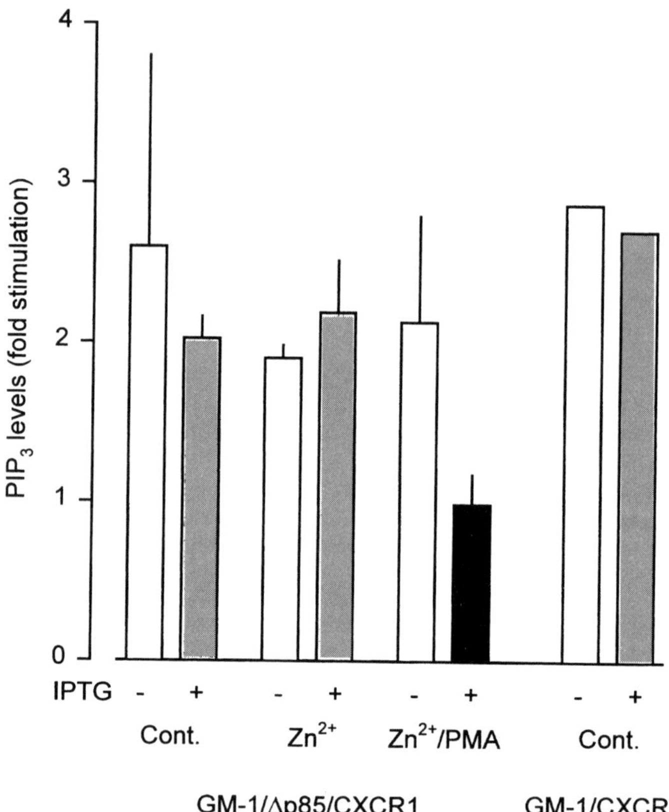

FIGURE 6. Expression of $\triangle$p85 inhibits IL-8–stimulated PIP$_3$ formation. GM-1 cells carrying a lac-switch system were transfected with CXCR1 (GM-1/CXCR1) alone or with CXCR1 and a dominant negative PI 3-kinase construct (GM-1/$\triangle$p85/CXCR1). Cells were treated ($\pm$) with IPTG alone (cont.) or in the presence of 100 μM ZnCl$_2$ (Zn^{2+}) or of 100 μM ZnCl$_2$ and 2 nM PMA (Zn^{2+}/PMA) for 4 h and then labeled with [^{32}P]orthophosphate for 70 min. Washed cells were stimulated for 15 sec with 1 μM IL-8 and lipids extracted, separated on TLC and quantified using a PhosphorImager. Duplicate determinations from two independent experiments.

inhibition of PIP$_3$ formation in agonist-stimulated neutrophils.[14] It is therefore conceivable, that neutrophil activation of PI 3-kinase$_\alpha$ is mediated by a tyrosine kinase.

Neutrophils show rapid tyrosine phosphorylations following challenge with fMet-Leu-Phe[59–64] and stimulus-dependent association of PI 3-kinase activity with anti-Lyn immunoprecipitates.[16,58,65,66] Radicicol, a potent tyrosine kinase inhibitor,[7] was found to prevent Lyn activation and PIP$_3$ formation, suggesting that the Src-related kinase is involved in PI 3-kinase activation.[14] However, the correlation of maximum

PI 3-kinase activity in Lyn-immunoprecipitates and of PIP_3 elevations in neutrophils is not satisfactory. In accordance with others[16] we observed a rapid peak of PIP_3 formation (10–20 sec) whereas maximum PI 3-kinase activity associated with anti-Lyn immunoprecipitates was detected at 30–60 sec.[14,16,51,58] Thus, the mechanism of PI 3-kinase$_\alpha$ activation in neutrophils remains to be established.

Expression of a dominant negative regulatory subunit of PI 3-kinase$_\alpha$ in GM-1 cells results in a marked suppression of PIP_3 formation. This finding is in line with the view that PI 3-kinase$_\alpha$ contributes significantly to the PIP_3 production stimulated by agonists of G-protein–coupled receptors.[14,65] PI 3-kinase$_\gamma$ is rapidly activated upon binding of $\beta\gamma$ subunits of heterotrimeric G-proteins to the regulatory subunit p101 and is independent of tyrosine phosphorylations.[15,22,56] Thus it is unlikely that a genistein target is located between the receptor and PI 3-kinase$_\gamma$, although a regulation of the enzyme by a tyrosine kinase–dependent mechanism can not be excluded. The role of PI 3-kinase$_\gamma$ in the regulation of PIP_3-dependent pathways in fMet-Leu-Phe–stimulated neutrophils is unclear. Our results show that at the highest concentrations used genistein does not fully inhibit the respiratory burst and the formation of PIP_3. The residual activity of the NADPH oxidase may indicate a genistein insensitive, PI 3-kinase$_\gamma$–mediated PIP_3 generation. Although considerable redundance in the signal transduction may exist, it is conceivable that distinct PI 3-kinase isoforms selectively regulate different PIP_3-dependent responses.

SUMMARY

Stimulation of the respiratory burst of neutrophil leukocytes with chemotactic agonists requires two concomitant signal transduction pathways. One is calcium dependent and leads to activation of phospholipase C, the other is calcium independent but sensitive to the fungal metabolite wortmannin, a specific inhibitor of phosphatidylinositide 3-kinase (PI 3-kinase). Two isoforms of PI 3-kinase have been characterized in neutrophils, the p85/p110 PI 3-kinase$_\alpha$ and the p101/p120 PI 3-kinase$_\gamma$. The relative contribution of the two PI 3-kinases in mediating chemoattractant-stimulated superoxide production and exocytosis in neutrophils is unclear. Here, we report that the protein tyrosine kinase inhibitor genistein markedly attenuates chemoattractant-stimulated phosphatidylinositol (3,4,5)-trisphosphate (PIP_3) formation in neutrophils. PI 3-kinase activity in untreated cells is bimodal showing a maximum production after 10–15 sec that protracts with a lower PIP_3 formation for approximately 2 min and returns to basal levels after 2–3 min. Genistein at 100 μM strongly inhibits PIP_3 elevation and the fMet-Leu-Phe–stimulated respiratory burst. The activity of purified PI 3-kinase, however, is not altered in the presence of genistein, suggesting that the genistein-sensitive intermediate is located between the G-protein–coupled receptor and PI 3-kinase. Expression of a dominant negative form of PI 3-kinase$_\alpha$ in GM-1/CXCR1 cells, a promyelolocytic cell line transfected with the G-protein–coupled receptor CXCR1, considerably reduces IL-8–stimulated PIP_3 formation. The present observations suggest that in phagocytes stimulated with agonists of G-protein–coupled receptors the bulk of PIP_3 is generated by PI 3-kinase$_\alpha$, which is activated through a genistein-sensitive target, presumably a protein tyrosine kinase.

REFERENCES

1. ALBELDA, S. M., C. W. SMITH & P. A. WARD. 1994. Adhesion molecules and inflammatory injury. FASEB J. **8:** 504–512.
2. BAGGIOLINI, M., F. BOULAY, J. A. BADWEY & J. T. CURNUTTE. 1993. Activation of neutrophil leukocytes: Chemoattractant receptors and respiratory burst. FASEB J. **7:** 1004–1010.
3. THELEN, M., B. DEWALD & M. BAGGIOLINI. 1993. Neutrophil signal transduction and activation of the respiratory burst. Physiol. Rev. **73:** 797–821.
4. KUKIELKA, G. L., C. W. SMITH, G. J. LAROSA, A. M. MANNING, L. H. MENDOZA, T. J. DALY, B. J. HUGHES, K. A. YOUKER, H. K. HAWKINS, L. H. MICHAEL, A. ROT & M. L. ENTMAN. 1995. Interleukin-8 gene induction in the myocardium after ischemia and reperfusion in vivo. J. Clin. Invest. **95:** 89–103.
5. COLLETTI, L. M., S. L. KUNKEL, A. WALZ, M. D. BURDICK, R. G. KUNKEL, C. A. WILKE & R. M. STRIETER. 1995. Chemokine expression during hepatic ischemia/reperfusion-induced lung injury in the rat. The role of epithelial neutrophil activating protein. J. Clin. Invest. **95:** 134–141.
6. CAMPS, M., A. CAROZZI, P. SCHNABEL, A. SCHEER, P. J. PARKER & P. GIERSCHIK. 1992. Isozyme-selective stimulation of phospholipase C-β2 by G protein βγ-subunits. Nature **360:** 684–686.
7. KATZ, A., D. WU & M. I. SIMON. 1992. Subunits βγ of heterotrimeric G protein activate β2 isoform of phospholipase C. Nature **360:** 686–689.
8. TRAYNOR-KAPLAN, A. E., A. L. HARRIS, B. L. THOMPSON, P. TAYLOR & L. A. SKLAR. 1988. An inositol tetrakisphosphate-containing phospholipid in activated neutrophils. Nature **334:** 353–356.
9. STEPHENS, L. R., K. T. HUGHES & R. F. IRVINE. 1991. Pathway of phosphatidylinositol(3,4,5)-trisphosphate synthesis in activated neutrophils. Nature **351:** 33–39.
10. VLAHOS, C. J., W. F. MATTER, R. F. BROWN, A. E. TRAYNOR-KAPLAN, P. G. HEYWORTH, E. R. PROSSNITZ, R. D. YE, P. MARDER, J. A. SCHELM, K. J. ROTHFUSS, B. S. SERLIN & P. J. SIMPSON. 1995. Investigation of neutrophil signal transduction using a specific inhibitor of phosphatidylinositol 3-kinase. J. Immunol. **154:** 2413–2422.
11. DEWALD, B., M. THELEN & M. BAGGIOLINI. 1988. Two transduction sequences are necessary for neutrophil activation by receptor agonists. J. Biol. Chem. **263:** 16179–16184.
12. CAMPS, M., C. HOU, D. SIDIROPOULOS, J. B. STOCK, K. H. JAKOBS & P. GIERSCHIK. 1992. Stimulation of phospholipase C by guanine-nucleotide-binding protein βγ subunits. Eur. J. Biochem. **206:** 821–831.
13. OKADA, T., O. HAZEKI, M. UI & T. KATADA. 1996. Synergistic activation of PtdIns 3-kinase by tyrosine-phosphorylated peptide and βγ-subunits of GTP-binding proteins. Biochem. J. **317:** 475–480.
14. PTASZNIK, A., E. R. PROSSNITZ, D. YOSHIKAWA, A. SMRCKA, A. E. TRAYNOR-KAPLAN & G. M. BOKOCH. 1996. A tyrosine kinase signaling pathway accounts for the majority of phosphatidylinositol 3,4,5-trisphosphate formation in chemoattractant-stimulated human neutrophils. N. Biol. Chem. **271:** 25204–25207.
15. STEPHENS, L., A. SMRCKA, F. T. COOKE, T. R. JACKSON, P. C. STERNWEIS & P. T. HAWKINS. 1994. A novel phosphoinositide 3 kinase activity in myeloid-derived cells is activated by G protein βγ subunits. Cell **77:** 83–93.
16. STEPHENS, L., A. EGUINOA, S. COREY, T. JACKSON & P. T. HAWKINS. 1993. Receptor stimulated accumulation of phosphatidylinositol (3,4,5)-trisphosphate by G-protein mediated pathways in human myeloid derived cells. EMBO J. **12:** 2265–2273.
17. HILES, I. D., M. OTSU, S. VOLINIA, M. J. FRY, I. GOUT, R. DHAND, G. PANAYOTOU, F. RUIZ-LARREA, A. THOMPSON, N. F. TOTTY, J. J. HSUAN, S. A. COURTNEIDGE, P. J. PARKER & M. D. WATERFIELD. 1992. Phosphatidylinositol 3-kinase: Structure and expression of the 110 kd catalytic subunit. Cell **70:** 419–429.

18. Hu, P., A. Mondino, E. Y. Skolnik & J. Schlessinger. 1993. Cloning of a novel, ubiquitously expressed human phosphatidylinositol 3-kinase and identification of its binding site on p85. Mol. Cell. Biol. **13:** 7677–7688.

19. Dhand, R., K. Hara, I. Hiles, B. Bax, I. Gout, G. Panayotou, M. J. Fry, K. Yonezawa, M. Kasuga & M. D. Waterfield. 1994. PI 3-kinase: Structural and functional analysis of intersubunit interactions. EMBO J. **13:** 511–521.

20. Hu, P. & J. Schlessinger. 1994. Direct association of p110β phosphatidylinositol 3-kinase with p85 is mediated by an N-terminal fragment of p110β. Mol. Cell. Biol. **14:** 2577–2583.

21. Stephens, L. R., T. R. Jackson & P. T. Hawkins. 1993. Agonist-stimulated synthesis of phosphatidylinositol(3,4,5)-trisphosphate: A new intracellular signalling system. Biochim. Biophys. Acta Mol. Cell Res. **1179:** 27–75.

22. Stephens, L. E., A. Eguinoa, H. Erdjument-Bromage, M. Lui, F. Cooke, J. Coadwell, A. Smrcka, M. Thelen, K. Cadwallader, P. Tempst & P. T. Hawkins. 1997. The Gβγ-sensitivity of a PI3K is dependent upon a tightly-associated adaptor, p101. Cell **89:** 105–114.

23. Stoyanov, B., S. Volinia, T. Hanck, I. Rubio, M. Loubtchenkov, D. Malek, S. Stoyanova, B. Vanhaesebroeck, R. Dhand, B. Nürnberg, P. Gierschik, K. Seedorf, J. J. Hsuan, M. D. Waterfield & R. Wetzker. 1995. Cloning and characterization of a G protein-activated human phosphoinositide-3 kinase. Science **269:** 690–693.

24. Thelen, M., M. P. Wymann & H. Langen. 1994. Wortmannin binds specifically to 1-phosphatidylinositol 3-kinase while inhibiting guanine nucleotide-binding protein-coupled receptor signaling in neutrophil leukocytes. Proc. Natl. Acad. Sci. USA **91:** 4960–4964.

25. Koyama, S., H. Yu, D. C. Dalgarno, T. B. Shin, L. D. Zydowsky & S. L. Schreiber. 1993. Structure of the PI3K SH3 domain and analysis of the SH3 family. Cell **72:** 945–952.

26. Theibert, A. B., V. A. Estevez, C. D. Ferris, S. K. Danoff, R. K. Barrow, G. D. Prestwich & S. H. Snyder. 1991. Inositol 1,3,4,5-tetrakisphosphate and inositol hexakisphosphate receptor proteins: Isolation and characterization from rat brain. Proc. Natl. Acad. Sci. USA **88:** 3165–3169.

27. Otsu, M., I. Hiles, I. Gout, M. J. Fry, F. Ruiz-Larrea, G. Panayotou, A. Thompson, R. Dhand, J. Hsuan, N. Totty, A. D. Smith, S. J. Morgan, S. A. Courtneidge, P. J. Parker & M. D. Waterfield. 1991. Characterization of two 85 kd proteins that associate with receptor tyrosine kinases, middle-T/pp60$^{c\text{-}src}$ complexes, and PI3-kinase. Cell **65:** 91–104.

28. Skolnik, E. Y., B. Margolis, M. Mohammadi, E. Lowenstein, R. Fischer, A. Drepps, A. Ullrich & J. Schlessinger. 1991. Cloning of PI3 kinase-associated p85 utilizing a novel method for expression/cloning of target proteins for receptor tyrosine kinases. Cell **65:** 83–90.

29. Yu, H., J. K. Chen, S. Feng, D. C. Dalgarno, A. W. Brauer & S. L. Schreiber. 1994. Structural basis for the binding of proline-rich peptides to SH3 domains. Cell **76:** 933–945.

30. Ye, Z.-S. & D. Baltimore. 1994. Binding of Vav to Grb2 through dimerization of Src homology 3 domains. Proc. Natl. Acad. Sci. USA **91:** 12629–12633.

31. Baldwin, G. S. & Q.-X. Zhang. 1993. Related GAP domains in inositol polyphosphate 5-phosphatase and the p85 subunit of phosphatidylinositol 3-kinase. Trends Biochem. Sci. **18:** 378–380.

32. Carpenter, C. L., K. R. Auger, M. Chanudhuri, M. Yoakim, B. Schaffhausen, S. Shoelson & L. C. Cantley. 1993. Phosphoinositide 3-kinase is activated by phosphopeptides that bind to the SH2 domains of the 85-kDa subunit. J. Biol. Chem. **268:** 9478–9483.

33. VOGEL, L. B. & D. J. FUJITA. 1993. The SH3 domain of p56^{lck} is involved in binding to phosphatidylinositol 3′-kinase from T lymphocytes. Mol. Cell. Biol. **13:** 7408–7417.

34. PLEIMAN, C. M., M. R. CLARK, L. K. T. GAUEN, S. WINITZ, K. M. COGGESHALL, G. L. JOHNSON, A. S. SHAW & J. C. CAMBIER. 1993. Mapping of sites on the Src family protein tyrosine kinases p55^{blk}, p59^{fyn}, and p56^{lyn} which interact with the effector molecules phospholipase C-γ2, microtubule-associated protein kinase, GTPase-activating protein, and phosphatidylinositol 3-kinase. Mol. Cell. Biol. **13:** 5877–5887.

35. PRASAD, K. V. S., O. JANSSEN, R. KAPELLER, M. RAAB, L. C. CANTLEY & C. E. RUDD. 1993. Src-homology 3 domain of protein kinase p59^{fyn} mediates binding to phosphatidylinositol 3-kinase in T cells. Proc. Natl. Acad. Sci. USA **90:** 7366–7370.

36. ZHENG, Y., S. BAGRODIA & R. A. CERIONE. 1994. Activation of phosphoinositide 3-kinase activity by Cdc42Hs binding to p85. J. Biol. Chem. **269:** 18727–18730.

37. RODRIGUEZ-VICIANA, P., P. H. WARNE, R. DHAND, B. VANHAESEBROECK, I. GOUT, M. J. FRY, M. D. WATERFIELD & J. DOWNWARD. 1994. Phosphatidylinositol-3-OH kinase as a direct target of Ras. Nature **370:** 527–532.

38. FRY, M. J. 1994. Structure, regulation and function of phosphoinositide 3-kinases. Biochim. Biophys. Acta Mol. Basis Dis. **1226:** 237–268.

39. WENNSTRÖM, S., P. HAWKINS, F. COOKE, K. HARA, K. YONEZAWA, M. KASUGA, T. JACKSON, L. CLAESSON-WELSH & L. STEPHENS. 1994. Activation of phosphoinositide 3-kinase is required for PDGF-stimulated membrane ruffling. Curr. Biol. **4:** 385–393.

40. BESSER, D., A. BARDELLI, S. DIDICHENKO, M. THELEN, P. M. COMOGLIO, C. PONZETTO & Y. NAGAMINE. 1997. Regulation of the urokinase-type plasminogen activator gene by the oncogene Tpr-Met involves GRB2. Oncogene **14:** 705–711.

41. AKIYAMA, T. & H. OGAWARA. 1991. Use and specificity of genistein as inhibitor of protein-tyrosine kinases. Methods Enzymol. **201:** 362–370.

42. GAROTTA, G., M. THELEN, D. DELIA, M. KAMBER & M. BAGGIOLINI. 1991. GM-1, a clone of the monoblastic phagocyte U937 that expresses a large respiratory burst capacity upon activation with interferon-γ. J. Leukocyte Biol. **49:** 294–301.

43. HAWKINS, P. T., A. EGUINOA, R.-G. QIU, D. STOKOE, F. T. COOKE, R. WALTERS, S. WENNSTRÖM, L. CLAESSON-WELSH, T. EVANS, M. SYMONS & L. STEPHENS. 1995. PDGF stimulates an increase in GTP-Rac via activation of phosphoinositide 3-kinase. Curr. Biol. **5:** 393–403.

44. DIDICHENKO, S. A., B. TILTON, B. A. HEMMINGS, K. BALLMER-HOFER & M. THELEN. 1996. Constitutive activation of protein kinase B and phosphorylation of p47^{phox} by membrane-targeted phosphoinositide 3-kinase. Curr. Biol. **6:** 1271–1278.

45. THELEN, M., A. ROSEN, A. C. NAIRN & A. ADEREM. 1990. Tumor necrosis factor alpha modifies agonist-dependent responses in human neutrophils by inducing the synthesis and myristoylation of a specific protein kinase C substrate. Proc. Natl. Acad. Sci. USA **87:** 5603–5607.

46. THELEN, M., M. WOLF & M. BAGGIOLINI. 1988. Activation of monocytes by interferonγ has no effect on the level or affinity of the nicotinamide adenine dinucleotide-phosphate oxidase and on agonist-dependent superoxide formation. J. Clin. Invest. **81:** 1889–1895.

47. FIECK, A., D. L. WYBORSKI & J. M. SHORT. 1992. Modifications of the E.coli Lac repressor for expression in eukaryotic cells: effects of nuclear signal sequences on protein activity and nuclear accumulation. Nucleic Acids Res. **20:** 1785–1791.

48. KLIPPEL, A., J. A. ESCOBEDO, M. HIRANO & L. T. WILLIAMS. 1994. The interaction of small domains between the subunits of phosphatidylinositol 3-kinase determines enzyme activity. Mol. Cell. Biol. **14:** 2675–2685.

49. HARA, K., K. YONEZAWA, H. SAKAUE, A. ANDO, K. KOTANI, T. KITAMURA, Y. KITAMURA, H.

UEDA, L. STEPHENS, T. R. JACKSON, P. T. HAWKINS, R. DHAND, A. E. CLARK, G. D. HOLMAN, M. D. WATERFIELD & M. KASUGA. 1994. 1-phosphatidylinositol 3-kinase activity is required for insulin-stimulated glucose transport but not for RAS activation in CHO cells. Proc. Natl. Acad. Sci. USA **91:** 7415–7419.

50. BAGGIOLINI, M., B. DEWALD & B. MOSER. 1994. Interleukin-8 and related chemotactic cytokines—CXC and CC chemokines. Adv. Immunol. **55:** 97–179.

51. TRAYNOR-KAPLAN, A. E., B. L. THOMPSON, A. L. HARRIS, P. TAYLOR, G. M. OMANN & L. A. SKLAR. 1989. Transient increase in phosphatidylinositol 3,4-bisphosphate and phosphatidylinositol trisphosphate during activation of human neutrophils. J. Biol. Chem. **264:** 15668–15673.

52. STEPHENS, L., T. JACKSON & P. T. HAWKINS. 1993. Synthesis of phosphatidylinositol 3,4,5-trisphosphate in permeabilized neutrophils regulated by receptors and G-proteins. J. Biol. Chem. **268:** 17162–17172.

53. HELDIN, C.-H. 1995. Dimerization of cell surface receptors in signal transduction. Cell **80:** 213–223.

54. WENNSTRÖM, S., A. SIEGBAHN, K. YOKOTE, A.-K. ARVIDSSON, C.-H. HELDIN, S. MORI & L. CLAESSON-WELSH. 1994. Membrane ruffling and chemotaxis transduced by the PDGF β-receptor require the binding site for phosphatidylinositol 3′ kinase. Oncogene **9:** 651–660.

55. VLAHOS, C. J. & W. F. MATTER. 1992. Signal transduction in neutrophil activation: Phosphatidylinositol 3-kinase is stimulated without tyrosine phosphorylation. FEBS Lett. **309:** 242–248.

56. YU, H., M. K. ROSEN & S. L. SCHREIBER. 1993.. ^{1}H and ^{15}N assignments and secondary structure of the Src SH3 domain. FEBS Lett. **324:** 87–92.

57. LEVITZKI, A. & A. GAZIT. 1995. Tyrosine kinase inhibition: an approach to drug development. Science **267:** 1782–1788.

58. COREY, S., A. EGUINOA, K. PUYANA-THEALL, J. B. BOLEN, L. CANTLEY, F. MOLLINEDO, T. R. JACKSON, P. T. HAWKINS & L. R. STEPHENS. 1993. Granulocyte macrophage-colony stimulating factor stimulates both association and activation of phosphoinositide 3OH-kinase and *src*-related tyrosine kinase(s) in human myeloid derived cells. EMBO J. **12:** 2681–2690.

59. BERKOW, R. L. & R. W. DODSON. 1990. Tyrosine-specific protein phosphorylation during activation of human neutrophils. Blood **75:** 2445–2452.

60. RICHARD, S., C. A. FARRELL, A. S. SHAW, H. J. SHOWELL & P. A. CONNELLY. 1994. C5a as a model for chemotactic factor-stimulated tyrosine phosphorylation in the human neutrophil. J. Immunol. **152:** 2479–2487.

61. ROLLET, E., A. C. CAON, C. J. ROBERGE, N. W. LIAO, S. E. MALAWISTA, S. R. MCCOLL & P. H. NACCACHE. 1994. Tyrosine phosphorylation in activated human neutrophils: Comparison of the effects of different classes of agonists and identification of the signaling pathways involved. J. Immunol. **153:** 353–363.

62. FIALKOW, L., C. K. CHAN, S. GRINSTEIN & G. P. DOWNEY. 1993. Regulation of tyrosine phosphorylation in neutrophils by the NADPH oxidase. Role of reactive oxygen intermediates. J. Biol. Chem. **268:** 17131–17137.

63. GRINSTEIN, S. & W. FURUYA. 1992. Chemoattractant-induced tyrosine phosphorylation and activation of microtubule-associated protein kinase in human neutrophils. J. Biol. Chem. **267:** 18122–18125.

64. BADWEY, J. A., R. W. ERICKSON & J. T. CURNUTTE. 1991. Staurosporine inhibits the soluble and membrane-bound protein tyrosine kinases of human neutrophils. Biochem. Biophys. Res. Commun. **178:** 423–429.

65. PTASZNIK, A., A. TRAYNOR-KAPLAN & G. M. BOKOCH. 1995. G protein-coupled chemoat-

tractant receptors regulate lyn tyrosine kinase Shc adapter protein signaling complexes. J. Biol. Chem. **270:** 19969–19973.

66. KHWAJA, A., B. HALLBERG, P. H. WARNE & J. DOWNWARD. 1996. Networks of interaction of p120^{cbl} and p130^{cas} with Crk and Grb2 adaptor proteins. Oncogene **12:** 2491–2498.

67. CHANMUGAM, P., L. FENG, S. LIOU, B. C. JANG, M. BOUDREAU, G. YU., J. H. LEE, H. J. KWON, T. BEPPU, M. YOSHIDA, Y. XIA, C. B. WILSON & D. HWANG. 1995. Radicicol, a potent tyrosine kinase inhibitor, suppresses the expression of mitogen-inducible cyclooxygenase in macrophages stimulated with lipopolysaccharide and in experimental glomerulonephritis. J. Biol. Chem. **270**(1): 5418–5426.

Influence of Heat Inactivation of Human Serum on the Opsonization of *Streptococcus mutans*

MICHELLE A. MOORE[a], ZAID W. HAKKI, RICHARD L. GREGORY,
LINDA E. GFELL, WAN K. KIM-PARK, AND MICHAEL J. KOWOLIK

Department of Oral Biology
1121 West Michigan Street
Indiana University School of Dentistry
Indianapolis, Indiana 46202-5186

INTRODUCTION

Streptococcus mutans has been implicated in numerous studies as the main etiological agent in dental caries[1] and there are two principle theories concerning the mechanism of host defense against this bacterium. The disruption of adherence of the cariogenic *S. mutans* to the tooth surface by salivary IgA[2] or the opsonization of bacteria by serum antibodies that enter the crevicular fluid can protect the host by facilitating phagocytosis.[3–6] Previous work has focused on the opsonization and phagocytosis of *S. mutans* by neutrophils *in vitro* since these methods were found as one of the principle means of host defense against bacteria.[7]

One mechanism of defense against caries is the serum (IgG) antibodies that pass through the gingival crevicular epithelium onto the tooth surface and opsonize *S. mutans* to be phagocytized by local neutrophils, inhibiting bacterial adherence and preventing the development of caries.[8] Some studies[3,4,9] used human or bovine serum to enhance neutrophil activation through opsonization. Human serum was denatured for 30 min at 57°C[10] or for 60 min at 57°C[11] to deactivate both the classical and alternative complement pathways or 3 min at 57°C to inhibit the alternative pathway but retain the classical pathway of complement activation.[9] Complement and antibody can attach to the surface of bacteria and activate complement receptors CR3, CR1, or by binding the Fc receptor of the phagocyte. This coating or opsonization enhances bacterial recognition by the neutrophils and increases phagocytosis.

The difference between the time intervals required for the heat inactivation of the complement in serum became of interest while trying to establish an efficient opsonization protocol for *S. mutans* bacteria. The deactivation process can be studied by the increase or decrease of neutrophil activation towards bacteria opsonized by the deactivated serum. This study was done to determine the minimum time of heat inactivation of human serum and methodology required to disrupt the complement cascade prior to its use as an effective opsonin. The assumption that bacterial opsoniza-

[a]Address all correspondence to: Michelle A. Moore, Department of Oral Biology, Indiana University School of Dentistry, 1121 West Michigan Street, Indianapolis, IN 46202-5186. Phone, 317-278-0222 and Fax, 317-278-0224.

tion will increase neutrophil activation *in vitro* is supported by all previously listed literature.

Activation can be quantitated by neutrophil chemiluminescence (CL), which reflects the burst of metabolic activity following phagocytosis. The respiratory burst of granulocytes is characterized by the generation of reactive oxygen metabolites and release of degradatory granule enzymes. This release is followed by the relaxation of activated oxygen radicals with photon emission, generating a light response as CL.[12] The light emission can be enhanced considerably by the chemiluminescent probe luminol, which is oxidized by the oxygen radicals from the respiratory burst.

For our study, strains of *S. mutans* were opsonized with human serum that had been denatured for 0, 30, and 60 min at 57°C. The strains were clinical isolates obtained from caries-active (CA) patients, caries-free (CF) individuals, and a laboratory strain (LS;TH16). The CA patients had decayed, missing, and filled teeth (DMFT) scores of at least 4 with no missing or filled teeth at the time of whole saliva collection. The aim of this study was to examine the denaturization process of human serum and establish the kinetic profile needed to disrupt the complement cascade while enhancing phagocytosis of *S. mutans* by opsonization.

MATERIALS AND METHODS

Isolation and preparation of S. mutans

Isolates of *S. mutans* were obtained from whole saliva and isolated on mitus salvarius sucrose bacitracin agar plates (Difco Laboratories Inc., Detroit, MI). Five isolates of *S. mutans* were obtained from CA patients (designated A2-4, A29-1, A17-5, A24-2, and A32-2) and five isolates from CF patients (I7-4, I2-4, I5-1, I6-3, and I4-1). An isolate of the laboratory strain (TH-16) was employed as a standard for this study. All bacteria were obtained from 24 h cultures in 10 ml of Todd Hewitt Broth (Difco) and washed twice by centrifugation for 10 min at $800 \times g$ in 10 ml of phosphate-buffered saline (PBS; Sigma Chemical Co., St. Louis, MO). The bacteria were resuspended in sterile PBS, counted by hematocytometer with Trypan Blue staining, and diluted to 1.0×10^7 bacteria/ml. The positive control *Staphylococcus aureus* was prepared in the same manner.

S. mutans enzyme-linked immunosorbent assay (ELISA) antigen was prepared by centrifugation of 24 h bacterial cultures at $7,000 \times g$ for 20 min. The bacterial pellet was washed twice with PBS and then resuspended in a 0.5% formaldehyde/PBS solution. Cells were incubated in the formaldehyde solution for 48 h at room temperature, then washed twice with PBS and resuspended in 0.1 M sodium carbonate/bicarbonate buffer (pH 9.6) to a OD reading of 0.5 absorbance at 660 nm.

Opsonization of S. mutans

Whole human blood was collected from healthy adult donors in sterile 10 ml vacutainer tubes with no additives (Fisher Scientific, Pittsburgh, PA), allowed to clot for 10 min, centrifuged at $700 \times g$ for 15 min, and the serum frozen in 0.5 ml aliquots. The aliquots were thawed 1 h prior to use in the experiment. Serum samples were heated to 57°C in a water bath for 0, 30, and 60 min time periods to inactivate complement. Opsonization of *S. mutans* was accomplished by incubating the bacteria in a 10% serum/PBS solution at 37°C for 30 min.

Isolation of Neutrophils

Whole blood was collected from healthy adult donors at the Central Indiana Regional Blood Center in Indianapolis. Blood (1 unit of 470 ml/experiment) was collected in citrate phosphate dextrose solution anticoagulant bags and centrifuged at $2,000 \times g$ at 4°C for 4 min. Buffy coat layers were drawn off and the neutrophils were isolated on a double dextran gradient (Hypaque-Ficoll Method-Histopaque, Sigma) by centrifugation at 21°C at $700 \times g$ for 35 min. After two washes in 10 ml of PBS and one wash with 10 ml of RPMI for 10 min at $200 \times g$, the neutrophils were resuspended in 10 ml of RPMI. Neutrophils were counted with Trypan blue staining (Sigma) on a hemocytometer and resuspended to a final concentration of 2.0×10^6 cells/ml.

Measurement of Chemiluminescence

Chemiluminescence (CL) was measured on a Model 1251 Luminometer (BioOrbit, Finland). 5.0×10^5 neutrophils (500 µl) and 5.0×10^6 bacteria (50 µl) with 350 µl of PBS were pipetted into cuvettes and incubated together at 37°C for 30 min. Then 100 µl of luminol at 2.0×10^{-6} M (Sigma) was dispensed by the luminometer (total reaction volume of 1 ml) and CL was measured and recorded for 120 min. All samples were assayed in triplicate for a minimum of ten separate experiments for each compared variable.

Determination of Bacterial Viability

One ml aliquots of bacteria were taken before and after opsonization. Enumeration of *S. mutans* was established on mitus salvarius-sucrose-bacitracin (MSSB) plates for caries free (CF), caries free–opsonized (CFO), caries active (CA), caries active–opsonized (CAO), laboratory strain (LS), and laboratory strain–opsonized (LSO) *S. mutans*. Aliquots were diluted 1:1,000 and spiral plated (Spiral Systems Co., Cincinnati, OH). Plates were incubated at 37°C for 48 h and colonies counted to determine viability.

ELISA Assays

A standard ELISA technique was used as previously described.[13] Plates were coated with whole cell ELISA antigen of *S. mutants* (100 µl), blocked with 200 µl of 2% bovine serum albumin (Sigma) in carbonate buffer and 100 µl of untreated or heat-inactivated human sera from known healthy adult donors was added. Horseradish peroxidase–labeled anti-human IgG antibody (100 µl; Sigma) and peroxidase substrate (σ-phenylenediamine dihydrochloride) containing 0.025% hydrogen peroxide (100 µl) were added sequentially. Color development occurred for 15–30 min and the reaction was stopped by adding 100 µl of 2 N H_2SO_4, and absorbances were measured using a Thermomax microplate spectrophotometer (Molecular Devices Corp., Menlo Park, CA) and statistically analyzed.

RESULTS AND DISCUSSION

Viability of S. mutans *in Experimental System*

S. mutans strains (CF I4-1, CF I7-4, CA A32-2, CA A17-5, and LS) were enumerated on MSSB agar plates; each plate inoculated with approximately 1×10^3 bacteria. Average viability was 82% before opsonization and 89% after incubation at 37°C for 30 min with human serum that had been denatured for 30 min at 57°C, (92% viability without serum), indicating no significant difference in viability between opsonized and nonopsonized bacteria (FIG. 1).

Effect of Heat Deactivation

CL data were obtained by using Luminometer cuvettes with the following samples: blank, *Staphylococcus aureus* as a positive control, CF bacteria strain (I2-4), opsonized CF bacteria (CFO), CA bacteria strain (A29-1), opsonized CA bacteria (CAO), LS bacteria (TH16), and opsonized LS bacteria (LSO) in each experiment.

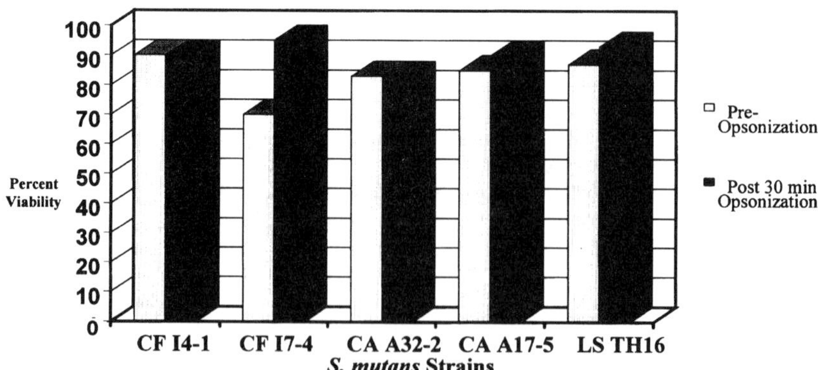

FIGURE 1. Viability of *S. mutans* before and after 30 min incubation in the presence of human serum. Percent viability calculated by comparing the number of bacteria plated (bacteria counted by hematocytometer with Trypan blue staining; equivalent to 100%) with *S. mutans* colonies on MSSB agar after 48 h of incubation at 37°C.

TABLE 1. CL Response as Represented by the Average Integrations (mV.min)

Time of Deactivation (min)	Positive Control	CF	CFO	CA	CAO	LS	LSO
0	549±147	624±43	1093±33	552±42	867±55	289±14	588±39
15	274±90	252±27	272±35	263±24	248±18	235±43	190±14
30	321±18	278±22	227±19	291±25	213±11	236±23	184±27
45	16,755±333	14,340±27	5,747±349	11,812±3	4,583±56	10,485±39	4,245±57
60	665±106	618±50	1,062±283	604±39	864±27	551±32	692±23
90	10,449±285	9,805±269	8,701±435	9,738±43	8,409±75	9,655±327	8,417±19

Human serum from the same subject, which was used to opsonize the bacteria, was heat inactivated for the respective time period, and neutrophils obtained from a single donor/separation were used for individual assays. TABLE 1 illustrates the average CL integrations measured by the luminometer in mV.min with neutrophil activation by *S. mutans*. The experiment consisted of eight identical samples of each serum deactivation time interval with three replicates of each variable. The data suggested significant serum opsonization at 0 min and 60 min heat deactivation ($p \leq 0.05$) for CF, CA, and LS *S. mutans* strains and is illustrated in FIGURES 2–4. The average percentage opsonization of *S. mutans* with human serum was compared. Data were determined by the difference in CL of opsonized and non-opsonized bacteria (FIG. 5).

Other experiments were conducted using luminometer cuvettes with the LS of *S. mutans* (TH-16) and comparing inactivation times directly and examining the degree of neutrophil stimulation by human serum alone and with the LS only (FIG. 6). Experimental samples examined were as follows: blank, neutrophils only (no serum or

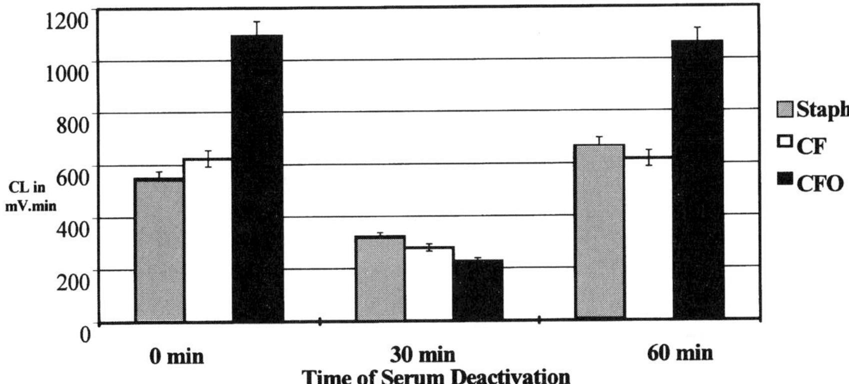

FIGURE 2. The effect of heat inactivation of serum on CL induced by CF strains of *S. mutans* represented by comparison of average 60-min integrations indicating neutrophil activation by CF bacterial strains by luminol-mediated chemiluminescence. The average integrations represented in this figure can be found in TABLE 1.

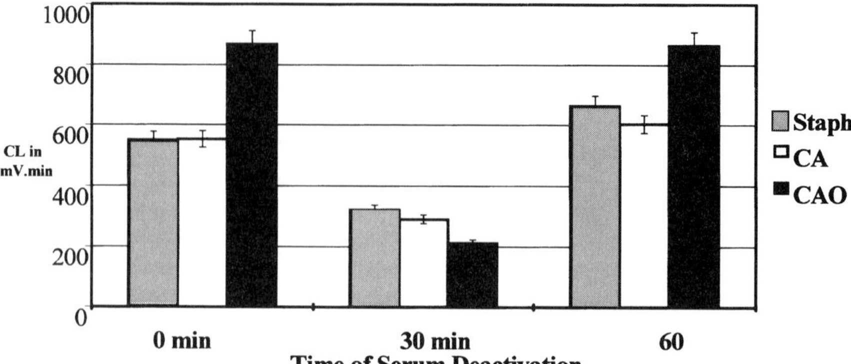

FIGURE 3. The effect of heat inactivation of serum on CL induced by CA strains of *S. mutans* represented by comparison of average 60-min integrations indicating neutrophil activation by CA bacterial strains by luminol-mediated chemiluminescence. The average integrations represented in this figure can be found in TABLE 1.

bacteria), cells plus nonopsonized LS bacteria, LS opsonized with 0 min–inactivated serum, LS opsonized with 30 min–inactivated serum, LS opsonized with 60 min–inactivated serum, 0 min–inactivated serum, 30 min–inactivated serum, and 60 min–inactivated serum. Human serum used to opsonize the bacteria was heat inactivated for the appropriate time period, and neutrophils were obtained from a single donor and were used for individual experiments. Data represent the average CL integration measured by the luminometer in mV.min following neutrophil activation by *S. mutans* in 10 experiments with three replicates of each variable.

All variables displayed a highly significant ($p \leq 0.001$) increase in CL with either

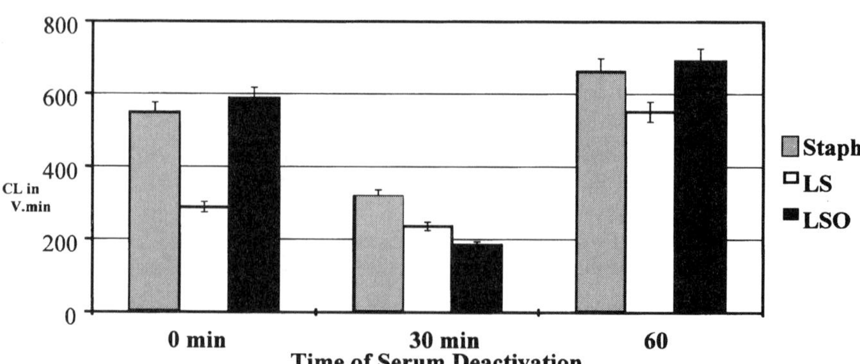

FIGURE 4. The effect of heat inactivation of serum on CL induced by LS (TH-16) strains of *S. mutans* represented by comparison of average 60-min integrations indicating neutrophil activation by CA bacterial strains by luminol-mediated chemiluminescence. The average integrations represented in this figure can be found in TABLE 1.

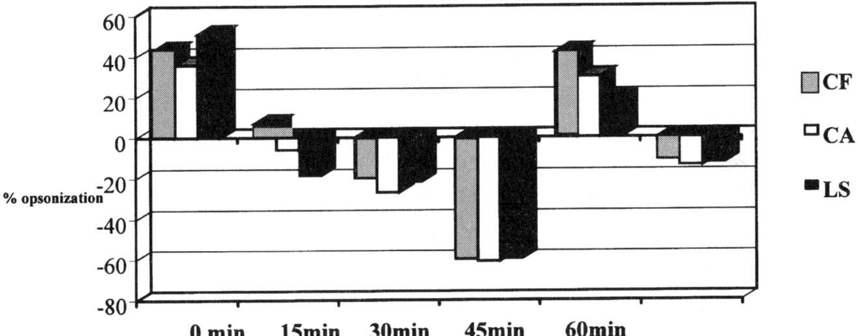

FIGURE 5. The effect of heat inactivation of human serum on its ability to opsonize *S. mutans* was compared by examining the change in CL (overall average integration for 60-min measurement at 37°C) and calculating the percentage of change (opsonization) from the non-opsonized control.

the addition of human serum alone or with serum-opsonized bacteria. There was no significant bacterial effect without the addition of serum, in fact there was a slight overall decrease in CL with 0 min heat inactivation. This is demonstrated by the overall CL integrations with and without TH16 *S. mutans*. Heat treatment significantly decreased the serum's ability to activate neutrophils, while it significantly ($p \leq$ 0.001) increased activation by opsonized TH16 *S. mutans*. There was a significant increase in CL response between 30 and 60 min inactivation times indicating a greater opsonization effect with 60 min heat inactivation of the serum.

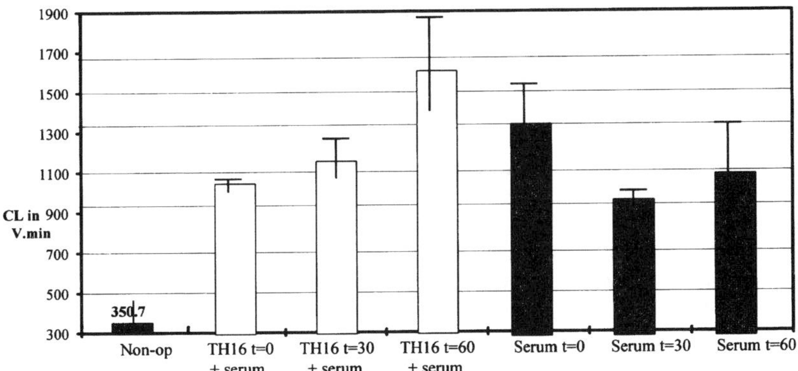

FIGURE 6. The effect of heat inactivation of serum was examined by comparing CL induced by LS *S. mutans* (TH-16). Average integrations are given in the figure. "t" indicates the time of heat inactivation of serum. Non-opsonized *S. mutans* only is represented by "Non-op". The TH-16 samples had both *S. mutans* and heat-inactivated serum, while the serum samples had heat-treated sera only.

Anti-S. mutans *Antibody Assays*

Standard ELISA assays were conducted in plates coated with TH-16, CA strains (A2-4, A29-1, A24-2, A17-5, A32-2) and CF strains (I4-1, I7-4, I6-3, I2-4, I5-1). Human serum was heat inactivated for 0, 30, or 60 min time intervals. There were significant increases in IgA antibody binding with heat inactivation of serum (60 > 30 > 0), but there was no significant increase in IgG or IgM antibody binding. In addition, the results indicated greater IgA and IgG antibody levels for CF strains of *S. mutans* than for CA strains ($p \leq 0.001$), but IgM antibody assays displayed no significant differences.

Complement Binding ELISA Assays

ELISA plates were coated with TH16 and heat-inactivated human serum from three subjects (MJK, MAM, and SWH) was added to respective wells. Goat anti-human C3b antibody was used to detect complement (C′) bound to *S. mutans*, then peroxidase-labeled anti-goat antibody was added followed by peroxidase substrate and absorbances recorded and compared. The data initially revealed a high degree of antibody crossreactivity between the goat anti-C3b and TH16 *S. mutans*. TH16 reactive anti-C′ was removed by incubating formalin-killed *S. mutans* at OD=0.5 with 10 ml of anti-C′ at 1:1,000 for 60 min at 37°C then 4°C overnight. When absorbances were adjusted by subtracting crossreactivity from both the antibody adsorbed and unadsorbed controls, significant decreases were present between 0 min and 30 min, 0 min and 60 min ($p \leq 0.05$), but no significant decreases were observed between 30 min and 60 min with any of the sera compared.

There was a significant decrease in C′ binding with the antibody adsorption ($p = 0.012$) when TH16 was compared in the absence of serum (mean absorbance 0.986 ± 0.030 without adsorption and 0.856 ± 0.010 with adsorption). A consistent decrease in complement binding with 30-min heat deactivation compared to 0 min ($p \leq 0.001$) with all three serum donors was observed with adsorbed and non-adsorbed anti-C′ antibody.

All significant differences held constant when the crossreactivity of *S. mutans* to anti-C′ was subtracted and the three sera compared together by standard *t* tests. The crossreactivity was examined by comparing average absorbances of all sera (three specific healthy donors) against TH16 alone. The crossreactivity was significantly decreased with heat inactivation of sera.

The results indicate that there was significantly increased CL with 60-min inactivation of the serum over the nonopsonized control. The data demonstrate that the inactivation of serum requires a minimum of 60 min at 57°C to disrupt the complement cascade and generate a substantial increase in chemiluminescence activity, while 30- and 15-min inactivations produced no significant increases over the control. Heat inactivation of human sera significantly decreased C3b binding to *S. mutans*, but could not explain the increased CL response after 60-min heat deactivation of the serum prior to *S. mutans* opsonization. IgA and IgM displayed a moderate increase in *S. mutans* binding with heat inactivation while IgG remained relatively constant.

C3b is the major opsonin of the complement system.[14] Heat inactivation of human sera for 30 min significantly decreased C3b binding to *S. mutans* ($p \leq 0.001$), but could not account for the significant increase in CL response and bacterial opsonization with 60-min heat treatment of the sera. These data indicate that there may be a change in antibody activity or serum proteins with 60-min heat inactivation. The marked opsonic and protective activities of IgM and IgG1 human antibody are closely related to their ability to bind complement and deposit C3 on bacterial surfaces,[15] but this does not account for possible alterations in direct antibody-antigen binding, which may occur with prolonged heat exposure. IgA and IgM antibodies displayed a moderate increase in *S. mutans* binding with heat inactivation, while IgG binding was relatively constant. This may contribute to the increase in CL and serum opsonization at the 60-min interval. Deactivation of serum for 15, 30, 45, and 90 minutes, prior to opsonization of the bacteria, resulted in ablated bacterial killing, when compared to the nonopsonized bacteria.

One possible explanation for the increase in chemiluminescence seen with 60-min heat inactivation of the serum may be that complement binds to *S. mutans* at antibody binding sites and inactivation of complement abrogates complement binding, allowing complete antibody binding to *S. mutans* antigens, and subsequently gives maximal opsonization and CL. This may provide early evidence that inactivation of serum requires a time of 60 min at 57°C to disrupt the complement cascade with respect to CL activity assays.

SUMMARY

Phagocytosis of bacteria, such as *Streptococcus mutans*, is important to host defense. One mechanism by which phagocytosis can be enhanced is by antibody or complement-mediated opsonization of bacteria. Many studies utilize opsonization of bacteria to enhance a cellular response, but little information has been found examining methodology or validity of the opsonization process following the denaturization of the serum. Human serum was inactivated by heat in order to disrupt the classical and alternative pathways of the complement cascade.[9] *S. mutans* isolated from human subjects were opsonized with heat-inactivated human serum before exposing them to viable neutrophils *in vitro*. Luminol-dependent chemiluminescence (CL) was used to measure neutrophil activation. Human serum used to opsonize the bacteria was denatured by incubation at 57°C for intervals of 30 and 60 min to inactivate complement. The results from the opsonization data indicated that there was significantly increased CL with 60-min inactivation of the serum (34% increase in mean integration mV.min; $p \leq 0.05$) over the nonopsonized control. This indicated a successful opsonization of the bacteria. In addition, the data demonstrate that the inactivation of serum requires a minimum of 60 min at 57°C to disrupt the complement cascade, while 30- and 15-min inactivations produced no significant increase in CL activity over the control. Standard sandwich ELISA assays, detecting complement binding to *S. mutans*, confirmed successful heat inactivation of serum showing a significant decrease ($p \leq 0.001$) in complement binding to *S. mutans* after 30 min, but could not explain the increased CL response after 60-min heat deactivation of the serum.

REFERENCES

1. LOESCHE, W. J. & L. H. STRAFFON. 1979. Longitudinal investigation of the role of *Streptococcus mutans* in human tissue decay. Infect. Immun. **26:** 498–507.

2. GREGORY, R. L., L. C. HOBBS, J. C. KINDLE, T. VANTO & H. S. MALMSTROM. 1990. Immunodominant antigens of *Streptococcus mutans* in dental caries-resistant subjects. Hum. Antibod. Hybridomas **1:** 132–136.

3. SCULLY, C. M. & T. LEHNER. 1979. Bacterial and strain specificities in opsonization, phagocytosis and killing of *Streptococcus mutans*. Clin. Exp. Immunol. **35:** 128–132.

4. SCULLY, C. M. & T. LEHNER. 1979. Opsonization, phagocytosis and killing of *Streptococcus mutans* by polymorphonuclear leukocytes, in relation to dental caries in the rhesus monkey (Macaca Mulatta). 1979. Arch. Oral Biol. **24:** 307–312.

5. SCULLY, C. M. 1980. Comparative opsonic activity for *Streptococcus mutans* in oral fluids, and phagocytic activity of blood, crevicular, and salivary polymorphonuclear leukocytes in rhesus monkeys. Immunol. **39:** 101–107.

6. SCULLY, C. M., M. W. RUSSELL & T. LEHNER. 1980. Specificity of opsonizing antibodies to antigens of *Streptococcus mutans*. Immunol. **41:** 467–473.

7. SHIGEOKA, A. O., R. T. HALL & H. R. HILL. 1979. Strain specificity of opsonins for group B streptococci types II and III. Infect. Immun. **23:** 438–435.

8. LEHNER, T., J. CALDWELL & R. SMITH. 1985. Local passive immunization by monoclonal antibodies against Streptococcal antigen I/II in the prevention of dental caries. Infect. Immun. **50**(3): 796–799.

9. RAINARD, P. & C. BOULARD. 1992. Opsonization of *Streptococcus agalactiae* of bovine origin by complement and antibodies against group B polysaccharide. Infect. Immun. **60:** 4801–4807.

10. HALL, M. A., M. S. EDWARDS & C. J. BAKER. 1992. Complement and antibody participation in opsonophagocytosis of type IV and V group B streptococci. Infect. Immun. **60:** 5030–5035.

11. HEMMING, V. G., R. T. HALL, P. G. RHODES, A. O. SHIGEOKA & H. R. HILL. 1976. Assessment of Group B streptococcal opsonins in human and rabbit serum by neutrophil chemiluminescence. J. Clin. Invest. **58:** 1379–1387.

12. KOWOLIK, M. J., C. G. CUMMING & M. GRANT. 1982. Interaction between human neutrophils and group B Streptococci (GBS) and group antigens, monitored by luminol-dependent chemiluminescence. J. Clin. Lab. Immunol. **8:** 55–58.

13. GREGORY, R. L., S. M. MICHALEK, S. J. FILLER, J. MESTECKY & J. R. McGHEE. 1985. Prevention of *Streptococcus mutans* colonization by salivary IgA antibodies. J. Clin. Immunol. **5:** 55–62.

14. KUBY, J. 1994. Immunology. 2nd edit. W. H. Freeman and Co. New York.

15. SHYUR, S., H. V. RAFF, J. F. BOHNSACK, D. K. KELSEY & H. R. HILL. 1992. Comparison of the opsonic and complement triggering activity of human monoclonal IgG1 and IgM antibody against Group B streptococci. J. Immunol. **148:** 1879–1884.

16. BJORKSTEN, B., P. K. PETERSON, J. VERHOEF & P. Q. QUIE. 1977. Limiting factors in bacterial phagocytosis by human polymorphonuclear leukocytes. Acta Pathol. Microbiol. Scand. **85:** 345–349.

17. CHESTNUTT, I. G., T. W. MACFARLANE, T. C. AITCHISON & K. W. STEPHEN. 1995. Evaluation of the *in vitro* cariogenic potential of *Streptococcus mutans* strains isolated from 12-year-old children with differing caries experience. 1990. Caries Res. **29:** 455–460.

18. DESOET, J. J. & J. DEGRAAFF. 1990. Monoclonal antibodies for enumeration and identification of mutans streptococci in epidemiological studies. Arch. Oral Biol. **35:** 165S–168S.

19. KELLY, C., P. EVANS, J. K.-C. MA, L. A. BERGMEIER, W. TAYLOR, L. J. BRADY, S. F. LEE, A. S. BLEIWEIS & T. LEHNER. 1990. Sequencing and characterization of the 185 kDa cell surface antigen of *Streptococcus mutans*. Arch. Oral Biol. **35:** 33S–38S.

20. MA, J. K.-C. & T. LEHNER. 1990. Prevention of colonization of *Streptococcus mutans* by topical application of monoclonal antibodies in human subjects. Arch. Oral Biol. **35:** 115S–122S.

21. PERRONE, M., L. E. GFELL, M. FONTANA & R. L. GREGORY. 1997. Antigenic characterization of fimbriae preparations from *Streptococcus mutans* isolates from caries free and caries susceptible subjects. Clin. Diag. Lab. Immunol. **4:** 291–296.

22. QUIE P. G. & E. L. MILLS. 1979. Bactericidal and metabolic function of polymorphonuclear leukocytes. Pediatrics **64:** 719–721.

23. RAINARD P. 1993. Activation of the classical pathway of complement by binding of bovine lactoferrin to unencapsulated *Streptococcus agalactiae*. Immunol. **79:** 648–652.

24. RUSSELL R. R. B. 1979. Wall-associated antigens of *Streptococcus mutans*. J. Gen. Microbiol. **114:** 109–115.

25. SMITH R. T., T. LEHNER & P. C. L. BEVERLY. 1984. Characterization of monoclonal antibodies to *Streptococcus mutans* antigenic determinants I/II, I, II and III and their serotype specificities. Infect. Immun. **46:** 168–175.

26. STAFFILENO L. K., M. HENDRICKS, R. LAPOLLA, C. BOHART, P. VANHOOK, J. I. ROSEN, J. WARNER, K. HOEY, D. WEGEMER, R. B. NASO, R. D. SUBLETT, B. WALDSCHMIDT, M. LEONG, G. B. THORNTON, T. LEHNER & J. A. HARON. 1990. Cloning of the amino terminal nucleotides of the antigen I/II of *Streptococcus sobrinus* and the immune responses to the corresponding synthetic peptides. Arch. Oral Biol. **35:** 47S–52S.

27. SWITALSKI L. M. & W. G. BUTCHER. 1993. An *in vitro* model for adhesion of bacteria to human tooth root surfaces. Arch. Oral Biol. **39:** 155–161.

Activation of the Neutrophil Respiratory Burst Requires Both Intracellular and Extracellular Calcium

W. K. KIM-PARK, M. A. MOORE, Z. W. HAKKI, AND M. J. KOWOLIK

Indiana University
Department of Oral Biology
1121 W. Michigan Street
Indianapolis, Indiana 46202-5186

INTRODUCTION

Extensive work has demonstrated the involvement of Ca^{2+} ion in the activation of various oxidases leading to the production of the reactive oxygen species in stimulated polymorphonuclear leukocytes (PMNs)[1–3] In addition, many researchers have shown that a receptor-mediated cell activator, FMLP or an activator of protein kinase C, phorbol myristate acetate (PMA), can alter the Ca^{2+} flux in non-excitable cells such as PMNs[4,5,6] by providing second messengers or activating membrane Ca^{2+} channels. The changes in Ca^{2+} flux, in turn, affect the activity of various oxidases when Ca^{2+}-mediated kinase activation causes phosphorylation of their subunits. Furthermore, it has been suggested that FMLP and PMA might produce reactive oxygen species via different mechanisms. Quin-2 buffered PMNs exhibited a significant inhibition of superoxide production with FMLP while the PMA-mediated pathway was not significantly affected by this intracellular Ca^{2+} chelation,[7] indicating the dependence of the FMLP-mediated pathway on intracellular Ca^{2+}. Since little information regarding the relative contributions of intra- or extracellular Ca^{2+} on the neutrophil respiratory burst exists, it was proposed to investigate if there was any difference in effects between the intra- and extracellular Ca^{2+}-mediated pathways on the stimulated respiratory burst in PMNs. In addition, selective inhibitors for various Ca^{2+}-dependent enzymes were tested in preincubation to identify any other pathways requiring different Ca^{2+} concentrations for their activation that might be masked under the experimental conditions. This might lead to the elucidation of more detailed mechanisms for regulating the respiratory burst with different stimulants, in terms of Ca^{2+} flux and enzyme activities, in temporal and spatial, yet orchestrated fashion, to generate reactive oxygen species in PMNs. The study was focused on manipulating Ca^{2+} levels intracellularly or extracellularly using specific Ca^{2+} chelators during pretreatment, followed by stimulant challenge to monitor Ca^{2+} availability during the respiratory burst.

In addition, it was proposed to determine whether human neutrophils have an N-methyl-D-aspartate (NMDA) Ca^{2+} channel, as chelation of extra- or intracellular Ca^{2+} by BAPTA or EGTA and subsequent stimulation with PMA or FMLP revealed that activation of NADPH oxidase and superoxide production can occur via a different Ca^{2+}-mediated cascade.[8] In excitatory cells (activated by membrane potential change), NMDA channels increase Ca^{2+} influx[9] followed by a subsequent activation of intracellular enzymes and second messenger system,[10,11] as well as diffusible messengers.[12,13] Glutamate congeners, including NMDA, bind to glutamate receptors (NMDA, quisqualate, and kainic acid sites), triggering Ca^{2+} influx and causing activation of various enzymes, including phospholipase C, phospholipase A_2, proteases, protein kinases, NOS (nitric oxide synthase), and phosphatases in neurons and macrophages.[10–12,14–16]

The presence of an NMDA receptor in neutrophils would potentially have a marked effect on the generation of free radical systems and thus host defense mechanisms.

MATERIALS AND METHODS

Buffy coats, separated from healthy human donor blood, was obtained from the Central Indiana Regional Blood Center. RPMI 1640, EGTA, PMA, luminol (5-amino-2,3-dihydro-1,4-phthalazinedione crystalline), D-2-amino-7-phosphonoheptanoate (AP7), glutamate, N-methyl-D-aspartate (NMDA), sodium vanadate, and HISTOPAQ-1119, were purchased from Sigma Chemical Co. (St. Louis, MO) and BAPTA was purchased from Cal Biochem. Reagent grade sodium fluoride was a gift from the Oral Health Research Institute of Indiana University School of Dentistry.

Neutrophils were harvested from the buffy coats by a standard method. Briefly, a double-dextran gradient, Histopaque-1119 (3 ml) and Histopaque-1077 (3 ml), was used to separate neutrophils by centrifugation at 20°C for 35 minutes. The lower band containing granulocytes was drawn off by pipette. After washing in 10 ml PBS, the cells were centrifuged at 950 RPM for 10 minutes and the supernatant was discarded. The washing procedure was repeated twice and the cells resuspended in 10 ml RPMI 1640 medium for counting. The average cell yield was 2.2×10^7 cells/ml in 10 ml of resuspended neutrophils. Viability of the harvested cells was determined by Trypan Blue staining. The harvested neutrophils were primed with either 10^{-11}M Formyl-Met-Leu-Phe (FMLP) or granulocyte macrophage colony–stimulating factor (GM-CSF) for 15 minutes during preincubation at 37°C, and luminol-dependent chemiluminescence (CL) generation following stimulation (10^{-7} M FMLP or PMA) was measured in millivolts (mV) over 60 minutes at 37°C.

Pretreatment of neutrophils with Ca^{2+} chelators or inhibitors of enzymes was performed for 15 minutes at 37°C during the preincubation phase. In control experiments, preincubation was with primers (10^{-11} M FMLP or GM-CSF) only. The dose-response study was determined using a serial dilution of drugs to find the optimal concentration of each drug and over a time profile between 0 to 90 minutes at 15-minute intervals. These procedures were repeated at least six times with three replicates of each variable in every run. Statistical analysis was made by the Student's *t* test in paired two-tail tests.

RESULTS

The yield of viable neutrophils and the identification of the cell type were determined microscopically by Trypan Blue staining. The average neutrophil percentage

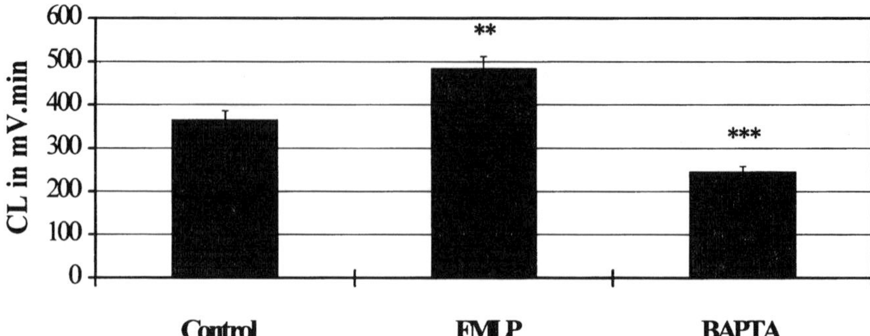

FIGURE 1. Effect on CL production of BAPTA pretreatment with FMLP as stimulant. The PMNs were preincubated with 12.5 μM BAPTA to chelate intracellular Ca^{2+} at 37°C for 15 min prior to stimulation with FMLP (10^{-7} M). Each bar is mean of 3 ± SEM. Similar results were produced in five other experiments. **$p<0.001$, ***$p<0.0001$.

in resuspension with RPMI 1640 medium was 95% of the cells with a 90–95% viability. For CL generation by FMLP (10^{-7}M) and PMA (10^{-7}M), the integrals were in the order of 500 and 1,000 mV, respectively in general. The optimal concentration of the primers was 10^{-11}M FMLP or GM-CSF while the optimal concentration of the stimulants was 10^{-7} M for either PMA or FMLP in this system. Preincubation time was 15 minutes and, following stimulation, the integration time was 60 minutes at 37°C. The preincubation with BAPTA followed by FMLP stimulation demonstrated a significant inhibition ($p<0.001$) of neutrophil CL production (FIG. 1) while the treatment potentiated PMA-stimulated CL production greatly ($p<0.001$) (FIG. 2). On the other hand, EGTA treatment inhibited CL production significantly ($p<0.001$) in both FMLP- and PMA-stimulated cells (FIGS. 3 and 4) indicating that both stimulants re-

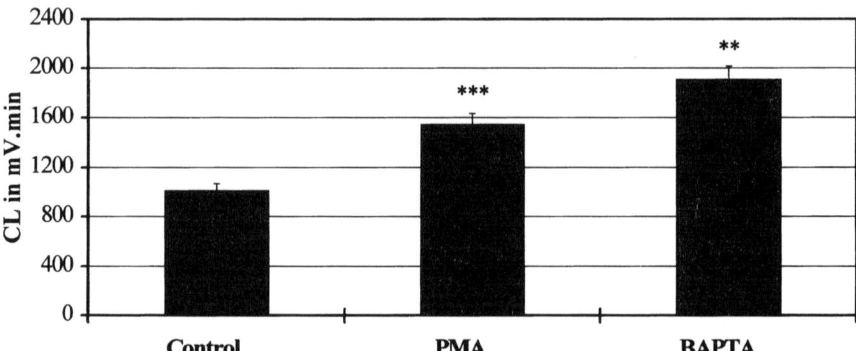

FIGURE 2. BAPTA potentiates CL production with PMA as stimulant. The PMNs were preincubated with 12.5 μM BAPTA at 37°C for 15 min prior to stimulation with PMA (10^{-7} M). Each bar is mean of 4 ± SEM. There was similar potentiation in five other experiments with PMA. **$p<0.01$, ***$p<0.005$.

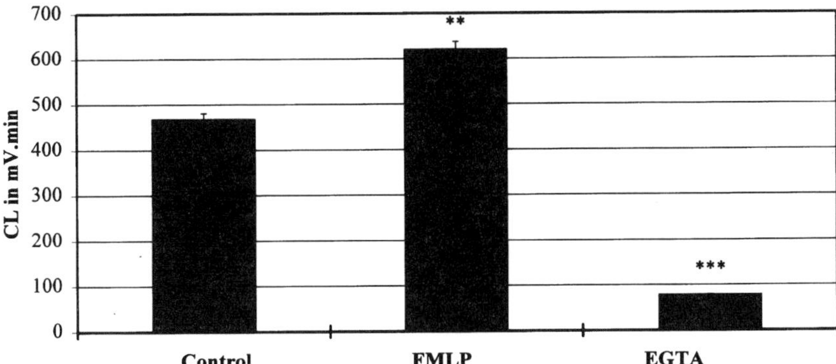

FIGURE 3. Effect on CL production EGTA pretreatment with FMLP as stimulant. 1.5 mM EGTA was preincubated with PMNs for 15 min to chelate extracellular Ca^{2+} prior to FMLP-mediated stimulation. Each bar is mean of 6 ± SEM. **$p<0.05$, ***$p<0.0001$.

quire extracellular Ca^{2+} for the activation of oxidases. Interestingly, the degree of inhibition of FMLP-mediated stimulation with EGTA was greater than with BAPTA (FIG. 5). When PMA and FMLP were both included simultaneously as stimulants, the activation seemed to be additive (FIG. 6).

A direct inhibition of endogenous phosphatase by sodium vanadate was compared to intracellular Ca^{2+} chelation with BAPTA when the cells were stimulated with PMA. The data showed that with sodium vanadate treatment, CL generation was stimulated by 124% of the control while BAPTA treatment increased it 48% from the control (data not shown). The control is primed cells only. A selective inhibitor of PKC, bisindolylmaleimide hydrochloride (BIMH, 0.2 μM), prevented PMA- or vanadate/PMA-mediated stimulation of CL significantly (58% and 44%, respectively) indicating that the stimulation was a net effect of kinase/phosphatase activation with PMA. The trend

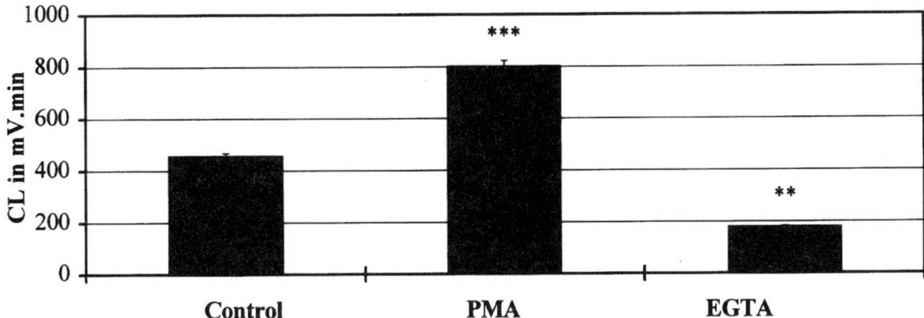

FIGURE 4. EGTA inhibits PMA-mediated stimulation of CL production. 1.5 mM EGTA was preincubated with PMNs for 15 min prior to PMA stimulation. The data were reproduced in five other experiments with similar inhibition with EGTA. **$p<0.05$, ***$p<0.0001$.

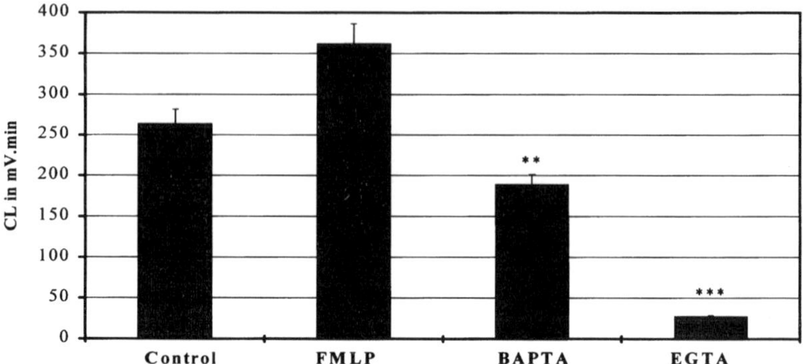

FIGURE 5. Comparative effects of BAPTA and EGTA on neutrophil stimulation. PMNs were pretreated with 12.5 μM BAPTA or 1.5 mM EGTA in preincubation media prior to FMLP stimulation during 60 min integration at 37°C. Extracellular Ca^{2+} chelation had more impact than intracellular Ca^{2+} chelation in inhibiting FMLP-mediated CL generation. Each bar is mean of 6 ± SEM from two experiments. Statistical comparisons were made to FMLP stimulation as control. **$p<0.05$, ***$p<0.0001$.

was the same with a selective inhibitor of tyrosine kinase (TK), genistein (0.2 μM) with stimulation by PMA, or vanadate/PMA, indicating the involvement of TK in the generation of superoxide cascade (TABLE 1).

Glutamate or NMDA alone did not stimulate CL generation in the primed cells, but the pretreatment with sodium vanadate stimulated it greatly. A competitive inhibitor for the NMDA receptor, AP7, prevented NMDA- or glutamate-mediated CL generation with control cells. In addition, AP7 and vanadate simultaneously reduced the vanadate-mediated stimulation of CL significantly. Furthermore, NMDA-mediat-

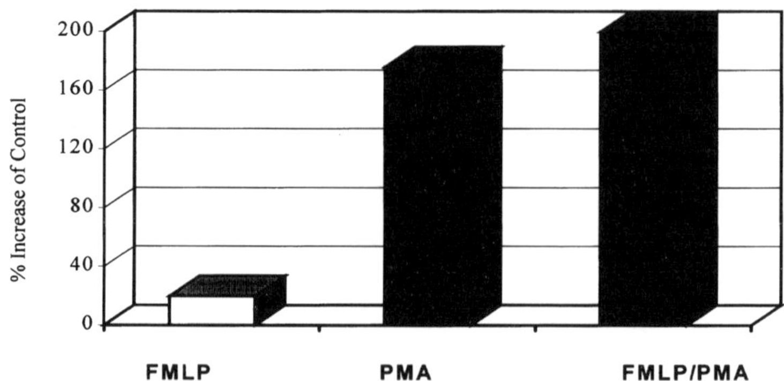

FIGURE 6. Additive effects between PMA and FMLP on CL production. PMA and FMLP simultaneously stimulated CL generation in additive manner. Each bar is mean of three sets of raw data.

TABLE 1. PMA with Kinase/Phosphatase Inhibitors on CL Generation

	Percentage Increase	Percentage Decrease
Control	0	0
PMA	147 ± 18.38	
PBA/BIMH		58 ± 0.707 (vs. PMA)
PMA/genistein		45.5 ± 1.06 (vs. PMA)
PMA/vanadate	4,497 ± 26.167	
PMA/vanadate/BIMH	2,482 ± 88.402	
PMA/vanadate/genistein	2,644 ± 153.111	

Note: The data are expressed as mean of 6 ± SEM. BIMH, bisindolylmaleimide hydrochloride; protein kinase C inhibitor, genistein; tyrosine kinase inhibitor, vanadate; sodium vanadate, tyrosine phosphatase inhibitor.

ed CL generation was EGTA sensitive, indicating that the NMDA cascade requires extracellular Ca^{2+}. Thus, NMDA-mediated CL generation was potentiated with vanadate and both kinase inhibitors reduced the vanadate-mediated potentiation (TABLE 2).

DISCUSSION

When the low concentration (10^{-11} M) of primers (FMLP or GM-CSF) was used during preincubation, it was predictable that priming would stimulate the cells upon subsequent stimulation. FMLP at the concentration of 10^{-11} M may be too weak to

TABLE 2. Effects of Glutamate Congeners on CL Generation

	Percentage Increase	Percentage Decrease
Control	0	0
Glutamate		18 ± 5.34
NMDA		5 ± 3.02
Glutamate/AP7		75 ± 1.732
NMDA/AP7		75 ± 1.414
Glutamate/EGTA		55 ± 4.05
NMDA/EGTA		56 ± 2.122
NMDA/BIMH		58.5 ± 1.06
NMDA/genistein		57.5 ± 1.06
Glutamate/vanadate	2,337 ± 507.12	
NMDA/vanadate	2,817 ± 91.94	
NMDA/vanadate/EGTA	415 ± 31.825	
NMDA/vanadate/BIMH	1,180 ± 45.97	
NMDA/vanadate/genistein	1,143 ± 23.34	
NMDA/vanadate/BI/gen	605.5 ± 18.03	

The data are expressed as mean of 6 ± SEM.

activate oxidases but sufficient to phosphorylate the p47 cytosolic component of oxidases without increasing the Ca^{2+} signal, leading to priming of the neutrophils, similar to another proven priming agent, GM-CSF.[17] Actual changes in transient Ca^{2+} levels were not assessed in this study, but the pharmacological manipulations of Ca^{2+} levels prior to measuring the changes in the respiratory burst were the major focus, using specific intra- and extracellular Ca^{2+} chelators. EGTA within the millimolar range and BAPTA in micromolar concentrations presumably chelated extracellular Ca^{2+} and intracellular Ca^{2+}, respectively, assuming the intracellular levels of Ca^{2+} to be approximately 10^{-7} M in the resting cell and 10^{-6} M in the stimulated cell[18] as compared to the millimolar range in the extracellular medium.

Firstly, in our experimental conditions, the neutrophils were shown to produce high levels of chemiluminescence with luminol, a cell-permeable CL substrate, as a measurement of respiratory burst with each stimulant. This method did not separate away the possible leakage of superoxide into the incubation media. Furthermore, the manipulations of Ca^{2+} levels in the cell or in the medium with specific Ca^{2+} chelators generated significant changes in CL production, indicating the pivotal role of intra- or extracellular Ca^{2+} in regulating the respiratory burst in human neutrophils. In addition, the PMA- and FMLP-mediated stimulation of CL production was clearly different in the dependency on the inositol-1,4,5-trisphosphate (IP_3)-mediated release of intracellular Ca^{2+}. BAPTA treatment leads to the chelation of intracellular Ca^{2+} in PMNs, yet permits the influx of Ca^{2+} from the extracellular medium when the cells are stimulated. Under these conditions, PMA-mediated stimulation of CL production was potentiated, indicating that PMA-mediated stimulation was not affected by the intracellular release of Ca^{2+} by IP_3, but bypasses the receptor-mediated PLC activation (which would generate DG and IP_3[19]) activating PKC directly. This is also a situation in which PMNs can activate their oxidases via the PKC cascade without any opposing intracellular effect that might be present if there were an excessive release of intracellular Ca^{2+}. The BAPTA-mediated intracellular Ca^{2+} chelation or pretreatment with vanadate would lead to a disinhibition of PKC activity by minimizing the endogenous phosphatase activity, resulting in a potentiation when PMA is used to stimulate the PMNs. The possibility of endogenous phosphatase activation by a transiently increased Ca^{2+} influx via the PMA-mediated cascade was tested with a selective inhibitor of phosphatase, sodium vanadate.

Surprisingly, millimolar concentrations of sodium vanadate potentiated CL generation to a greater degree than that of BAPTA treatment. Activation of endogenous phosphatase with transiently increased Ca^{2+} would tend to reduce (oppose) the PKC activity affecting the oxidases, when PMA generates intracellular Ca^{2+} levels sufficient to activate phosphatase. Therefore, the PMA-mediated stimulation of CL seen represented a net effect between the kinase/phosphatase cycles. The PKC-mediated stimulation of CL by PMA was evidenced by pretreating the PMNs with a selective inhibitor of PKC, Ro-31-8220, which prevented PMA-mediated stimulation and greatly reduced the respiratory burst of the cells pretreated with the vanadate. Others also demonstrated the inhibition of the PMA-mediated respiratory burst with staurosporine[20] and H-7[21] in PMNs. Furthermore, a selective inhibitor of TK, genistein, also inhibited PMA- or vanadate/PMA-mediated CL significantly, indicating that the PMA cascade can activate both kinases despite the involvement of phosphatase. The data indicate that the PMA-induced tyrosine phosphorylation is required for the activation of the respiratory burst. It is not clear whether this tyrosine phosphorylation is secondary to PKC activation to activate NADPH oxidase.[22] It was also demonstrated that PMA-mediated stimulation of the respiratory burst was inhibited by genistein in vanadate-treated PMNs. It is possible that a PMA-mediated Ca^{2+} influx is also responsible for activation of kinases and phosphatase. Conversely, FMLP-mediated stimulation of CL seems to be dependent on an IP_3-mediated release of stored Ca^{2+} because BAPTA-mediated chelation of intracellular Ca^{2+} caused a significant inhibition of CL production. A study using specific inhibitor(s) for IP_3-mediated release with FMLP would provide additional support for this argument. The inhibition with EGTA treatment followed by PMA or FMLP stimulation indicated that PMA or FMLP requires extracellular Ca^{2+} for the activation of oxidases to generate the respiratory burst in PMNs. The Ca^{2+} ionophore or inhibitor of the membrane Ca^{2+} channel (SKF 96365; a derivative of imidazole hydrochloride)[23] together with these stimulants would be additional candidates to test if extracellular Ca^{2+} is required for respiratory burst activation.

Another interesting observation on the inhibition of the FMLP pathway with BAPTA and EGTA was the difference in magnitude: EGTA treatment had more impact than BAPTA treatment in inhibiting FMLP-mediated stimulation of the respiratory burst. Several interpretations of the data are possible. (*1*) Without extracellular Ca^{2+}, FMLP may not stimulate membrane-bound PLC to generate second messengers, which in turn, will increase intracellular Ca^{2+} needed for the activation of oxidase(s) via the PKC cascade. (*2*) The contribution from cytosolic NADPH oxidase may be less than that of membrane-bound NADPH oxidase. Certainly, extracellular Ca^{2+} could initiate a cascade of sequential events or spatially different events that can be integrated as CL generation. Although FMLP-mediated receptor stimulation increases IP_3[19] and IP_3 has been implicated in the release of Ca^{2+} from intracellular stores in neutrophils,[24] FMLP-mediated PLC activation should not require intracellular Ca^{2+}. Furthermore, a possible synergism has been demonstrated between FMLP and PMA in the study. Since FMLP stimulates membrane-bound PLC to generate DG and IP_3,[19] the activator of PKC, PMA, would be synergistic (additive) with FMLP in stimulation of the respiratory burst in PMNs. Taken together, EGTA and the phosphatase inhibitor studies suggested that extracellular Ca^{2+} is required to stimulate the respiratory burst with PMA or FMLP but intracellular Ca^{2+} level might be critical to stimulation of the oxidases to produce respiratory burst with PKC- or other kinase-mediated pathways without any masking effect by the activated phosphatase. Considering the cross-talk between tyrosine phosphorylation of a subunit of NADHP oxidase and serine/threonine phosphorylation by PKC, which is essential for the activation of respiratory burst, phosphatase-mediated inactivation of tyrosine kinase can not be excluded. Indeed, vanadate-mediated disinhibition would apply to both PKC and TK. Our study with genistein supported the involvement of TK as well as PKC in activating the NADPH oxidase.

The study clearly demonstrated the heterogeneity in activation of the PMN oxidases that may have different components in different cellular location, to be activated in a different temporal fashion, providing evidence of complexity within the biochemical pathways in priming and activating neutrophils, through a Ca^{2+}-mediated cascade, via different stimuli.

Importantly, there are glutamate (NMDA) receptors in neutrophils regulating the

Ca^{2+} flux, in turn affecting the kinases/phosphatase cycle, depending on the concentration of Ca^{2+} at that moment. NMDA or glutamate alone did not alter CL generation, giving the impression that PMNs do not posses NMDA receptors. Initial speculation from this finding was that excessive Ca^{2+} influx via NMDA sites might be high enough to activate phosphatase in a dominant fashion, masking possible kinase activation. This was tested and proved, following AP7 and vandate treatment. The sodium vanadate–mediated inhibition of phosphatase might represent a disinhibition of protein kinase(s), and the significant reduction of the vanadate-mediated stimulation by AP7 or the kinase inhibitors provided evidence for the presence of the NMDA receptors and for the kinase/phosphatase cycle being crucial to regulation of superoxide generation in PMNs.

Since the NMDA receptor is a subreceptor of glutamate receptors, along with quisqualate and kainic acid sites (receptors), leading to an increase in Ca^{2+} influx in other cell types including neurons, it was an intriguing challenge to identify the existence of NMDA receptors in PMNs, which would regulate the respiratory burst via Ca^{2+} flux changes.

NMDA receptor desensitization via an excessive Ca^{2+} influx[25] was not ruled out in this study. It would be appropriate to determine the effect of different Ca^{2+} concentrations in the extracellular incubation media with NMDA. Importantly, the pretreatment with a competitive inhibitor, AP7, abrogated any CL generation by NMDA with the control cells, indicating the presence of NMDA receptors in these blood-derived cells (PMNs), which are regarded as non-excitable in contrast to neuronal cells.

Neither temporal and spatial profiles of the Ca^{2+}-mediated respiratory burst activation obtained by measuring the changes of Ca^{2+} concentration nor topographical observations of PMNs by confocal microscope were included in the study. It would be convincing for the study to measure any Ca^{2+} flux changes following each stimulant, which might regulate activities of oxidases or kinases. The study was focused on the pharmacological manipulation of the Ca^{2+} flux followed by biochemical assays, measuring the respiratory burst (as chemiluminescence) to determine the roles of intra- or extracellular Ca^{2+} in the stimulation of the various enzymes, including the oxidase, in PMNs.

SUMMARY

Activation of neutrophil oxidases, including NADPH oxidase, is Ca^{2+} dependent. The aim of this study was to determine the roles of intra- and extracellular Ca^{2+}, leading to generation of the respiratory burst, as monitored by luminol-dependent chemiluminescence (CL). All results were recorded as integrals (millivolt.min) and compared by a two-tail Student's t test. Preincubation of cells with chelators of intra- or extracellular Ca^{2+} inhibited N-Formyl-Met-Leu-Phe (FMLP)-stimulated burst activity ($p<0.01$). In contrast, stimulation by phorbol myristate acetate (PMA), while inhibited by extracellular Ca^{2+} chelation with EGTA ($p<0.001$), was potentiated by intracellular Ca^{2+} chelation with BAPTA ($p<0.01$). This suggests that the protein kinase C (PKC)–mediated burst may be diminished by intracellular Ca^{2+}-dependent phosphatase. A selective inhibitor of tyrosine phosphatase, sodium vanadate, potentiated CL generation by both FMLP and PMA, indicating a dominant phosphatase activation with transiently increased Ca^{2+}, masking the kinase-mediated respiratory burst. The selective inhibitors of PKC or tyrosine kinase prevented PMA and vanadate/PMA stimulation ($p<0.005$). Furthermore, the putative Ca^{2+} channel agonists glutamate (10^{-5}M) and N-methyl-D-aspartate (NMDA) (10^{-5}M) alone failed to influence CL output, but produced marked potentiation following pre-treatment with vanadate. Again this indicates a dominant activation of phosphatase triggered by the glutamate-mediated Ca^{2+} influx, so masking the kinase-dependent NADPH oxidase activity. A competitive antagonist of NMDA, AP7, significantly decreased vanadate-mediated CL in an EGTA-sensitive manner ($p<0.001$). The data confirm a requirement for intra- and extracellular Ca^{2+} in neutrophil respiratory burst activation via the kinase/phosphatase cycle, and an agonist effect by NMDA within the Ca^{2+} cascade mechanism.

ACKNOWLEDGMENT

The authors express sincere appreciation to Dr. Steven Edwards at the University of Liverpool for his critical review of this manuscript.

REFERENCES

1. HALLETT, M. B., S. W. EDWARDS & A. K. CAMPBELL. 1987. Control of oxygen radical production by luminol-dependent chemiluminescence: the roles of intracellular Ca^{2+}, oxygen and redox components. *In* Cellular Chemiluminescence. E. Von Dyke, Ed.: 173–92. CRC Press. Boca Raton, FL.
2. AL-MOHANNA, F. A. & M. B. HALLETT. 1988. The use of fura-2 to determine the relationship between cytoplasmic free Ca^{2+} and oxidase activation in rat neutrophils. Cell Calcium **9:** 17–26.
3. SADLER, K. L. & J. A. BADWEY. 1988. Second messengers involved in superoxide production by neutrophils: function and metabolism. *In* Phagocytes Defects II. Hematology/Oncology Clinics of North America. J. T. Curnutte, Ed.: 185–200. Sanders. Philadelphia, PA.
4. KANKAANRANTA, H., E. MOILANEN, K. LINDBERG & H. VAPAATALO. 1995. Pharmacological control of human polymorphonuclear leucocyte degranulation by fenamates and inhibitors of receptor-mediated calcium entry and protein kinase C. 1995. Biochem. Pharmacol. **50:** 197–203.
5. LUNDQVIST, H. & C. DAHLGREN. 1995. The serine protease inhibitor diisopropylfluorophosphate inhibits neutrophil NADPH-oxidase activity induced by the calcium ionophore inomycin and serum opsonised yeast particles. Inflamm. Res. **44:** 510–517.
6. LOPEZ, I., D. J. BURNS & J. D. LAMBETH. 1995. Regulation of phospholipase D by protein kinase C in human neutrophils. J. Biol. Chem. **270:** 19465–19472.
7. EDWARDS, S. W. 1991. Regulation of neutrophil oxidant production. *In* Calcium, Oxygen Radicals and Cellular Damage. C. J. Duncan Publishers. Cambridge University Press. Oxford.
8. KIM-PARK, W. K., M. A. MOORE, Z. W. HAKKI & M. J. KOWOLIK. 1996. Activation of the neutrophil respiratory burst requires both intracellular and extracellular calcium. Eur. J. Haematol. **59:** 12.

9. MacDermott, A. B., M. L. Mayer, G. L. Westbrook, S. J. Smith & J. L. Barker. 1986. NMDA-receptor activation increases cytoplasmic calcium concentration in cultured spinal cord neurons. Nature 331: 519–522.

10. Nicoletti, F., J. L. Meek, M. J. Iadarola, D. M. Chuang, B. L. Roth & E. Costa. 1986. Coupling of inositol phospholipid metabolism with excitatory amino acid recognition sites in rat hippocampus. J. Neurochem. 46: 40–46.

11. Seubert, P., J. Larson, M. Oliver, M. W. Jung, M. Baudry & G. Lynch. 1988. Stimulation of NMDA receptors induces proteolysis of spectrin in hippocampus. Brain Res. 460: 189–194.

12. Dumuis, A. M. Sebben, L. Haynes, J.-P. Pin & J. Bockaert. 1988. NMDA receptors activate the arachidonic acid cascade system in striatal neurons. Nature 336: 68070.

13. Garthwaite, J., S. L. Charles & R. Chess-Williams. 1988. Endothelium-derived relaxing factor release on activation of NMDA receptors suggests role as intercellular messenger in the brain. Nature 336: 385–388.

14. Bading, H. & M. E. Greenberg. 1991. Stimulation of protein tyrosine phosphorylation by NMDA receptor activation. Science 23: 912–914.

15. Bonfoco, E. D. Krainc, M. Ankarcrona, P. Nicotera & S. A. Lipton. 1995. Apoptosis and necrosis: Two distinct events induced, respectively, by mild and intense insults with N-methyl-D-aspartate or nitric oxide/superoxide in cortical cell cultures. Proc. Natl. Acad. Sci. USA 92: 7162–7166.

16. Fukunaga, K. & T. R. Sodering. 1990. Activation of Ca^{2+}/Calmodulin-dependent protein kinase II in cerebellar granule cells by N-methyl-D-aspartate receptor activation. Mol. Cell. Neurosci. 1(1): 133–138.

17. Hallett, M. B. & D. Lloyds. 1995. Neutrophil priming: the cellular signals that say "amber" but not "green." Immunol. Today 16: 264–268.

18. Pozzan, T., D. P. Lew, C. B. Wollheim & R. Y. Tsien. 1983. Is cytosolic ionized calcium regulating neutrophil activation? Science 221: 1413.

19. Majerus, P. W. T. M. Connolly, H. Deckmyn, T. S. Ross, T. E. Bross, H. Ishii, V. S. Bansal & D. B. Wilson. 1986. The metabolism of phosphoinositide-derived messenger molecules. Science 234: 1519–1526.

20. Dewald, B., M. Thelan, M. P. Wymann & M. Baggiolini. 1989. Staurosporine inhibits the respiratory burst and induces exocytosis in human neutrophils. Biochem. J. 264: 879–884.

21. Berkow, R. L., R. W. Dodson & A. B. Kraft. 1987. The effect of a protein kinase C inhibitor, H-7, on human neutrophil oxidative burst and degranulation. J. Leuk. Biol. 41: 441–446.

22. Phillips, W. A., S. Bassal & S. P. Green. 1995. Tyrosine phosphorylation: a signal for the activation of the phagocyte respiratory burst. Redox Rep. 1: 83–88.

23. Davies, E. V. & M. B. Hallett. 1995. A novel pathway for Ca^{2+} signaling in neutrophils by immune complexes. Immunology 85: 538–543.

24. Prestki, M., C. B. Wollheim & P. D. Lew. 1984. Ca^{2+} Homeostasis in permeabilized human neutrophils. J. Biol. Chem. 259: 13777.

25. Mayer M. L. & G. L. Westbrook. 1985. The action of N-methyl-D-aspartic acid on mouse spinal neurons in culture. J. Physiol 361: 65–90.

26. Koenderman, L., A. Tool, D. Roots & A. J. Verhoeven. 1989. 1,2-diacylglycerol accumulation in human neutrophils does not correlate with respiratory burst activation. FEBS Lett. 243: 399–403.

The Phagocyte in Human Gliomas

LORENZO LORUSSO AND M. L. ROSSI[a]

Department of Pathology
Walton Hospital
Liverpool L9 1AE United Kingdom

INTRODUCTION

The concept of "immune privilege" has historically been invoked to explain the observation that brain allografts were not rejected.[1,2] For a long time it was held that the central nervous system (CNS) was not endowed with lymphatic vessels and that the blood-brain barrier (BBB) acted as an "insulant" in this respect.[3] This belief has however recently been disavowed[4,5] as the very concept of "immune privileged site." Furthermore, astrocytes and microglia may play an active immune role as the former may express major histocompatibility complex (MHC) class I and II antigens whilst the latter secretes interleukin 1 (IL-1) and other cytokines, the triggers of the immune response.[6–8] Furthermore, tumor infiltrating lymphocytes and macrophages as well as reactive glial cells around tumors may produce cytokines that may have stimulatory or inhibitory effects on the very tumor cells.[9,10] Hence, macrophages, astrocytes, and microglia are capable of participating in a complex way to the immune reaction process.[11]

Already in 1936 Siris[12] had observed that rabbit antiserum against extracts of normal human brain and of glioblastoma exhibited the same reactivity profile in complement fixation tests, namely, they both recognized brain antigens. Since then several authors have demonstrated the existence of brain-specific antigens in glioma,[13,14] the latter also sharing large numbers of antigens with non-neoplastic glial cells.[15]

Particular attention has very recently also been paid to the presence and to the quantitation of mononuclear and microglial cells in intracranial tumors.[16–29]

The monocyte-macrophage system is a network of specialized phagocytic cells widely scattered throughout the body. These cells include peripheral blood monocytes, Kupffer cells, macrophages of lymph nodes and spleen, fixed macrophages of other tissues, and CNS microglia. There is evidence that peripheral blood monocytes originate from bone marrow precursors[30] and that tissue macrophages, including brain macrophages are derived from circulating monocytes that migrate from circulating monocytes into tissues where they become resident macrophages.[31]

Bone marrow precursors therefore maintain the pool of peripheral blood monocytes and tissue macrophages. However, some of the CNS macrophages derive from resident microglia.[32,33]

Microglia was recognized in 1932 by del Rio-Hortega by means of silver carbon-

[a]Address all correspondence to: Dr. M. L. Rossi, Department of Pathology, Walton Hospital, Rice Lane, Liverpool L9 1AE, U.K. Fax, 00 44 151 529 4540; Phone, 00 44 151 529 4573; Email, Rossi-M@wcnn.co.uk; and Web: http://ourworld.compuserve.com/homepages/marcorossi.

ate impregnation.[34,35] Microglia originates from mesenchyma and distributes to CNS white and gray matter[36] where, as resident macrophages, they comprise between 5 and 20% of the total glial cell population [glia proper and microglia].[37]

MONOCYTES AND MACROPHAGES

Morphological and Immunological Aspects

Monocytes originate from non-lymphoid precursors within bone marrow and circulate in peripheral blood with a half-life of 1–3 days.[38] Monocytes leave the peripheral circulation by margination and by migration into the extravascular pool. Monocytes have been identified in circulating human fetal blood from the fourth week of gestation.[39] During embryonic development, bone marrow–derived monocytes enter the brain and the retina and differentiate in microglia with its attendant morphological modifications. Monocytes preferentially enter the rat brain from the septum pellucidum and then migrate to diencephalon and telencephalon through the developing corpus callosum.[40] Macrophages in the developing rodent brain are morphologically different from those in the adult brain and express different antigens.[41] Experimental studies have demonstrated that programmed neuronal death is the stimulus that attracts monocytes to the developing nervous system and induces them to differentiate into macrophages and microglia.[42] Dying cells are postulated to act as chemotactic signal for monocytes and to stimulate monocytic recruitment for phagocytosis and removal of cellular debris.[43] Similarly, tissue macrophages originate from monocytes after they have migrated from the peripheral circulation as well as from the proliferation of macrophage precursors within tissues. Cells of the monocyte-macrophage system are heterogeneous in terms of their morphology, cytochemistry, function, and surface determinants. As promonocytes mature into monocytes and then into tissue macrophages, they increase in size, the nucleus/cytoplasmic ratio decreases, and the number of lysosomes and immunoglobulin G receptors increases. Monocytes do not contain phagocytosed material but may have cytoplasmic debris–free vacuoles when activated. Their presence is generally viewed as a non-specific sign of inflammation.[44] They also make their appearance after meningeal "irritation," e.g., as when induced by myelography or drugs.[45]

The maturation and differentiation of monocytes into macrophages is influenced by various processes including chemotactic agents,[46,47] lymphocytes,[48] bacterial endotoxins,[49] plasma proteins,[50] and cell surfaces.[51] Functionally, mature macrophages have greater ability to undergo phagocytosis and lymphocyte interaction than monocytes.[52] Macrophages are prominent in the leptomeninges and choroid plexus. Small numbers of macrophages are found in the cerebrospinal fluid (CSF), which indicates that there may be macrophage traffic through the choroid plexus to the CSF in normal brain.[43]

Macrophages secrete a variety of cytokines and growth factors (TABLE 1), including interleukin 1 and tumor necrosis factor (TNF) which can stimulate angiogenesis and glia proliferation.[53,54] Thus it is postulated that macrophages can contribute to the angiogenesis and gliogenesis of the developing CNS. In fact, it has been reported

TABLE 1. Cytokines Produced by the Monocyte/Macrophage/Microglia System in the CNS

Cytokine/Growth Factor	Cell	References
IL-1	Microglia, Macrophage	1,2
IL-6	Microglia, Macrophage	3,4
IL-8	Monocyte	5
IL-12	Macrophage	6
M-CSF	Macrophage, Microglia, Monocyte	7,8
GM-CSF	Macrophage	9
TNF-α	Microglia, Macrophage, Monocyte	10,11
γ-IFN	Microglia	16
MIP	Microglia	3,12
TGF-β	Macrophage, Microglia	13
PDGF	Macrophage, Microglia	14
NGF	Microglia	15

Abbreviations: IL, interleukin; M-CSF, macrophage colony-stimulating-factor; GM-CSF, granulocyte-macrophage colony-stimulating factor; TNF-α, tumor necrosis factor-α; γ-IFN, interferon-gamma; MIP, macrophage inflammatory protein; TGF-β, transforming growth factor -β; PDGF, platelet-derived growth factor; NGF, nerve growth factor.

References: (1) Griffin, N. S. T. *et al.* 1989. Proc. Natl. Acad. Sci. USA **86:** 7611–7622. (2) Strauss, S. *et al.* 1992. Lab. Invest. **66:** 223–230. (3) Merril, J. E. *et al.* 1991. FASEB J. **5:** 2391–2397. (4) Frei, K. *et al.* 1989. Eur. J. Immunol. **19:** 689–694. (5) Benveniste, E. N. 1992. J. Physiol. **263:** 1–16. (6) Trembleau, S. *et al.* 1995. Immun. Today **16:** 18. (7) Skerr, C. J. *et al. In* M. B. Sporn & A. B. Roberts, Eds.: Peptide Growth Factor and Their Receptors. 1990. Springer-Verlag. New York. (8) Gallo, P. *et al.* 1994. J. Neuroimmunol. **51:** 193–198. (9) Perry, V. H. *et al.* 1988. Trends Neurosci. **11:** 273–277. (10) Frey, K. *et al.* 1988. Ann N.Y. Acad. Sci. **540:** 218–227. (11) Morganti-Kossmann, M. C. 1992. Trends Pharmacol. Sci. **13:** 286–291. (12) Frey, K. *et al.* 1990. Ann. N.Y. Acad. Sci. **594:** 326–335. (13) Weller, M. *et al.* 1995. Brain Res. Rev. **21:** 128–151. (14) Giulian, D. 1993. Brain Behav. Immunol. **2:** 352–358. (15) Mallat, M. *et al.* 1995. Dev. Biol. **133:** 309–315. (16) Norenberg, M. D. 1994. J. Neuropathol. Exp. Neurol. **53:** 213–220.

that macrophages are present in the germinal matrix and subependymal zones and perivascular spaces throughout the brain and leptomeninges in frozen sections of autopsy brain tissue of 20 fetuses and infants from 18 weeks gestation to 8 postnatal months.[39]

The "brain macrophage" has also been referred to as the fifth cell type, e.g., after the oligodendrocyte, the astrocyte, the ependymal cell, and the resident microglia.[55] CNS "macrophages" include microglia, the only truly resident phagocytic parenchymal cell and, outside the BBB, macrophages of the meninges, supraependyma, epiplexus (Kolmer cell),[56] and perivascular regions.[57] The latter, otherwise known as perivascular cells or perivascular macrophages [PMs],[58] not to be confused with perivascular microglia (which are parenchymal microglia). PMs are separated from the CNS parenchyma[43] by the parenchymal basement membrane and by the glia limitans. This clear distinction between PMs and microglia did not become apparent until del Rio-Hortega.[35,59] PMs are immunophenotypically and morphologically distinct from microglia and from resident cells of the outer wall of the blood vessel, i.e., pericytes, smooth muscle cells, and fibroblasts.[57] Pericytes are indeed part of the vascular wall and are enclosed within a basal lamina, thus they are not CNS parenchymal cells.[60]

PMs are renewed from bone marrow precursors,[61] play a role in CNS immune responses, may express MHC class II antigens,[62] and may synthesize, together with T-cell, molecules such as B-7, a surface glycoprotein that has been implicated as a major participant in the stimulation of T cell proliferation and production of IL-2 and other cytokines[63–65] that may be involved in tumor cell recognition.[7] When one considers their location at the BBB interface, PMs are the first line of defense against human immunodeficiency virus (HIV) and other CNS infections.[57]

Various cytochemical, morphological, and immunological techniques have been used to identify cells of the monocyte-macrophage system. Immunocytochemical labeling of monocytes/macrophages with monoclonal antibodies (MAbs) is sensitive and specific.[16,66,67]

Macrophages bearing MHC class II (or HLA-Dr) and interleukin-2 receptors (IL-2R)[68,69] participate to the immune process as antigen presenting cells (APCs).[70] The other immune mechanisms include antibody-dependent cell-mediated immunity (ADCC) through the binding with Fc receptor of killer cells, and non-MHC restricted cytotoxicity.[71]

Antigen presentation by macrophages, the "professional" APCs, is a process involving two steps (signals 1 and 2). Signal 1 is antigen-specific and originates from the binding of the APC T cell receptor to the peptide-MHC complex. A similar mechanism is also involved for non-professional APCs, such as polymorphonuclear cells. Signal 2 is antigen-aspecific and is triggered by the B7 molecule exclusively expressed by professional APCs, which interacts with CD28 (or CTLA4) expressed on Th cells.[72] This is important because signal 1, in the absence of signal 2, as is the case for non-professional APCs, results in T cell inactivation, e.g., "T cell anergy."

In melanoma, a heightened expression of MHC class I by tumor cells may be a pointer towards good prognosis whilst a high expression of MHC class II may indicate a poorer prognosis.[73] Similarly, expression of MHC class II by glioma cells may be a negative prognostic factor.[74] Apart from its ADCC properties, macrophages may also process and digest, and present antigens in conjunction with -Dr class II antigens of their own membrane, e.g., antibody-independent cellular cytotoxicity. In addition, macrophages modulate the inflammatory and immune processes[75] by producing monokines (including interleukins,[76] colony stimulating factors,[77] complement factors) and cytolytic factor (such as TNF,[78] bioactive lipids including products of arachidonate metabolism,[79,80] and platelet activating factors,[81] which in turn may activate monocytes). To be cytotoxic after antigenic activation, macrophages and granulocytes require stimulation by complement factors, leukotrienes, or other cytokines whereas lymphocytes become cytotoxic or antibody-producing after antigenic challenge.

Macrophages may also be activated to release lysosomal enzymes following interaction with antigen-antibody complexes[82] and with lymphokines (gamma-interferon), and to operate selective targeted-phagocytosis and opsonin-mediated phagocytosis.[36] Other possible functions of CNS macrophages include ganglioside turnover, phospholipid catabolism, and apolipoprotein binding and secretion. Macrophages may also participate in homeostasis by processing and catabolizing neurotransmitters and hormones.[43]

MICROGLIA

Morphological and Immunological Aspects

Microglia is a stable cell population with rare mitoses and represents about 20% of the total glial pool. Microglia cells are more numerous in gray than white matter and in the former, different regions are endowed with greater numbers than others.[43,83]

Microglia was first recognized by Nissl who coined the name "Stabchenzellen" (rod cell). Nissl thought microglia to be reactive neuroglia and suggested that it had the capacity to migrate and phagocytose.[84] The phagocytic role of microglia in brain was questioned for quite some time[85] as blood-borne monocytes were thought to be the cells responsible for phagocytosis of damaged CNS.

The concept of the microglial cell as a resident mesenchymal element distinct from other non-neuronal cells, e.g., astrocytes and oligodendrocytes, was advanced by del Rio-Hortega[34,35] on the basis of studies of brains of developing animals impregnated with silver carbonate. He recognized that Ramon y Cajal's "third element"[86] consisted of two cell types, oligodendrocytes and microgliocytes. Hortega believed that microglia originated from the migration of the "embryonic corpuscles" from the pia mater into the brain during development. He considered its possible origin from mononuclear cells of the circulating blood, and asserted its ability to transform from ramified, "resting" cells into macrophages.[34] This last conclusion derived from observations he made on stab wounds in mature brains of a variety of animal species. Microglial response to these injuries led to development of migrating amoeboid microglia and then fully developed macrophages. The latter resembled the globose microglial cell that appears in the brain in embryonal and postnatal life.[83] In its mature and immature state, microglia has primarily an immune effector function and, together with resident macrophages, plays a major role in CNS defense and repair mechanisms.[87,88] This "early microglia" is endowed with mitotic activity.[89]

There is no information as to whether monocytes become macrophages or directly transform into microglia under the influence of astrocytes.[90–92] Microglia precursors migrate to the brain during development, before and during the formation of the BBB. Microglia becomes a permanent resident in the CNS after the formation of the BBB. Subsequently, microglial cells increase in number by a process of multiplication. Ameboid microglia, a transient population, transforms into ramified microglia, which persists into adulthood and is capable of transforming into active macrophages. Microglia cells of mature brain undergo division *in situ* but are also replaced by circulating monocytes.[93]

Microglia has immunophenotypic properties of monocytes and macrophages including the expression of the common leukocyte antigen and of class II MHC antigens.[94]

Reactive microglia demonstrates morphological changes when compared to resting resident microglia and newly expresses the ED1 epitope (a specific lysosomal marker), which is otherwise typically expressed by activated peripheral blood monocytes.[88]

A number of anti–monocyte-macrophage antibodies identify microglia but microglia-specific antibodies are not yet available.[67,95] MAbs are highly specific for human tissue macrophages and this has been exploited in the study of the histogenesis of microglia and its migration.

Microglia is already well differentiated in the 35th week human fetus whilst earlier it is less ramified.[39]

The microglia-monocyte-macrophage system appears to mature earlier than astroglia and removal of necrotic tissue by macrophages has been seen in fetal brain when astrocytic response is still minimal.

Microglia cells are small, elongated, and bipolar with two or three fingerlike branches. Electron microscopy shows that the cytoplasm is flattened and the nucleus elongated with dense peripheral chromatin. The Golgi apparatus is small and scattered lysosomal granules and isolated sheets of rough endoplasmic reticulum are present in the cytoplasm.[92] Microglia differs from oligodendroglia because it has few microtubules and structurally more complex dense bodies. Glycogen granules and attachment plaques are absent.[83]

The classical impregnation method with silver carbonate has remained unchanged.[34] Recently several, albeit non-specific, immunohistochemical and lectin methods to demonstrate microglia have been developed. Antibodies to microglia epitopes such as those against major histocompatibility complexes I and II,[96,97] leukocyte common antigen (OX-1),[98] a macrophage cytosolic protein (ED1),[90] IgG Fc receptor (G2),[99] and CR3 complement receptor (Mac-1, OX-42),[100] and MHC class I and II antigens (OX-18 and OX-6)[101] are commonly in use. Plant lectin Bandeiraea (Griffonia) simplicifolia agglutinin (BS-1)[102] and ricinus communis agglutinin-120 (RCA-1)[103] are good markers, but are more difficult to use routinely. Thiamine pyrophosphatase and nucleoside diphosphatase methods also clearly stain microglia,[104,105] but frozen or vibratome sections of aldehyde-fixed brain tissue are required because paraffin embedding destroys enzyme activity.

Microglia expresses the GD3 ganglioside and may thus be confused with its adult and perinatal progenitors.[106]

The microglia forms a network of antigen-presenting cells with a primary immune surveillance role[107] in the resting state.[108] However microglia can rapidly respond to CNS injury and become "activated" microglia, morphologically recognizable as the *rod cell* of Nissl.[84] Microglia first becomes activated but not phagocytic and expresses the ED1 epitope; subsequently it becomes phagocytic and ingests cellular debris and degeneration products. On the basis of these morphological and functional characteristics, it is possible to distinguish four different types of microglia: ameboid, ramified and quiescent, activated but not phagocytic, and phagocytic (as found in pathological areas).[55]

Microglia is involved in a variety of diseases of the CNS including HIV encephalitis,[109] Alzheimer's disease,[110] degenerative disorders,[111] multiple sclerosis,[112] head injury,[113] ischemia,[114,115] brain tumors,[116] and prion diseases.[117]

Immunobiology of Gliomas

About four decades ago, Burnet[118] and Jerne[119] independently put forward the concept of the immunological control of carcinogenesis, which became known as the "immunosurveillance" theory.[120] This postulates that neoplastic cells are antigenic and that they may be recognized by the immune system in a way similar to allograft rejection. In humans, immunosuppression is associated with an increased incidence of certain types of neoplasms and with an increased tumor burden.[121]

This concept contrasts with experimental data in immunodeficient animals, as in the athymic nude mice, where a higher incidence of malignancies or susceptibility to chemical carcinogens has not been observed.[122]

Exposure to certain carcinogens may be accompanied by systemic immunosuppression but this does not necessarily imply that they have tumorigenic potential.[123]

Most primary solid tumors are not highly immunogenic and therefore are less likely to be eliminated by the immune system.[124]

Recent human studies focusing on the local immune response have demonstrated that infiltrating tumor lymphocytes may participate in the control of tumor growth. It has been shown in animal models that the immunological status of tumor-infiltrating lymphoid cells is altered when compared with lymphoid cells in the spleen or peripheral blood of the same animal.[125]

The concept of local immunity may have particular relevance for the pathogenesis and biology of CNS tumors due to the fact that the brain differs immunologically from all other organs.[126,127] An immune response has been observed in the brain in multiple sclerosis and certain infections[128] and a heavy brain tumor lymphocytic infiltration after subcutaneous immunization with radiated autologous neoplastic cells has also been noted.[129]

Although an active interplay between CNS and immune system has recently been demonstrated,[130] anatomical and antigenic features may be responsible for the intrinsic weakness of the immune response in the CNS and for the difficulties in setting up an effective immunotherapy of CNS neoplasms: (*1*) The perivascular cells of the BBB limit access of chemoattractant proteins and humoral immune molecules, such as immunoglobulins, and of some of the immune effector cells.[4] (*2*) The absence of a true lymphatic system hampers the supply of immunocompetent effector cells, hence of antigen presentation.[130] (*3*) The MHC self recognition antigens are reduced in brain parenchyma around the neoplasm site. Class I MHC, which are required for recognition of foreign or neoplasm-associated cell surface antigen by cytotoxic T-lymphocytes, are absent from normal brain parenchyma and have been detected in only a fraction of glioma cells.[131] Class II MHC antigens are necessary for the activation of T-helper lymphocytes. HLA-Dr antigens, a subgroup of class II MHC antigens, are found only focally on the membrane of astrocytes in the white matter and in a small number of gliomas and glioma cells.[23,132] (*4*) Local antibody production has been attributed to migrated B lymphocytes[133,134] although B lymphocytes are few in number.[4,17,130] (*5*) Mechanisms mediating cellular cytotoxicity are impaired within the CNS. ADCC requires the initial recognition and binding of antibodies directed against tumor-associated antigens (TAA). These are antigens expressed on tumor cells that have the potential ability to lead to tumor rejection in an immunized host, before cytotoxic T-lymphocytes and macrophages are able to react with the Fc portion of antibody molecules.

APCs, such as macrophages and microglia, initiate a specific T cell response by simultaneous presentation of TAA and Class II MHC molecules to T-helper cells. A decrease in specific immune response in gliomas may be explained by reduced or modified expression of TAA.[135]

Beside the impaired local immune response, patients with malignant gliomas frequently show a decreased systemic immune response, in particular T-cell–mediated immunity. A reduced number of peripheral blood T-lymphocytes, particularly the CD4+ fraction of helper T cells,[136] a diminished reactivity to mitogens and antigenic stimuli, and a reduced production of IL-2 have also been described.[71,137]

On the basis of apparent limited brain immunoreactivity, the depressed intra-tumor immune response, and the reduced systemic cell–mediated immunity, it is clear that targeted immunobiological therapeutic strategies for the treatment of gliomas[138] are necessary to enhance the host response. This approach has a morphological substrate in the demonstration of mononuclear cell infiltrates in human gliomas.[17,139]

Macrophage/Microglia Network in Intracranial Tumors

Few morphological studies have addressed the presence of the macrophage/microglia system in brain tumors.[16–22,24–26,67,140] A preeminent perivascular mononuclear cell infiltrate in brain tumors had been shown almost 40 years ago.[141,142] Mononuclear cells are the majority of immunocompetent cells in high grade gliomas and macrophages account for up to 80% of this population.[16,17,67,133,143] Occasional natural killer cells and a few B-lymphocytes have also been evinced.[17,144–148] The first studies attempting to characterize and separately identify microglial cells from macrophages and lymphocytic subpopulations in gliomas were carried out on frozen samples due to the lack of antibodies suited to paraffin work.[16–27,67,149] Until recently, the main problem in reliably identifying monocytes, macrophages, and microglia was the lack of specific antibodies. Among the markers tested for monocytes are F4/80, CD11b, CD11c (the last on cryostat section by Ki-M1),[95,150,151] RM3/1, CD45RO (UCHL1 in common with macrophage).[67,95] For macrophages the markers are Ki-M1P (CD68), Ki-M6 (CD68 on cryostat section), CD13 and CD14 (antibodies to cryostat section only My7 and My4), and Y182A.[16,67,95,149,152] For microglia: EBM11 (CD68 in common with macrophage),[62] Ki-M1P (CD68), ED1 and ED2 which are not for parenchymal microglia, but rather for perivascular pericytes; ED3[67,83,95,140,149,157]; and the complement receptor CR3-32 HLA-Dr present in the monocyte/macrophage/activated microglia system.[67]

Most authors are in agreement on the abundance of macrophages in human brain neoplasms.[17,67,140,149,154,155] This is in agreement with experimental data.[153–155] A large number of infiltrating macrophages may positively correlate with the grade of malignancy in gliomas.[17,23,28,67,149] Roggendorf followed Kreutzberg criteria and distinguished the monocyte/macrophage pool of CNS neoplasms in four categories, finding the largest number of amoeboid microglia, ramified microglia, and macrophages in high-grade gliomas,[67] in line with early observations[116] and later ones.[16,17] Prominent microglial activation has been observed in cerebral non-

Hodgkin lymphomas (NHLs) and germinomas.[67] This is in agreement with Russell and Rubinstein's observation that these tumors have a large number of microglial cells.[156]

Further progress in the understanding the biology of microglia has recently been made with the introduction of MAbs recognizing epitopes of monocytes and macrophages in formalin-fixed paraffin-embedded sections.[62,92,157] CNS NHLs show an increased number of macrophages in the midst of the tumor as found in NHLs outside the CNS.[158] Gangliocytic tumors, e.g., gangliocytoma and neurocytoma, show very few microglia and macrophages perhaps because of a low concentration of IL-10.[67]

Rossi[17] studied the mononuclear cell infiltrate and the HLA-Dr expression by macrophages and tumor cells in a series of 386 frozen and 248 paraffin-embedded cranial and spinal intrinsic CNS tumors, with a panel of antibodies directed against macrophages, lymphocytes, and HLA-Dr antigens. Statistically significant differences in the *macrophage infiltrate in the tumor proper* between various tumors were found. Atypical meningiomas had the heaviest infiltrate when compared to all the other tumor groups. High grade astrocytomas (FIGS. 1–4) had a heavier infiltrate than low grade gliomas, benign meningiomas, pituitary adenomas, and schwannomas. The infiltrate in low grade gliomas was heavier than in pituitary adenomas; it was also heavier in benign meningiomas when compared with pituitary adenomas and schwannomas. *The perivascular macrophage infiltrate* was also heavier in atypical

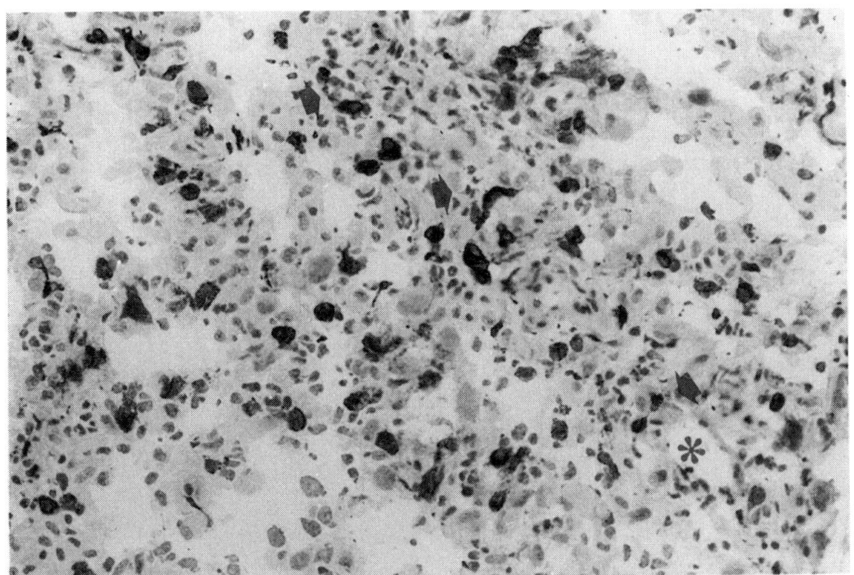

FIGURE 1. High grade astrocytoma (frozen section VICY1 × 400). Macrophage infiltrate around blood vessels (*arrows*) and within tumor proper. Note that tumor cells in the background are negative for HLA-Dr. Lumen of tangentially cut blood vessel highlighted by asterisk.

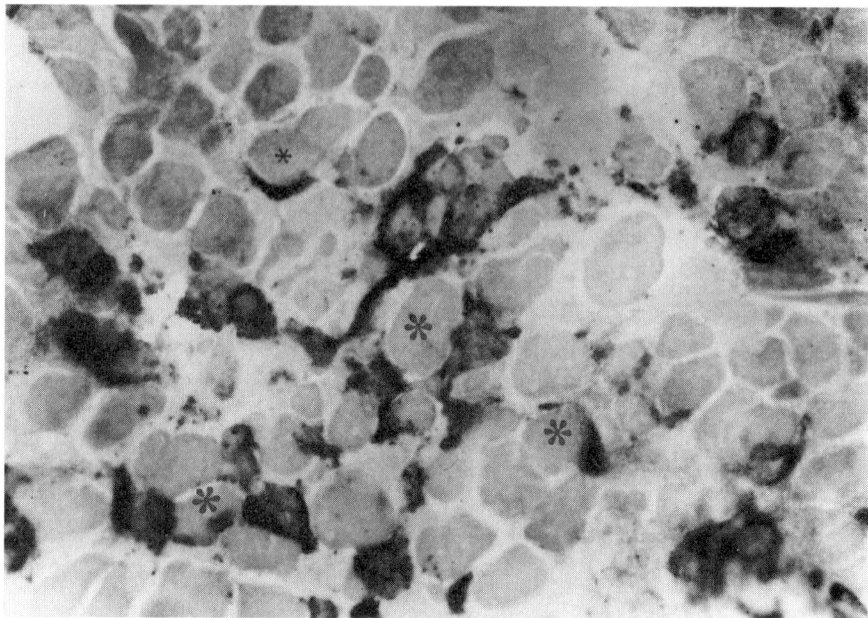

FIGURE 2. High grade astrocytoma (frozen section EBM11 × 800). Macrophages encircling individual tumor cells, the latter highlighted by asterisks.

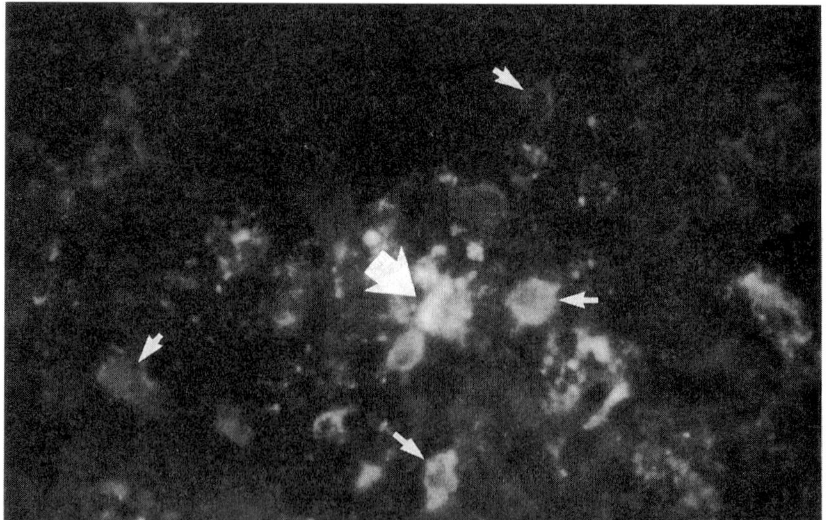

FIGURE 3. High grade astrocytoma (frozen section [immunofluorescence]: Y182a × 300). Compare the same field in the same section in FIGURE 4 when double immunostained for Fcγ receptor.

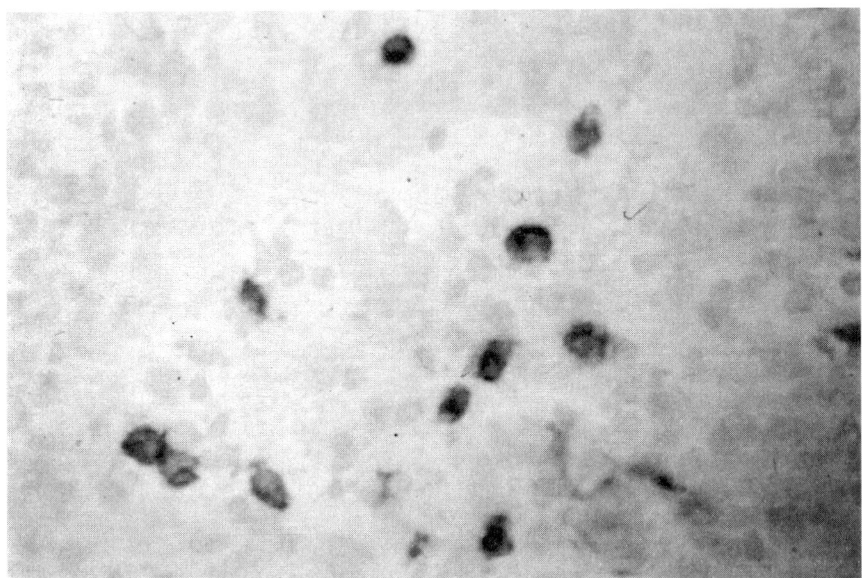

FIGURE 4. High grade astrocytoma (frozen section [immunoperoxidase]: 3G8 × 300). The same macrophages detected by Y182a (FIG. 3) (*arrow*) are also positive for Fcy receptor.

meningiomas as compared with all other tumors except carcinomas where there was no statistical difference. Benign meningiomas had a heavier infiltrate than high grade astrocytomas, low grade gliomas, and schwannomas. Carcinomas had a heavier infiltrate than low grade gliomas and schwannomas. The lymphocytic infiltrate consisted mostly of the CD8+ subset, was smaller than the macrophage infiltrate, was not present in all tumors, and was most extensive in atypical meningiomas. B lymphocytes and natural killer cells were scarcely represented if at all in all tumors.

Analysis of follow-up to demise of 68 high grade astrocytoma cases showed no correlation between the numbers of macrophages or CD8+ and CD4+ lymphocytes and survival. HLA-Dr antigen production by tumor cells (FIG. 5) was studied in 286 frozen tumors. These antigens were not expressed by oligodendrogliomas, subependymomas, medulloblastomas, and ganglion cell tumors. Meningiomas most frequently expressed them followed by astrocytomas and nerve sheath tumors. Comparison of the survival of HLA-Dr positive and negative high grade astrocytoma cases showed that the difference was not statistically significant. Rossi[17] concluded that macrophages are the predominant cells that infiltrate intracranial tumors followed by CD8+ lymphocytes and that there are significant differences in the extent of the infiltrate between various tumor groups mostly in relation to macrophages. However, there was no significant statistical correlation between survival and the various types of mononuclear cells infiltrating high grade astrocytomas or HLA-Dr expression by the same tumors. A variety of hypotheses could be put forward to explain these results in relation to macrophages, intra- or extradural tumor location, and tumor

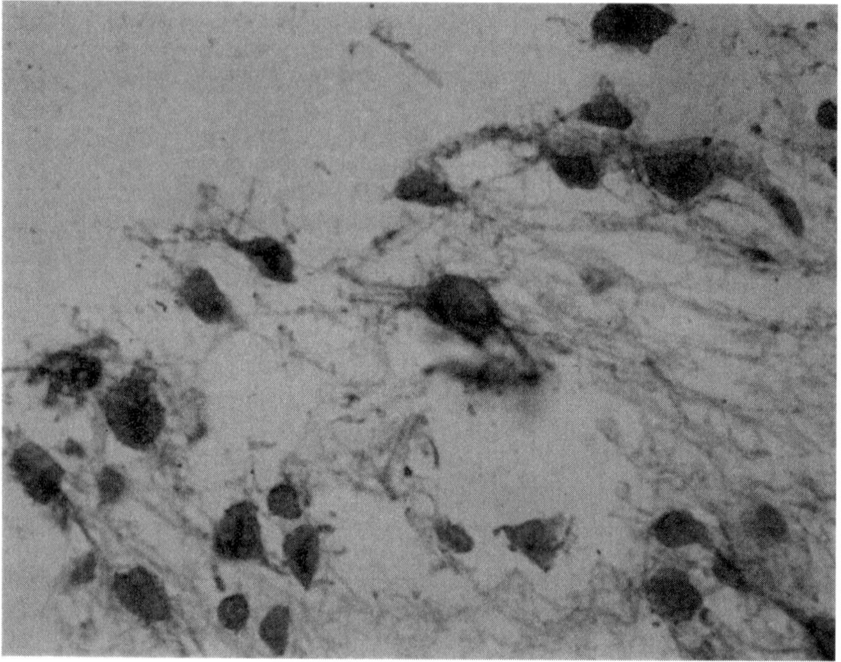

FIGURE 5. Low grade astrocytoma [Grade I/II] (frozen section: VICY1 × 650). Tumor cells positive for HLA-Dr in a grade II astrocytoma.

grade/behavior. Metastatic extradural carcinomas could be infiltrated by large numbers of macrophages as they are outside the BBB. However macrophages were present in perivascular spaces in large number in intradural metastatic carcinomas and high grade astrocytomas, this, one could assume, because these tumors lead to disruption of the BBB. Outside the BBB, atypical meningiomas may elicit a stronger immune response than their "benign" counterparts.[159] Similarly, a difference between the extent of the macrophage infiltrate in high and low grade gliomas could still be explained by saying that the BBB is "intact" or only slightly or partly permeable in low grade gliomas. HLA-Dr expression by tumors may be positively correlated with macrophage infiltration and microglia activation and the local presence of co-stimulatory molecules like B7 mainly in "benign" tumors (atypical meningiomas, "benign" meningioma and low grade astrocytoma). It may also be similarly correlated with the stronger positivity (e.g., with the number of HLA-Dr molecules) of pericytic cell and macrophages in the immediate vicinity of blood vessels.[71,153]

All of the above militates for an attempt at mounting an immune reaction against the tumor by macrophage/microglia, lymphocytes, and cytokines.[28] In "malignant" brain tumors the depression of immunoreactivity of macrophages and microglia is probably tumor-driven.[160,161] In fact, high grade gliomas secrete cytokines such as the immunosuppressive factor transforming growth factor-β (TGF-β) *in vitro* and *in vivo*. This factor downregulates macrophage/microglial cytotoxicity in a rat glioma model.[162,163] TGF-β has multiple effects on the immune system, most of which are inhibitory, i.e. it is an important mediator of tumor progression, suppression of immune-mediated tumor reaction, and its local expression in normal brain maintains the natural immune unresponsiveness.[78] Oncogenesis may be the most important role of TGF-β that may involve the induction of apoptosis in the T-cell compartment.[164] Future immunotherapeutic strategies for malignant gliomas will have to focus on blocking TGF-β activity or other immunosuppressive molecules at the site of neoplastic growth by means of gene therapy (oligonucleotide anti-sense).

Growth factors such as macrophage-colony stimulating factor could be used to stimulate the immune response with a resulting increase in infiltrating macrophages and microglial activity.[165–167] Another approach is the observation of the presence of necrosis, where there is a higher percentage of macrophages[16] especially in malignant gliomas; this may depend on insufficient blood supply and/or apoptotic mechanism;[168] apoptosis may indeed play a role in the growth of gliomas.[169] Recently the Fas/APO-1 protein was found in 11% of low grade, 50% of high grade astrocytomas, and in all glioblastoma investigated.[168] FAS/APO-1 is a member of the nerve growth factor (NGF)/TNF receptor superfamily called Fas/APO-1, a transmembrane protein[170,171] that plays a role in apoptosis in glioma cells because it is triggered by Fas after binding with a Fas ligand or anti-Fas monoclonal antibody. Immunohistochemical studies show a preferential Fas expression by perinecrotic tumor cells, many of which show morphological changes of apoptosis.[169] This protein is however not inhibited by TGF-β.[164,172] Combining macrophage-targeted immunotherapy with gene therapy may hold the key to the future.

REFERENCES

1. MEDAWAR, P. B. 1948. Immunity to homologous grafted skin. III The fate of skin homograft transplanted to the brain, to subcutaneous tissue and to the anterior chamber of the eye. Br. J. Exp. Pathol. **29:** 58–69.
2. BARKER, B. A. & R. E. BILLINGHAM. 1968. The role of afferent lymphatics in the rejection of skin homografts. J. Exp. Med. **128:** 197–221.
3. POLLACK, I. & R. D. LUND. 1990. The blood-brain barrier protects foreign antigens in the brain from immune attack. Exp. Neurol. **108:** 114–121.
4. FABRY, Z., C. S. RAINE & M. N. HART. 1994. Nervous tissue as an immune compartment: the dialect of the immune response in the CNS. Immunol. Today **15:** 21–28.
5. KIDA, S., O. R. WELLER, E. T. ZHANG, M. J. PHILLIPS & F. IANNOTTE. 1995. Anatomical pathways for lymphatic drainage of the brain and their pathological significance. Neuropathol. Appl. Neurobiol. **21**(3): 181–184.
6. FONTANA, A., W. FIERZ & H. WEKERLE. 1984. Astrocyte present myelin basic protein to encephalitogenic T-cell lines. Nature **307:** 273–276.
7. GRAEBER, M. B. & W. J. STREIT. 1990. Microglia: immune network in the CNS. Brain Pathol. **1:** 2–5.
8. WIKSTRAND, C. J. & D. D. BIGNER. 1980. Immunobiological aspects of the brain and human glioma. A review. Am. J. Pathol. **98:** 517–567.
9. SCHNEIDER, J., F. M. HOFMAN, M. L. J. APUZZO & D. R. HINTON. 1992. Cytokines and immunoregulatory molecules in malignant glial neoplasm. J. Neurosurg. **77:** 265–273.

10. CHATEL, M., C. LEBRUN & M. FRENAY. 1993. Chemotherapy and immunotherapy in adult malignant gliomas. Curr. Opin. Oncol. **5:** 464–473.

11. FREI, K., C. SIEPL, P. GROSCURTH, S. BODMER, C. SCHWERDEL & A. FONTANA. 1985. Antigen presentation and tumor cytotoxicity by interferon-gamma-treated microglial cells. Eur. J. Immunol. **17:** 1271–1278.

12. SIRIS, J. H. 1936. Concerning the immunological specificity of glioblastoma multiforme. Bull. Neurol. NY. **4:** 597–601.

13. HASS, W. K. 1966. Soluble tissue antigens in human brain tumor and cerebrospinal fluid. Arch. Neurol. **14:** 443–447.

14. DELPECH, B., A. DELPECH, J. CLEMENT & R. LAUMONIER. 1972. Etude immunochimique et immunologique des tumeurs du cerveau humain. Int. J. Cancer **9:** 374–382.

15. PIGUET, V., S. CARREL, A. C. DISERENS, J. P. MACH & N. DE TRIBOLET. 1985. Heterogeneity of the induction of HLA-Dr expression by human immune interferon on glioma cell lines and their clones. J. Natl. Cancer Inst. **76:** 223–228.

16. ROSSI, M. L., J. T. HUGHES, M. M. ESIRI, H. B. COAKHAM & D. B. BROWNELL. 1987. Immunohistological study of mononuclear cell infiltrate in malignant gliomas. Acta Neuropathol. **74:** 269–277.

17. ROSSI, M. L. 1992. Study of the cellular immune response in intracranial tumours. PhD. Thesis. Council for National Academic Awards. University of London.

18. ROSSI, M. L., M. M. ESIRI, N. R. JONES, H. B. COAKHAM, T. H. MOSS, F. F. CRUZ-SANCHEZ & M. P. CAREY. 1991. Characterization of the mononuclear cell infiltrate and HLA-Dr expression in 19 oligodendrogliomas. Surg. Neurol. **36**(2): 119–125.

19. ROSSI, M. L., J. R. BULLER, S. A. HEATH, M. P. CAREY, P. CARBONI, JR., G. KOUTSOUBELIS & H. B. COAKHAM. 1991. The monocyte/macrophage infiltrate in 35 medulloblastomas: a paraffin-wax study. Tumori. **77:** 36–40.

20. ROSSI, M. L., N. R. JONES, M. M. ESIRI, L. HAVAS, M. AL. IZZI & H. B. COAKHAM. 1991. Mononuclear cell infiltrate and HLA-Dr expression in intra and extradural secondary carcinomas. Pathol. Res. Practice **187:** 55–61.

21. ROSSI, M. L., N. R. JONES, M. M. ESIRI, L. HAVAS & H. B. COAKHAM. 1991. Mononuclear cell infiltrate, HLA-Dr expression and proliferation in 37 acoustic schwannomas. Histol. Histopathol. **5:** 427–432.

22. ROSSI, M. L., H. B. COAKHAM, J. R. BULLER & S. A. HEATH. 1991. Monocyte/macrophage infiltrate in 41 oligodendrogliomas: a paraffin-wax study. Pathol. Res. Practice **187**(2–3): 166–169.

23. ROSSI, M. L., N. R. JONES, G. F. KARR, M. M. ESIRI, L. HAVANS & H. B. COAKHAM. 1991. HLA-Dr expression by tumour cells compared with survival in high grade astrocytomas. Tumori. **77:** 122–125.

24. ROSSI, M. L., N. R. JONES, M. M. ESIRI, L. HAVAS, M. AL. IZZI & H. B. COAKHAM. 1990. Mononuclear cell infiltrate and HLA-Dr expression in 28 pituitary adenomas. Tumori. **76:** 543–547.

25. ROSSI, M. L., N. R. JONES, E. CANDY, J. A. R. NICOLL, J. S. COMPTON, J. T. HUGHES, M. M. ESIRI, T. H. MOSS, F. F. CRUZ-SANCHEZ & H. B. COAKHAM. 1989. The mononuclear cell infiltrate compared with survival in high grade astrocytomas. Acta Neuropathol. **78:** 189–193.

26. ROSSI, M. L., F. F. CRUZ-SANCHEZ, J. T. HUGHES, M. M. ESIRI, H. B. COAKHAM & T. H. MOSS. 1988. Mononuclear cell infiltrate and HLA-Dr expression in low grade astrocytomas: an immunohistological study of 23 cases. Acta Neuropathol. **76:** 281–286.

27. ROSSI, M. L., F. F. CRUZ-SANCHEZ, J. T. HUGHES, M. M. ESIRI & H. B. COAKHAM. 1988. An immunocytochemical study of the cellular immune response in meningiomas. J. Clin. Pathol. **41:** 314–319.

28. ROSSI, M. L., M. M. ESIRI & H. B. COAKHAM. 1992. Immune response in intracranial tumours: a review. Fun. Neurol. **7:** 351–375.

29. HART, M. N. & Z. FABRY. 1995. CNS antigen presentation. Trends Neuroscien. **11:** 475–481.
30. GORDON, S., P. R. CROCKER & L. MORRIS. 1986. Localization and function of tissue macrophages. *In* Biochemistry of Macrophages. Ciba Foundation Symposium **118:** 54–67.
31. KINNEY, H. C. & D. D. ARMSTRONG. 1997. Perinatal neuropathology. *In* Greenfield's Neuropathology. Sixth Edit. D. I. Graham & P. L. Lantos, Eds. **1:** 535–599. Edition Arnold. London.
32. FUJITA, S. & T. KITAMURA. 1976. Origin of brain macrophages and the nature of the microglia. *In* Progress in Neuropathology. A. M. Zimmermann, Ed. **3:** 1–50. Grune & Stratton. New York.
33. OEHMICHEN, M. & H. HUBER. 1976. Reactive microglia with membrane features of mononuclear phagocytes. J. Neuropathol. Exp. Neurol. **35:** 30–39.
34. DEL RIO-HORTEGA P. 1932. Microglia. *In* Cytology and Cellular Pathology of the Nervous System. W. Penfield, Ed. **2:** 481–534. Hoeber. New York.
35. DEL RIO-HORTEGA P. 1919. El tercer elemento de los centro nerviosos. Boll. Soc. Espanol. Biol. **9:** 68–120.
36. BERRY, M. & A. M. BUTT. 1997. Structure and function of glia in the central nervous system. *In* Greenfield's Neuropathology. Sixth Edit. D. I. Graham & P. L. Lantos, Eds. **1:** 63–83. Edition Arnold. London.
37. LAWSON, L. J., V. H. D. P. PERRY & S. GORDON. 1991. Heterogeneity in the distribution and morphology of microglia in the normal, adult mouse brain. Neuroscience **39:** 151–170.
38. HAYNES, B. F. & S. M. DENNING. 1993. Lymphopoiesis. *In* The Molecular Basis of Blood Disease. Second Edit. Stamatoyannopoulus *et al.*, Eds. W. B. Saunders Company. Philadelphia.
39. ESIRI, M. M., P. URRY & J. KEELING. 1990. Lipid-containing cells in the brain in sudden infant death syndrome. Dev. Med. Child. Neurol. **32:** 319–324.
40. DAVIS, E. J., T. D. FOSTER & W. E. THOMAS. 1994. Cellular forms and functions of brain microglia. Brain Res. Bull. **34:** 73–78.
41. THEELE, D. P. & W. J. STREIT. 1993. A chronicle of microglial ontogeny. Glia **7:** 5–8.
42. PERRY, V. H., D. A. HUME & S. GORDON. 1985. Immunohistochemical localization of macrophages and microglia in the adult and developing mouse brain. Neuroscience **15:** 313–326.
43. PERRY, V. H. & D. GORDON. 1988. Macrophages and microglia in the nervous system. Trends Neuroscien. **11:** 273–277.
44. RICEVUTI, G., P. BIDOLI, M. DANESINO, A. MAZZONE, M. PIACENTINI, G. P. RICEVUTI, M. L. ROSSI *et al.* 1983. Study of the inflammatory response in patients with advanced neoplasia by means of the skin window tecquiques and cytochemical methods. J. Rev. Lab. Med. **10:** 589–593.
45. FISHMAN, R. A. Composition of the cerebrospinal fluid. 1992. *In* Cerebrospinal Fluid in Diseases of Nervous System. Second Edit. R. A. Fishman, Ed.: 183–252. W. B. Saunders Company. Philadelphia.
46. MAURI, C., S. C. RIZZO, G. RICEVUTI, EDS. 1987. The Biology of Phagocytes in Health and Disease. Advances in the Bioscience. Pergamon Press. Oxford.
47. VERGHESE, M. W. & R. SNYDERMAN. 1989. Chemotaxis and chemotactic factor. *In* Human Monocytes. M. Zembala & G. L. Asherson, Eds.: 167–176. Academic Press. London.
48. BALKWILL, F. R. 1989. Cytokine in Cancer Therapy. Oxford University Press. Oxford.
49. LEVY, G. A. & E. H. COLE. 1989. The monocyte and disseminated intravascular coagulation. *In* Human Monocytes. M. Zembala & G. L. Asherson, Eds.: 429–438. Academic Press. London.
50. ROSS, G. D., M. J. WALPORT & N. HOGG. 1989. Receptors for IgG Fc and fixed C3. *In* Hu-

man Monocytes. M. Zembala & G. L. Asherson, Eds.: 123–140. Academic Press. London.

51. BERTON, G. & S. GORDON. 1983. Modulation of macrophage mannosyl-specific receptors by cultivation on immobilised zymosan. Effects of superoxide-anion release and phagocytosis. Immunology **49:** 705–715.

52. CLINE, M. J. 1978. Monocytes, macrophages and their disease in man. Invest. Dermatol. **71:** 56–58.

53. GIULIAN, D. & L. B. LACHMAN. 1985. Interleukin-1 stimulation of astroglial proliferation after brain injury. Science **228:** 497–499.

54. LEIBOVICH, S. J., P. J. POLVERINI, H. M. SHEPARD et al. 1987. Macrophage-induced angiogenesis is mediated by tumor necrosis factor-α. Nature **329:** 630–632.

55. KREUTZBERG, G. W., W. F. BLAKEMORE & M. B. GRAEBER. 1997. Cellular pathology of central nervous system. *In* Greenfield's Neuropathology. D. I. Graham & P. L. Lantos, Eds. Sixth Edit. **1:** 85–156. Edition Arnold. London.

56. ALLEN, D. J. 1975. Scanning EM of epiplexus macrophages (Kolmer cells) in the dog. J. Comp. Neurol. **161:** 197–214.

57. GRAEBER, M. B., W. J. STREIT & G. W. KREUTZBERG. 1989. Identity of ED2-positive perivascular cells in rat brain. J. Neurosci. Res. **22:** 103–106.

58. RAINE, C. S. Neurocellular anatomy. 1994. *In* Basic Neurochemistry. Fifth Edit. G. J. Siegel, B. W. Agranoff, R. W. Albers & P. B. Molinoff, Eds. **1:** 32. Raven Press. New York.

59. HICKEY, W. F., K. VASS & H. LASSMANN. 1992. Bone marrow-derived elements in the central nervous system: An immunohistochemical and ultrastructural survey of rat chimeras. J. Neuropathol. Exp. Neurol. **51:** 246–256.

60. GRAEBER, M. B. & W. J. STREIT. 1990. Perivascular microglia defined. Trends Neurosci. **13:** 366.

61. FRANKLIN, W. A., D. Y. MASON, K. PULFORD et al. 1986. Immunohistological analysis of human mononuclear phagocytes and dendritic cells by using monoclonal antibodies. Lab. Invest. **54:** 322–335.

62. GRAEBER, M. B., W. J. STREIT, D. BURINGER et al. 1992. Ultrastructural location of MHC class II positive perivascular cells in histologically normal human brain. J. Neuropathol. Exp. Neurol. **51:** 303–311.

63. FREEMAN, G. J., A. S. FREEDMAN, J. M. SEGIL, G. LEE et al. 1989. B7, a new member of the Ig superfamily with unique expression on activated and neoplastic B cells. J. Immunol. **143:** 2714–2722.

64. JUNE, C. H., J. A. LEDBETTER & C. B. THOMPSON. 1990. Role of the CD28 receptor in T cell activation. Immunol. Today. **11:** 211–216.

65. DE SIMONE, R., A. GIAMPAOLO, B. GIOMETTO et al. 1995. The costimulatory molecule B7 is expressed on human microglia in culture and in multiple sclerosis acute lesions. J. Neuropathol. Exp. Neurol. **54:** 175–187.

66. DAVEY, S. R., J. R. CORDELL, W. N. ERBER et al. 1988. A monoclonal antibody (Y182a) with specificity towards peripheral blood monocytes and tissue macrophages. J. Clin. Pathol. **41:** 753–758.

67. ROGGENDORF, W., S. STRUPP & W. PAULUS. 1996. Distribution and characterisation of microglia/macrophages in human brain tumors. Acta Neuropathol. **92:** 288–293.

68. HERMANN, F., S. A. CANNISTRA, A. LINDEMANN et al. 1989. Functional consequences of monocyte IL-2 receptor expression. Induction of IL1 beta secretion by IFN-Y and IL-2. J. Immunology **142:** 139–143.

69. PIZZOLO, G., F. VINANTE, A. RIGO et al. 1993. Il recettore per l'interleuchina 2 sulle cellule normali e neoplastiche. Suppl. Haematol. **78:** 8–12.

70. ADAMS, D. O. & T. A. HAMILTON. 1984. The cell biology of macrophage activation. Ann. Rev. Immunol. **2:** 283–318.

71. Tada, M. & N. de Tribolet. 1993. Recent advances in immunobiology of brain tumors. J. Neuro-Oncol. **17:** 261–271.

72. Lanzavecchia, A. 1993. A identifying strategies for immune intervention. Science **260:** 937–944.

73. Maudsley, D. J. & J. D. Pound. 1991. Modulation of MHC antigen expression by viruses and oncogenes. Immunol. Today **12:** 429–431.

74. Jennings, M. T., S. A. D. Ebrahim, H. T. Thaler, V. D. L. Jennings *et al.* 1989. Immunophenotypic differences between normal glia, astrocytomas and malignant glioma: correlation with karyotype, natural history and survival. J. Neuroimmunol. **25:** 7–28.

75. Zembala, M. & G. L. Asherson. 1989. Human Monocytes. Academic Press. London.

76. Cotran, R. S., V. Kumar & S. L. Robbins, Eds. 1989. Pathological basis of disease. Fourth Edit. W. B. Saunders Company. Philadelphia.

77. Hogg, N. 1986. Factor-inducer differentiation and activation of macrophages. Immunol. Today **7:** 65–66.

78. Weller, M. & A. Fontana. 1995. The failure of current immunotherapy for malignant glioma. Tumor-derived TGF-beta, T-cell apoptosis, and the immune privilege of the brain. Brain Res. Rev. **21:** 128–151.

79. Kurland, K. K., R. S. Bockman, H. E. Broxmeyer *et al.* 1978. Limitation of excessive myelopoiesis by the intrinsic modulation of macrophage-derived prostaglandin E. Science **199:** 552–556.

80. Stenson, W. F. & C. W. Parker. 1980. Prostaglandins, macrophages and immunity. J. Immunol. **125:** 1–5.

81. Bonney, R. J. & P. Davies. 1984. Possible autoregulatory functions of the secretory products of mononuclear phagocytes. Contemp. Top. Immunol. **13:** 99–218.

82. Ferreri, N. R., L. Beck & L. Spiegels. 1986. Beta-glucuronidase release from human monocytes induced with aggregated immunoglobulins of different classes. Cell. Immunol. **98:** 57–67.

83. Barron, K. D. 1995. The microglial cell. A historical review. J. Neurol. Scien. **134:** 57–68.

84. Nissl, F. 1899. Uber einige Beziehungen zwischen Nervenzellenrkrankungen und gliosen Erscheinungen bei verschiedenen Psychosen. Arch. Psychiat. **32:** 1–21.

85. Barron, K. D., E. D. Means, T. Feng & H. Harris. 1974. Ultrastructure of retrograde degeneration in thalamus of rat 2. Changes in vascular elements and transvascular migration of leucocytes. Exp. Mol. Pathol. **20:** 344–362.

86. Ramon Cajal S. 1952. Nevroglie. *In* Histologie du systeme nerveux de l'homme & des vertebres. Edicion preparada por el Instituto "Ramon y Cajal" con motivo del primer centenario de su fundador y maestro. **1:** 230–252. Instituto Ramon y Cajal. Madrid.

87. Gehrmann, J. & R. B. Banati. 1995. Microglial turnover in the injured CNS: activated microglia undergo delayed DNA fragmentation following peripheral nerve injury. J. Neuropathol. Exp. Neurol. **54:** 680–688.

88. Gehrmann, J., Y. Matsumoto & G. W. Kreutzeberg. 1995. Microglia: intrinsic immunoeffector cell of the brain. Brain Res. Rev. **20:** 269–287.

89. Leong, S. K. & E. A. Ling. 1992. Ameboid and ramified microglia: their interrelationship and response to brain injury. Glia **7:** 39–47.

90. Lassmann, H., M. Schmied, K. Vass & W. F. Hickey. 1993. Bone marrow derived elements and resident microglia in brain inflammation. Glia **7:** 19–24.

91. Sievers, J., R. Parwaresch & H. V. Woltge. 1994. Blood monocytes and spleen macrophages differentiate into microglia-like cells on monolayers of astrocytes: morphology. Glia **12:** 245–258.

92. Ling, E. A. & W. C. Wong. 1993. The origin and nature of ramified and ameboid neuroglia: a historical review and current concept. Glia **7:** 9–18.

93. LAWSON, L. J., V. H. PERRY & S. GORDON. 1992. Turnover of resident microglia in the normal adult mouse brain. Neuroscience **48:** 405–415.
94. DICKSON, D. W., L. A. MATTIACE, K. KURE & K. HUTCHINS. 1991. Microglia in human disease, with an emphasis on acquired immune deficiency syndrome. Lab. Invest. **64:** 135–156.
95. ULVESTEAD, E., K. WILLIAMS, S. MORK, J. ANTEL & H. NYLAND. 1994. Phenotypic difference between human monocytes/macrophages and microglial cells studied in situ and in vitro. J. Neuropathol. Exp. Neurobiol. **53:** 492–501.
96. STREIT, W. J., M. B. GRAEBER & G. W. KREUTZEBERG. 1989. Expression of Ia antigen on perivascular and microglial cells after sublethal and lethal motor neuron injury. Exp. Neurol. **105:** 115–126.
97. STREIT, W. J., M. B. GRAEBER & G. W. KREUTZEBERG. 1989. Peripheral nerve lesion produces increased levels of MHC antigens in the CNS. J. Neuroimmunol. **21:** 117–123.
98. GERHMANN, J. & G. W. KREUTZEBERG. 1995. Microglia in experimental neuropathology. *In* Neuroglial Cells. B. Ransom & H. Kettenmann, Eds. Oxford University Press. Oxford.
99. ULVESTAD, E., K. WILLIAMS, C. VEDELER *et al.* 1994. Reactive microglia in multiple sclerosis lesions have an increased expression of receptors for the Fc part of IgG. J. Neurol. Sci. **121:** 125–131.
100. GRAEBER, M. B., W. J. STREIT & G. W. KREUTZEBERG. 1988. Axotomy of the rat facial nerve leads to increased CR3 complement receptor expression by activated microglial cells. J. Neurosci. Res. **21:** 18–24.
101. MCLAURIN, J., G. ALMAZAN, K. WILLIAMS & J. P. ANTEL. 1995. Immortalization and characterization of rat microglial cells. Neuropathol. Appl. Neurobiol. **21:** 302–311.
102. STREIT, W. J. 1990. An improved staining method for rat microglial cells using the lectin from Griffonia simplicifolia (GSA I-B4). J. Histochem. Cytochem. **38:** 1683–1686.
103. MANNOJI, H., H. YEGER & L. E. BECKER. 1986. A specific histochemical marker (lectin Ricinus communis agglutinin-1) for normal human microglia, and application to routine histopathology. Acta Neuropathol. **71:** 341–344.
104. MURABE, Y. & Y. SANO. 1981. Thiamine pyrophosphatase activity in the plasma membrane of microglia. Histochemistry **71:** 45–52.
105. MURABE, Y. & Y. SANO. 1982. Morphological studies on neuroglia. VI. Postnatal development of microglial cells. Cell Tissue Res. **225:** 469–485.
106. WOLSWIJK, G. 1994. GD3 cells in the adult rat and optic nerve are ramified microglia rather than 0-2A adult progenitor cells. Glia **10:** 244–249.
107. PERRY, W. V., M. K. MATYSZASK & S. FEARN. 1993. Altered antigen expression of microglia in the aged rodent CNS. Glia **7:** 60–67.
108. STREIT, W. J., M. B. GRAEBER & G. W. KREUTZBERG. 1988. Functional plasticity of microglia: a review. Glia **1:** 301–307.
109. JORDAN, C. A., B. A. WATKINS, C. KUFTA & M. DUBOIS-DALCQ. 1991. Infection of brain microglia cells by human immunodeficiency virus type-1 is CD4 dependent. J. Virol. **65:** 736–742.
110. SHIGEMATSU, K., P. L. MCGEER, D. G. WALKER *et al.* 1992. Reactive microglia/macrophage phagocyte amyloid precursor protein produced by neurons following neural damage. J. Neurosci. Res. **33:** 549–558.
111. MCGEER, P. L., T. KAWAMATA, D. G. WALKER, H. AKIYAMA, I. TOOYAMA & E. G. MCGEER. 1993. Microglia in degenerative neurological disease. Glia **7:** 84–92.
112. RAINE, C. S. 1994. Multiple sclerosis: immune system molecules expression in the central nervous system. J. Neuropathol. Exp. Neurol. **53:** 328–337.
113. CLARK, J. M. 1974. Distribution of microglial clusters in the brain after head injury. J. Neurol. Neurosurg. Psychiatry. **37:** 463–474.

114. MORIOKA, T., A. N. KALHEUA & W. J. STREIT. 1993. Characterisation of microglial reaction after middle cerebral artery occlusion in rat brain. J. Comp. Neurol. **327:** 123–132.

115. GEHRMANN, J., R. B. BANATI, C. WIESSNERT, K-A. HOSSMANN & G. W. KREUTZBERG. 1995. Reactive microglia in cerebral ischaemia: an early mediator of tissue damage? Neuropathol. Appl. Neurobiol. **21:** 277–289.

116. PENFIELD, W. 1925. Microglia and the process of phagocytosis in glioma. Am. J. Pathol. **1:** 77–79.

117. SASAKI, A., J. HIRATO & Y. NAKAZATO. 1993. Immunohistochemical study of microglia in the Creutzfeldt-Jakob diseased brain. Acta Neuropathol. **86:** 337–344.

118. BURNET, F. M. 1959. The clonal selection theory of acquired immunity. Cambridge University Press. Cambridge.

119. JERNE, N. K. 1955. The natural-selection theory of antibody formation. Proc. Natl. Acad. Sci. U.S.A. **41:** 849–865.

120. BURNET, F. M. 1970. The concept of immunological surveillance. Prog. Exp. Tumor Res. **13:** 1–27.

121. FRAUMENI, J. R. & R. HOOVER. 1977. Immunosurveillance and cancer: epidemiological observation. Natl. Cancer Inst. Mongr. **47:** 121–126.

122. KRIPKE, M. L. 1988. Immunoregulation of carcinogenesis: past, present, and future. J. Natl. Canc. Inst. **80:** 722–727.

123. FOGH, J. & B. GIOVANELLA, EDS. 1978. The Nude Mouse in Experimental and Clinical Research. Academic Press. New York.

124. KLEIN, G. & E. KLEIN. 1977. Immunosurveillance against virus induced tumors and non-rejectability of spontaneous tumors: contrasting consequences of host versus tumor evolution. Proc. Natl. Acad. Sci. U.S.A. **74:** 2121–2125.

125. ANDERSON, T. M., Y. IBAYASHI & E. C. HOLMES. 1987. Modification of natural kill cell activity of lymphocytes infiltrating human lung cancer. Cancer Immunol. Immunother. **25:** 65–68.

126. MURPHY, J. B. & E. STURM. 1923. Conditions determining the transplantation of tissue in the brain. J. Exp. Med. **38:** 183–197.

127. FUCHS, H. E. & D. E. BULLARD. 1988. Immunology of transplantation in the central nervous system. Appl. Neurophysiol. **51:** 278–296.

128. LASSMANN, H., F. ZAMPRICH, K. ROSSLER & K. VASS. 1991. Inflammation in the nervous system: basic mechanism and immunological concepts. Rev. Neurol. **147:** 763–781.

129. SCHEINBERG, L. C., F. L. EDELMAN & W. A. LEVY. 1964. Is the brain "an immunological privileged site"? Arch. Neurol. **38:** 183–197.

130. WELLER, R. O., B. ENGELHARD & M. J. PHILIPS. 1996. Lymphocyte targeting of the central nervous system: a review of afferent and efferent CNS-immune pathways. Brain Pathol. **6:** 275–288.

131. LAMPSON, L. A. & W. F. HICKEY. 1986. Monoclonal antibody analysis of the MHC expression in human brain biopsies. J. Immunol. **136:** 4054–4062.

132. DE TRIBOLET, N., M. F. HAMOU, J. P. MACH *et al.* 1984. Demonstration of HLA-DR antigens in normal human brain. J. Neurol. Neurosurg. Psychiatry **74:** 417–418.

133. VON HANWEHR, R. I., F. M. HOFMAN, C. R. TAYLOR & M. L. J. APUZZO. 1984. Mononuclear lymphoid populations infiltrating the microenvironment of primary CNS tumors. J. Neurosurg. **60:** 1138–1147.

134. SAWAMURA, Y. & N. DE TRIBOLET. 1990. Immunobiology of brain tumours. Adv. Technol. Stand. Neurosurg. **17:** 3–64.

135. MONOD, L., Y. SAWAMURA & N. DE TRIBOLET. 1992. Immunotherapie des tumeurs du systeme nerveux central. Neurochirurgie **38:** 69–79.

136. CSERR, H. F. & P. M. KNOPF. 1995. Cervical lymphatics, the blood-brain barrier and the immunoreactivity of the brain: a new view. Immunol. Today **13:** 507–513.

137. BROOKS, W. H., M. G. NEYSKY, D. A. HORWITZ & D. E. NORMANSELL. 1990. Depressed cell-mediated immunity in patients with primary intracranial tumor. J. Exp. Med. **136:** 1631–1647.
138. JAECKLE, K. A. 1994. Immunotherapy of malignant gliomas. Semin. Oncol. **21:** 249–259.
139. BULLARD, D. E., G. Y. GILLESPIE, M. S. MAHALEY *et al.* 1986. Immunobiology of human gliomas. Semin. Oncol. **13:** 94–109.
140. ESIRI, M. M. & J. O'D. MCGEE. 1986. Monoclonal antibody to macrophages (EBM11) labels macrophages and microglial cells in human brain. J. Clin. Pathol. **39:** 615–621.
141. BERTRAND, I. & H. MANNEN. 1960. Etudes des reactions vasculaires dans les astrocytomes. Rev. Neurol. **102:** 3–19.
142. RIDLEY, A. & J. B. CAVANAGH. 1971. Lymphocytic infiltration in gliomas: evidence of possible host resistance. Brain **94:** 117–124.
143. GIOMETTO, B., F. BOZZA, F. FARESIN, L. ALESSIO, S. MINGRINO & B. TAVOLATO. 1996. Immune infiltrates and cytokines in gliomas. Acta Neurochir. **138:** 50–56.
144. SCHIFFER, D., G. CROVERI & C. PAUTASSO. 1974. Frequenza e significato degli infiltrati linfo-plasmacellulari nei gliomi umani. Tumori. **60:** 177–184.
145. UNDERWOOD, J. C. 1974. Lymphoreticular infiltration in human tumors: prognostic and biological implications: a review. Br. J. Cancer. **30:** 538–548.
146. JAMES, K., B. MCBRIDE & A. STUART. 1977. The macrophage and cancer. Eures. Symp. Edinburgh.
147. STAVROU, D., A. P. ANZIL, W. WEIDENBACH & H. RODT. 1977. Immunofluorescence study of lymphocytic infiltration in gliomas. Identification of T lymphocytes. J. Neurol. Sci. **33:** 275–282.
148. STEVENS, A., I. KLOTER & W. ROGGENDORF. 1988. Inflammatory infiltrates and natural killer cell presence in human brain tumors. Cancer **61:** 738–743.
149. PAULUS, W., W. ROGGENDORF & T. KIRCHNER. 1992. Ki-M1P as a marker for microglia and brain macrophages in routinely processed human tissue. Acta Neuropathol. **84:** 538–544.
150. WILLIAMS, A. E., S. RYDER & W. F. BLAKEMORE. 1995. Monocyte recruitment into the scrapie-affected brain. Acta Neuropathol. **90:** 164–169.
151. IWASAKI, Y., K. SAKO, I. TSUNODA & Y. OHARA. 1993. Phenotypes of mononuclear cell infiltrates in human central nervous system. Acta Neuropathol. **85:** 653–657.
152. PULDORF, K. A. F., E. M. RIGNEY, K. J. MICKLEM, M. JONES *et al.* 1989. KP1: a new monoclonal antibody that detects a monocyte/macrophage-associated antigen in routinely processed tissue sections. J. Clin. Pathol. **42:** 414–421.
153. MORIOKA, T., T. BABA, K. L. BLACK & W. J. STREIT. 1992. The response of microglial cells to experimental rat glioma. Glia **6:** 75–79.
154. MORANTZ, R. A., G. W. WOOD, M. FOSTER, M. CLARK & K. GOLLAHON. 1979. Macrophage in experimental and human brain tumours. Part 1: studies of the macrophages content of experimental rat brain. **50:** 298–304.
155. MORANTZ, R. A., G. W. WOOD, M. FOSTER, M. CLARK & K. GOLLAHON. 1979. Macrophage in experimental and human brain tumours. Part 2: studies of the macrophages content of human brain tumours. J. Neurosurg. **50:** 305–311.
156. RUSSELL, D. S. & L. J. RUBINSTEIN. 1989. Pathology of tumors of the nervous system. Edition Arnold. London.
157. RADZUN, H. J., M. L. HANSMANN, H. J. HEIDEBRECHT, S. BODEWADT-RADZUN, H. H. WACKER, H. KREIPE, H. LUMBECK, H. HERNANDEZ *et al.* 1991. Detection of a monocyte/macrophage differentiation antigen in routinely processed paraffin-embedded tissue by monoclonal antibody Ki-MP1. Lab. Invest. **65:** 306–315.
158. LENNERT, K. & A. C. FELLER. 1992. Histopathology of non-Hodgkin's lymphomas. Edition Springer. Berlin.

159. WOOD, G. W. & R. A. MORANTZ. 1979. Immunohistological evaluation of lymphoreticular infiltration in human CNS tumors. J. Natl. Cancer Inst. **62:** 485–490.

160. BODMER, S., K. STROMMER, K. FREI, C. SIEPL, N. DE TRIBOLET, I. HEID & A. FONTANA. 1989. Immunosuppression and transforming growth factor-beta in glioblastoma. Preferential production of transforming growth factor-beta 2. J. Immunol. **143:** 3222–3229.

161. STREIT, W. J. 1994. Cellular immune response in brain tumours. Neuropathol. Appl. Neurobiol. **20:** 175–216.

162. SCHEINEDER, J., F. M. HOFMAN, M. L. APUZZO & D. R. HINTON. 1992. Cytokines and immunoregulatory molecules in malignant glial neoplasms. J. Neurosurg. **77:** 265–273.

163. KIEFER, R., M. L. SUPLER, K. V. TOYKA & W. J. STREIT. 1994. In situ detection of transforming growth factor-beta mRNA in experimental rat glioma and reactive glia cells. Neurosci. Lett. **166:** 161–164.

164. WELLER, M., K. FREI, P. GROSCURTH, P. H. KRAMMER, Y. YONEKAWA & A. FONTANA. 1994. Anti-Fas/APO-1 antibody-mediated apoptosis of cultured human glioma cells. J. Clin. Invest. **94:** 954–964.

165. GIOMETTO, B., F. BOZZA, P. GALLO *et al.* 1992. Growth factor (M-CSF) and antigenic properties of macrophages in meningioma. J. Neuro-Oncol. **13:** 25–33.

166. GIOMETTO, B. & B. TAVOLATO. 1993. Immunologia dei tumori cerebrali. *In* Neuroimmunologia clinica. B. Tavolato, Ed. Il Pensiero Scientifico Editore. Roma.

167. JADUS, M. R., M. C. IRWIN, M. R. IRWIN, R. D. HORANSKY, S. SEKHON *et al.* 1996. Macrophage can recognise and kill tumor cell bearing the membrane isoform of macrophage colony-stimulating factor. Blood **87**(12): 5232–5241.

168. TACHIBANA, O., H. NAKAZAWA, J. LAMPE *et al.* 1995. Expression of Fas/APO-1 during the progression of astrocytoma. Cancer Res. **55:** 5528–5530.

169. LANTOS, P. L., S. R. VANDEBERG, P. KLEIHUES & M. B. S. LOPES. 1997. Tumours of the nervous system. *In* Greenfield's Neuropathology. Sixth Edit. D. I. Graham & P. L. Lantos, Eds. Vol. 2. Edition Arnold. London.

170. ITOH, N., S. YONEHARA, A. ISHII *et al.* 1991. The polypeptide encode by the cDNA for human cell surface antigen Fas can mediate apoptosis. Cell **66:** 233–243.

171. WATANABE-FUKUNAGA, R., C. I. BRANNAN, N. ITOH *et al.* 1992. The cDNA structure, expression and chromosomal assignment of the mouse Fas antigen. J. Immunol. **148:** 1274–1279.

172. WELLER, M., U. MALIPIERO, A. RENSING-EHL, P. BARR & A. FONATANA. 1995. Fas/APO-1 gene transfer for human malignant glioma. Cancer Res. **55:** 2936–2944.

Host Tissue Damage by Phagocytes

GIOVANNI RICEVUTI

Dipartimento di Medicina Interna e Terapia Medica
Sezione di Medicina Interna e Nefrologia
U.O. di Medicina Interna
Università degli Studi di Pavia
IRCCS Policlinico San Matteo
Pavia, Italy

INTRODUCTION

Cells that efficiently engulf a wide variety of microbes are termed professional phagocytes (TABLE 1).[1,2,44,46,47,78] This is to distinguish them from such non-specialized cells as fibroblasts, which may only make ineffective attempts to ingest foreign particles (TABLE 2).[78,93] Professional phagocytes (TABLE 1) include monocytes, macrophages, eosinophils, and polymorphonuclear leukocytes, also known as neutrophils (PMNs). Macrophages are long-living cells that are localized to various organs where they provide for a relatively stationary defense against organisms entering the body via the respiratory tract (alveolar macrophages), gastrointestinal tract (liver Kupffer cells and peritoneal macrophages), bloodstream (splenic macrophages and Kupffer cells), skin (Langherans cells), and lymphatics (lymph node macrophages).[47,78] Monocytes are formed in the marrow and can differentiate into macrophages to repopulate these areas. In addition, monocytes can leave the bloodstream to challenge local tissue invaders.[34,78]

The role of the eosinophil is not as well delineated but its major function is in defending the host against parasites.[78]

PMNs are qualitatively and quantitatively the most important phagocytic cells acting against acute bacterial infections.[49,50,65,71,78] They originate from the bone marrow and travel via the bloodstream. In response to the appropriate stimulus they leave the circulation and migrate towards the invading microorganisms and, given the appropriate conditions, they engulf and destroy them.[49,73] Chemotactic substances "guide" phagocytes to the infecting organisms. Antibody and complement can function as opsonins and enhance the ability of PMNs to engulf microbes and ingested organisms are killed by oxidative and nonoxidative systems.[87–93] Defects in the various aspects of PMNs function may be found in patients with recurrent, severe, or unusual infections.[3,7,8,17,22,46,47,49,65,81]

There is growing evidence that phagocytes may not only be considered as friends but also as foes as they may be involved in the causation of a variety of conditions.[3,14,16,18,24,30,34,38,41,44,47,50,53,65,68,73,74,78,80] Phagocytes play an important role in the inflammatory process as the first line of defense by producing toxic oxygen intermediates and proteolytic enzymes, and by modifying the expression of surface adhesion molecules. When engaged in "frustrated phagocytosis" they can cause tissue damage (TABLE 3).[3,24,44,46,68,71]

TABLE 1. The Phagocytic Network

Professional Phagocytes

Polymorphonuclear leukocytes
Mononuclear phagocytes

Variety of Phenotypes

Bone marrow: macrophages, monocytes, sinusoidal cells, lining cells
Bone tissue: osteoclasts
Gut and intestinal Peyer patches: macrophages
Connective tissue: histiocytes, macrophages, monocytes
Liver: Kupffer cells, monocytes
Lung: self-replicating macrophages, monocytes
Lymphoid tissue: free and fixed macrophages and monocytes
Nervous system: microglial cells (CD4+)
Spleen: free and fixed macrophages, sinusoidal lining cells, monocytes
Thymus: free and fixed macrophages, monocytes
Skin: resident Langerhans cells, dendritic cells, conventional macrophages

---

MECHANISMS OF TISSUE DAMAGE BY PHAGOCYTES

Tissue damage may be caused by phagocytes that normally flow through vessels, whereas they become adherent to the endothelium before diapedesis and cause damage to it and extravasal tissues.[7,11,17,22,31,35,44,47,50,60,65,74,80,81] Damage is mediated by the release of an impressive array of toxic products such as proteolytic enzymes, reactive oxygen radicals, and cationic proteins.[35,44,47,80] Primary, secondary, and tertiary granules of phagocytes are the source of these products and their release is facilitated by prior priming of phagocytes (TABLES 4 and 5).[34,54,74] Primers of exocytosis are both humoral and cellular. These primers are closely related to the process of phagocyte activation, which is one of the most important mechanisms involved in tissue damage by phagocytes.[87–93]

When activated, phagocytes adhere, an exuberant release of neutrophil metabolites occurs, and tissue damage is caused.[19,47,65,80] Therefore, phagocytes play a role

TABLE 2. The Phagocytic Network

Non Professional Phagocytes

Lymphocytes
NK and LGL cells
Platelets
Mast cells
Epithelial cells
Endothelial cells
Fibroblasts
HeLa cells
Erythrocytes

TABLE 3. Phagocyte Related Diseases

Alteration of cell rheology
Mechanical shear stress
Capillary obstruction
Release of free radicals
Release of leukotrienes and prostaglandins
Oxygen reperfusion injury
Cell-cell interaction
Priming
Inflammatory-immune injury and sepsis
Cigarette smoking
Cerebrovascular damage
Cerebrovascular ischemia
Atherosclerosis
Aging and senile dementia
DNA damage
Carcinogenesis
Bone resorption
Osteopetrosis
Cataractogenesis and retinopathy
Alcohol and doxorubicin cardiomyopathy
Porphyria, psoriasis, and dermal injury
Endothelial damage
Thrombosis and cid
Periodontal disease
Vasculitis

in maintaining homeostasis and in host defense but can also be mediators of damage in non-infectious diseases, especially when activated. When activation occurs, phagocytes begin to display highly characteristic pseudopodia, their metabolism is activated, superoxide radicals are formed, lysosomal release is triggered, and membrane adhesion energy processes increase.[74]

The main mechanisms involved in these conditions are priming and activation, upregulation and/or downregulation of adhesion molecules, cytokines release, release of lysosomal enzymes and of biological response modifiers, activation of the

TABLE 4. Neutrophil Mediated Inflammation

The acute inflammatory response is our first line of host defense. The vascular and tissue reactions that characterize the early stage of inflammation are remarkably similar in different kinds of injury and the neutrophil is the primary effector cell of this response.

(1) During inflammation a large number of neutrophil start to roll along and then firmly adhere to the endothelial cell at the site of injury.

(2) They migrate across the vessel wall into the surrounding tissue with the only purpose of ingesting and disposing of any unwanted material.

TABLE 5. Phagocyte Derived Inflammatory Mediators

The uncontrolled and overexuberant production of neutrophil's metabolites released into the surrounding milieu is partly responsible for the tissue damage often observed with acute inflammation and with chronic inflammatory disease.

Neutrophil-Derived Inflammatory Mediators

Eicosanoids, a group of potent pro-inflammatory lipids: LTs, PGs

Platelet-activating factors (PAF)

Neutrophil proteases and cationic protein contained in azurophil granules of neutrophils (e.g., defensins, elastase, cathepsin G and B, proteinase 3 and 4). There is evidence that the inappropriate release of these proteins is a contributing factor to tissue injury in SLE patients with glomerulonephritis

Cytokines: IL-1a and b, IL-6, IL-8, IFN, CSF TGF, TNF, etc.

arachidonic acid pathway and leukotriene release, and stimulation of cell-cell interaction.[87–93] In particular,[27,58,74] four mechanisms of activation have been identified to date: (*1*) via direct receptor stimulation by chemotactic substances such as LPS, endotoxins, complement, short-chain peptide sequences, cytokines, fatty acid products, and others; (*2*) by cell contact activation, a mechanism that can be effective in relation to endothelial cells; (*3*) by depletion of intrinsic deactivators such as adenosine and albumin; and (*4*) by mechanical shear stress.[74] Any of these pathways can convert a relatively benign circulating phagocyte into a mediator of cytotoxicity with no regard for innocent bystander cells.[87–93]

It is through the combination of exocytosis of ROI, kininogens, and vW factor that PMNs bridge inflammation, thrombosis, and atherosclerosis. In addition, ROI exocytosis causes lipoperoxydation.[1,6,7,10,15,17,24,25,30,31,33,51,65,74,78,80,81,83]

Free radicals are molecules or parts of molecules[17,46,47,60,66,77,83] that tend to be particularly reactive because they possess an unpaired electron in the outer orbit. They have been implicated in several pathological and physiological processes, including defense against infection, mutagenesis, and aging, but also cardiovascular biology.[3,47,65,68,69,74] Cardiovascular events that involve, or may involve, free radical–mediated processes include reperfusion arrhythmias,[16,22,29] reperfusion myocardial injury,[8,12,14,20,26,27,43,44,50,60,68,71,80,83–85] endothelial damage, and formation of atheroma.[22,32,33,35,44,46,50,66,71,74] Therefore, free radicals can react with each of the major classes of biological macromolecules and cause damage to proteins, nucleic acids, and lipids.[87–93] The reaction with certain amino acids may lead to the production of specific end products, such as protein carbonyls and bithyrosine, which can be used as markers of oxidative activity. It seems likely that many of the acute biological effects of free radicals will turn out to be mediated by the reaction with specific residues of proteins playing a crucial signaling role in cell function. Free radicals may interact either with purine or pyrimidine bases, or with the ribose phosphate backbone to produce strand breaks.[8,17,25]

The reaction of unsaturated aliphatic fatty acids with reactive oxygen species has already been referred to. Lipids are of particular interest as targets of free radical for several reasons: their susceptibility to radical-induced chain reactions, sometimes involving chain branching, their important role in biological membranes, and the increasing evidence for the involvement of partially oxidized lipids in atherogenesis by stimulating phagocytosis by macrophages, and possibly by stimulating the production of autoantibodies.[87–93]

The confirmation that reactive oxygen intermediates (ROI) are involved in the pathogenesis of arrhythmias may pave the way for the use of antioxidant drugs in their prevention.[17]

Free radicals produced by phagocytes have been implicated in some aspects of tumorigenesis by inducing genomic damage.[3,8,47,65,74,80]

Examples of phagocyte-related pathological conditions are listed in TABLE 3 according to the organ system.

PHAGOCYTE AND ENDOTHELIUM

Great interest has been aroused by the mechanism whereby inflammatory cells, especially activated PMNs damage vascular endothelium. Jacob and Vercellotti[12,34,35,43,44,47,50,53,65,74,80,86] believe granulocyte-mediated endothelial cytotoxicity is germane to a variety of clinical states, including immune complex vasculitis, some forms of adult respiratory distress syndrome, transient pulmonary dysfunction seen in hemodialyzed patients, and perhaps most importantly, atherosclerosis.[12,34,35,43,44,47,50,53,65,74,80,86] PMNs can lyse cultured endothelial cells, both by releasing toxic oxygen species and through proteolytic enzymes (TABLES 6 and 7). In the former case, oxygen species such as hydrogen peroxide, hydroxyl radical, and hypochlorous acid have all been shown to mediate granulocyte-induced endothelial damage *in vitro*. Jacob and Vercellotti[86] reported that lactoferrin amplifies endothelial damage by generating hydroxyl radicals, and that PAF primes PMNs to become endothelial cytotoxins.[87–93]

PMNs of peripheral blood form the first line of defense against foreign substances. Defense reactions against invaders include release of lysosomal constituents and the production of oxygen metabolites as a result of the respiratory burst associated with phagocytosis. The PMN however has little ability to differen-

TABLE 6. Phagocyte-Endothelial Interaction

In health, neutrophils do not adhere to endothelial cells or to connective tissue components. The adhesive interaction between neutrophil and endothelial cell is the hallmark of acute inflammation. In its capacity as a response to injury, inflammation must deal with at least two major circumstances:

- preservation of epithelial barrier function
- remodeling of tissue through removal of injured tissue
- ischemia reperfusion injury (myocardial infarction)
- direct mechanical injury
- physical injury (heat, radiation)
- chemical injury (irritants, toxins)
- immunological injury (autoimmune disease)

TABLE 7. Mechanisms of the Phagocyte Emigration

Neutrophil attraction and emigration is initiated by chemical signal (chemoattactants) sent by the tissue to the local microvasculature.

Neutrophil Chemoattractants

(1) Humoral factors

- complement fragment C5a des Arg
- fibrinopeptides
- fibrin degradation products

(2) Cellular factors

- IL-1
- IL-8
- TNF
- fMLP
- leukotriene B4

---

tiate between foreign and host antigens and, if normal host tissues are identified as damaged, the appropriate receptors on the plasma membrane of the PMN will be engaged eliciting its destructive potential.[2,3,30,43] Endothelial injury alters the physiological interaction between leukocytes and vessel wall increasing the adhesion of PMNs to endothelial cells. Damaged endothelium leads to the exposure of membrane receptors for immunoglobulin and complement fragments, thus further promoting PMN adherence.[1,4,5,9,13,16,18,19,22,27,30,31,33,34,37,40,46,73,76,78,83,86] Moreover, the recent demonstration that cultured endothelial cells synthesize platelet-activating factor (PAF), also a potent PMN activating factor, and release substances with chemotactic activity supports the concept that the endothelium is capable of generating mediators that can locally influence PMN function. It has also been shown that PMN activation may be triggered by 15 minutes of tissue ischemia followed by reperfusion. PMNs are potent effector cells that, once activated, are capable of releasing a variety of inflammatory mediators.[2,13,17,18,66] Granule constituents, reactive oxygen metabolites, and extracellularly released products of membrane phospholipases have been demonstrated to induce vascular injury or to alter vascular function *in vitro* and *in vivo*. Among the granule-based proteolytic enzymes, elastase has great potential for tissue destruction and may cause detachment, lysis, or derangement of endothelial cell barrier properties. It has recently been shown that PMN elastase detaches endothelial cells from culture substrates *in vitro* and that it degrades subendothelial matrices secreted by venous endothelial cells. In addition to its proteolytic activity, PMN elastase can provoke the release of endothelial adenine nucleotides by a process not involving the catalytic site. A substantial body of evidence suggests that platelets and PMNs interact potentiating each others effects on endothelial cells.[1,4,10,13,18,20,25,30,31,33,34,40,63,68,71,72,76,77,80,83] Platelets amplify PMN adherence to endothelial cells and may augment PMN cytotoxicity through the release of granule constituents such as serotonin or one of its metabolites. The concept of the reciprocal interaction between platelets and PMNs is strengthened by the observation that damaged endothelium may release PAF. This phospholipid, produced by a wide variety of cells including PMNs and platelets, is a pivotal mediator in the initiation and propagation of acute inflammatory responses, PMNs and platelet aggregation, increased adhesion of circulating leukocytes to endothelium, and in stimulating the respiratory oxidative burst.[87–93]

PHAGOCYTES AND ISCHEMIC HEART DISEASE

Research on the effects of PMNs on myocardial ischemia could lead to major breakthroughs in explaining the pathophysiology of ischemia and applications to the therapy of myocardial ischemia and related syndromes (TABLES 8 and 9). Recent studies suggest that PMNs play a role in the pathogenesis of acute myocardial ischemia and extension of myocardial injury.[1,3,4,6,9,22,24,27,41,44,46,47,48,50,53,58,60,65,71,74,83,86] High peripheral blood leukocyte counts and PMN activation correlate with the risk of acute ischemic coronary events in humans and reduction of circulating PMNs in the dog with rabbit-derived antiserum has resulted in smaller myocardial infarcts.[12,24,32,50,74]

Release of arachidonic acid metabolites like leukotrienes by activated PMNs may influence coronary vasomotor tone and modulate the response of the endothelium to various stimuli.[2,10,40] It has also been hypothesized that atherosclerotic plaques may activate complement and lead to PMN aggregation. The presence of the terminal C5b-9 complement complex was localized in atherosclerotic plaques indicating that complement activation had occurred *in situ* with subsequent membrane damage and tissue injury mediated by PMN activation.[50]

For this kind of damage to be caused, the microcirculation has, by right, to be involved through an increase in permeability and interaction with endothelial receptors.[87–93] These phenomena are more prominent as shear stress decreases and circulation slows down.[26,27,35,48,53,65,74,75,82]

TABLE 8. Phagocyte-Microcirculation Interaction

Vascular Change
The vascular change associated with inflammation are due to events initiated at the microvascular level:
Increase in permeability to plasma proteins and increase in the expression of endothelial cell adhesive
=
Edema formation and leukocyte accumulation
Mediators of increased microvascular permeability can act via a direct interaction with endothelial cells or via a mechanism that is dependent on the presence of neutrophil
Evidence for neutrophil-dependent edema formation was demonstrated in rabbit skin by Wedmore and Williams (1981). Evidence also suggests that reactive oxygen metabolites may play a central role (Shasby *et al.* 1982)

TABLE 9. Direct-Acting Mediators of Increased Microvascular Permeability

HA
5-HT
Arachidonate lipoxygenase products (LTC4, LTD4)
PAF
Substance P
Cytokines (IL-1, TNF, INF-g, IL-4)

NEUTROPHILS AND HEMOSTASIS

There is growing evidence that leukocytes are endowed with procoagulant activity as they release oxygen radical intermediates, kininogens, elastase, and cathepsin G, and by the proven interaction between PMNs, thrombin, and endothelium (TABLE 10).[1,2,4,6,9,13,18,27,31,32,33,50,65,74,76,81]

Phagocytes can cause inactivation of protein S through ROI and elastase, therefore leading to an increase in thrombin generation, which is one of the most important mechanisms of thrombosis in congenital cyanotic heart disease.[10,27,55,56]

Although a variety of cells, such as fibroblasts and smooth muscle, have been shown to constitutively express procoagulant activity (PCA), cells that are normally in contact with flowing blood express little or no PCA without prior stimulation. Recent studies have underscored that phagocytes play a primary role in thrombogenesis and that some leukocyte products augment the ability of endothelial cells to activate or support coagulation.[25] Leukocytes infiltrating an inflammatory site elaborate mediators that can stimulate the activation of blood coagulation on cell surfaces, increase vascular permeability, and enhance the expression of adhesion molecules of the integrin family on endothelial cell surfaces.[87–93] This sequence of events may permit the "percolation" of clotting substrates and proenzymes into an inflammatory site and encourage the migration of additional cells, such as phagocytes, to form a support network. Thrombin, fibrinopeptides, and fibrin degradation products express chemotactic and mitogenic properties that may aggravate the inflammatory response and influence the pattern of tissue repair. Phagocyte PCA has also been observed in several non-specific inflammatory disorders such as generalized Shwartzman reac-

TABLE 10. Thrombosis and Inflammation Are Overlapping and Interactive Processes

Activated neutrophils release cathepsin G, a direct activator of PLT.

Activated PLT can bind to PMNs by P-selectin and can activate PMNs by the release of various alpha-granule proteins:

- platelet-derived chemokines
- neutrophil-activating peptide-2 (NAP-2)
- platelet factor 4 (PF4)

tion, systemic lupus erythematosus, allograft rejection reaction, glomerulonephritis, sarcoidosis, hypereosinophilic syndrome, ARDS, bleomycin-induced pulmonary fibrosis, and others.[69] Both platelets and PMNs interact with the injured vessel wall and may contribute to thrombosis and vasospasm. Whereas platelet adhesion to the subendothelium and components of the media of the blood vessel, and PMN adhesion to the endothelium are relatively well understood, the interaction between platelets and PMNs is only now being recognized. Phagocytes, mainly PMNs, may influence thrombosis through different mechanisms such as release of biologically active substances and by interacting with platelets on the vessel wall. Leukocyte-derived products may be prothrombotic by activating platelet deposition and aggregation.[52,67] It is possible that the PMN–vessel wall interaction, which is modulated by platelets, may be due to the exposure of GMP-140 receptors (P-selectins) of activated platelets. The pathophysiological implication of platelet and PMN interaction in mural thrombus formation, vasoconstriction, and the development and progression of atherosclerosis and restenosis may be amplified. With the increasing awareness of the possible clinical relevance of these interactions, the concept of thrombosis as a pluricellular process has emerged.[1,4,18,52,65] Although platelets are specialized for hemostasis, they may also act as inflammatory cells do, by releasing substances with potential to influence the inflammatory response and by interacting with leukocytes and with vascular endothelial cells in modulating the inflammatory reaction.[87–93]

A hypothetical model of coagulation assembly on monocytes and HSV-infected endothelium in promoting cell adhesion and vascular injury proposes that both peripheral blood monocytes and HSV-infected endothelium can simultaneously activate the extrinsic coagulation pathway through binding and activation of the zymogen factor X.[1,74]

Although structurally unrelated, the two factor X receptors CD11b/CD18 on monocytes and gC receptor on HSV-infected endothelium recognize the same structural interacting motif in the ligand. Generation of thrombin after membrane assembly of the prothrombinase complex on both cell types feeds back to monocytes, platelets, and endothelium to induce chemotaxis, cell adhesion, platelet aggregation, and membrane expression of adhesion-promoting receptors, such as PADGEM/GMP-140. In this circumstance, in the presence of endothelial lesions and exposure of thrombogenic sites, phagocytes can become activated and platelet aggregates and emboli may form.[74] In these circumstances, thrombocytopenia has no effect on myocardial infarct size and the usual accumulation of platelets in the ischemic region does not take place in neutropenia.[74] This suggests that platelets are passively trapped between granulocytes, a feature that is in agreement with intravital microscopy observations.

Platelets may share in PMN activation through a biochemical pathway, possibly via the PAF. In this respect it is difficult to consider different pathologies as mediated by only one cell type. Platelets are most important in the development of thrombotic diseases, but their responses are highly influenced by other cells, such as PMNs, red blood cells, and the endothelium. PMNs are probably the most relevant cells in the early phases of inflammation and thrombosis but platelets too can take an active part in these processes.[4]

Platelet-PMN interactions may be explained[31] in terms of thromboregulation by

PMNs and by the "aid" platelets provide in regard to the accumulation of PMNs at the inflammatory site and their co-participation to the inflammatory process.

EXERCISE-INDUCED ASTHMA

Activation of PMNs has been associated with normal immune function, inflammation, and exercise-induced muscle damage.[42] Exercise challenge provokes bronchoconstriction in most asthmatics and experimental data suggest an important role for phagocytes, eicosanoids, and other molecules released by phagocytes in mediating this process. The following mechanisms have been suggested: (*1*) vascular engorgement due to airway temperature changes; (*2*) mediator release due to hypertonicity of airway lining fluid; (*3*) stimulation of neural reflexes and neuropeptide release with possible increase of all three by structural and functional damage to the airway epithelium. The intensity of exercise and conditions of the inspired air are the main determinants of the bronchoconstrictor response to exercise in asthmatics, with some contribution from the underlying level of bronchial hyperresponsiveness.[87–93] Phagocytes and mast cells are involved in this process by releasing leukotrienes, prostaglandins, eosinophilic cationic proteins, histamine, and PAF. In addition, in patients suffering from EIA it is easy to observe an increase in serum PMN chemotactic activity and complement receptor expression in PMN and monocyte, but their response to exogenous chemotactic stimulation is decreased. In addition, unregulated peripheral blood PMNs following exercise show markedly enhanced capacity for LTB4 generation.

PHAGOCYTES AND THE BRAIN

Cells of the macrophage lineages are ubiquitously distributed in the body, including the central nervous system. They represent an essential host defense system to protect from infections. Recently, Piani and co-workers indicated that brain macrophages may also be responsible for tissue destruction, including loss of neurons and demyelination.[87–93] The mechanisms involved in macrophage-mediated neurotoxicity are not yet well defined. Recently, confirming previous reports, Piani and colleagues[87–90] found that activated microglial cells produce and secrete ROI, which are effective in mediating neurotoxicity. In experimental disease models, ROI have been implicated in the pathogenesis of the deleterious effects of severe head injury as well as cerebral ischemia and reperfusion. Oxygen scavengers, such as SOD and catalase, have been shown to minimize brain damage by reducing edema, minimizing breakdown of the blood-brain barrier, and preventing seizures. The major pathway for microglia-mediated neurotoxicity *in vitro* in cocultures of microglia and cerebellar neurons appears to involve cytotoxic molecules interacting with the NMDA subtype of the glutamate receptor on neurons. Furthermore, mechanisms that primarily impair the regulatory circuits (glutamate uptake by astrocytes) may lead to the activation of harmful macrophage effector mechanisms when these would otherwise have been only subliminally activated.

PHAGOCYTES, ADHESION MOLECULES, THE 5-LIPO-OXYGENASE PATHWAY PRODUCTS, AND VASCULAR DISEASES

PMNs provide an effective defense against bacterial and fungal infections, but they are also important in the pathogenesis of tissue damage in non-infectious diseases. It has been shown that complement-stimulated PMNs are able to aggregate, adhere to endothelium, and damage endothelial cells both *in vivo* and *in vitro*.[5,17,23–25,28,29,31,32,34,35,40,41,44,46,47,49,53,54,58,61–63,65,67–69,71,72,76,79,83–85] Intravascular activation of PMNs can therefore cause vascular endothelial injury, an important step in the pathogenesis of atherosclerosis.[64] Moreover, PMNs aggregation may cause leukostatic plugs leading to microvascular occlusion.[67] Recent experimental and clinical observations have begun to define the molecular antigenic determinants on the surface of leukocytes that contribute to the adhesion process (TABLE 11).[35,46,47,64,67,68] These studies have established the critical role *in vivo* of CD11/CD18 leukocyte adhesion molecules (TABLE 12), a family of cell surface glycoproteins consisting of three heterodimers sharing a common β subunit with a distinct α subunit (CD11a, CD11b, CD11c). CD11b/CD18 and CD11a/CD18 receptors are particularly important in respect of adhesion to endothelial cells.[50,65,67,70]

The potential role of intravascular PMN aggregation as an effector mechanism for endothelial damage in human vascular injury (TABLE 13) has elicited considerable interest and is supported by *in vitro* studies[67] and by the observation of PMN aggregates in the blood of animals *in vivo*.[4,20–22,47,50,70] It has also been hypothesized that atherosclerotic plaque material may activate complement and lead to PMN aggregation.[4,22,50,67,71]

The presence of the terminal C5B-9 complement complex has been localized in atherosclerotic plaques indicating that complement activation has occurred *in situ* with subsequent membrane damage and tissue injury mediated by PMN activation.[44,46,50,66,71] Our data show that PMN aggregability is increased in the coronary sinus of patients with angiographically documented coronary disease as compared to control subjects with normal coronary vessels. Local release of eicosanoid arachidonic acid derivatives, such as leukotrienes and thomboxane A2, by activated PMNs may influence coronary vasomotor tone and modulate endothelial response to various stimuli.[7,24,27,32,48] Available information on the biological effect of eicosanoids has led to the postulation that they have a role in vascular and non-vascular processes and in a host of human conditions such as allergic diseases, asthma, psoriasis, ARDS,

TABLE 11. Adhesion Molecules

Intimate cell-cell contact or adhesion is crucial for the normal functioning for all multicellular organisms.

Adhesion molecules are structures expressed (constitutively or not) on the surface of cells.

They are responsible for recognition by and attachment to other cells, extracellular matrix components, or even synthetic surfaces.

In this context, adhesion molecules are essential to many stages of life—from embryonic development to host defense and wound healing.

TABLE 12. Classification of the Adhesion Molecules

Integrins:	CD11a/CD18 or LFA-1
CD11b/CD18 or MAC-1	CD11c/CD18 or p150,95
Immunoglobulins:	ICAM-1 or CD54
ICAM-2	VCAM-1
Selectins:	LAM-1
ELAM-1	P-Selectin
Carbohydrates	Phospholipids

neonatal pulmonary hypertension, allergic rhinitis, gout, rheumatoid arthritis, inflammatory bowel disease,[40] and so forth.[87–93]

Leukotrienes are very potent "proinflammatory" mediators able to induce contraction of smooth muscle of bronchi and gastrointestinal system and induce vasoconstriction as well as increase endothelial cell permeability.[23,40,44,68]

Vasoconstriction has been demonstrated by the ability of leukotriene C4 and leukotriene D4 to increase systemic vascular resistance in a rat model and to diminish coronary flow in isolated guinea pig heart.[23,40,50,68] The effects of intravenous injection of a small dose (3 nmol) of leukotriene D4 in patients with normal coronary arteries have recently been tested.[14,40,48,50] These authors found a progressive increase in coronary vascular resistance that peaked at 15 min after injection and returned to baseline values after 20 min. Such an increase was associated with greater myocardial oxygen extraction, whereas myocardial oxygen consumption did not change. The vasoconstrictor effect of leukotriene C4 on coronary arteries is synergistic with that of thromboxane A2 released by platelets. Experimental data show that the decrease in coronary flow produced by the combination of both substances is greater than the simple sum of the effects caused by the two eicosanoids administered separately. In our study, PMNs were separated from blood samples taken from patients with coronary artery disease and subjects with normal coronary arteries. Af-

TABLE 13. Phagocytes as an Effector Mechanism for Endothelial Damage in Human Vascular Injury

Pathology of Microvascular Endothelium

INFLAMMATION AND IMMUNITY

Endothelial cell undergo changes at the sites of inflammatory reactions.

These changes are

- functional: altered regulation of platelet and coagulation; enhanced adhesion of specific leukocyte classes
- morphological towards a phenotype comparable to that of high endothelial venules in lymphoid tissue

These changes are driven by cytokines and the altered endothelial cell properties depend on the cytokines to which the cells are exposed

ter stimulation with calcium ionophore A23187 the supernatant was analyzed for leukotriene C4 by radioimmunoassay. Two measurements were obtained for each patient, one after stimulation of PMNs obtained from blood samples taken from aorta and the other after stimulation of PMNs from the coronary sinus, to assess whether the passage through the coronary circulation modifies the response of leukocytes to the same stimulus.

Our results show that in patients with coronary artery disease,[22,23,47,49,50,63,66] PMNs obtained from the coronary sinus release a lower amount of leukotriene C4 than PMNs isolated from aortic blood, whereas no difference is found in subjects with normal coronary vessels. Moreover, a significant correlation is found between the extent of coronary disease and the percent reduction of leukotriene C4 generation by PMNs isolated from the coronary sinus as compared to PMNs separated from aortic blood.

A possible explanation is that PMNs could be activated during transit over the atheromatous plaques of coronary arteries and that they could produce leukotriene C4. Prior activation in the coronary arteries may account for the lower release of C4 leukotriene by PMNs separated from the coronary sinus of patients with coronary artery disease. Chronic endothelial injury and coronary artery stenosis lead to the accumulation of platelets and white blood cells, which can release potent mediators of vasoconstriction.[23] Production of leukotriene C4 by PMNs may contribute to the development of the inappropriate vasoconstriction that occurs as a result of the endothelial dysfunction associated with the atherosclerotic involvement of coronary vessels.[87-93]

Recent studies of ischemic heart disease suggest that immunologically mediated processes often accompany cardiac injury and contribute to their pathogenesis. Murine models of myocarditis have provided insights into the mechanisms whereby autoimmune responses to cardiac antigens arise and cause pathological changes. It is now evident that phagocytic cells, antigen presenting cells, T lymphocytes, cytokines, and antibodies may all contribute to cardiac injury.[43] Furthermore, murine models have demonstrated that both the propensity to develop autoreactivity following cardiac injury and the vulnerability of the heart to these responses are under genetic control.

PHAGOCYTES AND PTCA

Circulating PMNs defend the body against invading microbes by releasing a complex assortment of agents and toxins.[2,8,9,29,30,37,44,53,60,83] The potentially destructive armamentarium of PMNs may also act as mediator of inflammatory tissue damage and may also play a critical role in the pathogenesis of vascular injury.[35] Proteolytic enzymes like elastase and reactive oxygen metabolites like superoxide anion discharged by activated PMNs have direct cytotoxic effects and are able to destroy human endothelial cells.[3] The purpose of one of our previous studies[19,20,21,22,46,47,50,63,67,71] was to ascertain whether PMN activation would take place after coronary angioplasty (PTCA) in humans. We concluded by hypothesizing that the release of toxic substances by PMNs during PTCA may amplify the endothelial damage caused by balloon dilatation of the vessel. Moreover, PMNs may potentiate platelet activation,[4,13,18,31] which commonly occurs after PTCA as a result of arterial injury and which is thought to play an important role in the pathogenesis of restenosis.[14,33,37]

Balloon dilation induces arterial injury that is mild and superficial in the area where the balloon has contact with the arterial wall but deep in the region of a split or tear.[87–93] In the dilated region vascular injury with endothelial denudation and exposure of subendothelial structures and collagen fibrils trigger the immediate deposition and aggregation of platelets.[23] Although the mechanisms of restenosis are not completely understood, they appear to be related to the hemorrheological response to the therapeutic injury induced by the balloon on the vessel.[23] PMN activation, which follows PTCA, may aggravate endothelial damage through the release of proteolytic enzymes and the generation of oxygen free radicals and may further stimulate platelets, thus having a potential bearing on the subsequent development of restenosis. Oxygen radicals have also been implicated in the pathogenesis of the "stunned myocardium"[12,24–26,41,52,53] and the persistent post-ischemic myocardial dysfunction despite restoration of blood flow. Engler and Covell[26,27] recently reported that marked reduction in the number of circulating PMNs by leukopak filtration significantly enhances recovery of postischemic myocardial function in a canine model and concluded that activated PMNs are the direct cause of "stunned myocardium." It is interesting to note that Wijns and colleagues[84] found that coronary occlusion during PTCA was associated with profound alterations in diastolic function that persisted after restoration of myocardial blood flow. Activation of PMNs and release of oxygen radicals may account for these still unexplained observations in patients undergoing balloon angioplasty.

PHAGOCYTES AND RHEUMATOID ARTHRITIS

There is considerable evidence that PMNs, lured to the joint space by a complex series of cellular and molecular signals, are responsible for a substantial portion of the joint destruction seen in rheumatoid arthritis.[57] Rheumatoid arthritis (RA) is a chronic, symmetrical polyarticular disease of joints, characterized by pain, swelling, and stiffness as well as redness and warmth of multiple joints. Inflammation in the rheumatoid joint affects diverse structures.

Synovial pannus, which consists of hypertrophic synovium, is predominantly infiltrated by mononuclear leukocytes. Immune complexes formed by rheumatoid factor and anti-collagen antibodies in the joint may activate complement, leading to C5a generation and chemoattraction of PMNs.[87–93]

The joint space in RA is filled almost exclusively with PMNs and the hyaluronan synovial fluid is much less viscous. PMN counts in rheumatoid synovial fluid may exceed $100,000/mm^3$, and turnover may be more than a billion cells per day in a 30-ml joint effusion.[36]

Recent data suggest an expanded model of inflammation in which PMN–endothelial interactions also play an important role in the pathogenesis of the rheumatoid joint by the CD11b/CD18 adhesion molecules. The endothelium therefore represents both a barrier and a regulatory checkpoint for PMN migration. For instance, in response to classic chemoattractants such as FMLP and C5a, expression and activity of

CD11b/CD18 are upregulated on PMNs, leading to PMN–endothelial interaction. Once in the joint space, PMNs may bind to and phagocytose soluble immune complexes, resulting in prostaglandin and leukotriene production, PMN degranulation, and respiratory burst. Premature activation may result in the release of PMN proteinase granules and toxic oxygen metabolites directly into the synovial fluid by "regurgitation during feeding" mechanism. The "rheumatoid PMN" is fundamentally different, functionally and in its molecular expression from the "non-rheumatoid" PMN.[3,17,30,36,40,45,46,51,54,57,58,65,78,80]

PHAGOCYTES AND CARDIOPULMONARY BYPASS

Activated PMNs release highly active enzymes, such as myeloperoxidase and lactoferrin, which can be involved in tissue destruction mediated by oxygen free radicals. Cardiopulmonary bypass has been reported to activate PMNs.[10,39,56,80,81] Borowiec and collaborators demonstrated that bypass circuits coated with heparin reduce release of PMN factors in experimental studies.[10]

In their study, heparin-coated circuits (HC) were compared with noncoated circuits (C). In the HC group the heparin dose was reduced to 75% (225 IU/kg). Group C had the standard dose of 300 IU/kg. No preoperative differences in myeloperoxidase and lactoferrin in peripheral blood were observed between the two groups.

At the end of the bypass procedure there was a significant increase of these enzymes in both groups ($p < 0.001$) followed by a later decrease. In group HC however, the release of myeloperoxidase was significantly lower than in group C (215 ± 24 versus 573 ± 133 μg/L, mean ± standard error of the mean). Release of lactoferrin was significantly lower in group HC than in group C both at the end of cardiopulmonary bypass (659 ± 79 versus $1,448 \pm 121$ μg/L) and 3 hours after bypass (224 ± 37 versus 536 ± 82 μg/L). PMNs as well as total numbers of leukocytes continued to increase until 1 hour after bypass ($p < 0.001$) and then showed a slow decrease. It was concluded that the use of heparin-coated circuits reduced the release of PMN factors because of lower activation of leukocytes.

Patients undergoing coronary bypass grafting[55,56] present different phagocyte-dependent complications in relation to the different treatment with bubble or membrane oxygenators. Cardiac performance, assessed on the basis of the postoperative need for inotropic support, was significantly better in the membrane oxygenator group. After perfusion lasting more than 2 hours, respiratory function, measured as alveolar-arterial oxygen pressure gradient, was less compromised in that group and renal function, quantified as postoperative rise in serum creatinine was less disturbed. Cerebral function, studied in terms of psychometric test results and concentrations of adenylate kinase in cerebrospinal fluid, did not differ between bubble and membrane oxygenator groups. In investigations concerning changes in inflammatory activity during bypass, complement activation could not be related to the clinical parameters mentioned. Release of PMN lactoferrin and myeloperoxidase was greater in the bubble oxygenator group and correlated with impaired cardiac and renal performance but not with pulmonary or cerebral dysfunction.

Activation of phagocytes could also occur during surgical procedures. Wanscher and coworkers[79] studied degranulation of PMNs following minor surgery and the contributory role of temporary limb ischemia in 22 otherwise healthy patients undergoing elective arthroscopy under general anesthesia with and without tourniquet. Apart from an increase in lactate levels following tourniquet release, there was no difference in the complement split product C3d, cortisol, leukocyte, or creatinine kinase levels between the two groups. There was post-operative increase in plasma $E\alpha 1$–proteinase inhibitor concentration, whereas lactoferrin values decreased 4 h following tourniquet deflation. Anesthesia and minor surgery are followed by post-operative release of elastase by PMNs. This is not related to complement activation and is apparently unaffected by 50 min of lower limb ischemia. Anesthesia and minor surgery do not cause lactoferrin release.

PHAGOCYTES AND VASCULITIS

Vasculitis can be defined as an inflammatory reaction affecting blood vessels.[73] It is typically associated with PMN and mononuclear leukocyte infiltration and often with necrosis of the vessel wall itself. Vasculitis is often widespread and associated clinically with systemic disease and injury to many organs. PMNs appear to be one of the principal effector cells in patients with systemic vasculitis and are also the target of autoantibodies that are almost always found in the serum of patients with these diseases.[87–93]

PHAGOCYTES, SEPTIC SHOCK, AND CHRONIC UREMIA

In septic shock, activation of PMN and complement system significantly contributes to the pathophysiology of the condition. Toxicity effects due to interleukin-2 (IL-2) strongly resemble the clinical picture seen during septic shock. Experimental data[2,3,25,30,38,39,80,81] suggest that activation of PMNs initiates endothelial cell damage, which subsequently leads to activation of the complement cascade. This latter system then contributes to the hemodynamic changes and capillary leakage seen in IL-2–treated patients.[87–93]

Neutrophils are activated during sepsis[38] as well as during hemodialysis. To find out whether PMNs are further activated during hemodialysis with cellulosic and non-cellulosic membranes, Horl and co-workers compared the plasma levels of the main PMN components in patients with chronic uremia who were undergoing regular hemodialysis treatment and patients with acute renal failure with and without sepsis. During hemodialysis with cuprophane dialyzers, plasma-granulocyte elastase complexed with α-proteinase inhibitor and lactoferrin levels increased in patients who were undergoing regular hemodialysis treatment, but these levels increased further in patients with acute renal failure who did not have sepsis. Maximal PMN degranulation was observed in patients with acute renal failure and sepsis. There was only mild degranulation in all three groups during dialysis with dialyzers made of polysulphone. Horl's data demonstrate that PMN activation is increased in patients with acute renal failure and that it is further increased by superimposed sepsis. Cellulose-containing dialysis membranes cause further PMN activation.

PHAGOCYTES AND RENAL ISCHEMIC-REPERFUSION INJURY

Renal ischemic-reperfusion injury (IRI) frequently occurs in transplanted as well as native kidneys[61] and effective treatment still remains elusive. Leukocytes and their products may be important in the pathogenesis of renal IRI. Do leukocyte adhesion molecules mediate renal reperfusion injury?

With recent evidence implicating leukocytes and oxygen free-radicals in renal reperfusion injury, there has been renewed interest in delineating the role of leukocyte adhesion molecules in these processes.[87–93] In animal experiments, administration of monoclonal antibodies to leukocyte adhesion molecules has attenuated reperfusion damage in many organs, including heart, liver, and skeletal muscle.[85] Adhesion receptors on leukocytes and their corresponding ligands have recently been identified. In the heart, considerable evidence supports the role of CD11/CD18, ICAM-1, and of the selectin receptors in IRI.

However, on the basis of experimental studies in animal models, even though renal IRI appears to be ICAM-1 mediated, the role of the CD11/CD18 pathway appears to be minimal. In addition, available evidence does not support the concept that L-selectin has significant involvement in renal IRI.

PHAGOCYTES AND OSTEOPETROSIS

Osteopetrosis[59] comprises of a group of rare metabolic diseases of skeletal development that are characterized by a generalized increase in skeletal mass resulting from reduced osteoclast-mediated bone resorption. Specific immune regulators and growth factors that influence osteoclast ontogeny and/or activation have been implicated in the pathogenesis of some of the naturally occurring mutations associated with osteopetrosis in animals. Most recently, loss-of-function experiments using transgenic mice with targeted disruptions of the c-src or c-fos proto-oncogenes have resulted in different osteoclast abnormalities producing osteopetrosis. Cytokines are polypeptides, produced by a variety of immune cells including lymphocytes, macrophages, and other phagocytic cells, which mediate cellular communication and effector functions within the immune system. More recently, cytokines have been shown to have biological effects on various non-immune cells, including those of the skeleton. Various abnormalities in cellular and humoral immunity involving lymphocytes, PMNs, macrophages, and monocytes have been reported in osteopetrotic animals and children. Another important development concerning the role of the immune system in the pathogenesis of osteoclast dysfunction in osteopetrosis is related to recently demonstrated defects in inflammation-primed macrophage activation, a cascade that involves the conversion of serum vitamin D–binding protein (DBP) to a potent macrophage activating factor (DBP-MAF). This factor is a potent stimulator of macrophage function (e.g., superoxide production and phagocytosis) and is able to stimulate osteoclastic bone resorption.

TABLE 14. Phagocyte, Inflammation, and Tissue Damage

A rapid increase in leukocyte adhesion to endothelial cells is one of the first events in the acute inflammatory response and in the pathogenesis of vascular disease.

A subgroup of cell surface glycoproteins (the CD11/CD18 complex) play a major role in the leukocyte adhesion process; in particular the CD11b/CD18 receptors can be upregulated from intracellular granules by chemotactic factors such as C5a, IL-8, and PAF

"New" concept: neutrophils are not short-lived cells incapable of significant protein synthesis, but there are a variety of substances that can elicit the neutrophil to produce many substances

CONCLUSION

On the basis of clinical, biochemical, and novel data on the inflammatory process now available, it can be concluded that phagocytes form a wide network that, although having in common the primordial mechanism of phagocytosis, specialize in different organs so as to be able to take up specific functions pertinent to that organ. In this light, as these cells remain fully capable of releasing toxic substances, they can cause damage to the host itself whilst attempting to defend it against a variety of noxae (TABLE 14). This holds true for all phagocytes but it is especially important for professional phagocytes such as PMNs and monocytes especially when these are primed or activated. Pathological conditions where these cells are predominantly involved include ischemic cardiovascular conditions (TABLE 15), where, as these cells cross the vessels to reach ischemic tissue, they also damage the endothelium. The same cells may also compound and participate to the pathogenesis of other conditions including ARDS and other respiratory disorders, cancerogenesis (especially at the level of the gastrointestinal tract), and many more (TABLE 3).

SUMMARY

Evidence continues to accumulate on the importance of neutrophils (PMNs) and phagocytes in the causation of tissue and endothelial injury that frequently accompanies the inflammatory response. Increased production of superoxide anions in combination with decreased endothelial antioxidant activity may contribute to the development of vascular disease including atherosclerosis, vasospasm, diabetic vascular complications, tissue damage in ischemia-reperfusion, and hypotension. Free radi-

TABLE 15. Phagocytes Are Involved in the Vascular Damage

Some data suggest a role for inflammation in the pathophysiology of unstable angina.

Patients with unstable angina have an increased expression of granulocyte and monocyte CD11b/CD18 adhesion receptors, indicating that an inflammatory reaction takes place in the coronary tree of patients with unstable angina.

cals generated in the vascular wall may act directly on smooth muscle or interact with each other thus producing biologically active endogenous mediators. Derangement of macrophage function may occur in conditions characterized by protein malnutrition, thus leading to failure to develop a specific immunoresponse and to an increase in the production of oxygen intermediate radicals, which may cause tissue damage. A local inflammatory response followed by endothelial cell activation could also facilitate migration of immunocompetent cells into the parenchyma of grafted organs and stimulate dendritic cells in the graft. There is now convincing evidence that excessive and prolonged production of NO contributes to tissue damage in septicemia, ischemia/reperfusion injury, and other inflammatory conditions. There is also increasing evidence that the complement system plays an important role in tissue damage in association with phagocytes, e.g., in ischemia/reperfusion injury, carcinogenesis, and aging. It can therefore be surmised that phagocytic cells may act both as "friends" and as "foes" and that they are important mediators of tissue damage in a variety of conditions.

REFERENCES

1. ALTIERI 1993. Coagulation assembly on leukocytes in transmembrane signaling and cell adhesion. Blood **81:** 569–579.
2. BAARS, J. W., C. E. HACK, J. WAGSTAFF, A. J. EERENBERG-BELMER, G. J. WOLBINK, L. G. THIJS, R. J. STRACK VAN SCHIJNDEL, H. L. VAN DER VALL & H. M. PINEDO. 1992. The activation of polymorphonuclear PMNs and the complement system during immunotherapy with recombinant interleukin-2. Br. J. Cancer **65**(1): 96–101.
3. BABIOR, D. M., R. S. KIPNESS & J. I. CURNUTTE. 1973. Biological defense mechanisms: the production by leukocytes of superoxide, a potential bactericidal agent. J. Clin. Invest. **52:** 741–747.
4. BAZZONI, E., A. DEJANA & A. DEL MASCHIO. 1991. Platelet-neutrophil interactions. Possible relevance in the pathogenesis of thrombosis and inflammation. Haematologica **76:** 491–499.
5. BENOWITZ, N. L. 1988. Pharmacologic aspects of cigarette smoking and nicotine addiction. N. Engl. J. Med. **319:** 1318–1330.
6. BERK, B. C., W. S. WEINTRAUB & R. W. ALEXANDER. 1990. Elevation of C-reactive protein in "active" coronary artery disease. Am. J. Cardiol. **65:** 168–172.
7. BERLINER, S., S. SCLAROVSKY, G. LAVIE, J. PINKHAS, M. ARONSON & J. AGMON. 1986. The leukergy test in patients with ischemic heart disease. Am. Heart J. **111:** 19–22.
8. BOLLI, R. 1991. Oxygen-derived free radicals and myocardial perfusion injury: an overview. Cardiovasc. Drugs Ther. **5:** 249–268.
9. BOOGAERTS, M. A., O. YAMADA, H. S. JACOB & C. F. MOLDOW. 1982. Enhancement of granulocyte-endothelial cell adherence and granulocyte-induced cytotoxicity by platelet release products. Proc. Natl. Acad. Sci. USA **79:** 7019–7023.
10. BOROWIEC, J., S. THELIN, L. BAGGE, L. NILSSON, P. VENGE & H. E. HANSSON. 1992. Heparin-coated circuits reduce activation of granulocytes during cardiopulmonary bypass. A clinical study. J. Thorac. Cardiovasc. Surg. **104**(3): 642–647.
11. BOYUM, A. 1968. Isolation of mononuclear cells and granulocytes from human blood. Scand. J. Clin. Lab. Invest. **97:** 77–110.
12. BRAUNWALD, E. & R. A. KLONER. 1982. The stunned myocardium: prolonged, postischemic ventricular dysfunction. Circulation **66:** 1146–1149.

13. CAMUSSI, G., M. AGLIETTA, F. MALAVASI, C. TETTA, W. PIACIBELLO, F. SANAVIO & F. BUS-SOLINO. 1983. The release of platelet-activating factor from human endothelial cells in culture. J. Immunol. **1:** 2397–2403.

14. CHESEBRO, J. H., J. Y. T. LAM, L. BADIMON & V. FUSTER. 1987. Restenosis after arterial angioplasty: a hemorrheologic response to injury. Am. J. Cardiol. **60:** 10B–16B.

15. COHEN, M. S., D. M. ELLIOT, T. CHAPLINSKI, M. M. PIKE & J. E. NIEDEL. 1982. A defect in the oxidative metabolism of human polymorphonuclear leukocytes that remain in circulation early in hemodialysis. Blood **60:** 1283–1289.

16. CURTIS, M. J., M. K. PUGSLEY & M. J. A. WALKER. 1993. Endogenous chemical mediators of ventricular arrhythmias in ischaemic heart disease. Cardiovasc. Res. **27:** 703–719.

17. DE BONO, D. P. 1994. Free radicals and antioxidants in vascular biology: the roles of reaction kinetics, environment and substrate turnover. Med. **87:** 445–453.

18. DEL MASCHIO, A., V. EVANGELISTA, G. RAJTAR, Z. M. CHEN, C. CERLETTI & G. DE GAETANO. 1990. Platelet activation by polymorphonuclear leukocytes exposed to chemotactic agents. Am. J. Physiol. **258:** H870–H879.

19. DE SERVI, S., A. MAZZONE & G. RICEVUTI. 1990. Granulocyte activation after coronary angioplasty in humans. Curculation **82:** 140–146.

20. DE SERVI, S., A. MAZZONE, G. RICEVUTI, A. FIORAVANTI, E. BRAMUCCI, L. ANGOLI, S. GHIO & G. SPECCHIA. 1990. Granulocyte aggregation after coronary angioplasty in human. Circulation **82:** 140–144.

21. DE SERVI, S., A. MAZZONE, G. RICEVUTI, A. FIORAVANTI, E. BRAMUCCI, L. ANGOLI, S. GHIO & G. SPECCHIA. 1990. Granulocyte aggregation after coronary angioplasty in human. Circulation **82:** 140–144.

22. DE SERVI, S., G. RICEVUTI & A. MAZZONE. 1991. PMNs function in coronary artery disease. Am. J. Cardiol. **68:** 64B–68B.

23. DE SERVI, S., G. RICEVUTI & A. MAZZONE. 1991. Transcardiac release of leukotriene C4 by neutrophils in patients with coronary artery disease. Am. Coll. Cardiol. **17:** 1125–1128.

24. DINERMAN, J. L., J. L. MEHTA & T. G. P. SALDEEN. 1990. Increased neutrophil elastase release in unstable angina pectoris and acute myocardial infarction. Am. Coll. Cardiol. **15:** 1559–1563.

25. EDWARDS, F. & R. RICKLES. 1992. The role of leukocytes in the activation of blood coagulation. Sem. Hematol. **29:** 202–212.

26. ENGLER, R. & J. W. COVELL. 1987. Granulocytes cause reperfusion ventricular dysfunction after 15-minute ischemia in the dog. Circ. Res. **61:** 20–28.

27. ENGLER, R. L., M. D. DAHLGREN, D. MORRIS, M. A. PETERSON & G. SCHMID-SCHOENBEIN. 1986. Role of leukocytes in the response to acute myocardial ischemia and reflow in dogs. Am. J. Physiol. **251:** 314–319.

28. ENGVALL, E., K. JONSSON & P. PERLMANN. 1971. Enzyme-linked immunosorbent assay. II. Quantitative assay of protein antigen, immunoglobulin G, by means of enzyme-labelled antigen and antigen-coated tubes. Biochim. Biophys. Acta **251:** 427–435.

29. ENTMANN, M. L., K. YOUKER, S. B. SHAPPELL, C. SIEGEL, R. ROTHLEIN, W. J. DREYER, F. C. SCHMALSTIEG & C. W. SMITH. 1990. Neutrophil adherence to isolated canine myocytes. J. Clin. Invest. **85:** 1497–1506.

30. EVANGELISTA, V., G. RAJTAR, G. DE GAETANO, J. G. WHITA & C. CERLETTI. 1991. Platelet activation by fMLP-stimulated polymorphonuclear leukocytes: the activity of cathepsin G is not prevented by antiproteinase. Blood **77:** 2379–2388.

31. FAINT. 1992. Platelet-neutrophil interactions: their significance Blood Rev. **6:** 83–91.

32. HAMMERSCHMIDT, D. E., C. S. GREENBERG, O. YAMADA, P. R. CRADDOCK & H. S. JACOB. 1981. Cholesterol and atheroma lipids activate complement and stimulate granulocytes. A possible mechanism for amplification of ischemic injury in atherosclerotic states. J. Lab. Clin. Med. **98:** 68–77.

33. HARKER, L. A. 1987. Role of platelets and thrombosis in mechanism of acute occlusion and restenosis after angioplasty. Am. J. Cardiol. **60:** 20–28.
34. HARLAN, J. M. 1987. Consequence of leukocyte-vessel wall interactions in inflammatory and immune reactions. Sem. Thromb. Hemostas. **13:** 434–444.
35. HARLAN, J. M. 1985. Leukocyte-endothelial interactions. Blood **65:** 513–525.
36. HOLLINSWORTH, E. R., C. SIEGEL & W. A. CREASEY. 1967. Granulocyte survival in synovial exudate of patients with rheumatoid arthritis and other inflammatory joint diseases. Yale J. Biol. Med. **39:** 289–296.
37. HOLMES, D. R., JR., R. E. VLIESTRA, H. C. SMITH, G. W. VETROVEC, K. M. KENT, M. J. COWLEY, D. P. FAXON, A. R. GRUENTZIG, S. F. KELSEY, K. M. DETRE, M. J. VAN RADEN & M. B. MOCK. 1984. Restenosis after percutaneous transluminal coronary angioplasty (PTCA): A report from the PTCA registry of the National Heart, Lung, and Blood Institute. Am. J. Cardiol. **53:** 77C-81C.
38. HORL, W. H., R. M. SCHAFER, M. HORL & A. HEIDLAND. 1990. Neutrophil activation in acute renal failure and sepsis. Arch. Surg. **125**(5): 651–654.
39. KLEMPNER, M. S., J. I. GALLIN, J. E. BALOW & D. P. VAN KAMMEN. 1980. The effect of hemodialysis and C5a des arg on neutrophil subpopulations. Blood **55:** 777–783.
40. LEWIS, K. F. AUSTEN & R. J. SOBERMAN. 1990. Leukotrienes and other products of the 5-lipoxygenase pathway. N. Engl. J. Med. **323:** 645–655.
41. LUCCHESI, B. R. 1987. Role of neutrophils in ischemic heart disease: Pathophysiologic role in myocardial ischemia and coronary artery reperfusion. *In* Thrombosis and Platelets in Myocardial Ischemia. J. L. Mehta, Ed.: 35–48. Davis. Philadelphia, PA.
42. MAKKER, S. T. HOLGATE. 1994. Mechanisms of exercise-induced asthma. Eur. J. Clin. Invest. **24:** 571–585.
43. MALKIEL, A., P. KUAN & B. DIAMOND. 1996. Autoimmunity in heart disease: mechanisms and genetic susceptibility. Molec. Med. Today **2:** 336–342.
44. MALECH, H. L. & J. I. GALLIN. 1987. Neutrophils in human diseases N. Engl. J. Med. **317:** 687–694.
45. MANSSON, B., P. GEBOREK, T. SAXNE & S. BJORNSSON. 1990. Cytidine deaminase activity in synovial fluid of patients with rheumatoid arthritis: relation to lactoferrin, acidosis, and cartilage proteoglycan release. Ann. Rheum. Dis. **49**(8): 594–597.
46. MAURI, C., A. NOTARIO & G. RICEVUTI, EDS. 1989. Pathophysiology of phagocytes and clinical aspects of phagocytic disease. Int. J. Immunopath. Pharmac. (special issue) **2:** 55–128.
47. MAURI, C., S. C. RIZZO & G. RICEVUTI, EDS. 1987. The Biology of Phagocytes in Health and Disease. Pergamon Press. New York.
48. MAYROVITZ, H., M. WIEDEMAN & R. TUMA. 1977. Factors influencing leukocyte adherence in microvessels. Thromb. Haemost. **38:** 823–831.
49. MAZZONE, A. & G. RICEVUTI. 1990. Interaction between morphine and granulocyte aggregation in myocardial ischaemia. Cardiovasc. Drugs Therapy **4:** 303–304.
50. MAZZONE, A., G. RICEVUTI, S. DE SERVI & A. NOTARIO. 1989. Granulocytes and myocardial ischemia. Int. J. Immunopath. Pharmac. **2:** 123–128.
51. McPHAIL, L. C. & R. SNYDERMANN. 1983. Activation of the respiratory burst enzyme in human polymorphonuclear leukocytes by hemoattractants and other soluble stimuli. Evidence that the same oxidase is activated by different transductional mechanisms. J. Clin. Invest. **72:** 192–201.
52. MERHI, J., J. Y. T. LAM, L. L. LACOSTE, J. G. LATOUR, R. GUIDOIN & D. WATERS. 1993. Effects of thrombocytopenia and shear rate on neutrophil and platelet deposition on endothelial and medial arterial surfaces. Arterioscler. Thromb. **13:** 951–957.
53. MEHTA, J., J. DINERMAN, P. MEHTA, G. P. SALDEEN, D. LAWSON, W. H. DONNELLY & R. WALLIN. 1989. Neutrophil function in ischemic heart disease. Circulation **79:** 549–556.

54. NEUMANN, S., G. GUNZER, N. HENRICH & H. LANG. 1984. PMN elastase assay: Enzyme immunoassay for human polymorphonuclear elastase complexed with alpha-1-proteinase inhibitor. J. Clin. Chem. Clin Biochem. **22:** 693–697.

55. NILSSON, L., H. TYDEN, O. JOHANSSON, U. NILSSON, G. RONQUIST, P. VENGE, T. ABERG & S. O. NYSTROM. 1990. Bubble and membrane oxygenators—comparison of postoperative organ dysfunction with special reference to inflammatory activity. Scand. J. Thorac. Cardiovasc. Surg. **24**(1): 59–64.

56. NILSSON, L., U. NILSSON, P. VENGE, O. JOHANSSON, H. TYDEN, T. ABERG & S. O. NYSTROM. 1990. Inflammatory system activation during cardiopulmonary bypass as an indicator of biocompatibility: a randomized comparison of bubble and membrane oxygenators. Scand. J. Thorac. Cardiovasc. Surg. **24**(1): 53–58.

57. PILLINGER, M. & S. B. ABRAMSON. 1995. The neutrophil in rheumatoid arthritis. Rheum. Dis. Clin. North Amer. **21:** 691–714.

58. PLOW, E. F. 1982. Leukocyte elastase release during blood coagulation. A potential mechanism for activation of the alternative fibrinolytic pathway. J. Clin. Invest. **69:** 564–571.

59. POPOFF, G. & B. SCHNEIDER. 1996. Animal models of osteopetrosis: the impact of recent molecular developments on novel strategies for therapeutic intervention. Molec. Med. Today **2:** 349–358.

60. PRZYKLENK, K. 1988. Oxygen-derived free radicals and "stunned myocardium." Free Radical Biol. Med. **4:** 39–44.

61. RABB. 1994. Cell adhesion molecules and the kidney. Am. J. Kidney Dis. **23:** 155–166.

62. RICEVUTI, G., R. BAIGUERA, A. MAZZONE, S. ROSSINI, F. FASANI, M. C. TUMMINELLO & D. PENSATO. 1987. Effects of phosphatidylserine on immunologic indices in aged patients. Ann. N.Y. Acad. Sci. **496:** 731–734.

63. RICEVUTI, G., S. DE SERVI, A. MAZZONE, L. ANGOLI, S. GHIO & G. SPECCHIA. 1990. Increased neutrophil aggregability in coronary artery disease. Eur. Heart J. **11:** 814–818.

64. RICEVUTI, G. & A. MAZZONE. 1989. Definition of CD 11a,b,c, and CD 18 glycoproteins on chemotactically deficient granulocyte membranes in patients affected by myeloid disorders. Acta Haematologica **81:** 126–130.

65. RICEVUTI, G. & A. MAZZONE. 1989. The revisited neutrophils. Inflammation **13:** 475–482.

66. RICEVUTI, G., A. MAZZONE, S. DE SERVI & P. FRATINO. 1989. New trends in coronary artery disease: the role of granulocyte activation. Atherosclerosis **78:** 261–265.

67. RICEVUTI, G., A. MAZZONE & A. NOTARIO. 1989. Membrane glycoproteins in superoxide release from neutrophils. Proceedings of NATO advanced research workshop. A. Crastes de Paulet, L. Bouste Blazy & R. Paoletti, Eds. Bendor, October 5-8, 1988. Plenum Press. New York.

68. RICEVUTI, G., A. MAZZONE & A. NOTARIO. 1989. The pathophysiology of phagocytes. Int. J. Immunopath. Pharmac. **2:** 99–113.

69. RICEVUTI, G., L. PACCHIARINI, A. MAZZONE, D. ROTA SCALABRINI, G. GRIGNANI & S. C. RIZZO. 1987. Activation of arachidonic acid metabolism during aggregation of polymorphonuclear granulocytes. Hemat. Rev. Comm. **1:** 329–339.

70. RICEVUTI, G., S. DE SERVI & A. MAZZONE. 1990. Increased neutrophil aggregability in coronary artery disease. Eur. Heart J. **11:** 814–819.

71. RICEVUTI, G., A. MAZZONE, D. PASOTTI, S. DE SERVI & G. SPECCHIA. 1991. Role of granulocytes in endothelial injury in coronary heart disease in humans. Atherosclerosis **91:** 1–14.

72. RINDER, H. M., J. L. BONAN, C. S. RINDER, K. A. AULT & B. R. SMITH. 1991. Activated and unactivated platelet adhesion to monocytes and neutrophils. Blood **78:** 1760–1769.

73. SAVAGE, A. & J. REES. 1994. Role of neutrophils in vasculitis *In* Immunopharmacology of Neutrophils. P. G. Hellewell & T. J. Williams, Eds.: 249–275. Academic Press, Inc.

74. SCHMID-SCHONBEIN, G. 1988. Granulocyte: friend and foe. NIPS **3:** 144–147.

75. SRIVASTAVA, C. H., T. A. RADO, D. BAUERLE & H. E. BROXMEYER. 1991. Regulation of human bone marrow lactoferrin and myeloperoxidase gene expression by tumor necrosis factor-alpha. J. Immunol. **146**(3): 1014–1019.

76. TOOTHILL, V. J., J. A. VAN MOURIK, H. K. NIEWENHUIS, M. J. METZELAAR & J. D. PEARSON. 1990. Characterization of the enhanced adhesion of neutrophil leukocytes to thrombin-stimulated endothelial cells. Immunology **145**: 283–291.

77. VAN GELDER, B. F. & E. C. SLATER. 1962. The extinction coefficient of cytochrome c. Biochim. Biophys. Acta **58**: 593–597.

78. WADE, G. L. MANDELL. 1983. Polymorphonuclear leukocytes: dedicated professional phagocytes. Am. J. Med. **74**: 686–693.

79. WANSCHER, M., S. ANTONSEN, P. TOFT, L. KJAER-NIELSEN, F. KNUDSEN & H. R. JORGENSEN. 1992. The influence of tourniquet ischaemia on post-operative degranulation of polymorphonuclear granulocytes. Eur. J. Anaesthesiol. **9**(3): 217–222.

80. WEISS, S. J. 1989. Tissue destruction by neutrophils. N. Engl. J. Med. **320**: 365–377.

81. WEISSMANN, G., J. E. SMOLEN & H. M. KORCHAK. 1980. Release of inflammatory mediators from stimulated neutrophils. N. Engl. J. Med. **303**: 27–34.

82. WEKSLER, B. B., E. A. JAFFE, M. S. BROWER & O. F. COLE. 1989. Human leukocyte cathepsin G and elastase specifically suppress thrombin-induced prostacyclin production in human endothelial cells. Blood **74**: 1627–1634.

83. WERNS, S. W. & B. R. LUCCHESI. 1988. Leukocytes, oxygen radicals, and myocardial injury due to ischemia and reperfusion. Free Radical Biol. Med. **4**: 31–37.

84. WIJNS, W., P. W. SERRUYS, C. J. SLAGER, J. GRIMM, H. P. KRAYENBUEHL, P. G. HUGENHOLTZ & O. M. HESS. 1986. Effect of coronary occlusion during percutaneous transluminal angioplasty in humans on left ventricular chamber stiffness and regional diastolic pressure-radius relations. J. Am. Coll. Cardiol. **7**: 455–463.

85. WINN, D., D. MIHELICIC, N. B. VEDDER, S. R. SHARAR & J. HARLAN. 1993. Monoclonal antibodies to leukocytes and endothelial adhesion molecules attenuate ischemic-reperfusion injury. Behring Inst. Mitt. **92**: 229–237.

86. JACOB, H. S., P. R. CRADDOCK, D. E. HAMMERSCHMIDT & C. F. MOLDOW. 1980. Complement-induced granulocyte aggregation. An unsuspected mechanism of disease. N. Engl. J. Med. **302**: 789–797.

87. GRUPPO ITALIANO DI CITOMETRIA (G. RICEVUTI IN COLLABORAZIONE CON B. BRANDO E E. SOMMARUGA.) 1993. Nationwide quality control trial on lymphocyte immunophenotyping and flow cytometer performance in Italy. Cytometry **14**: 294–306.

88. MAZZONE, A., S. DE SERVI, G. RICEVUTI, I. MAZZUCCHELLI, G. FOSSATI, D. PASOTTI, E. BRAMUCCI, L. ANGOLI, F. MARSICO, G. SPECCHIA & A. NOTARIO. 1993. Increased expression of neutrophil and monocyte adhesion molecules in unstable coronary artery disease. Circulation **88**: 358–363.

89. DE SERVI, S., A. MAZZONE, G. RICEVUTI, G. FOSSATI, I. MAZZUCCHELLI, D. GRITTI, L. ANGOLI & G. SPECCHIA. 1996. Clinical and angiographic correlates of leukocyte activation in unstable angina. 860–866.

92. NOTARIO, A., R. PAOLETTI & G. RICEVUTI. 1996. Abstract Book of the 2nd International Congress on Phagocytes: Biological and Clinical aspects. Pavia, (September 4-7, 1996). Eur. J. Haemat. Supplementum **57**(59): 1–84.

93. PIANI, D., B. CONSTAM, K. FREI & A. FONTANA. 1994. Macrophages in the brain: friends or enemies? NIPS **9**: 80–84.

Index of Contributors

Altieri, S., 274–278
Ambrosini, B., 21–28
Arangino, V., 21–28
Azzarà, A., 29–52

Baldi, A., 284–294
Ballantyne, C. M., 243–265
Barbacane, R. C., 223–232
Barni, S., 194–199, 274–278
Bellosta, S., 322–329
Bernini, F., 322–329
Birdsall, H. H., 243–265
Bobbio-Pallavicini, E., 295–303
Borin, P., 358–362
Borregaard, N., 62–68
Boulay, F., 69–84
Bratt, J., 163–169
Brouchon, L., 69–84

Caldiroli, E., 130–134
Capelli,E., 194–199, 279–283
Capodici, C., 1–12
Cassatella, M. A., 233–242
Cataldo, I., 223–232
Ceroni, M., 279–283
Civallero, M., 279–283
Conti, P., 223–232
Cosentino, M., 130–134
Craig, S. R., 200–214

De Amici, M., 295–303
De Ponti, F., 130–134
De Toni, S., 358–362, 363–367
Del Giacco, G. S., 21–28
Del Giacco, S. R., 21–28
Didichenko, S. A., 368–382
Dunzendorfer, S., 135–146, 330–340

Edwards, S. W., 341–357
Entman, M. L., 243–265

Fedele, D., 363–367
Ferrante, P., 53–61
Fietta, A. M., 130–134
Fontana, G., 363–367
Fossati, G., 274–278, 284–294
Frangogiannis, N., 243–265
Frigo, G. M., 130–134
Gasmi, L., 341–357
Gasperini, S., 233–242
Gennaro, R., 147–162
Gerzeli, G., 194–199, 274–278
Gfell, L. E., 383–393
Ghiani, A., 21–28
Giacobbe, O., 295–303
Giannini, E., 69–84
Gregor, A., 200–214
Gregory, R. L., 383–393
Gritti, D., 295–303
Guerini, F., 53–61

Hakki, Z. W., 383–393, 394–404
Han, G., 1–12
Harlan, J. M., 311–321
Hybertson, B. M., 266–273

Introna, M., 93–116
Ironside, J. W., 200–214

Kähler, C. M., 135–146, 330–340
Kiechl, S., 135–146
Kim-Park, W. K., 383–393, 394–404
Kowolik, M. J., 383–393, 394–404
Kumar, A. G., 243–265

Lapolla, A., 363–367
Leaver, H. A., 200–214
Lecchini, S., 130–134
Lee, Y. M., 266–273
Lindsey, M. L., 243–265

Lombardini, S., 21–28
Lorusso, L., 405–425

Manca, E., 21–28
Mantovani, A., 93–116
Marino, F., 130–134
Marinu-Aktipi, K., 279–283
Mazzucchelli, I., 284–294
Mendozzi, E., 53–61
Moore, M. A., 383–393, 394–404
Moroni, M., 295–303
Moulding, D. A., 341–357
Musu, D., 21–28

Naik, N., 69–84
Nano, R., 194–199, 274–278, 279–283
Notario, A., 284–294, 295–303

Palmblad , J., 13–20, 163–169
Paoletti, R., 322–329
Pillinger, M. H., 1–12
Pinelli, T., 274–278
Piva, E., 358–362, 363–367
Placido, F. C., 223–232
Plebani, M., 358–362, 363–367
Porta, C., 295–303
Prati, U., 274–278

Quayle, J. A., 341–357

Ramamoorthy, C., 311–321
Reale, M., 223–232
Reinisch, N., 135–146, 330–340
Repine, J. E., 266–273
Ricevuti, G., ix–x, 426–448
Roda, K., 53–61
Rolandi, M. L., 284–294
Romeo, D., 147–162
Rossen, R. D., 243–265
Rossi, M. L., 405–425
Roveda, L., 274–278
Russo, M. P., 233–242

Samuelsson, J., 13–20
Sarasella, M., 53–61
Schepetkin, I., 170–193
Schratzberger, P., 135–146, 330–340
Segal, A. W., 215–222
Servidio, G., 358–362
Sharar, S. R., 311–321
Shatwell, K. P., 215–222
Smith, C. W., 243–265
Sozzani, S., 93–116
Speciale, L., 53–61
Su, B. H., 200–214

Taddei, M., 130–134
Taramelli, D., 53–61
Tardif, M., 69–84
Thelen, M., 368–382
Trakatellis, M., 223–232

Vedder, N. B., 311–321
Venkataprasad, N., 117–129
Verhoeven, A. J., 85–92

Ward, P., 304–310
Watson, F., 341–357
Weissmann, G., 1–12
Whittle, I. R., 200–214
Wiedermann, C. J., 135–146, 330–340
Willeit, J., 135–146
Williams, J. R., 200–214
Winn, R. K., 311–321

Yap, P. L., 200–214
Youker, K. A., 243–265

Zanetti, M., 147–162
Zonta, A., 274–278